Fourth Edition

Health Care Delivery
in the United States

D92$1950II

Fourth Edition

Health Care Delivery in the United States

Anthony R. Kovner, Ph.D.
and Contributors

with a Foreword by
Founding Editor **Steven Jonas,** M.D.

Springer Publishing Company
New York

Copyright © 1990 by Springer Publishing Company, Inc.

Springer Publishing Company, Inc.
536 Broadway
New York, NY 10012

90 91 92 93 94 / 5 4 3 2

Library of Congress Cataloging-in-Publication Data

Health care delivery in the United States / Anthony R. Kovner [editor]
  with contributors ; founding editor, Steven Jonas. — 4th ed.
      p.   cm.
  Includes bibliographical references.
  ISBN 0-8261-2076-8
  1. Medical care—United States.   I. Kovner, Anthony R.
II. Jonas, Steven.
  [DNLM: 1. Delivery of Health Care—United States.   2. Health
Services—United States.   W 84 AA1 H376]
RA395.A3H395   1990
362.1'0973—dc20
DNLM/DLC
for Library of Congress   90-9449
                                                              CIP

Printed in the United States of America

Contents

Foreword to the Fourth Edition

A New Chapter

Health Care Delivery in the United States has a new editor, my professional colleague and friend, Dr. Anthony Kovner. Dr. Kovner was my first choice as my successor. When he accepted our invitation to take on this responsibility in the Spring of 1987, I was thrilled. Dr. Kovner has a thorough knowledge of health care delivery in the United States and a fine record of teaching, service, research, and publication in the field. He pledged at that time that he would continue the most important traditions of the book: comprehensiveness, an emphasis on description of things as they are, objectivity with a measured allowance for presentation of the authors' viewpoints, and readability. At the same time, he promised to bring in new blood.

Dr. Kovner has succeeded admirably. He has done the book proud, and the result is what I hoped it would be. I am confident that our readers, who have purchased more than 60,000 copies of this book in the first 13 years of its existence, will agree with my assessment of Dr. Kovner's work.

An Old Chapter

Having been associated with this book since I first conceived it in 1974, I am impressed with how much things change in the health care delivery system, yet how much they stay the same. There are many subjects covered in this fourth edition that were either nonexistent or not considered important enough for inclusion in the first edition, published in 1977. These new subjects reflect both new problems and proposed new solutions to them. However, the new problems are but subsets of the major issues that the U.S. health care delivery system faces. And the major issues have changed little if at all since at least 1932.

Dr. Kovner begins Chapter 1 of the fourth edition with the same quote from the *Final Report of the Committee on the Costs of Medical Care* with which I began Chapter 1 of each of the first three editions of this book. Reading it is both instructive and depressing. It could have been written yesterday. Although in 1990 we are spending about 200 times what we spent in 1932, a multiplier that far exceeds the results of inflation during the period, now as then "the problem of providing satisfactory medical service to all the people of the United States at costs which they can meet is a pressing one." Still "many persons do not receive service which is adequate either in quantity or quality." The result remains "a tremendous amount of preventable physical pain and mental anguish, needless deaths, economic inefficiency, and social waste."

There have been enormous advances in both biomedical and epidemiological knowledge since 1932. Hundreds of billions of dollars of capital have been invested in biomedical research, the construction of hospitals and other health care facilities, and the training and education of millions of physicians, nurses, and other health care professionals. Hundreds of billions of dollars are now spent every year using the capital base.

Much that is beneficial for the population is done. Yet the major problems remain: a significant minority of the population does not receive "medical service . . . which is adequate either in quantity or quality"; costs are ever more out of control; and there still is a tremendous amount of "preventable . . . pain . . . anguish . . . death . . . and . . . waste."

The opening paragraph of the *Final Report* concludes that "these conditions are . . . largely unnecessary. The United States has the economic resources, the organizing ability and the technical expertise to solve this problem." One must agree with the first sentence. But 60 years or so later, one must wonder if the second is completely true. We certainly have the economic resources. But do we have the organizing ability and the technical expertise? If we do, why has a nation that has flown to the moon, created the most powerful military force the world has ever known, and developed a marvelous system for growing food and creating an abundance of consumer goods that benefits many, though certainly not all, of its people not been able to solve the listed health and health care problems?

In my view, the answer is political. We do have the organizing ability and the technical expertise. Our achievements in other realms prove it. But you will note that the word "politics" does not appear in the much-quoted paragraph from the *Final Report*. And that is where the central obstacles to change lie: in the political realm.

We have not yet been able to create and mobilize the political will to bring about the changes in the system that are necessary to solve the listed problems. The same forces that labeled the *Final Report* a "Communist plot" when it was published and who then opposed major change in the organization of services—in particular the role, function, and mode of payment of the physician—oppose major change now. We will be able to do nothing significant to solve the cited problems until we deal with those forces.

This book is primarily descriptive, not prescriptive. Thus, it serves the needs of both those who simply want to know what the U.S. health care delivery system is like and how it works and those who would take the descriptions provided and develop their own prescriptions for change. Before one can usefully say what might be or what ought to be, one must know what *is*. That is the need that this book meets. The rest, dear reader, is up to you.

> STEVEN JONAS, M.D., M.P.H.
> *Professor, State University of New York*
> *Stony Brook, N.Y.*

Preface

Health Care Delivery in the United States is intended as an introduction for those studying to be clinicians or managers and for those who wish to know more about health care and how it is delivered in this country.

Deuschle noted in his preface to the first edition:

> The book is basically descriptive in nature, examining the various elements in the delivery system and elucidating their interactions; it succeeds in describing this labyrinthine system lucidly and comprehensively. It does not neglect the economic ramifications . . . nor the political controversies. . . . The book is up to date in terminology and thus will help meet the urgent need of health workers to communicate with one another and with the public at large.

The mission of this fourth edition is identical to that of the preceding three; we hope we have achieved a similar measure of success.

Since publication of the first edition in 1977, the book's contributors have tried to reflect the changing health care delivery system. Although some of the nomenclature has varied, all four editions have had chapters on the concept of health care, data, manpower, nursing, ambulatory care, hospitals, mental health, financing, government, planning, and control of quality. Long-term care has merited its own chapter since the second edition in 1981. Technology assessment and futures were first presented in the third edition and are now in the fourth as well.

This current edition includes new chapter-length discussions of governance and management, comparative health systems, and ethics. These are all major topics that now deserve separate treatment. More health care is being provided in organizations that are governed and managed. How health care is organized and paid for in other countries, particularly Canada, is becoming highly significant in the discussion of American health policy. And ethical questions in health care are important in political elections and in discussions of how to allocate limited health care resources in response to virtually unlimited demand.

The topics of HMOs, home care, and corporatization remain important but as integral elements of the overall system. They are therefore discussed within their relevant contexts. HMOs are covered in Chapter 6, "Ambulatory Care," and in Chapter 10, "Financing for Health Care." Home care is discussed in Chapter 8, "Long-Term Care." Corporatization is discussed in Chapter 16, "Governance and Management," and in Chapter 19, "Futures."

As with earlier editions, we hope this book continues to be found useful by both students and professionals.

ANTHONY R. KOVNER, PH.D.
Professor, Robert F Wagner Graduate
School of Public Service
New York University
New York, N.Y.

Acknowledgments

The editor wishes to acknowledge the prompt and effective effort of all chapter authors and the creativity, knowledge, and cooperation of the editor of the first three editions, Steven Jonas.

Contributors

H. David Banta directs a project on future health care technology in the Hague, Netherlands for the World Health Organization. He was previously Assistant Director of the Office of Technology Assessment, United States Congress and Deputy Director of the Pan American Health Organization. Dr. Banta received his M.D. from Duke and his M.P.H. and M.S.Hyg. from Harvard.

Charles Brecher, Professor of Public and Health Administration at New York University, teaches courses on urban politics and health policy analysis. He is co-director of the Setting Municipal Priorities Project, which for the past five years has issued annual reviews of policy and financial issues in New York City. He has a Ph.D. in political science from the City University of New York and has written books and articles in the field of public expenditure analysis, health policy, and manpower policy.

Steven Jonas is Professor of Community and Preventive Medicine, School of Medicine, State University of New York at Stony Brook. The Founding Editor of *Health Care Delivery in the United States,* he has authored/coauthored 5 books and more than 100 professional articles and book reviews on health policy, medical education reform, and the role and function of health-promotion/disease-prevention services in the health care delivery system. For the general public he has authored/coauthored three books and numerous articles on exercise, health, and nutrition. Dr. Jonas received his M.D. from Harvard and his M.P.H. from Yale. He is a past president of the Association of Teachers of Preventive Medicine, a Fellow of the American College of Preventive Medicine, an associate editor of the *American Journal of Preventive Medicine* and of *Preventive Medicine,* and Editor of the *Springer Series on Medical Education.*

James R. Knickman, Professor of Public Administration, teaches health economics, evaluation of health programs, and policy analysis at New York University. His research interests focus on applications of quantitative methods in public policy analysis. He is currently doing research in the area of long-term-care financing. In addition, he is directing a project assessing potential policy solutions to the problem of homelessness among New York families. Professor Knickman served as Special Assistant for Health Policy in New York City's Office of Management and Budget. He received his Ph.D. in public policy analysis from the University of Pennsylvania.

Lorrin M. Koran, Professor of Psychiatry (Clinical) at Stanford University Medical Center, is the Acting Medical Director of the Charter Hospital at Stanford. His research interests include relationships between mental disorders and physical disease, characteristics of the mental health services delivery system, and the treatment of obsessive-compulsive disorder. Dr. Koran has served as Special Assistant to the Director of the National Institute of Mental Health. He received his M.D. from Harvard Medical School.

Anthony R. Kovner is Professor of Public and Health Administration at the Robert F. Wagner Graduate School for Public Service at New York University. He has been a senior manager in two hospitals, a nursing home, a group practice, and a neighborhood health center, as well as a senior health care consultant of a large industrial union. An organizational theorist by training, his research interests include health services management and governance. He has edited three textbooks and written a book and numerous articles on health services management, hospital governance, health regulation, and hospital budgeting. Dr. Kovner is a senior program consultant for the Robert Wood Johnson Foundation. He received his M.P.A. from Cornell University and his Ph.D. in public administration from the University of Pittsburgh.

Christine Kovner is Assistant Professor of Nursing at New York University. She has worked as a public health nurse, a home care coordinator, and a director of inservice in nursing at a small acute-care hospital. Her research interests are in the area of nursing resource use and cost of nursing care of the elderly. She received her M.S.N. from the University of Pennsylvania and her Ph.D. in nursing from New York University.

Roger Kropf, Associate Professor of Public Health Administration at New York University, is a specialist in health planning and management information systems. He is the senior author of *Strategic Analysis for Hospital Management,* which examines strategic planning in hospitals and how management information systems can be used to improve decision-making. He serves on the editorial board of the *Journal of Ambulatory Care Mangement.* Professor Kropf received a Ph.D. from the Maxwell School of Citizenship and Public Affairs at Syracuse University.

Robert S. Lawrence is Charles S. Davidson Associate Professor of Medicine, Chief of Medicine at Cambridge Hospital, and Director of the Division of Primary Care at Harvard Medical School. He has been the medical director of a rural neighborhood health center network and the developer of training programs in primary care internal medicine. He teaches ambulatory care, clinical interviewing, and preventive medicine to medical students and internal medicine residents at Harvard Medical Center. His research interests include patients' health beliefs and symptom interpretation, determinants of health-promoting behavior, and strategies for integrating preventive medicine into primary care practice. He received his B.A. and M.D. from Harvard University.

Hila Richardson is the Senior Director for Long Term Care at the New York City Health and Hospitals Corporation. Previously, she was the Associate Director of the Rural Hospital Program, a national demonstration sponsored by the Robert Wood Johnson Foundation and based at New York University's Program in Health Policy and Management. Dr. Richardson also was on the staff of the Institute of Medicine and has held several nursing positions. She has held teaching positions at the University of Virginia School of Nursing, Columbia University School of Public Health, and New York University School of Graduate Public Administration. Dr. Richardson received a B.S. in Nursing from the University of Virginia, an M.P.H. from Johns Hopkins University, and a Dr. P.H. from Columbia University.

Victor G. Rodwin is Associate Professor of Public and Health Administration and Associate Director of the Advanced Management Program for Clinicians (AMPC) at New York University. He coordinates the Kellogg Seminar in Health Policy and Management and teaches courses in politics and comparative health systems. He has also served as adviser to the Director of the French National Health Insurance Fund (CNAMTS) and has taught comparative health systems at the University of California at Berkeley and the University of Paris IX (Dauphine). He is the author of *The Health Planning Predicament: France, Quebec, England, and the United States* and a coauthor of *The End of an Illusion: The Future of Health Policy in Western Industrialized Nations*. Professor Rodwin received an M.P.H. and a Ph.D. in planning from the University of California at Berkeley.

Dena J. Seiden is Ethicist at Elmhurst General Hospital in Queens, New York and a principal of Medical Ethics Consulting Services in New York City. She has worked as consulting ethicist to the Kaiser-Permanente Health Plan and to St. Luke's-Roosevelt Hospital Center. She teaches ethics at the Wagner School of Public Service at New York University and the Columbia School of Public Service. She is a former health care manager with 13 years of experience. Ms. Seiden received her Master's in Philosophy from Union Theological Seminary and expects to receive her doctorate from Union in 1990.

Steven S. Sharfstein is currently Executive Vice President and Medical Director at The Sheppard and Enoch Pratt Hospital and Clinical Professor of Psychiatry at the University of Maryland. He spent 13 years with the National Institute of Mental Health, where he was Director of the Mental Service Programs and also held positions in consultation liaison and behavioral medicine on the campus of the National Institutes of Health. From 1983 to 1986 he was Deputy Medical Director of the American Psychiatric Association. He has written on a wide variety of clinical and economic topics and has published more than 75 professional papers, 14 book chapters, and 6 books, including (as coauthor) *Madness and Government: Who Cares for the Mentally Ill?*, a history of the federal community mental health centers program. Trained in psychiatry at the Massachusetts Mental Health Center from 1969 to 1972, Dr. Sharfstein also received an M.P.A. from the Kennedy School of Government in 1973.

Kenneth E. Thorpe is Associate Professor of Health Economics in the Department of Health Policy and Management, Harvard School of Public Health. He has also served as consultant to the Rand Corporation and the Subcommittee on Health Insurance for the New York State Council on Health Care Financing, where he aided in the development of New York's new hospital payment system. His primary research interests include evaluations of the impact of public policies on hospital and nursing home behavior. Recent projects include an evaluation of the cost and access implications of alternative hospital payment methodologies in New York's (Medicare) waiver program and the impact of DRG payment on hospital readmission rates, as well as his ongoing research evaluating the RUG-II nursing home payment system in New York. Most recently, his research has focused on the effects of proposed employer health insurance mandates and expansions of Medicaid. He received his M.A. in public policy analysis from Duke University and his Ph.D. from the Rand Graduate School.

Beth C. Weitzman, Assistant Professor of Public and Health Administration, teaches courses in quality assessment and community health and medicine at New York University. She has extensive experience as an evaluator of both educational and health programs. Her research interests focus on policies and programs affecting children, adolescents and the poor, particularly in regard to health care quality and utilization. Recent research studies have focused on families at risk of homelessness and on the relationship between health insurance and health status and utilization for working poor women. Professor Weitzman holds an MPA and PhD from New York University.

Fourth Edition

Health Care Delivery
in the United States

1

Introduction

Anthony R. Kovner

The State of Health Care Delivery in the United States

In the last edition of this book, Jonas cites a study of health care delivery made almost 60 years ago, which summarized its findings in these terms:

> The problem of providing satisfactory medical service to all the people of the United States at costs which they can meet is a pressing one. At the present time, many persons do not receive service which is adequate either in quantity or quality, and the costs of service are inequitably distributed. The result is a tremendous amount of preventable physical pain and mental anguish, needless deaths, economic inefficiency, and social waste. Furthermore, these conditions are . . . largely unnecessary. The United States has the economic resources, the organizing ability and the technical expertise to solve this problem. [Committee on the Costs of Medical Care, p. 2]

This statement is applicable to the health care delivery system in the United States today.

If this is the problem, what then should we do about it, and would the remedy be worse than what we have? According to Easterbrook (1987),

> The U.S. approach costs more than other systems, but it also produces the most sophisticated care; an outcome which should not be dismissed as coincidental. Of the socialized nations only Canada is thought to have medicine equal to ours, and its conversion from an enterprise system is most recent. European socialized approaches are possible in part because the money-hungry American system produces breakthroughs others can buy or duplicate. [p. 74]

Although many would disagree with the above statement, according to a 1987 Cambridge Report nationwide survey;

While Americans appear to be satisfied with the performance of their health-care system, two out of three say they would favor national health insurance funded by tax dollars. At the same time, however, they appear unwilling to pay what a program might realistically cost. Fewer than 20% say they would be willing to spend more than $50 a year in higher taxes or insurance premiums to help pay for care for people who can't afford it. [Pokorny p. 3]

Others, like Abramowitz (1988), argue that government should promote market competition:

United States health care delivery over the next five to ten years will see tremendous competition, resulting in wider choices for consumers, declining profit margins for virtually all providers, and tottering market shares for traditional providers. The times will increasingly favor managed fee-for-service medicine incorporating pre-admission certification, and HMOs and PPOs will proliferate. These trends will eventually shrink excess capacity eliminating marginal providers and causing cost growth to steadily grow, at the same time enabling the quality of health care to rise—assuming of course that the "right" providers leave the market. [Abramowitz, p. 42]

The above quotations suggest that (1) the United States has serious problems of cost, access, and quality of health care; (2) how serious these problems are depends on who is answering the question: most of the poor, minority, and rural Americans or most of the rest, which is the majority of the population; (3) how we can solve these problems and the consequences of different approaches is a matter for dispute among the informed (as well the uninformed); I would argue further that most Americans are indifferent to and uninformed about these matters.

How well the country is doing in health care delivery depends on the standard we wish to compare ourselves against, as well as how we define health. Certainly, Americans consume a great deal of health care, much of which is medically unnecessary. Interventions such as physician office visits do not always result in predictable measurable improvements in health status. Does this mean we should make fewer physician and emergency room visits? Not necessarily.

The infant death rate and life expectancy are two common standards for comparing a population's health status. In 1960 the U.S. mortality rate for infants under 1 year of age was 26.0 per 1,000 live births (U.S. Bureau of the Census). In 1987 the rate had decreased by over half, to 10.6. The 1987 infant mortality rate in Japan was 5.2 deaths per 1,000 live births (Iglehart).

With regard to life expectancy, women live longer than men. In the United States in 1960 life expectancy was 66.6 years for men and 73.1 years for women. By 1987 life expectancy had risen to 71 years for men and 78 years for women.

In Japan in 1986 the average life expectancy for men was 74.2 years, 80.9 years for women.

On the expenditure side, in 1960 Americans spent $27 billion on health care, which was 5.3% of our gross national product (U.S. Bureau of the Census). In 1987 we spent $439 billion, which was 11.0% of our GNP. Japan's health care expenditures represented 6.7% of the GNP in 1986 (Iglehart). For 1987, approximately $2,130 per year was being spent for health care for each American, while the Japanese, in 1986, were spending $831 for each person. And over 35 million Americans lack health insurance, while all Japanese have some form of health insurance.

Do these figures mean that health care for most Americans is not as good as that for most Japanese? Not necessarily. The figures say nothing about the quality of health care, its distribution, its appropriateness, or the way in which care is given. One's answer also depends on how "good health care" is defined. Is emphasis placed on access to care, utilization of care, preventable death and disability, or on perceptions of how care is given by clinicians in organizations? Quality of care also has to do with the standard against which care is measured. Are we comparing the quality of care for all Americans to that of Japanese in 1990? Are we comparing the quality of health care for all Americans in 1990 to that in 1960? Or are we comparing the quality of care used by white Americans in 1990 to that used by black Americans? Different answers will be given to ratings of quality depending on which specific question is asked.

Harris and Associates have surveyed Americans, British, and Canadians on these matters. According to their 1988 poll, Americans are significantly less happy with their health care system than either the British or Canadians are with theirs (Blendon). Only 54% of Americans report being "very satisfied" with their last physician encounter, compared with 73% of Canadians and 63% of British. And only 57% of Americans who were hospitalized in the 12 months prior to the survey say they were "very satisfied" with their hospital stays. This compares to 71% for Canadians and 67% for British. The majority of Americans say they would prefer a system like the Canadian health care system to the one they currently have.

In analyzing the results of the Harris survey, Blendon (1989, p. 7) concludes that

> a new (or perhaps newly recognized) climate of public opinion about health care is taking shape in the 1990s . . . of Americans say they want a fundamental break with their current health care policies and a much more central role played by the federal government in remedying America's health problems.

Blendon is discussing two different questions. First, how satisfied are insured Americans with the health system? Second, how dissatisfied are the more than 35 million Americans who lack adequate health insurance? Prior to the 1988 Harris survey, it was commonly accepted that Americans, if they had adequate health insurance, were more or less satisfied with the system, particularly in contrast to the British. Those lacking health insurance have been dissatisfied for many years, but they have lacked the political power to bring about change.

To what extent are the significant differences that exist among Americans confined to the health sector? Aren't there similar inequities between poor black and most white Americans in education, housing, income, and consumption in general? Why aren't more Americans more concerned about these kinds of inequities, and when, if ever, will we become more concerned? How will we become more concerned if we don't know about the seriousness of the problems? Thirty-six million American adults read below the eighth-grade level, and 45% of Americans never read books. In addition, 46.7% of black children are below the poverty line (Lapham, Pollan, & Etheridge).

This book will not authoritatively answer questions such as (1) who should pay for the care of the nation's uninsured poor; (2) who should pay for extended nursing home care or in-home care for elderly patients; (3) how should health care costs be controlled; and (4) how should quality of care be assured. These are "value" questions, not "fact" questions. Reasonable men and women presented with the same facts on these issues will come up with different answers. Reasonable people may also differ on whether these issues need to be resolved now or in the near future, on what will be the consequences of not doing anything significantly different, and on the consequences of implementing an Option A versus an Option B, C, or D.

This book does present the elements of the health care delivery system, and it analyzes how they function. We describe the people who use health care and the people who provide health care, as well as the organizations in which they work. We examine how different parts of the health care delivery system function, and we discuss assessment of the current and future health care delivery system.

What Is Health Care, and Who Is Served?

The United States had a population of more than 247 million Americans in 1987. The population resides in an area greater than 3.6 million square miles. So we are one of the largest countries in the world, based on either population or area. Unlike that of most European and other developed countries, the American population is heterogeneous—that is, we are made up of people from a wide variety of cultures, races, and ethnic groups, and we are dispersed over a large land mass. This has implications for the types of health care and the ways in which they should be provided. For example rural Eskimos in Alaska, middle-class working people in the suburbs, and blacks who live in our large cities have differing needs in different geographic situations.

In Chapter 2 the many definitions of health, disease, and illness are discussed, including their biological, psychological, and social components. Health has its personal and community aspects. And health care can be viewed as a right or as a privilege.

In Chapter 3 we present the principal quantitative measures used to describe the health and illness of the population. Vital statistics are routinely compiled on births, deaths, sickness and health status, and utilization of care by populations. Data concerning health and health care are expressed in terms of numbers and rates. They include demographic characteristics, sickness and health status, and utilization of health services.

Who Provides Health Care in What Kinds of Organizations?

Health care is provided by doctors and nurses and by more than 200 different occupational groups, ranging from physical therapists to lab technicians. Chapters 4 and 5 examine the professionals, particularly physicians and nurses, who provide most of the care. Health care is increasingly being provided in larger and more complex organizations, which are governed and managed. Chapters 6 through 9 examine four leading types of health care organizations: ambulatory care, hospitals, long-term care, and mental health. Some of these types of organizations overlap. For example, health maintenance organizations (HMOs) commonly provide inpatient hospital care, ambulatory care, and mental health services. Mental health organizations and hospitals commonly provide inpatient and outpatient care.

What Are Some Important Ways of Analyzing the Health Care System?

An important way of analyzing the health care sector is by looking at how services are financed. This includes how much money is spent on health care, what the money buys, where the money comes from, and how the money is paid out. Chapter 10 looks at these areas; Chapter 11 examines cost containment. Containing health care costs has been an important national problem for at least 25 years. To ameliorate this problem, we must first understand the factors accounting for increasing costs and then review efforts to control costs, which so far have focused on the hospital. It may then be possible to learn what has succeeded, what has failed, and why.

The government's role in health care is more extensive than that of financing and containing costs; government agencies also regulate providers and provide health services directly. Federal, state, and local governments have different and overlapping health care roles. These are examined in Chapter 12.

Planning is important for health care organizations and is addressed in Chapter

13. As with financing, planning can be analyzed at the various governmental or institutional levels. Techniques for planning health care include measuring health status, analyzing consumer preferences, and measuring and evaluating utilization. Quality control and technology assessment, covered in Chapters 14 and 15, respectively, are concerned with the benefits of health care, sometimes in relationship to their costs. Technology assessment includes evaluating efficacy, safety, and cost-effectiveness by identifying, testing, synthesizing, and disseminating results. The computerized axial tomography (CAT) scanner and the electronic fetal monitor are two technological developments that have recently been thoroughly assessed in this way.

The quality of care is increasingly being measured as we learn more about the relationship between medical and other interventions and related health outcomes. The quality of health care comprises the patient's health status and attitudes to care and the structures, processes, and outcomes of care. Simply defining what is meant by high-quality care does not guarantee its implementation. Approaches to assuring quality health care include licensing, accreditation and certification, and review of care by organizations such as Professional Review Organizations (PROs) that target inappropriate utilization relative to agreed-upon standards of care. How are policy and administrative decisions made in health care organizations? Chapter 16, "Governance and Management," explores this question by focusing on the role, structure, and function of governing boards and the role, function, and training of health care organization managers.

Chapter 17 looks at health systems in other countries. There is a large literature on the comparative analysis of health care systems, but Americans have rarely attempted to draw lessons from the experience of other countries. This, however, shows signs of changing as Americans have recently looked to the Canadian system with regard to containment of costs. Canada has adequate health insurance for all high levels of health status and has achieved notable success in controlling the growth of health care costs. And of course, other countries can and do learn from the American experience, for example, in the area of quality assessment and assurance.

Health care ethics, addressed in Chapter 18, is a relatively recent academic discipline. Among the major topics in health care ethics are informed consent, do-not-resuscitate orders, forgoing of life-sustaining systems, treatment of multiply handicapped newborns, abortion, confidentiality, allocation of scarce resources, equity of access, and issues relating to the care of AIDS patients.

What Is the Present and Future of Health Care Delivery in the United States?

The authors of this book present the reader with the facts and issues in 18 chapters. In Chapter 19 we review these facts and ask you to consider what should be done to alter health care delivery in the United States in the years ahead. We hope that you will care about these issues, discuss them, and work with us to retain the best in the American system while creating better ways to deliver good-quality health care at reasonable costs to all Americans.

References

Abramowitz, K. S. "The Future of Health Care in America." *MGM Journal,* July/August 1988, p. 42.

Blendon, R. J. "Three Systems: A Comparative Survey." *Health Management Quarterly, 11*(1), 2, 1989.

Committee on the Costs of Medical Care. *Medical Care for the American People.* Chicago: University of Chicago Press, 1932. Reprinted, Washington, D.C.: USDHEW, 1970.

Deuschle, K. W. "Foreword." In S. Jonas (Ed.), *Health Care Delivery in the United States* (pp. x–xi). New York: Springer Publishing Co., 1977.

Easterbrook, G. "The Revolution." *Newsweek,* January 26, 1987, pp. 40–74.

Iglehart, J. K. "Japan's Medical Care System." *New England Journal of Medicine, 319*(17), 1166, 1988.

Lapham, L., Pollan, M., & Etheridge, E. *The Harper's Index Book.* New York: Henry Holt, 1987.

Pokorny, G. "Report Card on Health Care." *Health Management Quarterly, 10*(1), 3, 1988.

U.S. Bureau of the Census. *Statistical Abstract of the United States* (108th ed.), Washington, D.C.: U.S. Government Printing Office, 1988.

2

What Is Health Care?

H. David Banta

It seems a truism that the purpose of health care is to promote health, yet most observers of the health care system would agree that it deals primarily with disease and not with health. The education of health professionals, physicians in particular, focuses on physical pathology and derangements of biophysiologic functioning (Jonas; Millis), and medical practice is almost exclusively concerned with the diagnosis and treatment of disease.

This chapter will argue for a broader conception of health and health care. It is doubtless easier to care for disease than to promote good health; moreover, such activities as health education lack the drama associated with the crisis-care technology of university hospitals. One must also recognize the limitations of knowledge in the psychological and social spheres. Yet health care providers must deal with people's real needs. The growth of self-care and alternative systems of care indicates considerable discontent with the present patterns of health care practice (Sidel & Sidel). A particular problem in the modern world is that of translation; with international movement of people, the possibilities of misunderstanding between health care provider and patient are growing (Ebden, Carey, Bhatt, & Harrison).

This chapter will also point out some of the limitations of contemporary health and medical knowledge. Much of present-day health care is based on old, never-proven technology. In many cases this technology is probably not effective, and it is often costly (see Chapter 15). Although physical cures are possible in some cases, what most people need is caring.

Health care must deal with the nature of society and its members. For example, an aging population raises new challenges, including rehabilitation and supports for functioning in the home and community for an ever-larger group of chronically disabled people.

Finally, the chapter will take a modest look into the future. The health care system is in a state of rapid change, and health care providers, especially physicians, are being criticized from all sides. Medicine and health must be defined socially because, as society changes, its state of health and its view of what constitutes health changes as well.

What Are "Health" and "Disease"?

Health, disease, and *illness* are terms we use often without thinking about precise definitions. It is easy to think of health as being the lack of disease, or of illness and disease as being interchangeable terms. In fact, health and disease are not simply opposites, and disease and illness do not mean precisely the same thing (Kass).

The Greeks made a philosophical distinction between the concepts of health and disease. As Sigerist (p. 57) said, "The [ancient Greek] physicians had an explanation for health. Health, they believed, was a condition of perfect equilibrium. When the forces or humors or whatever constituted the human body were perfectly balanced, man was healthy. Disturbed balance resulted in disease. This is still the best general explanation we have." The cult of Asklepios, however, concentrated on disease and miracle cures, and with the rise of Christianity, the idea of disease was given a preferential place. The Greek idea of health as a perfect balance had little meaning to the masses of that day, living as they did in poverty, sickness, and oppression. Later, scientific medicine began to develop, but the idea of miracle cures persisted, as it does in present-day medicine. It is a seductive dream: a cure that can compensate for the abuses the individual and society have perpetuated, correcting at a stroke the effects of cigarette smoking or of breathing polluted air over a period of years.

Webster's Unabridged Dictionary reflects this conflict, defining *health* as "physical and mental well-being," but continuing, "freedom from defect, pain, or disease." Health statistics, of course, are actually disease statistics, and health care is often disease care. Jago (1975) lists 43 uses of *health* as an adjective, most of which add to the confusion. Examples include *health status, health center,* and *health worker.*

The World Health Organization (WHO) (1944, p. 29) defines *health* as a "state of complete physical, mental, and social well-being, and not merely the absence of disease or infirmity." This definition has been criticized as being utopian (Dubos; Kass). Perhaps its greatest weakness is that it has no reference to cultural concepts of disease and health. It completely excludes death as a natural endpoint of life. For example, how one comes to terms with death and suffering must be a part of one's health. Perhaps a more functional definition is that proposed by Kass (1981), namely, "the well-working of the organism as a whole" (p. 4).

Disease also is frequently defined rather ambiguously. *Webster's* suggests

"uneasiness or distress," and more sweepingly, "any departure from health."
Blakiston's New Gould Medical Dictionary (1956) terms *disease* "a failure of the
adaptive mechanisms of an organism to counteract adequately the stimuli and
stresses to which it is subject, resulting in a disturbance in function or structure of
any part, organ, or system of the body."

Whereas *disease* is a biomedical concept, *illness* is a state of being. As Cassell
(1976, p. 48) says, "Disease, then, is something an organ has; illness is something a man has." Illness has social and psychological as well as biomedical
components. One can have a disease without feeling ill, as in asymptomatic
hypertension; and one can surely be ill without being diseased.

Other definitions of health have stressed life functioning, seeing health as the
"state of optimum capacity for effective performance of valued tasks" (Parsons,
1958, p. 168) or as "personal fitness for survival and self-renewal, creative social
adjustment, and self-fulfillment. The most exacting test of one's health is to stay
alive and to retain the capacity for self-repair and self-renewal" (Hoyman,
p. 189).

Health status indicators have been developed to measure functioning as an
outcome of health care (Kaplan, Bush, & Berry; McPeek, Gilbert, & Mosteller;
Mushkin & Dunlop). It is interesting to note, considering the argument that death
must be part of a definition of health, that people surveyed find some states of
life worse than death (Williams).

Biological Factors in Health

Health is obviously dependent upon biological factors. Genetic endowment of
the individual is the starting point, but health is to a large extent the result of the
complex interaction of this soma with the environment (Burnett). The environment includes physical surroundings, social factors (largely beyond the control
of the individual), and personal lifestyle.

The environment is a crucial determinant of health. In 1857 the tuberculosis
death rate in Massachusetts was 450 per 100,000; by 1890, the figures had fallen
to 250; by 1920, to 114; and by 1938, to 35.6 (Sigerist, p. 46). Yet the first
specific antituberculosis therapy was not in general use until after 1938, convincing evidence that the prevalence of a disease can decline dramatically without
effective medical care, apparently from environmental factors.

An analysis of falling death rates and increasing population in England and
Wales since 1841 has shown that these changes considerably preceded any direct
medical intervention. Death rates in England and Wales fell from about 22 per
1,000 in 1841 to around 6 per 1,000 in 1971. McKeown (pp. 93–94) concludes
that 92% of the fall between 1848 and 1901 and 73% from 1901 to 1971 resulted
from a reduction in the number of deaths from infectious diseases. Most of this
reduction was due to a falling number of deaths from tuberculosis. Death rates

from respiratory tuberculosis fell steadily beginning in 1838, although chemotherapy did not begin until 1948. After 1948, however, the fall in the death rate increased, indicating an effect of chemotherapy. McKeown also examined the death rates for bronchitis, pneumonia, and influenza, which, after tuberculosis, were the greatest causes of mortality in the infectious disease era. The death rate for these conditions has been little affected by the introduction of antibiotics; rather, McKeown concludes, improvement in nutrition has been the most important influence. He estimates that hygienic measures, such as improvement in water supplies and sewage disposal, were responsible for about one-fifth of the reduction. Moreover, McKeown states, "With the exception of vaccination against smallpox, whose contribution was small, the influence of immunization and therapy on the death rate was delayed until the 20th century, and had little effect on national mortality trends before the introduction of sulphonamides in 1935. Since that time it has not been the only, or probably the most important influence" (p. 94). (The issue will be addressed further in "The Efficacy of Health Care," later in this chapter).

Diseases caused by microorganisms have been the scourge of humans throughout recorded history and have been the largest biological determinant of death and disability. Now, although infectious diseases persist, they are of limited importance for most of the population of the United States. Diseases of the circulatory system now account for more than 50% of the deaths in the United States annually. Chronic diseases have other important effects, such as the limitations of activity due to arthritis. Overall, chronic diseases have become the most prevalent and troublesome.

Chronic diseases are largely dependent on biological factors as well, although no specific etiology (such as a microorganism) can be identified for most such conditions (Burnett, pp. 2–3). The importance of genetic factors to the basic biological makeup of the individual is being recognized. It is becoming increasingly apparent that congenital causes of sickness, disability, and death have been relatively unresponsive to changes in environment and medical care. We now know beyond question that diet, air and water pollution, occupational hazards, and cigarette smoking are critical in the genesis of chronic disease. For example, epidemiological studies indicate that up to 90% of cancers are related to environmental factors, including smoking and nutrition. (Office of Technology Assessment, 1982)

However, the importance of genetics has probably been underestimated even in these cases. For example, a number of studies have demonstrated that there is a genetic basis for alcoholism (Reich). Those who contract lung cancer from smoking cigarettes probably have a genetic predisposition. The essential point is that the interaction between genetic factors and the environment in producing individual disease is enormously complex, and much research is needed to elucidate the relationship.

Psychological Factors in Health

The biomedical model of health and disease has been challenged increasingly in recent years. As Engel (p. 591) says, this model "assumes disease to be fully accounted for by deviations from the norm of measurable biological variables. It leaves no room within its framework for the social, psychological, and behavioral dimensions of illness." Yet, as Engel says, treatment directed at a biochemical abnormality does not necessarily restore health. This is because of discrepancies between the physical measurements and the psychological and social variables.

Currently, research is demonstrating that the organism must be approached as a whole being, not just as the sum of physical parts. Derangements in psychic functioning have been shown to cause physical health problems, including death. For example, a large body of research has demonstrated the effects of bereavement (Osterweis, Solomon, & Green), leading Engel to ask, "Is grief a disease?" His answer is, "Yes, if the grieving person is functioning badly" (p. 601).

At the same time, the health care provider's behavior and "the relationship between patient and physician powerfully influence therapeutic outcome for better or for worse. These constitute psychological effects which may directly modify the illness experience or indirectly affect underlying biochemical processes" (Engel, p. 599). Research on the placebo effect demonstrates this fact. The placebo effect apparently involves endogenous morphinelike substances that create changes in the central nervous system and in the activation centers in the brain. This research points out that it may be possible to tap the organism's own healing mechanisms directly (Lipkin).

There also are different psychological perceptions of what constitutes health and illness (White, 1971). The negative stimuli that affect behavior range from vague feelings of uneasiness to severe pain. Although health care providers react quickly to a patient's pain, they often tend to dismiss the vague anxieties of careseekers unless physiological evidence for malfunction can be found. However, such vague feelings are often indicative of real illness: It has been shown that such self-perceptions and symptoms may predict mortality (Daly & Tyroler; Singer, et al.). An individual's perceptions are influenced by physiological determinants, such as chemical imbalances or hunger, as well as by psychological factors. Perception is also affected by sociocultural factors (see following section).

An important part of the perceptual influences on health in today's world are the expectations that people bring with them when coming into contact with the health care system. Medicine is overvalued by the public, and this is at the root of many problems facing the health care field, such as malpractice. A society bent on instant gratification does not accept pain or death as part of living. Yet it is likely that "right living" and social change, rather than medicine, are the keys to achieving a healthier population (Berkman & Breslow).

Social Factors in Health

Since health and illness are defined functionally, sickness can be seen as a social role that carries with it certain rights and obligations (Parsons, 1951; Susser). Sick people are exempt from many normal social obligations and are not considered entirely responsible for their own state. Even when they have brought an illness upon themselves—as in a careless accident or lung cancer caused by cigarette smoking—they are not assumed to be solely responsible for the process of getting well. However, the sick role does entail responsibilities. Sick people are expected to cooperate in their treatment and to attempt to return to normal functioning as soon as possible.

With increasing cost-consciousness in the health care sector, one hears more and more proposals that would require people who are thought to have brought disease upon themselves to pay a higher price. For example, a smoker would pay a higher health insurance premium. This approach has been rightly called "blaming the victim" for problems that often have contributing social causes. Smoking, for example, is often related to work frustrations, rage, or seductive advertising. Such behavior is often more common in the lower socioeconomic classes (Berkman & Breslow; Prager et al.), which means that such policies would discriminate against the less fortunate in the society.

Other cultures have conceptions of health and disease entirely different from those of the United States (Mechanic, pp. 129–130). Even in this country, perceptions of disease and use of health care services vary greatly according to class (Koos; Kunitz) and ethnic group. Zaborowski (1952), in what has become a classic paper, examines the meaning of pain in Jews, Italians, and "Old Yankees" in an American hospital and finds rather remarkable differences.

The role of value systems and social structures should be evident, as the example of other countries helps to make clear. People in developing countries may suffer from malaria and schistosomiasis without assuming the sick role (Susser). Every physician is familiar with people who function well despite organic disease that, all else being equal, should be incapacitating. It becomes the responsibility of the physician or other health care provider to encourage independence.

Furthermore, the lack or presence of certain social factors can influence the development of disease. For example, social networks influence the development of physical and mental illness (Berkman & Breslow, p. 121). Significant life changes, such as bereavement or divorce, are associated with pregnancy complications; but in one study women with good psychosocial resources were shown to have only one-third the complication rate of others (Nuckolls, Cassel, & Kaplan). A growing body of research leads to the generalization that social and psychological supports are associated with better health outcomes, at least in part because they can ameliorate the effects of stress (Asher; Elliott & Eisdorfer; Mumford, Schlesinger, & Glass).

Society generally views the medical profession as acting at the organic level in curing and preventing disease. But medicine also must function at the psychological level, giving reassurance and care to those who seek help; and at the social level, legitimizing the sick role and perhaps helping to arrange social supports. Further, society's categorization of health and disease changes over time. Within recent memory, social problems such as suicide and drug addiction have been redefined and are now considered to be illnesses (Mechanic, pp. 192–194). Broadening the conception of ill health in this way has dangers that will be discussed later (Illich; Szasz).

Personal and Community Health Services

Given our broad definition of health, we may examine health services in a broad context as well. Health services have been defined as (1) those services delivered by personnel engaged in medical occupations, such as physicians and nurses, plus other personnel working under their supervision; (2) the physical capital involved, such as hospitals; and (3) the other goods and services, such as drugs and bandages (Fuchs, 1966). Weinerman (p. 273) defined the health services system as "all of the activities of a society which are designed to protect or restore health, whether directed to the individual, the community, or the environment."

A critical distinction must be made between health care and medical care. Medical care is generally thought of as care provided by a physician, restricted in scope, focusing on pathophysiological and social problems, and containing a strong element of "caring."

Health and health care services, on the other hand, may generally be divided into two broad categories: personal and community. Personal health care services deal directly with individuals for the maintenance of health or the control or cure of illness. Community health services are directed toward population groups. The public today takes for granted the provision of pure drinking water and sanitary sewage disposal, but pure water supply has probably had a greater impact on health than any other factor except nutrition. Other community health services include solid waste disposal; food, milk, and drug control and inspection; fluoridation of water; and control of air and noise pollution.

A number of health services—which can be called "combined" services—have aspects of both community and personal health services. Mass immunization programs, by protecting each immunized individual, protect the community as a whole. "Herd immunity" prevents epidemics. This is especially true of diseases caused by obligatory human parasites like the now-eradicated smallpox virus. Other such combined community and individual services include tuberculosis and venereal disease case-finding and treatment programs, which gradually reduce the total number of sources of infection to healthy persons, thereby contributing to community health.

A definition of health care must take into account its boundaries and its providers. There are more than 16 health workers for every physician in the United States, yet when most people think of health care, they think of physicians. If health care is to live up to a dynamic definition, the contributions of such providers as social workers, technicians, and administrators will need to be recognized. Physicians have been slow to acknowledge these contributions, yet they too are beginning to be aware of the importance of teamwork in health care and of the need for special efforts to foster such teamwork.

Likewise, if health care is in part aimed at improving or assisting social functioning, it must grapple in some way with societal problems. Rudolph Virchow, the great German pathologist, who as a youth fought on the barricades against Bismarck's government, described his profession in these words: "Medicine is a social science and politics is nothing else but medicine on a large scale" (Sigerist, p. 93). In a day when cancer is the second greatest cause of death in the United States, and 40% of cancer could probably be controlled by changing the environment, it is counterproductive for a physician to provide personal care while ignoring a workplace where patients are exposed to carcinogens or a refinery whose fumes may be causing cancer in a nearby residential area. Kass (1981) answers this dilemma by stressing that the physician is not the only person responsible for health but that the physician's responsibility for societal problems is similar to that of other citizens.

There is also the danger of defining health care too broadly, so as to encompass all areas of life. Medicine has always displayed an eagerness to appropriate many of humankind's vast panoply of problems, especially if they can be transliterated into medical nomenclature. When therapeutic success eluded such practitioners, they simply redoubled their efforts. This phenomenon has been labeled "creeping medical imperialism" (Sederer, p. 268). Although the patient generally initiates contact, seeking assistance, and must be assumed to be in control of her or his own life, medicine increasingly fosters a dependency role (Mechanic, pp. 15, 169). This situation is made more acute in an era of chronic disease, in which patients need care at frequent intervals for a period of years. Illich (1976) has coined the phrase "social iatrogenesis" to describe what happens when an individual loses control of his or her own life through health care. There is also a risk in the tendency to broaden the definition of mental illness, taking away an individual's autonomy and personhood by calling him or her "sick" (Szasz). Taken to the extreme, an example is the use of psychiatry in the Soviet Union, where dissidents are often mislabeled mentally ill and incarcerated. It is these considerations that led Cassell (1977) to conclude that the job of medicine is not merely to save life but also to preserve autonomy.

Health Care as a Right

As early as 1787, Thomas Jefferson wrote:

> Without health there is no happiness. And attention to health, then, should take the place of every other object. The time necessary to secure this by active exercises should be devoted to it in preference to every other pursuit. I know the difficulty with which a strenuous man tears himself from his studies at any given moment of the day; but his happiness, and that of his family depend on it. The most uninformed mind, with a healthy body is happier than the wisest valetudinarian. [Foley, p. 402]

With the growing affluence of the United States, this kind of thinking has become more and more prominent. Although high-quality health care is certainly not available to the entire population, it is generally accepted that this country is in the process of putting the concept into operation, despite setbacks during the Reagan years.

The idea of "health care as a right" is different from "health as a right." Health is primarily the concern of the individual; one can strive for it, but the health care system cannot provide it. However, *health care* for all is a realizable goal. The United States has been slow, however, to take the necessary steps. Until the enactment of Medicare in 1965, no unit of government had taken general responsibility for aiding nonindigent individuals when they were ill. The roots of this inattention can be found in the American ethic of freedom and equality. Harlow (White, 1971, p. 56) says it well: "There has been a stubborn insistence on protecting the individual's freedom by making him responsible for his own tragedy."

A significant percentage of people in the United States can be said to have a right to health care already. Most workers in this country have work-related health insurance. Of course, a time of high unemployment points out the fallacy of using this mechanism to assure access to health care. In addition to workers' insurance, in 1982 almost 30 million people had a right to care under the Medicare program (Office of Technology Assessment, 1984, p. 27), and millions more poor people had access through Medicaid. However, in the mid-1980s there were approximately 35 million Americans who had no health insurance, about 19% of the population. The growth of for-profit hospitals and "preferred provider organizations," along with Reagan administration health care cutbacks, will worsen access for large parts of the population (Kinzer). A study of California hospitals has shown that patient transfers, or "dumping," has increased dramatically as a result of lack of insurance coverage (Himmelstein et al.).

Many who endorse the concept of health care for everyone are not sure how to put it into effect. It is simply not feasible to make available everything any individual could want at all times. Likewise, health care providers cannot have everything they want to do a good job. Limits must be set to avoid falling into the "bottomless pit" of medical expenditure (Fuchs, 1974). Some form of rationing of health care seems inevitable (Jennett). One would hope that denying access to underprivileged people would not become a mechanism for rationing.

The Value We Place on Health

It is commonly felt among health professionals that all possible services should be provided by the health care system. But are people willing to support health services to that extent? Health is certainly an important value, but it is not the only value. Achilles recognized this in the *Iliad:* "Either, if I stay here and fight beside the city of the Trojans, my return home is gone, but my glory shall be everlasting; but if I return home to the beloved land of my fathers, the excellence of my glory is gone, but there will be a long life left for me, and my end in death will not come to me quickly" (Homer, p. 209). Achilles chose to stay and die. The modern analogue might be the skydiver or skier who intentionally takes a risk for the sake of the thrill derived from the sport. To the extent that the public is aware of risk factors, one could say that the person who smokes cigarettes, eats saturated fats, or refuses to wear seatbelts is deciding that other values are more important than good health.

Society can invest more in justice, beauty, or knowledge, just as it invests in health (Fuchs, 1974). Health economists deal with the problem of limited resources for such investments by speaking of marginal benefit and marginal cost. Is the added benefit of a day in the hospital, for example, worth the added cost? What are our values and priorities? Every physician confronts conflicting values every day in practice. A person may continue to indulge in unhealthy behavior, even though knowing the risks, because the values of the person make that behavior more important than theoretical future health consequences. Such problems can be dealt with only by active, public intervention in matters that society generally considers personal.

However, our society already intervenes rather aggressively in human behavior, particularly through the economic system. Navarro (1975) says, "A far better strategy than self-care and changes in life-style to improve the health of the individual would be to change the economic and social structure that . . . conditioned and determined that unhealthy individual behavior to start with" (p. 352). He uses the example of an unhealthy diet, citing the well-known nutritionist Dr. Jean Mayer, who maintains that the food conglomerates have a primary responsibility for the poor diet of U.S. citizens. These conglomerates are interested primarily in perpetuating the most profitable eating patterns through advertisements for snack foods and fast-food restaurants.

It may not be necessary to intervene actively in affecting values and behavior in all cases. Workplaces can be engineered for safety. Beef can be produced with less saturated fat. Cigarettes can be made that are safer; in fact, the amount of tar and nicotine in the average cigarette has been reduced approximately 25% over the past 20 years. Air bags can be installed in all cars. Although the balance between public health and personal freedom is difficult to attain, society cannot afford to be passive in the face of mounting evidence of risk factors that could in many cases be controlled. Some interventions are necessary to protect the public, as when vaccination was made compulsory, over the objections of a vocal minority.

Clearly, both personal and governmental action is needed. This country needs a health policy that deals with four elements seen to affect health: human biology, environment, lifestyle, and health care organization (Lalonde). As Sigerist (1970) says,

> The people's health is the concern of the people themselves. They must be enlightened in matters of health. They must want it and take an active part in its administration. And since the protection of health is a task of great magnitude, the people will endeavor to fulfill it collectively through the state and its organs. That is why health is a primary concern of the people *and* of government. [p. 102]

The Efficacy of Health Care

There have been some remarkable improvements in health in the United States since 1900. The purpose of this section is to analyze the contribution of health and medical care to those improvements. Such measures as life expectancy and infant mortality rates are useful in understanding the reason for the improvements. Unfortunately, readily available statistics are all related to mortality, whereas data on morbidity are difficult to obtain and verify. Furthermore, there are not as yet any generally accepted direct measures of health itself. Thus, for long-term historical analysis of health levels, we are forced to rely on mortality data.

Between 1900 and 1980 in the United States, both the overall (crude) death rate and infant mortality rate fell, while life expectancy from birth rose (see Table 2.1). However, while crude mortality declined almost 50% during that period, the infant mortality rate declined by about 87%. In fact, the major portion of the decline in the crude mortality rate is due to the remarkable drop in mortality that occurred generally in the younger age groups in the population. Table 2.2 shows the 1980 age-specific mortality rates as percentages of the 1900 age-specific mortality rates. The death rate for the 1- to 4-year-old age group in 1980 was only 3% of the rate in 1900, whereas for people over age 85 in 1980 it was still more than 60% of the 1900 rate. Note too the large gap in percentage improvement between the 15-to-35 age group and the 45-to-65 age group.

TABLE 2.1 Mortality Rate, Infant Mortality Rate, and Life Expectancy from Birth, U.S., 1900–1970

Year	Crude mortality rate (per 1,000 pop.)	Infant mortality rate per 1,000 live births[a]	Life expectancy from birth (in years)
1900	17.2	(99.9)	47.3
1920	13.0	85.9	54.1
1940	10.8	47.0	62.9
1960	9.5	26.0	69.7
1970	9.5	20.0	70.9
1980	8.8	12.6	73.7

[a]Data available only from 1915.
Source: Data for 1900–1960 derived from R. D. Grove and A. M. Hetzel, *Vital Statistics Rates in the United States, 1940–1960* (National Center for Health Statistics, U.S. Dept. of Health, Education and Welfare, 1968), Tables 38, 51, and 53. Data for 1970 and 1977 are from Health Services Research), Tables 9, 10, and 11.

This evidence is corroborated if one looks at mortality data in another way. Table 2.3 shows the average number of years of life remaining at specific ages in 1900 and in 1982 and the percentage change in life expectancy at specified ages between those two years. The percentage increase in life expectancy is a large one. Further, in 1982, one could expect to live 27.2 years longer from birth than

TABLE 2.2 Age-Specific Mortality Rates, U.S., 1900 and 1980

Age group (years)	Age-specific mortality rate (per 1,000 pop.) 1900	Age-specific mortality rate (per 1,000 pop.) 1980	1980 rate as % of 1900 rate
1–4	19.8	0.6	3.0
5–14	3.9	0.3	7.7
15–24	5.9	1.2	20.3
25–34	8.2	1.4	17.1
35–44	10.2	2.3	22.6
45–54	15.0	5.8	38.7
55–64	27.2	13.5	49.6
65–74	56.4	30.0	53.2
75–84	123.3	60.9	49.4
85 and over	260.9	159.8	61.3

Source: Statistical Abstract of the United States, 1974 (Bureau of the Census, U.S. Dept. of Commerce, 1974), Table 83.

TABLE 2.3 Average Remaining Lifetime in Years at Specified Ages, U.S., 1900 and 1982, and Percent Change Between 1900 and 1982

Age in years	Life expectancy		Years difference	% change
	1900	1982		
0	47.3	74.5	27.2	57.5
5	55.0	69.1	14.1	25.6
15	46.8	59.3	12.5	26.7
25	39.1	50.0	10.9	27.9
35	31.9	40.6	8.7	27.3
45	24.8	31.5	6.7	27.0
55	17.9	23.2	5.3	29.6
65	11.9	16.8	4.9	41.2
75	7.1	10.1	3.0	42.3
85	4.0	6.1	2.1	52.5

Source: Statistical Abstract of the United States, 1971, 1974 and 1978 (Bureau of the Census, U.S. Dept. of Commerce, 1971 and 1974 and 1978). (See p. 70 in 1978 edition.)

one could in 1900. However, upon reaching age 65, one could expect to live only 4.9 years longer than one could have in 1900. Tables 2.2 and 2.3 thus indicate that the most important factor in the fall in the crude mortality and the rise of life expectancy from birth is the decrease in the infant mortality rate. If many more individuals survive the first year of life and then live into their 60s and 70s, the overall life expectancy of any one group of such fortunate infants is going to rise.

The leading causes of death changed significantly between 1900 and 1985. In 1900, the five leading causes of death were, in order, influenza and pneumonia, tuberculosis, gastritis, heart disease, and stroke. In 1985, the five leading causes of death were heart disease, cancer, stroke, personal injury, and chronic obstructive pulmonary disease. In 1900, three of the five leading killers were infectious diseases. In 1985, none of the top five were infectious diseases. But for each of the leading killers in that year, cigarette smoking and/or alcohol abuse was a major risk factor.

Since the improved life expectancy in 1985 resulted primarily from the marked change in infant and child mortality that took place during the period it is worthwhile to look specifically at the major killers of infants and young children early in the century. They were the major infectious diseases, including infantile diarrhea, tuberculosis, typhoid fever, measles, diphtheria, and influenza and pneumonia. Most of the decline in infant mortality has resulted from the decline in infectious diseases. Some diseases were probably affected most by nutrition, as in the case of tuberculosis. Others, such as infantile diarrhea and typhoid fever, were probably more affected by environmental sanitation. Diphtheria was on the decline prior to the development of a vaccine, but the vaccine probably contributed greatly to the near disappearance of the disease. Finally, pneumonia was probably affected by improved environment. As mentioned earlier, McKeown (1976) was unable to demonstrate a significant effect on mortality of the introduction of antibiotics. Thus, personal health services do not appear to have made an important contribution to the fall in infant mortality.

Infant mortality is a useful index to consult in considering other influences on health, such as social class. Maternal age and parity, birth weight of the infant, rapidity of childbearing, loss by the mother of a previous child, paternal social class, and the region of the country in which the child is born have all been shown to be related to infant mortality (Morris, pp. 60, 241). The infant mortality rate is sensitive to environmental conditions, such as housing, sanitation, and pure food and water (Rosen). The birth weight of the infant, one of the factors in infant mortality, has itself been related to a number of factors, including stress and smoking during pregnancy (Hemminki & Starfield).

The infant mortality rate at least gives a useful indication of the commitment of a society to health, especially that of its children. Table 2.4 shows the relationship of the U.S. rate to other countries, from 1950 to 1985. The U.S. rate has declined but not as rapidly as that of other countries; therefore, it has fallen from a position of sixth to last among the countries shown in the table. In part, the relatively high infant mortality in the United States is due to the experience of the lower socioeconomic and nonwhite racial groups. In 1980, the black infant mortality rate was 22.1 per 1,000; the white infant mortality rate was 11.5 per 1,000 (National Center for Health Statistics, p. 183). Most of the factors known to influence infant mortality can be changed for the better by enlightened social policy, but some of these, such as child spacing by birth control, can be approached through medical care itself.

Improved medical care certainly has had a positive effect on infant mortality. An analysis of infant deaths in New York City found that adequacy of prenatal care was strongly associated with higher infant birth weight and survival, and it was estimated that adequate health services could reduce the overall 1968 rate of 21.9 per 1,000 live births as much as 33%, to 14.7% per 1,000 (Kessner). More recent analyses have confirmed this basic finding (Showstack, Budetti, & Minkler; Sokol).

However, the value or efficacy of health care in general has come under increasing scrutiny (see Chapter 15). The rapidly rising costs of medical care have fostered a climate of questioning the value of the care provided, and such critics as McKeown (1976) and Illich (1976) have been widely quoted. It has been estimated that only 10 to 20% of procedures employed by health professionals have objective, controlled clinical trials to support the view that they will be helpful (Office of Technology Assessment, 1978; White, 1968). Clinical physicians will counter the evidence with "clinical experience." Physicians, however, have unconscious reasons for wishing a therapy to succeed, and each sees a limited spectrum of the population and its problems (Mechanic, p. 11).

TABLE 2.4 Infant Mortality Rates in Selected Countries 1950–1985

Country	1950–1955		1980–1985		% Change 1950–55 to 1980–85
	Rate[a]	Rank	Rate[a]	Rank	
Australia	24	4	10	12	–57
Belgium	45	14	11	17	–76
Canada	36	11	9	9	–75
Denmark	28	8	8	5	–71
Finland	34	10	6	1	–82
France	45	14	9	9	–80
German Dem. Rep.	58	18	11	17	–81
German Red. Rep.	48	16	11	17	–77
Hong Kong	79	20	10	12	–87
Iceland	21	2	6	1	–71
Ireland	41	12	10	12	–76
Japan	51	17	6	1	–88
Luxembourg	43	13	9	9	–79
Netherlands	24	4	8	5	–66
Norway	23	3	8	5	–65
Spain	62	19	10	12	–83
Sweden	20	1	7	4	–65
Switzerland	29	9	8	5	–72
United Kingdom	28	6	10	12	–64
United States	28	6	11	17	–61

[a]Rate represents deaths under 1 year of age per 1,000 live births.
Source: United Nations Children's Fund (quoted in National Leadership Commission on Health Care, Health Care Expenditures and Utilization Chartbook. Washington, DC, 1987, p. 1.

The practitioner is unable to avoid bias or to compare therapies to a control, and these are essential aspects of a controlled clinical trial. Perhaps the greatest problem overall is the dearth of scientific evidence on efficacy and safety (Office of Technology Assessment, 1978).

The technology most questioned is what Thomas called "half-way technology"—technologies that deal with the symptoms of a condition without affecting the underlying disease process. These technologies, such as renal dialysis, respirators, and cardiac monitors and pacemakers, have come to dominate modern medicine. A mechanical orientation traced to Descartes has developed. As Freymann 1974, (p. 172) says, "Cartesian mechanism and dualism encourage the naive faith that because the universe is composed of elemental particles, the total explanation of its complex systems can be found in information derived from these particles. There are many examples of this faith in medical literature." The resources of the physical and chemical sciences have intensified this "engineering" approach during this century. One of the greatest dangers of this approach is that technology is used to define illness and to determine who qualifies for care. One result of this is pointed out by Engel (1981, p. 592): "The frustration of those who find what they believe to be their legitimate health needs inadequately met by too technologically oriented physicians is misinterpreted as 'unrealistic expectations' when it is actually a genuine discrepancy between illness as actually experienced and as it is conceptualized in the biomedical mode."

This mechanistic orientation toward diagnosis and treatment has tended to obscure those activities aimed at improving functioning of the chronically physically and mentally disabled. With an aging population, the need for such activities will grow (Stout & Crawford). Rehabilitation has not traditionally been accorded great importance in health care in relation to diagnosis and therapy, and it is often seen in the same mechanistic way. In fact, rehabilitation, especially for elderly people, is mainly a low-technology activity involving multidisciplinary teams. Psychosocial aspects are particularly important in the elderly because of the prevalence of depression and cognitive losses (Lewis). Effective rehabilitation can enable elderly people to improve their independence and live in their preferred setting (Cohen). Mechanical technologies, such as prosthetics and simple robots, can play a role in such activities, but they must then be evaluated rigorously.

The efficacy of many health service interventions can be questioned (Cochrane). Although the physician has a number of functions, prescribing or selecting technology seems to play the dominant role in the minds of both public and provider. A major challenge for the future is to expand greatly the scientific basis for medical treatment (see Chapter 15).

The Caring Function

Health professionals sometimes become so involved in delivering services that they neglect medicine's traditional role, caring for people. As Sigerist (1970) says,

> Disease, then, is a biological process. . . . But this process takes place in man, and thus always involves the mind. . . . Disease, a destructive process that threatens life, may destroy only a few cells that can easily be replaced, but it may destroy the entire organism and with it the individual. For this reason, man suffers and is afraid: disease reminds him that he is mortal, that he must die sooner or later, and if the illness is serious, it may be very soon. . . . Elementary fears, age-old views, come from the depth of the unconscious, breaking through the thin crust of education. [p. 93]

Although care has a long history, it is little spoken of in today's technological world of medicine. However, there are studies that support the importance of care. It has been shown that patients who demonstrate acceptance—measured by a scale including trust in the surgeon, optimism about the outcome, and confidence in their ability to cope—healed faster in a trial involving eye surgery (Frank). Caring itself can be an effective method of therapy (Haggerty; Mechanic, pp. 129–130). In an earlier section of this chapter I summarized the extensive evidence that psychological and social supports affect outcomes.

Studies of primary care settings have indicated that a large majority of patients present either with psychological problems or with physical complaints that a physician is trained to regard as trivial (Mechanic, p. 119). Yet caring is really the essence of health care. As stated in the conclusions of the 1972 Sun Valley Forum on National Health, "Medical Cure and Medical Care,"

> Traditionally, medical care has served as much to relieve pain and anxiety and system function as it has to effect cures. Medical care is a highly personalized service with both physical and psychologic elements; these are highly related in the consumer's motivation to seek service and in the physician's ability to achieve cooperation by his advice and to change behavior to be conducive to health. There was widespread agreement that both the "curing" and "caring" functions are central to high-quality care, and that models for delivering health services must allow for the effective integration of both concerns. [p. 232]

Literature on "compliance" with health providers' advice confirms the importance of caring elements in practice (DeMatteo & DiNicola; Haynes). The relationship is most effective when it is a partnership, which requires open communication, mutual understanding, rapport, and trust.

At the end of life, caring is also important. If death is accepted as the inevitable end, inappropriate therapies such as respirators, artificial nutrition, and hydration will not be used when they cannot be effective. It is increasingly acceptable to withhold such therapies in dying patients (Emanuel; President's Commission). Do-not-resuscitate orders are based on judgments of either no medical benefit or a resulting poor quality of life (Tomlinson & Brody). More than three-quarters of the states now have enabling legislation recognizing the Living Will, in which people describe how they wish to be treated when dying (Emanuel). A growing alternative to hospital terminal care is the hospice, in which palliative care and extensive support services are provided to patients whom curative interventions can no longer be expected to benefit (Bulkin & Lukashoc).

The Future of Health Care

Health care is in a crisis (Engel). We have developed a health care system characterized by large institutions and specialists practicing narrow, technological medicine (Szasz). Naturally, this system has its value and should not be entirely abandoned. Further advances that have been predicted include human gene therapy, understanding the genetic origin of many diseases, regeneration of tissues, slowing of aging, and increased epidemiological knowledge resulting from data banks. This technological system is failing to meet many human needs, however, and is largely ignoring opportunities for disease prevention and health promotion. The recent trend toward further institutionalization and the movement of profit-making firms into the health care sector can only exacerbate these problems (see Chapter 18).

The physician is not to be envied. Confidence in physicians has fallen (Burnham, 1982). The physician is expected to be a "double agent," both taking care of a sick person *and* representing the interests of society, especially in holding down financial costs (Burnham, 1977). Pines and Maslach say that

> . . . the source of the problem is not the individual but the structure and the environment of the helping professions themselves. . . . The helping professions are asked to be warm and caring, on the one hand, and objective, on the other. If they fail to meet these high expectations and treat their patients or clients in ways that are considered indifferent, rude, or even dehumanizing, people are quick to criticize them and complain about the individuals who staff society's service institutions. [p. 246]

Kass (1981) feels that the solution to this problem is for health care professionals to focus on their true goal, the promotion and preservation of health.

The biomedical model needs to be expanded to become a social model (Kickbusch). Elements of a social model would include recognition of the limitations of the professional model of health, acceptance that health may not be the highest goal, promotion of self-reliance as an expression of human dignity and development, and recognition that there is more than one form of curing or healing. The social model requires one to see that major health problems are closely linked to social values and economic interests and that social integration and social support are central to health and well-being. This is closely related to the biopsychosocial model described by Engel (1981). Another essential element of it is approaching a person as a whole, that is, practicing holistic medicine. In an aging society, rehabilitation and home care, as well as death care, will need additional emphasis.

If the traditional system is unable or unwilling to deal with people's problems in a warm and caring way, the public will either force it to change or will find other types of providers who can meet those needs (Starr). As noted earlier, the increasing popularity of self-care and alternative healers already seems to indicate a growing dissatisfaction.

The Future of Humanity

Earlier sections of this chapter have argued that the concept of health depends greatly on psychological, social, and cultural factors. Thus, the future of health and health care is intertwined with our view of ourselves and how we act on that view. Enduring traits of the American character include self-reliance and independence, propensity to participate in local affairs, innovativeness, and a sense of efficacy and optimism (Inkeles). Recent changes include growing social tolerance, a decline of the Protestant ethic, and decreasing political confidence. Society is becoming increasingly secular, empirical, and "this worldly" (Kahn & Weiner, pp. 38–39). At the same time, the public is more accepting of spiritual and transcendental experience and more critical of the growth-and-consumption ethic of business (Harman). Alternative methods of therapy, such as religious and secular healing, healing by the laying on of hands, and the use of imagery, are gaining visibility (Sheik; Sobel).

Some of the implications for health care include a broadened definition of health, reduced status for professionals, recognition that the whole society is the environment that affects health, a blurring of the distinction between mental and physical illness, changing attitudes toward death, and control over medical technology (Harman).

Summary and Conclusions

This chapter has argued for a broadened concept of health and health care and has supported the idea of health care as a right. Health care is seen as a combination of curative medicine, caring, and attention to social factors. Curing and caring are part of the tradition of health care, but the health care professions have paid relatively little attention to the benefits that could result from changes in the physical and social environment.

It is important to emphasize that treating disease is not the same as creating health. Dubos (1971) sees health as a mirage that will continue to recede just beyond reach, and he believes that this is good:

> Human life implies adventure, and there is no adventure without struggles and dangers. . . . Attempts at adaptation will demand efforts, and these efforts will often result in failure. . . . Disease will remain an inescapable manifestation of his struggles. While it may be comforting to imagine a life free of stresses and strains in a carefree world, this will remain an idle dream. Man cannot hope to find another Paradise on earth, because Paradise is a static concept while human life is a dynamic process. [p. 278]

References

Asher, C. "The Impact of Social Support Networks on Adult Health." *Medical Care, 22,* 349, 1984.

Berkman, L., & Breslow, L. *Health and Ways of Living.* New York: Oxford University Press, 1983.

Blakiston's New Gould Medical Dictionary, 2nd Ed. New York: Blakiston Division, McGraw-Hill, 1956.

Bulkin, W., & Lukashok, H. "Rx for Dying: The Case for Hospice." *New England Journal of Medicine, 318,* 376, 1988.

Burnett, M. *Genes, Dreams, and Realities.* New York: Basic Books, 1971.

Burnham, J. "The Physician as a Double Agent." *New England Journal of Medicine, 297,* 278, 1977.

Burnham, J. "American Medicine's Golden Age: What Happened to It?" *Science, 215,* 1474, 1982.

Cassell, E. *The Healer's Art.* Philadelphia: Lippincott, 1976.

Cassell, E. "Autonomy and Ethics in Action." *New England Journal of Medicine, 297,* 333, 1977.

Cochrane, A. *Effectiveness and Efficiency.* London: Nuffield Provincial Hospitals Trust, 1971.

Cohen, B. S. "Geriatric Rehabilitation." *American Family Physician, 360,* 133, 1984.

Daly, M., & Tyroler, H. "Cornell Medical Index Response as Predictor of Mortality." *British Journal of Preventive & Social Medicine, 26,* 159, 1972.

DeMatteo, M. R., & DiNicola, D. D. *Achieving Patient Compliance: The Psychology of the Medical Practitioner Role.* New York: Pergamon Press, 1982.

Dubos, R. *Mirage of Health.* New York: Harper & Row, 1971.

Ebden, P., Carey, O. J., Bhatt, A., & Harrison, B. "The Bilingual Consultation." *Lancet, 1,* 347, 1988.

Elliott, G., & Eisdorfer, C. (Eds.). *Stress and Human Health.* New York: Springer Publishing Co., 1982.

Emanuel, E. J. "Should Physicians Withhold Life-Sustaining Care from Patients Who Are Not Terminally Ill?" *Lancet, 1,* 106, 1988.

Engel, G. "The Need for a New Medical Model: A Challenge for Biomedicine." In A. Caplan, H. T. Engelhardt, & J. McCartney (Eds.), *Concepts of Health and Disease* (pp. 589–607). Reading, MA.: Addison-Wesley, 1981.

Foley, J. P. (Ed.). *Jeffersonian Cyclopedia: A Comprehensive Collection of the Views of Thomas Jefferson* (Vol. I). New York: Russell and Russell, 1967.

Frank, J. "Mind-Body Interactions in Illness and Healing. Paper Presented at the May Lectures, "Alternative Futures for Medicine," Airlie House, Airlie, VA, April 4, 1975.

Freymann, J. *The American Health Care system: Its Genesis and Trajectory.* New York: Medcom Press. 1974.

Fuchs, V. "The Contribution of Health Services to the American Economy." *The Milbank Memorial Fund Quarterly, 44,* 65, 1966.

Fuchs, V. *Who Shall Live?* New York: Basic Books, 1974.

Haggerty, R. "The Boundaries of Health Care." In D. S. Sobel (Ed.), *Ways of Health* (pp. 45–60). New York: Harcourt, Brace, Jovanovich, 1979.

Harman, W. "New Images of Man: What to Do Until the New Paradigm Arrives." Paper Presented at the May Lectures. "Alternative Futures for Medicine," Airlie House, Airlie, VA, April 4, 1975.

Haynes, R. B. "A Critical Review of the "Determinants" of Patient Compliance with Therapeutic Regimens." In D. Sackett & R. B. Haynes (Eds.), *Compliance with Therapeutic Regimens* (pp. 26–39). Baltimore, MD: Johns Hopkins University Press, 1976.

Hemminki, E., & Starfield, B. "Prevention of Low Birth Weight and Pre-Term Birth." *Milbank Memorial Fund Quarterly/Health and Society, 56,* 339, (1978).

Himmelstein, D., Woolhandler, S., Harnly, M., Bader, M., Silber, R., Backer, H., & Jones, A. "Patient Transfers: Medical Practice as Social Triage." *American Journal of Public Health, 74,* 494, 1984.

Homer. *The Iliad.* Translated by R. Lattimore. Chicago: University of Chicago Press, 1951.

Hoyman, H. "The Spiritual Dimensions of Man's Health in Today's World." In D. Belgum (Ed.), *Religion and Medicine.* Ames, IA: Iowa State University Press, 1967.

Illich, I. *Medical Nemesis.* New York: Pantheon Books, 1976.

Inkeles, A. "Continuity and change in the American character." In S. M. Lipset (Ed.), *The third century* (pp. 389–416). Stanford, CA: Hoover Institution Press, 1979.

Jago, J. " 'Hal'—Old word, new task: Reflections on the words 'Health' and 'Medical.' " *Social Science and Medicine, 9,* 1, 1975.

Jennett, B. *High Technology Medicine, Benefits and Burdens.* London: The Nuffield Provincial Hospitals Trust, 1984.

Jonas, S. *Medical Mystery: The Training of Doctors in the United States.* New York: W. W. Norton, 1979.

Kahn, H., & Weiner, A. *The Year 2000.* New York: Macmillan, 1967.

Kaplan, R. M., Bush, J., & Berry, C. "Health status: Types of validity and index of well-being." *Health Services Research, 11,* 478, 1976.

Kass, L. "Regarding the end of medicine and the pursuit of health." In A. Caplan, H. T. Engelhardt, & J. McCartney (Eds.), *Concepts of Health and Disease, Interdisciplinary Perspectives* (pp. 3–30). Reading, MA: Addison-Wesley, 1981.

Kessner, D., *Infant Death: An Analysis by Maternal Risk and Health Care.* Washington, D.C.: Institute of Medicine, National Academy of Sciences. 1973.

Kickbusch, I. "Involvement in Health: A Social Concept of Health Education." *International Journal of Health Education, 24* (Suppl.), 3, 1981.

Kinzer, D. "Care of the Poor Revisited." *Inquiry, 21,* 5, 1984.

Koos, E. *The Health of Regionville.* New York: Hafner, 1954.

Kunitz, S., "Changing Health Care Opinions in Regionville, 1946–1973." *Medical Care, 13,* 549, 1975.

Lalonde, M. *A New Perspective on the Health of Canadians.* Ottawa, Canada: Government of Canada, 1974.

Lewis, C. B. "Rehabilitation of the Older Person: A Psychosocial Focus." *Physical Therapy, 64,* 517, 1984.

Lipkin, M. "Psychological Aspects of Evaluation of Outcome." In H. D. Banta (Ed.), *Resources for Health* (pp. 90–98). New York: Praeger, 1982.

McKeown, T. *The Role of Medicine: Dream, Mirage, or Nemesis.* London: The Nuffield Provincial Hospitals Trust, 1976.

McPeek, B., Gilbert, J., & Mosteller, F. "The End Result: Quality of Life." In J. Bunker, B. Barnes, & F. Mosteller (Eds.), *Costs, Risks, and Benefits of Surgery* (pp. 170–175). New York: Oxford University Press, 1977.

Mechanic, D. *Politics, Medicine, and Social Science.* New York: Wiley, 1974.

Millis, J. *A Rational Policy for Medical Education and Its Financing.* New York: The National Fund for Medical Education, 1971.

Morris, J. *Uses of Epidemiology.* Edinburgh, Scotland: Churchill Livingstone, 1975.

Mumford, E., Schlesinger, H., & Glass, G. "The Effects of Psychological Intervention on Recovery from Surgery and Heart Attacks: An Analysis of the Literature." *American Journal of Public Health, 72,* 141, 1982.

Mushkin, S., & Dunlop, D. *Health: What Is It Worth?* New York: Pergamon Press, 1979.

National Center for Health Statistics. *Health United States and Prevention Profile 1983* (USDHEW Publication No. PHS 84-1232). Hyattsville, MD: U.S. Government Printing Office, 1983.

Navarro, V. "The Industrialization of Fetishism or the Fetishism of Industrialization: A Critique of Ivan Illich." *International Journal of Health Services, 5,* 347, 1975.

Nuckolls, K. B., Cassel, J. C., and Kaplan, B. H. "Psychosocial assets, life crisis and the prognosis of pregnancy." *American Journal of Epidemiology, 95,* 431, 1972.

Office of Technology Assessment, Congress of the United States. *Assessing the Efficacy and Safety of Medical Technologies.* Washington, D.C.: U.S. Government Printing Office, 1978.

Office of Technology Assessment, Congress of the United States. Cancer Risk, Assessing and Reducing the Dangers in our Society. Boulder, CO: Westview Press, 1982.

Office of Technology Assessment, Congress of the United States. *Medical Technology and Costs of the Medicare Program.* Washington, D.C.: U.S. Government Printing Office, 1984.

Osterweis, M., Solomon, F., & Green, M. (Eds.). *Bereavement, Reactions, Consequences and Care.* Washington, D.C.: National Academy Press, 1984.

Parsons, T. *The Social System.* Glencoe, IL: The Free Press, 1951.

Parsons, T. "Definitions of Health and Illness in the Light of American Values and Social Structure." In E. Jaco (Ed.), *Patients, Physicians, and Illness.* Glencoe, IL: The Free Press, 1958.

Pines, A., & Maslach, C. *Experiencing Social Psychology.* New York: Knopf, 1979.

Prager, K., et al. "Maternal Smoking and Drinking Behavior before and during Pregnancy." In National Center for Health Statistics, *Health United States and Prevention Profile, 1983* (USDHEW Pub. No. PHS 84-1232). Hyattsville, MD: (pp. 33–39). U.S. Government Printing Office, 1983.

President's Commission for the Study of Ethical Problems in Medicine. *Deciding to Forego Life-Sustaining Treatment.* Washington, D.C.: U.S. Government Printing Office, 1983.

Reich, T. "Biologic-Marker Studies in Alcoholism." *New England Journal of Medicine, 318,* 180, 1988.

Rosen, G. *A History of Public Health.* New York: MD Publications, 1958.

Sederer, L. "Moral Therapy and the Problem of Morale." *American Journal of Psychiatry, 134,* 267, 1979.

Sheikh, A. (Ed.). *Imagination and Healing.* Farmingdale, N.Y.: Baywood, 1984.

Showstack, J., Budetti, P., & Minkler, D. "Factors Associated with Birthweight: An Exploration of the Roles of Prenatal Care and Length of Gestation." *American Journal of Public Health, 74,* 1003, 1984.

Sidel, R., & Sidel, V. "Toward the Twenty-first Century." In V. Sidel & R. Sidel (Eds.), *Reforming Medicine, Lessons of the Last Quarter Century* (pp. 267–284). New York: Pantheon Books, 1984.

Sigerist, H. *Medicine and Human Welfare.* College Park, MD: McGrath Publishing Co., 1970.

Singer, E., et al. "Mortality and Mental Health: Evidence for the Midtown Manhattan Re-Study." *Social Science and Medicine, 10,* 517, 1976.

Sobel, D. S. (Ed.). *Ways of Health.* New York: Harcourt Brace Jovanovich, 1979.

Sokol, R., "Risk, Antepartum Care and Outcome: Impact of a Maternity and Infant Care Project." *Obstretrics and Gynecology, 56,* 150, 1980.

Starr, P. *The Social Transformation of American Medicine.* New York: Basic Books, 1982.

Stout, R. W., & Crawford, V. "Active-life Expectancy and Terminal Dependency: Trends in Long-term Geriatric Care over 33 Years." *Lancet, 1,* 281, 1988.

Sun Valley Forum on National Health. "Medical Cure and Medical Care" (Summary). *Milbank Memorial Fund Quarterly, 50,* 231, 1972.

Susser, M. "Ethical Components in the Definition of Health." In A. Caplan, H. T. Engelhardt, & J. McCartney, (Eds.), *Concepts of Health and Disease, Interdisciplinary Perspectives* (pp. 93–105). Reading, MA: Addison-Wesley, 1981.

Szasz, T. *The Manufacture of Madness.* New York: Harper & Row, 1970.

Tomlinson, T., & Brody, H. "Ethics and Communication in Do-Not-Resuscitate Orders." *New England Journal of Medicine, 318,* 43, 1988.

U.S. Bureau of the Census. *Statistical Abstract of the United States,* 1984. Washington, D.C.: U.S. Government Printing Office, 1984.

Weinerman, E. R. "Research on Comparative Health Service Systems." *Medical Care, 9,* 272, 1971.

White, K. "International Comparisons of Health Services Systems." *Milbank Memorial Fund Quarterly, 46,* 117, 1968.

White, R. *Right to Health: The Evolution of an Idea.* Ames, IA: The University of Iowa Press, 1971.

Williams, A. "Economics and the Rational Use of Medical Technology." In F. F. H. Rutten, & S. J. Reiser (Eds.), *The Economics of Medical Technology* (pp. 109–120). New York: Springer-Verlag, 1988.

World Health Organization. "The Constitution of the World Health Organization." *WHO Chronicle, 1,* 29, 1944.

Zaborowski, M. "Cultural Components in Responses to Pain." *Journal of Social Issues, 8,* 16, 1952.

3

Population Data for Health and Health Care

Steven Jonas

Quantitative analysis provides a basic means of describing, and thus understanding, the population served by our health care delivery system. Quantitative analysis of populations—especially in terms of number, health status, and health care services utilization—elucidates the population's place in and relation to the delivery system.

Most of the data in this chapter will be 2 to 4 years out of date by the time this book is published. This is because of the nature of most data gathering and reporting, on the one hand, and book writing and publishing, on the other. The data that are presented here relate, particularly to change and rates of change. These are major issues for any health care delivery system.

Quantitative Perspectives

There are three major quantitative perspectives from which a population can be viewed in relation to health and health care services. First is the *number* of people and what are called *demographic* characteristics (from the Greek, "describing the people"). Among the important demographic characteristics are geographic distribution, age, sex, marital status, and such social characteristics as ethnicity, income, education, employment, and measures of social class.

Second are the *health status* and the *sickness status* of the population. With the current level of sophistication of data gathering and analysis, it is much easier to characterize the latter than the former. The ill-health status of the population is described by measures of mortality (death) and morbidity (sickness). Mortality and morbidity may be counted for the population as a whole, in which case the numbers or rates are defined as *crude*. Alternatively, mortality and morbidity may be counted by cause or by demographic characteristics used in describing segments of the population.

The third quantitative perspective for viewing a population is *utilization of health services:* who uses how many of what kinds of services, when, and where. Utilization can be measured from two points of view: that of the consumer and that of the provider. For example, visits to physicians by patients can be reported in terms of how many visits the average patient makes to a physician each year. The same set of events can be reported in terms of how many patient visits the average physician provides each year. An excellent review of patient-perspective utilization research has been carried out by Hulka & Wheat (1985).

When one knows how many people there are, what their health and sickness status is, and the levels at which they utilize services, one has quantitatively characterized a population in relation to its health and health care fairly well.

Numbers and Rates

Population, health status, and utilization data all can be presented in two forms: as numbers and as rates. A *number* represents simply a count of conditions, individuals, and events. A *rate* has two parts, a numerator and a denominator. The numerator is the number of conditions, individuals, or events counted. The denominator is (usually) a larger group of conditions, individuals, and events from among which the numerator is drawn.

It is customary to give the rate as applying during a particular time period. For example, one could count 1,000 deaths occurring in a particular population during a year. This *number* of deaths becomes a *rate* if one counts the population, finds that number to be 100,000, and then says that the mortality *rate* is 1,000/100,000 per year. The rate can be expressed as a percentage (in this case, 1%), as a rate per thousand (in this case, 10), or as any other formulation that is useful.

The multipliers are usually in powers of 10. The magnitude is usually chosen to make the rate a number of reasonable size. Thus, the more infrequent the event being counted by the numerator, the larger the denominator. For example, crude death rates for a whole population, from all causes, are usually given as per 1,000 of the population. Rarer, cause-specific mortality rates are given as per 100,000 or even as per 1 million. This is done so that the rate will not appear as a fractional number.

Denominators as well as numerators can be fairly specific. In discussing deaths from lung cancer related to cigarette smoking, for example, a rate can be determined for the number of deaths per year from lung cancer in males over age 45 who have smoked two or more packs of cigarettes per day for 20 years or more (the numerator), per all males over 45 who have smoked two or more packs of cigarettes per day for 20 years or more (the denominator). Usually, however, the units of the numerator and the denominator in health indices are different. For example, in cause-specific mortality rates, the unit for the numerator is deaths by cause, and the unit for the denominator is persons.

Although rates are usually fractions, they will occasionally be whole numbers. For example, in measuring total morbidity in a population, one may find that the number of diagnosed disease conditions is greater than the number of people. The rate then is usually given with a denominator of 1; for example, "In the population of a central African city there are 2.5 disease conditions per person." This usage also occurs in utilization rates; for example, "The annual physician-visit rate in the United States is about 5.0 per person."

A very important use of rates is to measure changes over time, as when the death rate for condition X goes down from one year to the next. Health care service utilization rates are not usually given in terms of numerators and denominators. Hospital admission rates that are specific for a particular hospital, for example, are not usually given as per person but simply as per unit of time, as follows: "In 1989, the admission rate for hospital Y was 1,000 per month." This practice prevails because the sizes of the populations served by most providers are not known.

The Purposes of Quantification

Description. There are two major purposes for quantification of health care delivery system data. First, quantification *describes* the population under consideration. Demographic characteristics such as location (do many people live near marshes in which malaria-carrying mosquitoes live?) and age distribution (are there many infants and/or old people?) give some indication of the population's relative disease risk. Disease-specific mortality and morbidity rates point out the major health and illness problems in the population. The infant mortality rate gives some indication of both general health levels and the availability of medical care. The distribution by place, age, sex, ethnic group, and social class of crude and disease-specific mortality and morbidity rates shows which population subgroups are being affected by what diseases.

Utilization data show how the population uses the health care delivery system. As we noted, utilization of health services can be viewed from the consumer's perspective: how many times the average person sees a physician per year and what the sources of care are. It can also be viewed from the point of view of the provider: how many patient visits the average physician provides in a year. Further, data can be subdivided according to the various demographic characteristics of the population. For example, the average annual per-person physician visit rates can be reported by age, sex, and geographic distribution of a group of patients admitted to a particular hospital during a year.

In addition, demographic analyses of the providers themselves, both individuals and institutions, can be done. One can determine the average number of visits provided annually by physicians according to their age, practice location, and specialty. Thus, *descriptively,* quantification tells us how many of what kind of people are at risk, what kinds of diseases and conditions of ill health they

have, how those problems are distributed in the population, and who goes where
for how many of what kinds of health services, delivered by which types of
providers.

Program Planning. The second purpose of quantification in health care
delivery is for *program planning,* as it might be carried out by a hospital, a health
maintenance organization, a city health services administration, or a private
physician. Description can reveal the existence of problems. If there is the will
and the money to do something about them, data also can be used to help design
solutions. Once new programs are under way, data can be used to evaluate their
effects and effectiveness. Thus, data are necessary for logical program planning,
as they are in most fields of human endeavor. However, it must be remembered
that they are not sufficient. Before the use of data has any real meaning for
planning, the agencies and institutions that control the health care delivery
system must first make a policy decision to undertake program planning and to
implement a suitable plan. We discuss the problems of health care program
planning in the United States in Chapter 13.

To illustrate the use of data for this purpose, let us take the hypothetical case of
planning a hospital for a medical school in a suburban/semirural area. A program
is to be designed for this hospital. The program is to help meet the health care
needs of the community as well as the educational and research needs of the
medical school. (The three functions of any medical school, in theory at least,
are patient care [service], teaching, and research. It is to be hoped, of course,
that these three functions can be coordinated in a positive way for the benefit of
each one).

The first step in rationally planning for a new medical school hospital would
be to delineate a proposed service area. One would count population, determine
population density, examine modes of transportation, and evaluate existing
health care resources, particularly the more complex and sophisticated ones
already in use. Some of the specific questions are as follows:

- How many people are there, and where are they located?
- What are the rates of population change?
- What are the age, sex, and marital status distributions?
- What are the social class and ethnic characteristics?
- What is the sickness and health profile?
- What are the existing health care resources, and how are they used?
- What do existing providers see as their needs?
- How do they view the new facility, and how will they relate to it?

The answers to these and many other similar questions define the health and
health care needs of the population to be served. They also characterize the
existing health care resources. In planning any new health care facility, it is

essential to know how it is going to relate functionally to existing providers, both individual and institutional. The data can then be used to identify and quantify both the met and the unmet health and health care needs of the population. Only when that has been done can rational planning for a new program and facility be undertaken.

Amalgamating, classifying, and analyzing all of these data are the bases for rational program planning. The data afford the opportunity to make intelligent decisions on facility design, location, services and service priorities, space allocation, administrative structure, community relations, staffing and personnel policies, teaching and research programs, capital cost, expense budget, and so on. In general, one can say that intelligent decisions in health services planning depend on intelligent use of health and health care data. Unfortunately, that does not always happen in the United States.

A particular problem with health and health care data occurred during the early 1980s. The Reagan administration sharply reduced federal data-gathering and data-analysis activities (Mundinger). This meant that less information was published, especially on population characteristics such as health status. Moreover, what was published was increasingly delayed. The reader of this chapter will notice that certain data—census and vital statistics, for example—are reasonably up to date. However, other data are some years behind (and farther behind than they used to be). Certain classes of data presented in previous editions of this book are now simply unavailable. It is to be hoped that this situation will be corrected.

Population

Number

The Constitution of the United States requires that a census of the nation be taken at least once every 10 years (U.S. Bureau of the Census, p. 1). The original purpose of the census was to provide the basis for the apportionment of seats in the House of Representatives of the U.S. Congress. A census has been carried out every 10 years since 1790. Although every effort is made for completeness, the Census Bureau has estimated that in 1980 it undercounted by between 1 and 2% (U.S. Bureau of the Census, p. 1). In addition to the decennial censuses, the Census Bureau makes interim estimates on various parameters, based on information gathered from population samples and a variety of other sources. The U.S. resident population as of July 1, 1987, was estimated to be 243,249,000 (U.S. Bureau of the Census, Table 2). In addition, there were about 2 million U.S. citizens (excluding military personnel) living abroad (U.S. Bureau of the Census, Table 4).

Births, deaths, immigration, and emigration produce changes in population size. During the 1970s and 1980s, the population growth rate averaged about 1.0% per year. During the 1960s the population grew at the rate of about 1.3% per year. This decline stems primarily from a decrease in the birth rate. The bearing on health services of such matters as population size, growth rate, and birth rate should be obvious.

Demographic Characteristics

In 1986, 76.6% of the population lived in what are called *metropolitan statistical areas* (MSAs) (U.S. Bureau of the Census, Table 30). The figures for 1950 and 1970 were 56% and 69%, respectively. The definition of an MSA is determined by the federal Office of Management and Budget, an agency of the executive branch (U.S. Bureau of the Census, p. 872). As of January 1980, an MSA included (1) at least one city with a population of 50,000 or more, or (2) a Census Bureau–defined urbanized area of at least 50,000 inhabitants and a total MSA population of at least 100,000 (75,000 in New England). In addition, an MSA has to include the county in which the central city is located, as well as adjacent counties that are determined to be metropolitan in character.

As of 1986, it was estimated that the U.S. population was 49% male and 85% white, with a median age of 31.8 (32.7 for whites, 26.9 for blacks) (U.S. Bureau of the Census, Table 20). The median age was up from 28 in 1970. In 1983, 26.6% of the population was under 17, and 12.1% was age 65 and over, up from 9.8% in 1970 (U.S. Bureau of the Census, Table 20). In 1986 about 66% of males and 61% of females over 18 were married (U.S. Bureau of the census, Table 47). In 1980 about 2.5 million Americans were inmates of institutions (up from 2.1 million in 1970). Over 1.4 million were in homes for the aged, about 150,000 lived in homes for the mentally handicapped, and about 61,000 were residents in tuberculosis and other chronic-disease hospitals (U.S. Bureau of the Census, Table 74). See Table 3.1 for a comparison of U.S. demographic characteristics for 1970 and 1986.

Social-class status is often thought to be a valuable parameter by which to cross-tabulate population, health/illness, and utilization data.[1] Unlike the government of England, however, the U.S. government has not developed a social-class index by which it cross-tabulates its demographic data. Thus, we are forced to use ethnicity and income as rough indicators of social class. This is unfortunate because social class is really determined by the combination of several factors, including income, education, employment, and dwelling place. A great deal of such information is in fact collected by the government, but an index has not been created.

---

[1] A detailed discussion of this very important subject, with an extensive bibliography, is presented in *The Health Gap*, edited by Robert Kane, M.D. (New York: Springer Publishing Co., 1975). See also Office of Health Resources Opportunity, *Health Status of Minorities and Low Income Groups* (DHEW Pub. No. HRA 79-627) (Washington, D.C.: U.S. Government Printing Office, 1979).

Table 3.1. Demographic Characteristics, U.S. Population, 1986, with Selected Comparisons for 1970

Characteristic	1986	1970
Number (millions)	243	203
Living in an MSA	77%	69%
Male	49%	49%
White	85%	87%
Median age	31.8	28
Living in institutions (millions)	2.5 (1980)	2.1
Marriage rate (per thousand)	9.9	10.6
Divorce rate (per thousand)	4.8	3.5

Sources: U.S. Bureau of the Census. *Statistical Abstract of the United States: 1971,* Tables 14, 15, 21; *1987,* Tables 20, 30, 74. Washington, D.C.: U.S. Government Printing Office, 1971, 1988.

The information we have been presenting so far comes from the "Population" section of the *Statistical Abstract of the United States: 1988* (U.S. Bureau of the Census). Additional information necessary to develop a comprehensive profile is contained in the "Education," "Social Insurance and Human Services," "Labor Force, Employment, and Earnings," and "Income Expenditures, and Wealth" sections of the same publication.

Vital Statistics

How They Are Collected

In public health, "vital statistics" traditionally consist of births, deaths, marriages, and divorces. In the United States, primary responsibility for collecting these data lies with the states. Not all states collect all categories of data. In most states that do collect them, the Department of Health is responsible, and it regularly publishes at least some of the data collected on a routine basis. Where possible, state health departments rely on county and other local health departments to do the actual counting. The locally accumulated data are then organized at the state level and transmitted to the federal level. The district government for Washington, D.C., carries out such responsibilities in that city.

The National Center for Health Statistics (NCHS) established a National Death Index (NDI) in 1979 (NCHS, 1983a, p. 12). The NDI is a central computerized index of death-record information compiled from magnetic tapes provided by the vital statistics offices of the states. The NDI contains a standard set of information that identifies each death. This information is used to search files for death records. It is available to research investigators and can assist them in finding out whether persons in their studies may have died. It provides the names of the states in which those deaths occurred and the numbers of the death certificates. Arrangements can then be made to obtain such information as cause of death.

The collection of mortality data in the United States did not begin on an annual basis until 1900. At that time 10 states and the District of Columbia became "death registration states" and forwarded the results to the federal government (U.S. Bureau of the Census, p. 57). Until 1946 the Census Bureau assembled the vital statistics at the national level. From 1946 to 1960 the work was performed by the Bureau of State Services of the U.S. Public Health Service. Since 1960 the NCHS, in the Department of Health and Human Services, has carried out the function.

Beginning in 1915, 10 states and the District of Columbia also formed a "birth registration area," collecting birth data on an annual basis. By 1933 all states were in both the birth and death registration areas. (Fetal deaths have been counted annually since 1922.) The corresponding "marriage registration area" was first formed in 1957. By 1987 it included 41 states, the Virgin Islands, Puerto Rico, and the District of Columbia. The "divorce registration" area was established in 1958; by 1987 it covered 31 states and the Virgin Islands (U.S. Bureau of the Census, p. 58).

The NCHS calculates vital statistics rates based on the actual number of persons counted by the Census Bureau on April 1 of each decennial year, as well as the midyear estimates made for other years. Cause-specific mortality data are classified according to the *International Classification of Diseases, Ninth Revision, Adapted for Use in the United States* (NCHS, 1979), the so-called ICDA-9. The ICDA-9 Clinical Modification (ICDA-9-CM) is an extension of the ICDA-9, which is required for use in all hospitals in the United States receiving federal funds.

Natality

In 1987, approximately 3.8 million babies were born in the United States *(Monthly Vital Statistics Report)*. The annual rate was 15.7 live births per 1,000 population rate, up from the lowest rate recorded in recent years, 14.6 in 1975–1976. The birth rate had been steadily dropping from a post-World War II high of 25, achieved in 1955 (U.S. Bureau of the Census, Table 81). The fertility rate (the number of births that 1,000 women would have in their lifetime if, at each year of age, they experienced the birth rates occurring in the specified year) for 1980–1984 was 1,819. That was down from the post-World War II high of 3,690 in 1955–1959 but up slightly from the low of 1,738 recorded in 1976 (U.S. Bureau of the Census, Table 82). If the death rate were to remain stable over a long period and there were no immigration, with this birth rate the U.S. population would actually diminish in size.

Mortality

Crude Death Rate. For 1987 the crude death rate (total deaths per 1,000 population) in the United States was 8.7 (*Monthly Vital Statistics Report*, p. 1). This compares with a rate of 9.5 for the 1960s and between 8.8 and 8.5 for the 1970s (U.S. Bureau of the Census, Table 110).

Mortality data are rather neatly reported. There is one primary reporting authority, usually the local health department or, if none exists, the state health department acting in its place. Death is a well-defined event in the vast majority of cases, although with recent advances in medical technology the possibility of dispute has arisen. Since both hospitals and funeral directors are legally required to report all deaths, with rather serious penalties for failure to comply, we can assume that most deaths are reported.

Determination of a cause of death has presented some problems from time to time. In most cases it is left up to the physician to certify that the patient is dead. Physicians have varying diagnostic styles, opinions, and abilities. Furthermore, there have been changes in the technical definitions of causes of death over time.[2] For example, is diabetes or coronary artery disease the cause of death in a patient who dies from a heart attack that resulted from the complications of diabetes? The reporting authorities have rules to cover these instances. Most physicians follow them, but difficulties occasionally arise.

Much data on differential death rates by the basic demographic variables of age, color, and sex can be found in the *Monthly Vital Statistics Report, Vital Statistics of the United States,* the *Statistical Abstract,* and special studies published in *Vital and Health Statistics,* Series 20. Mortality is relatively high during the first year of life, drops to a relatively low level until the mid-40s, and then begins to climb again (U.S. Bureau of the Census, Table 111).

For the total population, males have a higher mortality rate than do females at all ages. As the population ages in toto, the preponderance of females over males in the older age groups increases. Although the crude death rate for nonwhites is lower than for whites, the age-specific death rates for nonwhites are higher than for whites at all ages until 85. The crude death rate is lower for nonwhites because the nonwhite population is younger.

Cause-specific Mortality Rates. In 1987 the 10 leading causes of death (excluding the diagnostic categories of "symptoms and ill-defined conditions" and "all other diseases") were, in order, heart disease, cancer, stroke, personal injury, chronic obstructive pulmonary disease, influenza and pneumonia (primarily pneumonia), diabetes mellitus, suicide, cirrhosis of the liver, and kidney

[2]For a detailed discussion of this problem, see "Estimates of Selected Comparability Ratios Based on Dual Coding of 1976 Death Certificates by the Eighth and Ninth Revisions of the International Classification of Diseases," *Monthly Vital Statistics Report, 28*(11) (Suppl.), February 1980.

disease (*Monthly Vital Statistics Report,* Table 6). Homicide was the 11th leading cause of death. In 1960 the 10 leading causes of death were heart disease, cancer, stroke, personal injury, certain diseases of early infancy, influenza and pneumonia, diabetes mellitus, congenital anomalies, cirrhosis of the liver, and suicide. Homicide was well down on the list (U.S. Bureau of the Census, Table 117).

Infant Mortality. The infant mortality rate is the number of deaths under the age of 1 year among children born alive, divided by the number of live births. As was pointed out in Chapter 2, infant mortality appears to be related to a variety of socioeconomic, environmental, and health care factors. Some authorities (Morris, pp. 56ff., 267; Rosen, p. 342) consider it to be a fairly sensitive indicator of general health levels in a population. In 1987 the infant mortality rate in the United States was 10 per 1,000 live births (*Monthly Vital Statistics Report,* p. 1). The rate has been declining steadily since 1940, when it was 47 (Grove & Hetzel, Table 38). In fact, the infant mortality rate has been falling since it was first recorded in this country at 99.9 in 1915.

The most striking feature of the U.S. infant mortality rate is that, although it has consistently fallen over the years, the rate for blacks has just as consistently remained almost double the white rate (U.S. Bureau of the Census, Table 113). Detailed examinations of the relationships among ethnicity, other factors, and infant mortality are contained in *Vital and Health Statistics* (NCHS, 1981) and in a publication of the Office of Health Resources Opportunity (pp. 35–39).

A classic study of factors related to infant mortality is the work of Kessner et al. (1973) sponsored by the National Academy of Sciences. They found that in 140,000 births in New York City, with the infectious diseases that formerly took the lives of many infants mainly under control, "generally, adequacy of [health] care . . . is strongly and consistently associated with infant birth weight . . . and survival" (p. 1). Kessner and his co-authors also concluded from their study that

> the survival of infants of different ethnic groups varies widely; . . . there is consistent association between social classes as measured by the educational attainment of the mothers and infant birth weight and survival; . . . within categories of mothers' educational attainment, there are consistent trends relating the adequacy of care . . . to infant survival; . . . there is a gross misallocation of services by ethnic group and care when the risks of the women are taken into account." [pp. 2–3]

Almost 20 years later the results of this study are apparently still valid.

Marriage and Divorce

In 1987 the marriage rate stood at 9.9 per 1,000 population (*Monthly Vital Statistics Report,* p. 1), down from 10.6 in 1970 (U.S. Bureau of the Census,

Table 126). The divorce rate, which had stood at 3.5 per 1,000 population in 1970 (U.S. Bureau of the Census, Table 126), was 4.8 in 1987, close to 50% of the marriage rate. Detailed analysis of marriage and divorce statistics can be found in *Vital and Health Statistics,* Series 21, "Data on Natality, Marriage and Divorce."

Morbidity

Morbidity refers to sickness, illness, and disease. Like mortality, morbidity data can be expressed in both numbers and rates. It can be cross-tabulated with the broad range of demographic characteristics. Morbidity data are extremely important in characterizing the health status of a population. Mortality data alone are not adequate for that purpose, for several reasons. Many diseases and conditions of ill health that are widely prevalent in the population do not appear in mortality figures. This is particularly so in a country such as the United States, in which communicable disease, with a few exceptions, is not a major problem.

Such significant but nonfatal conditions include arthritis, low-back pain, the common cold, mild emotional and sexual problems, and the like. There are other diseases that may kill but do so rarely in relation to their appearance in the population. Included in this category are sexually transmitted disease (STD) other than acquired immune deficiency syndrome (AIDS), duodenal ulcer, and gallbladder disease. When looking at morbidity, one learns not only which are the important diseases and the patterns of their distribution in the population but also how they affect people in terms of limitation of activity.

To understand morbidity data, we must understand the terms *incidence* and *prevalence. Incidence* is the number of new cases of the disease in question occurring during a particular period, usually a year. *Prevalence* is the total number of cases existing in a population during a time period or at one point in time *(point prevalence).*

Reporting morbidity is not nearly as simple as reporting mortality. When is a person sick? Who decides—the physician? the patient? The problems of perception of illness and of the sick role were referred to in the preceding chapter. Furthermore, although it is thought that the determination of cause of death by physicians is reasonably reliable, the accuracy of physician diagnosis in illness is more questionable (Koran).

Although the law requires that all deaths be reported, only certain categories of sickness, the infectious diseases, must be reported. The list appears in a publication of the Centers for Disease Control of the U.S. Public Health Service called *Morbidity and Mortality Weekly Report.* Among the 34 infectious diseases only 5 can be considered significant in the United States: AIDS, gonorrhea, hepatitis, syphilis, and tuberculosis (Centers for Disease Control). Clearly, there are no reporting requirements for many categories of disease important in the United States.

It is known that physicians fail to report certain diseases even when legally required to do so. Some private physicians will not report venereal disease in private patients on the grounds of avoiding "embarrassment." Tuberculosis reporting, other than from institutions, is inhibited by the possible economic consequences: Some employers automatically fire persons with tuberculosis. (Although the disease is one of low infectivity, it is commonly thought to be highly contagious, even by some health professionals.) Many physicians fail to report cases of the common childhood viral infections because they consider them to be "inconsequential."[3] The reporting of both AIDS and seropositivity for the human immunodeficiency virus (HIV) is an extremely complex and controversial subject (Dickens; Walters).

In mortality, there is only one possible source of data. It isn't the patient. In morbidity, however, both providers and patients can obviously be data sources; as a result, quite different pictures of the same reality can be obtained. Providers can report morbidity by diagnostic categories and also by patient chief complaints; that is, what the patient reports to the physician as being the problem. Patients don't usually come to a physician saying "I've got diabetes mellitus, Doc" but rather something like "I've been feeling kind of weak, and I'm drinking a great deal of water and urinating a lot."

Patients can also report chief complaints directly in a population survey. From a chief-complaint profile for a population, obtained from either source, some estimates of the morbidity patterns can be obtained. One advantage of deriving information directly from patients is that certain patients with certain types of illnesses will never come to medical attention. Thus, morbidity surveys that gather information only from providers will not give a complete picture.

Other than reportable communicable disease data published by the Centers for Disease Control in *Morbidity and Mortality Weekly Report*, the regular source of morbidity data in the United States is the NCHS, which includes the Health Examination Survey (since 1970 the Health and Nutrition Examination Survey [HANES]), the Health Interview Survey, the Hospital Discharge Survey, and the National Ambulatory Medical Care Survey. The results of these surveys are published periodically in both *Vital and Health Statistics* and *Monthly Vital Statistics Report*. Together, these activities constitute the National Health Survey (NCHS, 1963). Series 1 of *Vital and Health Statistics* contains the general methodological and historical accounts. Detailed descriptions of all of the surveys can be found in Appendix I of *Health United States 1984* (NCHS, 1984).

Data also are collected on the *incidence of morbid conditions*. In 1986 the incidence of acute conditions was 190 per 100 persons per year, up about 85%

---

[3]For example, we can estimate that just before the introduction of the measles vaccine in the mid-1960s, the measles reporting rate was around 10%. Almost all children get measles before their fifth birthday. There were about 4 million births annually in the United States at that time, but only 400,000 cases of measles were reported annually. Since, on the average, 4 million children were getting the disease each year, the reporting rate was about 10%.

from the rates in the two previous years (NCHS, 1987, p. 3). Most common were influenza (29%), respiratory conditions (22%), injuries (14%), infective and parasitic diseases (12%), and digestive system conditions (3%). Persons sought medical attention for these conditions about 58% of the time. Acute conditions were associated with about 764 days of restricted activity per 100 persons per year (NCHS, 1987, Table A). About 14% of the population experienced limitation in all activity due to chronic conditions (NCHS, 1987, Table C). The major chronic conditions causing limitations in activity in 1986 were heart conditions, arthritis and rheumatism, impairments of back or spine, sinusitis, hypertension, and impairments of lower extremities and hips (NCHS, 1987, Table 57).

The Hospital Discharge Survey (HDS) reports on morbidity and mortality as it occurs in hospitals. This is an example of provider-perspective data and affords a rather accurate illness profile of patients in hospitals. It must be remembered, however, that the overwhelming majority of ill persons do not require hospitalization. Thus, the morbidity profile of the population as a whole does not match that seen in hospitals. The results of the HDS appear in *Vital and Health Statistics,* Series 13, and in a publication called *Advance Data from Vital and Health Statistics,* published on an irregular basis.

The HDS is carried out on a sampling basis in nonfederal, short-stay hospitals (hospitals with six or more beds and an average length of stay of 30 days or less). In 1986 approximately 71% of discharges from those hospitals were accounted for by seven diagnostic groups: diseases of the circulatory system, 16%; childbirth, 11%; diseases of the digestive system, 11%; injury and poisoning, 9%; diseases of the respiratory system 9%; diseases of the genitourinary system, 8%; and cancer, 7% (*Advance Data,* 1987, Table 5). The five most common specific diagnoses are females with deliveries; heart disease; malignant neoplasm (cancer); fractures, all sites; and cerebrovascular disease.

The National Ambulatory Medical Care Survey (NAMCS) (NCHS, 1974a,b) was developed in the 1970s as a component of the National Health Survey. It concentrates on private physicians' offices, which in 1980 accounted for about 80% of all physician's office visits (NCHS, 1983b). The data are collected using a stratified random sample of all office-based allopathic and osteopathic physicians in the contiguous United States, excluding anesthesiologists, pathologists, and radiologists. Simple questionnaires on each patient seen during a given period are filled out. Morbidity, patient demographic data, and utilization data are collected, as well as data on practice characteristics. NAMCS data were collected and published annually until 1984 and trienially after 1984. The data presented here were the most recent available at the time of writing.

In the NAMCS, morbidity data are collected from two perspectives: (1) the patient's reason for coming to the office and (2) the physician's diagnosis. In 1981 the 10 leading patient reasons for coming to the office were general medical exam, routine prenatal exam, postoperative visit, symptoms referable to the throat, reason not specified, blood pressure test, cough, head cold, upper respiratory infection, and back symptoms (*Advance Data,* 1983, Table 5). These account for 27% of all visits. The 10 leading physicians' diagnoses were essential hypertension, normal pregnancy, health supervision of infant or child, upper respiratory infection, general medical exam, middle-ear infection, diabetes mellitus, special investigations, follow-up exam, and sebaceous gland (on the skin) disease (*Advance Data,* 1983). In addition to general survey data such as these, NAMCS also publishes a variety of special studies in *Advance Data* and *Vital and Health Statistics* (NCHS, 1980, pp. 12–13). These reports cover the several medical physician specialties, patient demographic characteristics, and diagnostic categories.

Health Status

In 1979 the Office of the Assistant Secretary for Health (OASH) of the U.S. Department of Health and Human Services published the first national health status report, *Healthy People: The Surgeon General's Report on Health Promotion and Disease Prevention* (1979). Subsequently, the Office of Disease Prevention and Health Promotion (ODPHP), part of OASH, published *Promoting Health and Preventing Disease: Objectives for the Nation* (fall 1980). A total of 216 objectives were established for dealing with 15 major diseases and conditions that can be prevented by using existing knowledge and techniques. The 15 were grouped into three sets of 5: preventive health services for such conditions as high blood pressure and sexually transmitted disease, health protective services for such problems as toxic agent control and occupational safety and health, and health promotion programs to deal with such conditions as cigarette smoking and sedentary life-style. Implementation plans were published in 1983 (ODPHP, 1983), the *Prospects for a Healthier America* in 1984 (ODPHP, 1984), and *A Midcourse Review* in 1986 (ODPHP, 1986). As of 1988, ODPHP was preparing a new set of objectives for the year 2000.

In support of this new effort, in 1985 the NCHS carried out a Health Promotion/Disease Prevention (HPDP) Survey as part of the ongoing Health Interview Survey (NCHS, 1988a). The HPDP Survey was to be repeated in 1990. As well as being published in *Vital and Health Statistics,* Series 10, results also appear from time to time in *Advance Data.*

Key findings include the following (NCHS, 1988a, pp. 2, 5–8): In 1985 about one-fourth of U.S. adults were 20% or more above desirable body weight, 85% of adults had had a blood pressure measurement in the previous year, about 30% of people 18 or older regularly smoked cigarettes, 13% of men and 3% of women drank more than 2 oz of alcohol per day, and fewer than 5% of adults exercised regularly at an intensity level high enough to reduce the risk of heart disease. The cited volume contains an extensive bibliography.

Although we know a great deal about how to characterize the health and illness status of our population, many aspects of this process are still not well understood. For example, we have yet to solve completely the problem of constructing a health status index for individuals that would be broadly useful and easily determined (Andersen; Balinsky & Berger; Bergner et al.; Boyle & Torrance; Bush et al., Kaplan et al., Sackett et al.). Bergner (1985) published a mid-1980s state of the art review.

Utilization of Health Care Services

We come now to the third health data perspective: how the population utilizes the health care delivery system. We have pointed out that in quantifying utilization of health services, the same series of events can be counted from either the patient's or the provider's perspective. The results of the two types of counts are not always the same. Thus, when discussing utilization, one has to be careful to distinguish the two approaches.

It should be noted that reliable utilization data is regularly reported only for services provided by licensed M.D.s and D.O.s (doctors of osteopathic medicine) in licensed allopathic (M.D.-staffed) and osteopathic hospitals. There is an unknown amount of "alternative therapy" provided in this country by such healing disciplines as chiropractic, naturopathy, homeopathy, accupuncture/accupressure therapy and its variants, and "holistic health" practices. The practitioners of these disciplines do not report utilization, they are not surveyed, and much of their service is not reimbursed by insurance companies. Thus, it is not possible at present to make even a reliable estimate of the volume of this care.

Utilization of Ambulatory Services

As we have noted, the Health Interview Survey (HIS) provides patient-perspective data for the utilization of ambulatory services. According to the HIS, in 1986 there were about 5.4 physician visits per person (NCHS, 1987, Table D). This figure includes telephone contacts, which account for about 13% of all "visits" reported by patients. Three visits per person were made to a physician's office, 0.8 took place in hospital, and 0.9 in other locations. About 75% of the population made at least one visit to a physician. In general, females made more visits than did males, and as might be expected, the visit rate increased with age. In 1986 about 58% of the population over the age of 2 years made at least one visit to the dentist.

There are several sources for provider data on the utilization of ambulatory services. The most comprehensive is the NAMCS, explained previously. The NAMCS provides data on visits by age, race, sex, geographic region, metropolitan/nonmetropolitan living area, type of physician, and duration of visit. It also supplies data on morbidity.

The other major source of provider-perspective ambulatory service utilization data is the AHA's annual publication *Hospital Statistics,* published each summer. For 1987 the AHA reported about 311 million outpatient visits, including 83.5 million visits to hospital emergency units. The balance were made to clinics and other units, such as outpatient hemodialysis and rehabilitation services (AHA, Table 5A). *Hospital Statistics* provides considerable detail on these data by such variables as number of beds, ownership, type, geographical region, and medical school affiliation (AHA, Tables 3, 5–9, 12, 13).

Utilization of Hospital Services

Turning to utilization of hospital services, the HDS reported that for 1986 there were 143.1 reported discharges per 1,000 persons from short-stay hospitals,[4] approximately 34.2 million discharges (*Advance Data,* 1987, Table 2). The average reported length of hospital stay was 6.4 days, representing a continuing downward trend that began in the early 1970s. Other classes of data provided by the HDS are utilization according to various hospital characteristics, morbidity (discussed previously), and an analysis of surgery.

NCHS also provides patient-perspective hospital utilization data through the HIS. NCHS points out that because of "differences in collection procedures, population sampled, and definitions," the results from the HIS and the HDS are not entirely consistent (NCHS, 1979a, p. 1). For 1986, the HIS reported significantly fewer discharges from short-stay hospitals than did the HDS: about 27.9 million discharges, 118 per 1,000 population, with an average length of stay of 6.6 days (NCHS, 1987, Table 77).

Hospital utilization data is, of course, also published in the AHA's *Hospital Statistics.* For 1987 the 6,821 AHA-registered hospitals, with a total of 1.27 million beds, reported 34.4 million admissions, an occupancy rate of slightly under 69%, and an average daily census of 873,000 (AHA, Table 1). In the same year the 5,659 hospitals that the AHA classifies as "nonfederal, short-term" admitted 31.6 million patients to their 961,000 beds. The occupancy rate was 64.9%, and the average daily census was about 624,000. *Hospital Statistics* contains voluminous data on these variables and many others, including fiscal parameters, according to hospital type, size, ownership, geographical location, and the like.

Certain provider-perspective hospital utilization data also appear in *Health: United States,* a compendium of much government and nongovernment health

---

[4]The HDS definition of a short-stay hospital is one that has "six beds or more for inpatient use and an average length of stay of less than 30 days" (*Advance Data,* 1987, p. 13). In the past the HDS used a different definition. The current one is the same as that used by the AHA.

and health care data published annually by NCHS since the mid-1970s (see, for example, NCHS, 1988b).

Conclusion

Much data concerning the population, its health, and how it uses the health care delivery system are collected in the United States, although they are somewhat less comprehensive, less frequently published, and less readily available in the 1980s than they were in the 1960s and 1970s. As we have seen, there is some inconsistency among these data. This inconsistency may result in part from lack of coordination in data-collection efforts. Furthermore, there is the obvious gap between the provider perspective and the patient perspective on the counts of events.

There have been criticisms of the federal statistical collection, reporting, and analysis system. A 1979 study by the Office of Technology Assessment[5] found "federal data collection activities . . . to be overlapping, fragmented, and often duplicative" (p. iii). In brief, the report recommended that a "strengthened coordinating and planning unit within [HHS]" be established that "would embody three basic characteristics: sufficient authority to impose decisions on agencies; the necessary statistical and analytical capabilities to conduct activities requiring technical expertise and judgement; and adequate resources to build a viable core effort" (p. 55). This recommendation has apparently not yet been followed.

Regardless of problems with the system, however, we do know a great deal about health, disease, and illness in the United States and about the functioning of the U.S. health care delivery system. There are gaps in our knowledge, to be sure; some of them would have been filled if the provisions of the National Health Resources Planning and Development Act (P.L. 93-641, Sec. 1513,b,1) relating to data had been carried out. They were not. These requirements called for the mandatory national collection of data on (1) population health status, (2) health care delivery system utilization, (3) effects of the health care delivery system on health, (4) health care delivery resources, and (5) environmental and occupational exposure factors relating to health.

Implementation of this provision of the law would constitute the biggest step forward in health-data assemblage since the organization of the vital-statistics system. Despite these problems with the data themselves, however, what we need to remember above all is that data mean little unless they are put to proper use.

[5]This report is especially valuable to students of the federal data system and its users. It not only describes data collection activities and the way they are organized and supervised but also presents and analyzes all of the statutory authorities establishing them.

References

Advance Data. "1983 Summary: National Ambulatory Medical Care Survey." March 16, 1983.

Advance Data. "1986 Summary: National Hospital Discharge Survey." September 30, 1987.

American Hospital Association. *Hospital Statistics, 1988 Edition.* Chicago: AHA, 1988.

Andersen, R. "Health Status Indices and Access to Medical Care." *American Journal of Public Health, 68,* 458, 1978.

Balinsky, W., & Berger, R. "A Review of the Research on General Health Status Indexes." *Medical Care, 13,* 283, 1975.

Bergner, M. "Measurement of Health Status." *Medical Care, 23,* 696, 1985.

Bergner, M., et al. "The Sickness Impact Profile: Validation of a Health Status Measure." *Medical Care, 14,* 57, 1976.

Boyle, M. H., & Torrance, G. W. "Developing Multiattribute Health Indexes." *Medical Care, 22,* 1045, 1984.

Bush, J. W., et al. "Health Indices, Outcomes, and the Quality of Medical Care." In R. Yaffee & D. Zalkind (Eds.), *Evaluation in Health Services Delivery.* New York: Engineering Foundation, 1975.

Centers for Disease Control. *Morbidity and Mortality Weekly Report, 37*(19), May 20, 1988.

Dickens, B. M. "Legal Rights and Duties in the AIDS Epidemic." *Science, 239,* 580, 1988.

Grove, R. D., & Hetzel, A. M. *Vital Statistics Rates in the United States: 1940–1960.* Washington, D.C.: National Center for Health Statistics, 1968.

Hulka, B. S., & Wheat, J. R. "Patterns of Utilization: The Patient Perspective." *Medical Care, 23,* 438, 1985.

Kaplan, R. M., et al. "Health Status Index: Category Rating versus Magnitude Estimation for Measuring Levels of Well-Being." *Medical Care, 17,* 501, 1979.

Kessner, D. M., et al. *Infant Death: An Analysis by Maternal Risk and Health Care.* Washington, D.C.: Institute of Medicine, National Academy of Sciences, 1973.

Koran, L. "The Reliability of Clinical Methods, Data and Judgments." *New England Journal of Medicine, 293,* 695, 1975.

Monthly Vital Statistics Report, 36(12), March 21, 1988.

Morris, J. N. *Uses of Epidemiology.* Baltimore: Williams and Wilkins, 1964.

Mundinger, M. N. "Health Service Funding Cuts and the Declining Health of the Poor." *New England Journal of Medicine, 313,* 44, 1985.

National Center for Health Statistics. "Origin, Program and Operation of the U.S. National Health Survey." *Vital and Health Statistics,* Series 1, No. 1, August 1963.

National Center for Health Statistics. "National Ambulatory Medical Care Survey: Background and Methodology: United States—1967–1972." *Vital and Health Statistics,* Series 2, No. 61, April 1974. (a)

National Center for Health Statistics. "The National Ambulatory Medical Care Survey: Symptom Classification." *Vital and Health Statistics,* Series 2, No. 63, May 1974. (b)

National Center for Health Statistics. *Health Resources Statistics: Health Manpower and Health Facilities,* 1976–77 (DHEW Pub. No. PHS 79-1509). Hyattsville, MD.: NCHS, 1979. (a)

National Center for Health Statistics. *Ninth Revision International Classification of Diseases, Adopted for Use in the United States.* Hyattsville, MD.: NCHS, 1979. (b)

National Center for Health Statistics. "The National Ambulatory Medical Care Survey." *Vital and Health Statistics*, Series 13, No. 44, April 1980.

National Center for Health Statistics. "Infant Mortality Rates: Socioeconomic Factors." *Vital and Health Statistics*, Series 22, No. 14, 1981.

National Center for Health Statistics. *Health United States, 1983* DHHS Pub. No. PHS 83-1200. Hyattsville, MD.: NCHS, 1983. (a)

National Center for Health Statistics. "Physician Visits: Volume and Interval since Last Visit, United States, 1980." *Vital and Health Statistics*, Series 10, No. 144, June 1983. (b)

National Center for Health Statistics. *Health United States 1984* (DHHS Pub. No. PHS 85-1232). Hyattsville, Md.: NCHS, 1984.

National Center for Health Statistics. "Current Estimates from the National Health Interview Survey, United States, 1986." *Vital and Health Statistics*, Series 10, No. 164, October 1987.

National Center for Health Statistics. "Health Promotion and Disease Prevention, U.S., 1985." *Vital and Health Statistics*, Series 10, No. 163, February 1988. (a)

National Center for Health Statistics. *Health United States, 1987* (DHHS Pub. No. PHS 88-1232) Hyattsville, MD: NCHS March 1988. (b)

Office of the Assistant Secretary for Health. *Healthy People: The Surgeon General's Report on Health Promotion and Disease Prevention* (DHEW Pub. No. PHS 79-55071). Washington, D.C.: U.S. Government Printing Office, 1979.

Office of Disease Prevention and Health Promotion. *Promoting Health/Preventing Disease: Objectives for the Nation.* Washington, D.C.: U.S. Government Printing Office, 1980.

Office of Disease Prevention and Health Promotion. "Public Health Service Implementation Plans for Attaining the Objectives for the Nation." *Public Health Reports*, Sept.–Oct. 1983 (Suppl.).

Office of Disease Prevention and Health Promotion. *Prospects for a Healthier America.* Washington, D.C.: U.S. Government Printing Office, 1984.

Office of Disease Prevention and Health Promotion. *The 1990 Health Objectives for the Nation: A Midcourse Review.* Washington, D.C.: U.S. Government Printing Office, 1986.

Office of Health Resources Opportunity. *Health Status of Minorities and Low Income Groups* (DHEW Pub. No. HRA 79–627). Washington, D.C.: U.S. Government Printing Office, 1979.

Office of Technology Assessment. *Selected Topics in Federal Health Statistics.* Washington, D.C.: U.S. Government Printing Office, 1979.

Rosen, G. *A History of Public Health.* New York: MD Publications, 1958.

Sackett, D. L., et al. "The Development and Application of Indices of Health: General Methods and a Summary of Results." *American Journal of Public Health, 67,* 423, 1977.

U.S. Bureau of the Census. *Statistical Abstract of the United States: 1988.* Washington, D.C.: U.S. Government Printing Office, 1987.

Walters, L. "Ethical Issues in the Prevention and Treatment of HIV Infection and AIDS." *Science, 239,* 597, 1988.

4

Health Manpower: With an Emphasis on Physicians

Steven Jonas

With this chapter we begin our consideration of the personnel and institutional inputs to the health care delivery system in the United States. The emphasis in this chapter is on physicians. The medical profession is only one of many occupations required to make the health care delivery system work. However, primarily because of the licensing laws, it is the physicians who are the dominant actors in the system (see also chapters 6 and 14). Nursing, the largest single occupational category, is covered separately in Chapter 5.

The health care industry is labor-intensive. Thus, the education and use of health professionals is a critical variable in determining the distribution, efficiency, economy, and cost of the industry and its products. Manpower is of course not a variable standing on its own. Financing, organization, and delivery of health services; regulatory requirements; biomedical research; and consequent technological developments all affect the size and use of the health manpower pool.

The health care field has enjoyed a long period of expansion. Since World War II both the number and types of health care workers have increased greatly. There was also continuous growth in funding of services and programs from both the private and public sectors (see Chapter 10). Until the mid-1970s it was not really necessary to make hard choices among programs. More money always seemed to be available. However, by the 1980s the open-ended flow of third-party payments for certain types of health services had begun to diminish somewhat. Until then few observers of the system raised questions concerning efficiency, efficacy, and cost-effectiveness. Nor had many considered the cost implications of adding the new types of personnel. But many new health services, particularly those employing high technology, require many additional large manpower inputs.

In the first and second editions of this book, this chapter was written by Ruth S. Hanft. Certain portions of her work are used in this chapter. Her contributions are acknowledged with many thanks.

The development of the new health care occupations has been spurred by the development of new technologies and services. As a result, costs have been significantly increased. In the 1980s these factors became major concerns. For example, "health care rationing" became an important issue (Daniels; Engelhardt; Fuchs, 1984; Green; Hayward; Miller & Miller; Strauss et al.). It will certainly have an effect on health care workforce issues.

Increases in the size of the manpower pool and the development of new types of manpower tend to increase the total supply of services. The traditional constraints of the economic market do not operate in the health care field (Fein, 1967; Fuchs, 1974, 1984; see also Chapter 10). In certain circumstances, health manpower can create its own demand by prescribing the use of its services for patients. Physicians are known to create a major portion of the demand for their own services (Dyckman; Fuchs & Kramer; Maloney & Reemtsma; Reinhardt, 1975; Wennberg & Lapenas), as do certain other types of health manpower. Thus, increases in manpower supply may well increase the demand for services.

From the late 1970s onward, a number of health manpower problems were being discussed in government, by the public, and among experts in the field (Bureau of Health Professions, 1983, 1985, 1986; GMENAC; Goldsmith; Health Policy Agenda; Health Resources Administration; Institute of Medicine, 1978; Jonas, 1984a; New York State Education Department; Record et al.; Reed and Evans; Schwartz et al., 1980, 1988a & b, U.S. Senate). The problems discussed included the following:

- How large a manpower pool is needed? How is the problem of physician oversupply (see below) to be dealt with?
- Why is the ratio of manpower to hospital beds higher in the United States than in any other industrialized country?
- How can the distribution of manpower by both specialty and geography be improved?
- What is a primary care physician? How many are needed? How many specialists?
- Should the trend toward further specialization of professional and allied health manpower be encouraged or halted?
- Will "physicians' extenders" (e.g., physicians' associates and clinical nurse practitioners) be substitutes for physicians? Or will they be used instead to expand and enhance services and possibly add to health sector costs? Or will the growth in the number of physicians foreclose use of the new direct-care professions?
- Should the methods of financing education for the health professions be altered? Should the government continue to subsidize the education of high-earning professionals when it subsidizes the training of other professions only minimally?

As long ago as 1978, Mick noted that a number of these issues had already been with us for some time. In this chapter we will deal with some of them and discuss the available information that can be used in analyzing them.

Number and Types of Health Workers

In 1986, more than 8 million people were working in the health care industry (see Table 4.1). This total excludes the large but unknown number of housekeeping, kitchen, and maintenance personnel who work primarily in institutions. It also excludes persons in health-related occupations who are working in what the U.S. Bureau of the Census classifies as nonhealth industries. They include pharmacists working in drugstores, school nurses, and nurses working in private households.

The range of skills required in the industry is vast. It overlaps those of many other industries. There are many sites of employment: hospitals, nursing homes, private offices, ambulatory health care centers of various types, health maintenance organizations, research laboratories and foundations, patients' homes, elementary and secondary schools, colleges and universities, manufacturing plants, hospital supply and pharmaceutical companies, prisons, custodial institutions, and ships.

By mode of functioning, health care providers may be divided into three major groups: independent practitioners, dependent practitioners, and supporting staff. This model is similar to that developed by Freidson in *Professional Dominance: The Social Structure of Medical Care* (1970) (see especially Chapter 5). The definitions are useful, but it should be noted that the lines separating the three groups are not always precise.

The independent practitioner group consists of those health care providers allowed by law to deliver a delimited range of services to any persons who want them, without supervision or authorization of the practitioner's work by third parties. Among the independent practitioners are physicians (osteopathic and allopathic), dentists, chiropractors, optometrists, and podiatrists.

The law allows the dependent practitioner group to deliver to persons a delimited range of services, often of a particular type specified by law, under the supervision and/or the authorization of independent practitioners. The dependent category includes nurses; psychologists; social workers; pharmacists; physician assistants; dental hygienists; and speech, physical, and occupational therapists. However, in certain situations for certain patients, many of the workers in these occupations may and can assume the role of independent practitioner.

The definition of the line between the independent and dependent groups is the source of many conflicts at present. There has been a growing demand for independent practice status, particularly in the nursing profession (see Chapter 5). The Federal Rural Clinics Act (P.L. 95-210) took a step in this direction. It

Table 4.1 Persons Employed in Selected Health Service Sites, in thousands, According to Place of Employment: United States, Selected Years, 1970–1986[a]

Place of employment	1970[b]	1975	1980	1981	1982	1983	1984	1985	1986
Totals	4,246	5,945	7,339	7,617	7,810	7,874	7,934	7,910	8,129
Offices of physicians	477	618	777	811	898	888	896	894	896
Offices of dentists	222	331	415	423	415	441	468	480	497
Offices of chiropractors[c]	19	30	40	46	53	54	61	59	66
Hospitals	2,690	3,441	4,036	4,186	4,341	4,348	4,288	4,269	4,368
Nursing and personal care facilities	509	891	1,199	1,230	1,217	1,342	1,362	1,309	1,339
Other health service sites	330	634	872	921	886	801	859	899	963

[a]Data are based on household interviews of a sample of the civilian noninstitutionalized population.

[b]April 1, derived from decennial census; all other data years are annual averages from the Current Population Survey.

[c]Data for 1980–1982 are from the American Chiropractic Association; data for all other years are from the U.S. Bureau of Labor Statistics.

Note: Totals exclude persons in health-related occupations who are working in non-health industries, as classified by the U.S. Bureau of the Census, such as pharmacists employed in drugstores, school nurses, and nurses working in private households. Totals include federal, state, and county health workers.

Sources: U.S. Bureau of the Census: 1970 Census of Population, occupation by industry. *Subject Reports.* Final Report PC(2)-7C. Washington, D.C.: U.S. Government Printing Office, October 1972; U.S. Bureau of Labor Statistics: *Labor Force Statistics Derived from the Current Population Survey: A Databook, Vol. I.* Washington, D.C.: U.S. Government Printing Office, September 1982: *Employment and Earnings, January 1983–87.* Vol. 30, No. 1; Vol. 31, No. 1; Vol. 32, No. 1; Vol. 33, No. 1; Vol. 34, No. 1. Washington, D.C.: U.S. Government Printing Office, January 1983–1987; American Chiropractic Association: Unpublished data.

reduced the supervision required of nurse practitioners and physician assistants working in certain rural clinics for reimbursement of services under Medicare and Medicaid.

Supporting staff, rather than providing a range of services to patients, carry out specific work tasks authorized by and under the supervision of independent and/or dependent practitioners. The work of supporting staff may or may not be regulated by laws directly pertaining to them. However, if there are not special laws, supporting staff work under the legal authority provided for their supervisors.

This group includes clerical, maintenance, housekeeping, and food-processing workers; research workers; administrators; record keepers; nurse's aides; dental assistants; and technicians, primarily laboratory and radiological. In certain situations some of these persons may assume the role of dependent practitioner. The struggles over status and responsibility between certain categories of supporting staff and dependent practitioners sometimes mirror those between independent and dependent practitioners.

According to the U.S. Bureau of the Census (1986, Table 140), in 1985 the major health occupation groups were as follows: 2.7 million nurses and nurses aides; 492,000 physicians; 131,000 dentists; 172,000 pharmacists; 257,000 therapists, including physical, speech, and occupational; and 416,000 laboratory and radiology technicians (see Table 4.2). The changes in supply over time for the major categories of independent and dependent providers are shown in Table 4.3, which also shows the variations in geographical distribution of the major health professions. Note the major changes for physicians, dentists, nurses, and veterinarians and the smaller changes for pharmacists and optometrists. Most health care workers are female. However, most physicians, dentists, other independent health care practitioners, as well as administrators and other persons in policymaking positions, are male.

The United States has one of the highest physician-to-population ratios in the world. In 1985 it was 220 per 100,000. The types of health professionals in the United States are also more varied than they are elsewhere. In the independent category, for example, osteopathic physicians, podiatrists, and optometrists are virtually unknown in most other countries. The variety of allied categories is also unique to the United States.

Physician Supply

As shown in Table 4.4, in 1985 there were about 535,000 physicians in the United States. Table 4.5 shows that the growth has been rapid since 1970. (The numbers in Tables 4.4 and 4.5 are not consistent. Please see the note to Table 4.4.) In 1970 the physician-to-population ratio was 156 per 100,000. According

Table 4.2 Employed Persons in Selected Health Occupations: 1985[a]

Occupation	Number (thousands)	% Female	% Black
Total	5,715	77.0	13.2
Health diagnosing occupations[b]	728	14.8	3.2
Physicians[c]	492	17.2	3.7
Dentists	131	6.5	2.6
Health assessment and treating occupations[b]	2,006	85.6	7.0
Registered nurses	1,447	95.1	6.8
Pharmacists	172	29.8	3.2
Dietitians	81	93.9	19.3
Therapists	257	76.2	7.2
Managers, medicine and health	106	59.2	8.1
Health technologists and technicians[b]	1,115	83.4	13.6
Clinical laboratory	295	75.5	11.0
Dental hygienists	56	99.5	2.0
Radiology	121	73.8	7.5
Licensed practical nurses	402	96.9	19.6
Health service occupations	1,760	89.9	24.5
Dental assistants	168	99.0	3.6
Health aides, except nursing	350	85.6	17.8
Nursing aides, orderlies, and attendants	1,242	89.9	29.2

[a]Covers civilians 16 years old and over. Annual averages based on data collected by Bureau of the Census as part of Current Population Survey.
[b]Includes other occupations not shown separately.
[c]Medical and osteopathic.
Source: U.S. Bureau of Labor Statistics, *Employment and Earnings,* January 1986.

to estimates made in the early to mid-1980s, it was generally expected to exceed 230 per 100,000 by 1990 (Bureau of the Health Professions, 1986; GMENAC, p. xv; Stambler, 1979; Luft & Arno, 1986). As noted above, it had already reached 220 per 100,000 in 1985.

The majority of physicians work in patient care, and of those the majority are in office-based practice. The largest specialist group is general and family practice. Except for a mild drop in the mid-1970s, its numbers have remained fairly constant. The numbers of internists and pediatricians have been increasing faster than the increase in physicians overall. The number in obstetrics and "other specialties" have just about kept pace with the overall rise; the number in surgery has been increasing at a slower rate. However, of physicians in office-based practice, the proportion of family and general practitioners dropped from 27% in 1970 to 16% in 1985. This is against a backdrop of repeated warnings of the dangers of overspecialization issued by myriad observers since the 1930s.

Table 4.3 Active Health Personnel and Number per 100,000 Population,[a] According to Occupation and Geographic Region: United States, 1970, 1980, and 1985

Year and occupation	Number of active health personnel	United States	North-east	Geographic region Midwest	South	West
1970						
Physicians[b]	290,862	142.7	185.0	127.5	114.8	158.2
Doctors of medicine[c]	279,212	137.0	178.7	118.2	111.5	154.8
Doctors of osteopathy	11,650	5.7	6.3	9.3	3.3	3.4
Dentists[b]	95,680	47.4	58.9	46.3	35.3	54.9
Optometrists	18,400	9.0	9.7	10.3	6.6	10.5
Pharmacists[c]	112,570	55.4	60.1	57.5	50.6	52.9
Podiatrists	7,110	3.5	6.0	3.6	1.6	3.0
Registered nurses	750,000	368.9	491.2	367.5	281.8	355.9
Veterinarians	25,900	12.7	8.3	16.1	11.8	15.0
1980						
Physicians[b,d]	409,917	182.4	224.8	165.8	157.1	200.1
Doctors of medicine[c,d]	393,407	174.9	216.1	153.3	152.8	195.8
Doctors of osteopathy	16,510	7.5	8.7	12.5	4.3	4.3
Dentists[b]	121,240	54.9	65.2	53.1	44.4	63.7
Optometrists	22,330	10.1	10.2	11.2	8.0	12.3
Pharmacists[c]	142,780	64.7	60.8	67.7	65.0	64.6
Podiatrists	8,880	4.0	6.3	3.9	2.5	4.1

Registered nurses[d]	1,272,900	560.0	736.0	583.6	443.4	533.7
Associate and diploma	908,300	399.9	536.0	429.2	316.5	351.1
Baccalaureate	297,300	130.9	161.0	127.8	103.8	148.1
Master's and doctorate	67,300	29.6	39.0	26.7	23.0	34.6
Veterinarians	36,000	16.3	10.8	19.9	16.0	18.5
1985						
Physicians[b]	489,834	206.8	262.5	189.7	177.8	212.0
Doctors of medicine[c]	470,434	198.5	252.5	175.8	172.7	207.3
Doctors of osteopathy[e]	19,400	8.3	10.0	13.9	5.1	4.7
Dentists[b]	135,500	56.9	67.9	58.7	46.1	61.4
Optometrists	23,900	9.9	9.9	11.1	7.7	12.0
Pharmacists[c]	159,200	66.3	64.4	77.8	67.4	52.0
Podiatrists[e]	9,700	4.2	6.9	4.2	2.6	3.9
Registered nurses	1,531,200	641.4	805.5	702.2	524.3	594.9
Associate and diploma	1,016,670	425.8	542.4	479.6	348.0	371.2
Baccalaureate	419,200	175.6	209.4	185.1	145.0	181.1
Master's and doctorate	95,310	39.9	53.7	37.9	31.4	42.8
Veterinarians	41,600	17.4	12.5	21.0	17.1	18.5

[a] Ratios for physicians and dentists are based on civilian population; ratios for all other health occupations are based on resident population.
[b] Excludes doctors of medicine in federal service; excludes dentists in military service; 1985 total for physicians includes 1984 data for doctors of osteopathy.
[c] Excludes U.S. possessions.
[d] Revised figures.
[e] Data are for 1984.

Source: Division of Health Professions Analysis, Bureau of Health Professions: *Supply and Characteristics of Selected Health Personnel* (DHHS Pub. No. HRA 81-20) Health Resources Administration. Hyattsville, Md., June 1981; Bureau of Health Professions: *Fifth Report to the President and Congress on the Status of Health Personnel in the United States.* Health Resources and Services Administration. (DHHS Pub. No. HRS-P-OD-86-1) Rockville, Md., 1986; unpublished data.

Table 4.4 Active Physicians, According to Type of Physician, and Number per 10,000 Population: United States and Outlying U.S. Areas, Selected 1950–85 Estimates and 1990 and 2000 Projections[a]

Year	All active physicians	Doctors of medicine	Doctors of osteopathy	Active physicians per 10,000 population
1950	219,900	209,000	10,900	14.1
1960	259,400	247,300	12,200	14.0
1970	326,500	314,200	12,300	15.6
1971	337,400	325,000	12,400	16.1
1972	348,300	335,500	12,800	16.4
1973	355,700	342,500	13,200	16.4
1974	370,000	356,400	13,600	16.9
1975	384,500	370,400	14,100	17.4
1976	399,500	385,000	14,500	17.9
1977	405,900	390,800	15,100	18.0
1978	424,000	408,300	15,700	18.6
1979	440,400	424,000	16,400	19.1
1980	457,500	440,400	17,100	19.7
1981	466,600	448,700	18,000	19.9
1982	483,700	465,000	18,700	20.5
1983	501,200	481,500	19,700	21.1
1984	—	—	20,800	—
1985	534,800	512,900	21,900	22.0
1990 (projection)	587,700	559,500	28,200	23.5
2000 (projection)	696,600	656,100	40,400	26.0

[a]Data based on reporting by physicians and medical schools.
Note: Population estimates include residents in the United States, Puerto Rico, and other U.S. outlying areas; U.S. citizens in foreign countries; and the armed forces in the United States and abroad. For 1990 and 2000, the Series II projections of the total population from the U.S. Bureau of the Census are used. Estimation and projection methods are from the Bureau of Health Professions. The numbers for doctors of medicine differ from American Medical Association figures because physicians not classified by activity status and whose addresses are unknown are allocated into the totals.
Source: Bureau of Health Professions: *Fifth Report to the President and Congress on the Status of Health Personnel in the United States* (DHHS Pub. No. HRS-P-OD-86-1) Health Resources and Services Administration, Rockville, Md., 1986; unpublished data.

Geographic Distribution

Physicians are distributed very unevenly on a geographic basis. As shown in Table 4.6, Mississippi has the lowest ratio of physicians per 100,000 population (118), and Massachusetts has the highest (302). The issue of geographic maldistribution (Hudson & Nourse) has been of concern for quite some time and is certainly of contemporary concern as well. Wennberg (1984) has shown that variations in physician supply have an important influence on the patterns of practice. For example, where there are more surgeons, there is more surgery, regardless of, and without noticeable impact on, the health status of the population. This situation obviously has important implications for both cost containment and quality assurance.

Part of the geographic variation in practice patterns found by Wennberg (1984) is explained by the fact that high physician-to-population ratios are naturally related to the location of the major tertiary-care medical centers. These centers in part serve patients who reside out of state. However, the most important cause of the difference in physician-to-population ratios lies in the complex set of factors that make some areas of the country particularly attractive to physicians and others particularly unattractive.

Comparing physician-to-population ratios for areas as large as states can blur the size of the geographic inequities in physician distribution within states by averaging out high- and low-distribution areas (New York State Education Department, pp. 1–2). These disparities can be substantial. In New York State an apparent 12% physician oversupply is reduced to 1% if the heavy concentration of physicians in New York City is removed from the calculations. Within the city itself there is an enormous variation, as between the Upper East Side in Manhattan and East New York in Brooklyn.

There are many factors contributing to the geographic imbalances in physician supply, such as

- The content of the training programs at the undergraduate and graduate medical education levels, including the site of clinical training.
- The procedures used in the selection of medical students, where the students were raised, and what their interests are (Balinsky; National Center for Health Services Research).
- The social and cultural amenities of given geographic areas (Steinwald & Steinwald).
- The peer contact available in different areas, including the existence of medical schools, area health education centers, and contact with other physicians, particularly through organized group practice arrangements.
- Geographic disparities in fees for the same services (Institute of Medicine, 1976).
- Age, sex, and specialty considerations, as well as the general population shift toward the Sunbelt (Steiber).

One program designed to encourage physicians to locate in underserved areas is the National Health Service Corps (NHSC) (Comptroller General; Mullan; Smith & Gerard). It places physician and nonphysician health manpower in areas designated as having shortages. The NHSC provides scholarship support for

Table 4.5 Physicians, According to Activity: United States, Selected Years, 1970–1985[a]

Activity	1970	1975	1980	1983	1984	1985
Doctors of medicine	328,020	388,626	462,276	513,040	530,585	545,986
Professionally active	304,926	335,608	409,992	464,114	476,995	490,410
Nonfederal	278,855	309,410	393,407	442,969	457,364	470,434
Patient care	252,778	285,345	358,470	403,956	414,914	426,721
Office-based practice	187,637	211,776	269,001	305,755	316,757	325,836
General and family practice	50,415	45,863	47,265	50,804	51,466	53,181
Internal medicine	22,841	28,070	40,276	46,974	50,936	52,333
Pediatrics	10,203	12,559	17,204	19,887	21,223	22,025
General surgery	17,975	19,613	22,262	23,561	23,876	24,519
Obstetrics and gynecology	13,732	15,469	19,306	22,101	22,815	23,256
Other specialty	72,471	90,202	122,688	142,428	146,441	150,522
Hospital-based practice	65,141	73,569	89,469	98,201	98,157	100,885
Residents and interns	45,514	53,150	59,127	69,763	69,506	71,302
Full-time hospital staff	19,627	20,419	30,342	28,438	28,651	29,583
Other professional activity[b]	26,077	24,065	34,937	39,013	42,450	43,713

Federal	26,071	26,198	16,585	17,950	19,631	19,976
Patient care	20,566	22,325	13,513	13,992	15,256	15,877
Office-based practice	2,819	1,841	679	1,382	931	961
Hospital-based practice	17,747	20,484	12,834	12,610	14,325	14,916
Residents and interns	5,173	4,089	2,323	2,485	3,024	3,149
Full-time hospital staff	12,574	16,395	10,511	10,125	11,301	11,767
Other professional activity[b]	5,505	3,873	3,072	3,958	4,375	4,099
Inactive	19,533	21,360	25,609	36,703	37,671	38,646
Information not available	357	25,790	20,285	12,223	12,795	13,950
Unknown address	3,204	5,868	6,390	3,195	3,124	2,980

[a]Data based on reporting by physicians.
[b]Includes medical teaching, administration, research, and other.
Note: Federal and nonfederal doctors of medicine in the 50 states and the District of Columbia are included.
Sources: Haug, J. N., Roback, G. A., & Martin, B. C.: *Distribution of Physicians in the United States, 1970.* Chicago: American Medical Association, 1971; Goodman, L. J., & Mason, H. R.: *Physician Distribution and Medical Licensure in the U.S., 1975.* Chicago: American Medical Association, 1976; Department of Statistical Analysis: *Physician Distribution and Medical Licensure in the U.S., 1978.* Chicago: American Medical Association, 1980; Bidese, C. M., & Danais, D. G.: *Physician Characteristics and Distribution in the U.S.* Chicago: American Medical Association, 1982; Roback, G. A., & Eiler, M. A.: *Physician Characteristics and Distribution in the U.S.* Chicago: American Medical Association, 1983; Eiler, M. A.: *Physician Characteristics and Distribution in the U.S.* Chicago: American Medical Association, 1984; Randolph, L. L.: *Physician Characteristics and Distribution in the U.S. 1985 and 1986.* Chicago: American Medical Association, to be published. (Copyrights 1971, 1976, 1980, and 1983–86: Used with the permission of the American Medical Association.)

Table 4.6 Nonfederal Physicians, per 10,000 Civilian Population, According to Geographic Division, State, and Primary Specialty: United States, 1975 and 1985

| | Total physicians[a] | | Doctors of medicine[b] | | | |
| | | | Patient care[c] | | Primary care[d] | |
Geographic division and state	1975	1985	1975	1985	1975	1985
United States	15.3	20.7	13.5	18.0	4.1	5.4
New England	19.1	26.7	16.9	22.9	4.6	6.2
Maine	12.8	18.7	10.7	15.6	3.8	5.4
New Hampshire	14.3	18.1	13.1	16.7	4.6	5.6
Vermont	18.2	23.8	15.5	20.3	5.2	6.5
Massachusetts	20.8	30.2	18.3	25.4	4.7	6.4
Rhode Island	17.8	23.3	16.1	20.2	4.4	5.5
Connecticut	19.8	27.6	17.7	24.3	4.7	6.4
Middle Atlantic	19.5	26.1	17.0	22.2	4.5	5.9
New York	22.7	29.0	20.2	25.2	5.1	6.3
New Jersey	16.2	23.4	14.0	19.8	4.1	5.5
Pennsylvania	16.6	23.6	13.9	19.2	4.0	5.4
East North Central	13.9	19.3	12.0	16.4	3.7	5.0
Ohio	14.1	19.9	12.2	16.8	3.7	4.8
Indiana	10.6	14.7	9.6	13.2	3.8	4.6
Illinois	14.5	20.5	13.1	18.2	4.1	5.5
Michigan	15.4	20.8	12.0	16.0	3.2	4.5
Wisconsin	12.5	17.7	11.4	15.9	4.0	5.4
West North Central	13.3	18.3	11.4	15.6	3.8	5.2
Minnesota	14.9	20.5	13.7	18.5	4.6	6.5
Iowa	11.4	15.6	9.4	12.4	3.5	4.3
Missouri	15.0	20.5	11.6	16.3	3.3	4.7
North Dakota	9.7	15.8	9.2	14.9	4.1	5.8
South Dakota	8.2	13.4	7.7	12.3	3.4	5.0
Nebraska	12.1	15.7	10.9	14.4	4.2	5.3
Kansas	12.8	17.3	11.2	15.1	3.9	5.2
South Atlantic	14.0	19.7	12.6	17.6	3.7	5.2
Delaware	14.3	19.7	12.7	17.1	3.8	4.7
Maryland	18.6	30.4	16.5	24.9	4.2	6.5
District of Columbia	39.6	55.3	34.6	45.6	7.2	10.3
Virginia	12.9	19.5	11.9	17.8	3.8	5.4
West Virginia	11.0	16.3	10.0	14.6	3.3	4.4
North Carolina	11.7	16.9	10.6	15.0	3.5	4.7
South Carolina	10.0	14.7	9.3	13.6	3.3	4.5
Georgia	11.5	16.2	10.6	14.7	3.3	4.3
Florida	15.2	20.2	13.4	17.8	3.9	5.3
East South Central	10.5	15.0	9.7	14.0	3.2	4.5
Kentucky	10.9	15.1	10.1	13.9	3.6	4.8
Tennessee	12.4	17.7	11.3	16.2	3.2	4.7
Alabama	9.2	14.2	8.6	13.1	3.0	4.2
Mississippi	8.4	11.8	8.0	11.1	3.1	4.2

Table 4.6 *Continued*

| Geographic division and state | Total physicians[a] | | Doctors of medicine[b] | | | |
| | | | Patient care[c] | | Primary care[d] | |
	1975	1985	1975	1985	1975	1985
West South Central	11.9	16.4	10.5	14.5	3.5	4.5
Arkansas	9.1	13.8	8.5	12.8	3.4	4.8
Louisiana	11.4	17.3	10.5	16.1	3.3	4.5
Oklahoma	11.6	16.1	9.4	12.9	3.2	4.0
Texas	12.5	16.8	11.0	14.7	3.6	4.5
Mountain	14.3	17.8	12.6	15.7	4.1	5.0
Montana	10.6	14.0	10.1	13.2	4.5	5.4
Idaho	9.5	12.1	8.9	11.4	4.0	4.8
Wyoming	9.5	12.9	8.9	12.0	4.1	4.6
Colorado	17.3	20.7	15.0	17.7	4.6	5.6
New Mexico	12.2	17.0	10.1	14.7	3.4	4.8
Arizona	16.7	20.2	14.1	17.1	4.2	5.1
Utah	14.1	17.2	13.0	15.5	3.8	4.4
Nevada	11.9	16.0	10.9	14.5	3.6	4.6
Pacific	17.9	22.5	16.3	20.5	5.2	6.6
Washington	15.3	20.2	13.6	17.9	4.7	6.3
Oregon	15.6	19.7	13.8	17.6	4.6	6.1
California	18.8	23.7	17.3	21.5	5.5	6.7
Alaska	8.4	13.0	7.8	12.1	3.5	5.6
Hawaii	16.2	21.5	14.7	19.8	4.9	7.0

[a]Includes active nonfederal doctors of medicine and doctors of osteopathy in all other specialties not shown separately. Doctors of osteopathy data are for 1984.
[b]Excludes doctors of osteopathy; states with large numbers are Florida, Michigan, Missouri, New Jersey, Ohio, Pennsylvania, and Texas.
[c]Excludes doctors of medicine in medical teaching, administration, research, and other nonpatient care activities.
[d]Includes doctors of medicine in patient care office-based general practice and family practice, internal medicine, and pediatrics.
Sources: Compiled by Health Resources and Services Administration, Bureau of Health Professions, based on data from the American Medical Association: *Physician Distribution and Licensure in the U.S., 1975* and *Physician Characteristics and Distribution in the U.S., 1986 Edition.*

students in the health professions in return for service after completion of training (Health Resources and Services Administration, 1984, 1986). The health professionals are then assigned to Health Manpower Shortage Areas (HMSAs) and Medically Underserved Areas (MUAs) for time proportional to the duration of their scholarship aid. The program is sponsored jointly by the federal government and the community of placement, with the latter providing the facility.

There is some evidence that the program has influenced its graduates to locate in rural areas (Stamps & Kuriger).

There is evidence that with the increased supply of physicians, geographic spillover is occurring. Data show that board-certified physicians are moving into certain nonmetropolitan areas (Newhouse et al; Schwartz et al., 1980; Williams), although by one method of estimation there will still be subspecialist shortages in many of the smaller cities (Schwartz et al., 1988a). Hemenway (1982) examined the various factors taken into account when considering the optimal location of physicians. Estes (1982) pointed out that the Schwartz and Williams studies of dispersal did not consider what the optimum number and location might be, just that doctors are moving; nor did they consider the situation in the really small towns. A comparative study of U.S., British, and Swedish efforts to deal with the problem of physician geographic distribution showed that none was completely successful (Rosenthal & Frederick).

Physician Oversupply

> . . . The University in this city now numbers 1100 medical students. Considering the number of universities . . . and the large number of students in attendance almost everywhere, it becomes a serious question what is to become of [the students] after their graduation. The country is now more supplied with physicians, and if the increase continues for a number of years in the same ratio it is difficult to conceive in what way the medical men will earn their daily bread.

The United States in the 1980s? No, Germany in the 1880s ("JAMA 100 Years Ago", p 1123). The problem is not a new one. However, it is still with us. In the United States, at the same time that geographical distribution is quite uneven and remains a serious problem, there appears to be a general oversupply of physicians (American College of Surgeons; Bailey; Bureau of Health Professions, 1985, 1986; "Doctor Surplus"; GMENAC; Harris; Igelhart; Luft & Arno). (There are a few observers who disagree with this estimation [Schloss; Schwartz et al., 1988b].) In the ordinary free market, this is a fact that those interested in efficiency and cost containment would welcome. However, the marketplace for health services is not an ordinary one because physicians, the major controllers of service supply, have a strong influence over the creation of demand (Lave et al.; Reinhardt, 1975).

In the 1960s the widespread opinion had been that the United States faced a serious physician shortage in terms of numbers alone (Carnegie Commission on Higher Education; National Advisory Commission on Health Manpower; Peterson & Pennell; Surgeon General's Consultant Group). Another view identified the problem not as to absolute supply of physicians but in terms of what physicians do, what specialties they are in, and where they are located geographically (Castleton; Fein; Navarro; Senior & Smith).

In 1959 the federal Bane Commission recommended that medical schools increase the output of medical graduates to 11,000 per year by 1975 and then level off after that (Fordham, 1980). If its recommendations had been followed, the country would probably not be facing the current physician oversupply. The medical school expansion that followed the Bane report overshot the mark, however. There were about 15,000 graduates in 1975. Moreover, the Bane Commission had predicated its projections on a predicted population of 235 million (not the actual 1975 total of 213 million). To anticipate and deal with these problems would have required careful, *national* planning, hard to do in this country (Blum).

At any rate, as the end of the 1970s approached, it became increasingly apparent that the various federal and state initiatives undertaken in the 1960s and early 1970s to increase the supply of physicians had indeed worked too well. Annual medical school output approximately doubled in the 20 years from 1967 to 1987, to an estimated 15,800 (AMA, 1988, Table 6), after having grown by less than 2,000 in the previous 20 years. The production of new graduates peaked at 16,327 in 1984.

The GMENAC Report

In 1976 concern in Congress over the issue of physician manpower planning led to the creation of the Graduate Medical Education National Advisory Committee (GMENAC). Placed under the auspices of the Department of Health, Education and Welfare, GMENAC was to advise the secretary on five major questions:

1. What number of physicians is required to meet the health care needs of the nation?
2. What is the most appropriate specialty distribution of these physicians?
3. How can a more favorable geographic distribution of physicians be achieved?
4. What are the appropriate ways to finance the graduate medical education of physicians?
5. What strategies can achieve the recommendation formulated by the committee?

The committee was able to answer the first question definitively but not the others. It summarized its findings in one paragraph:

There will be *too many* physicians in 1990. There will be substantial *imbalances* in some specialties. There will continue to be a marked *unevenness* in the geographic distribution of physicians. The country may be training *too many* nonphysician providers for 1990. The factors influencing specialty choice are *complex*. The actual cost of graduate medical education is *unknown*. Economic motivation in specialty and geographic choice is *uncertain*.

GMENAC developed a new method for studying physician supply requirements. Previous studies had used gross physician-to-population rates to make
their estimates. GMENAC used a sophisticated, predictive needs formula for
each specialty. Epidemiological knowledge became the basis for predicting
actual demand in terms of diseases and conditions. Then well-defined estimates
of the supply of physician time and number of physicians required to meet the
demand were made. The committee also developed a new method for predicting
what the actual physician supply would be.

GMENAC predicted that by 1990 there would be 536,000 M.D.s and D.O.s,
but only 466,000 would be required according to the epidemiologically based
estimates. In 1985, as we have seen, there were already between 490,000 and
535,000 active physicians, depending upon how the counts were made (see
Tables 4.4 and 4.5). For the year 2000 the estimated surplus was 145,000. It was
estimated that more than half of the 1990 surplus would be graduates of foreign
medical schools catering to U.S. citizens. Table 4.7 shows the predicted shortages, balances, and surpluses by specialty.

The committee's major recommendations were as follows:

- Medical schools should significantly reduce class size, and no new medical
  schools should be opened.
- The entry of foreign medical graduates into the United States should be
  severely restricted.
- The production of nonphysician primary care providers should be stabilized, but more research on the role and function of these professionals
  should be done.
- Some voluntary planning efforts should be undertaken by the various
  specialties.
- Medical workforce planning should focus on small-area geographical and
  specialty requirements.
- Ambulatory care and training should be emphasized.
- New reimbursement methods, designed to help achieve health policy objectives, should be developed.

There are also many other supporting recommendations.

Subsequent to GMENAC

In the 5 years following the publication of the GMENAC report, little happened
in a planned way pursuant to its recommendations. The number of first-year
medical students declined slightly, from 17,320 in 1981 to 16,779 in 1987
(AMA, 1988, Table 6), a far cry from the 17% reduction called for by GME-
NAC. Moreover, in 1988 there were still over 3,000 more residency training
positions offered in the official National Resident Matching Program (NRMP)

Table 4.7 Ratio (%) of Projected Physician Supply to Estimated Requirements—1990

	Ratio (%)	Require-ments	Surplus/ (Shortage)
Shortages:			
Child psychiatry	45	9,000	(4,900)
Emergency medicine	70	13,500	(4,250)
Preventive medicine	75	7,300	(1,750)
General psychiatry	80	38,500	(8,000)
Hematology/oncology internal medicine	90	9,000	(700)
Dermatology	105	6.950	400
Gastroenterology internal medicine	105	6,500	400
Near balance:			
Osteopathic general practice	105	22,000	1,150
Family practice	105	61,300	3,100
General internal medicine	105	70,250	3,550
Otolaryngology	105	8,000	500
General pediatrics and subspecialties	115	36,400	4,950
Urology	120	7,700	1,650
Orthopedic surgery	135	15,100	5,000
Ophthalmology	140	11,600	4,700
Thoracic surgery	140	2,050	850
Infectious diseases internal medicine	145	2,250	1,000
Obstetrics/gynecology	145	24,000	10,450
Plastic surgery	145	2,700	1,200
Allergy/immunology internal medicine	150	2,050	1,000
Surpluses:			
General surgery	150	23,500	11,800
Nephrology internal medicine	175	2,750	2,100
Rheumatology internal medicine	175	1,700	1,300
Cardiology internal medicine	190	7,750	7,150
Endocrinology internal medicine	190	2,050	1,800
Neurosurgery	190	2,650	2,450
Pulmonary internal medicine	195	3,600	3,350
Physical medicine and rehabilitation[a]	75	3,200	(800)
Anesthesiology[a]	95	21,000	(1550)
Other:			
Nuclear medicine[a]	n.a.	4,000	n.a.
Pathology[a]	125	13,500	3,350
Radiology[a]	155	18,000	9,800[a]
Neurology[a]	160	5,500	3,150

[a]The requirements in these six specialties were estimated crudely after a review of the literature. They should be considered as very rough approximations, and tentative.
Source: Graduate Medical Education National Advisory Committee. *Report.* Washington, D.C.: U.S. Department of Health and Human Services. Vol. 1, p. 5, 1980.

than were filled through the match (Graettinger). For the 15,776 U.S. medical school seniors graduating with M.D. degrees more than, 19,500 positions were open. Even with D.O., Canadian, and other foreign graduates applying, there were plenty of vacancies. The recommended cuts had not been made in graduate training programs either.

By 1985 it was becoming more difficult for U.S.-citizen foreign medical graduates (USFMGs) to enter U.S. graduate training but not because of any particular planned program. In 1985 the examination for entry into residency training following graduation with the M.D. degree was significantly stiffened. On the first administration of that test, the pass rate for USFMGs dropped to the almost inconceivably low level of 4% (Association of American Medical Colleges, 1985). It rose on subsequent administrations of the exam to about 50% (Ferguson). Nevertheless, by 1988 the number of USFMGs applying through the official NRMP for residency positions was only slightly more than half of what it had been in 1984 (Graettinger).

By 1985, projections of physician supply had become even gloomier than GMENAC's. Using a different methodology, the Bureau of Health Professions (1986) of the Department of Health and Human Services predicted that by 1990 the supply of active physicians would be 587,700. This was about 50,000 more than GMENAC had predicted. In fact, the 535,000 figure that GMENAC had predicted for 1990 was reached in 1985 (Table 4.4). By the mid-1980s there were "no more doctors needed" signs hanging out in many communities, especially in affluent suburbs and high-priced central-city areas. An increasing number of hospital medical staffs were closing themselves to newcomers and trying to deal with the legal (antitrust) consequences of so doing. Between 1975 and 1985 the average number of physician office visits per week declined by over 25%, from 110.8 to 74.9 ("The Office Physician's").

Future Developments

In dealing with this situation, one can try to rely on market forces. This is, in general, what has been tried to date; it has not been very effective. If market mechanisms were effective, the physician pool would expand or contract in relation to changes in supply and demand, as happens in other sectors of the economy. In medicine, market forces fail because of lack of consumer information, artifical licensure and certification barriers, the nonprofit nature of most of the hospital sector, the ability of the provider to influence the demand for services, rapid changes in technology, and consumer expectations (Fuchs, 1974; Reinhardt, 1975).

There have been a variety of predictions of what will happen in the future (Bailey; Freedman; GPEP; Jonas, 1984b; Maloney & Reemtsma):

- There will be a gradual increase in the proportion of physicians in salaried service. This will occur as newer graduates, in particular, look for relative job and income security, compared to that found in an increasingly competitive private practice sector. (This was already occurring as of 1986 [Riffer]).

- There will be some decline in the number of hours worked per week by physicians (Freiman & Marder, 1984). How much this will offset the physician surplus remains to be seen. (As of 1986, this had not yet begun to occur, even as the visits-per-week average declined significantly [Gonzalez and Emmons, Table 4].)

- There may be a decline in the average real income of physicians; however, as physicians in the growing salaried sector learn trade unionism, with the powerful, licensure-protected weapons they have, they may be able to prevent this from happening (Marcus). (It happened that in 1986 physician real income rose for the first time since 1983 [Gonzalez & Emmons, p. 120].)

- The corporatization of American medicine will be abetted.

- There may be a broadening of the array of services offered by physicians, especially where private practice remains active and competition is heavy. This broadening could include more convenient hours, less time in the waiting room, improved doctor-patient communication, health-promotion/disease-prevention services, and sociomedical services.

- There will be a gradual decline in the number of USFMGs entering the system. (This has already occurred, as noted above.)

- There may be some unemployed licensed M.D.s and D.O.s: the inadequate, the poorly trained, and the ones who simply do not want to move to where the jobs are. (There is anecdotal evidence that this has occurred, but hard data are difficult to come by.)

- There will not be any coordinated national planning, either at the medical school entry level or the graduate (residency) training level. (So far, this prediction has been borne out.)

Foreign Medical Graduates

From the mid-1950s until the early 1980s the United States was a major importer of foreign-born physicians (Stevens et al.). The use of foreign medical graduates (FMGs) had provoked considerable debate (Butter; Kleinman et al., 1974, 1975a, 1975b; Saywell et al.; Stevens et al.). A number of reports expressed concern about the dependence of the U.S. health care system on FMGs, the "brain drain" from underdeveloped nations, and the quality of the education of FMGs (Association of American Medical Colleges, 1974; National Advisory Commission on Health Manpower). The Health Professions Educational Assistance Act of 1976 (P.L. 94-484) put severe restrictions on the entry into the United States of foreign-born FMGs who intended to become permanent residents. By the early 1980s the flow had been reduced to a trickle.

Another phenomenon began to cause growing concern in the late 1970s. It was the influx of a significant number of U.S. citizens who earned their medical degrees abroad (Imperato, 1984a; Mulvihill & Rosner; Relman; Stillman et al.; Weinberg & Bell). This phenomenon had begun on a small scale in the 1920s. Until the mid-1970s, most U.S. students studying medicine abroad attended university medical schools. Most of the students in those schools were their own country's nationals. There was just one independent proprietary medical school serving a predominantly U.S.-citizen student body, at Guadalajara in Mexico.

However, in the mid-1970s, there was an extraordinary crush of applicants to U.S. medical schools, even with the rapid increase in the number of available places. In response, a number of new foreign proprietary medical schools were established to cater mainly to U.S. citizens (Bloom). They were located primarily in Puerto Rico, other Caribbean islands, and Mexico. The adequacy of the undergraduate training and the ability of their students to obtain residency training was in question from the time of their founding (Imperato, 1984b). Nevertheless, mechanisms designed to limit licensure of less than adequately trained physicians who happened to be U.S. citizens proved difficult to develop. The courts would not accept state laws designed to exclude graduates of certain foreign medical schools with provisions and requirements that did not extend to graduates of all foreign medical schools.

There was one feature that distinguished the curricula of most of the foreign medical schools catering almost exclusively to U.S. citizens from those schools that educate primarily their own nationals. It is the use of U.S. hospitals for the so-called clinical clerkships that come in the third and fourth years of medical school. Because they are often situated on small Caribbean islands, most of the U.S.-citizen foreign medical schools do not have the clinical facilities to run clerkships on site. In the late 1970s, some of them began making arrangements with U.S. hospitals to provide this training (Pierson; Riddle). Often these hospitals were not teaching hospitals, at either the undergraduate or the graduate level. Quality and supervision of the educational experiences thus were often questionable. It was this feature that enabled state licensing boards to develop controls for U.S.-born FMGs that would pass muster in the courts.

The New York State Board of Regents, the body responsible for medical licensure in that state, took the lead in developing this approach (Jonas, 1981, 1984b). The board established a system of quality controls for the clerkships provided in New York State hospitals, and foreign medical schools had to meet certain minimum standards to ensure that they were properly preparing their students for the clerkships. As it turned out, few schools were able to meet the requirements for approval to place their students in clerkships in New York State hospitals. A number of other states adopted similar regulations (Jonas, 1985).

By the late 1980s the influx of USFMGs had diminished sharply (Graettinger). There were several reasons for this, some of which were commented on by Ferguson (1987):

- Word of the physician oversupply situation and the possibility of a future decline in relative physician income began to spread among the public. Medicine started to become less attractive as a career. This was reflected in the decline in the ratio of applicants to available places in U.S. medical schools from 2.7 in 1976 to 1.8 in 1986 (AMA, 1988, Table 5).
- The decline in the U.S. medical school applicant/acceptee ratio made it much easier for otherwise qualified applicants to gain admission to a U.S. medical school. In fact, in 1988 the Association of American Medical Colleges felt that the problem of the diminishing applicant pool was serious enough to warrant holding a conference devoted solely to consideration of the situation (Association of American Medical Colleges, 1988).
- Despite the surplus of available residency places in the NRMP, only about one-third of USFMGs entering the match in 1988 obtained residencies (Graettinger, Table 1). In contrast, more than 85% of U.S. graduate match applicants obtained places.
- The number of U.S.-citizen foreign medical schools, the number of available U.S.-hospital clinical clerkship positions, and the number of U.S. citizens attending those schools that remained in business are all declining.

Thus, in part by default, the USFMG problem seems to be on the way to solution, at least in terms of the reduction in numbers recommended by GMENAC.

Education and Training of Health Professionals

The education and training of health professionals is a major industry in the United States. There are more than 1,600 educational institutions at the technical, baccalaureate, and graduate levels. They provide health sciences education in one or more of the 200 or so health-related occupations that exist in the United States. There are many issues, of course. In this section, we will focus primarily on medical education and its problems. The next chapter reviews nursing education in some depth. For an excellent recent overview of health sciences education in general, including dentistry, pharmacy, allied health, and public health (strangely not including health administration), see the *Handbook of Health Education* by Christine McGuire and colleagues (1983).

There are many sites for training health professionals. Allopathic and osteopathic physicians, dentists, veterinarians, optometrists, pharmacists, podiatrists, and nurses all train in both independent and university-based colleges and professional schools. Nurses also train in hospitals, although this arrangement has declined sharply since the 1960s. These various schools are found in both the public and private sectors, with a growing trend toward public schools and university-based institutions. In the past 20 years most of the expansion of medical and osteopathic schools has come through state university institutions and the expansion of nursing programs through state and locally supported community colleges.

Medical Education

As of 1987 there were 127 fully accredited allopathic medical schools in the United States (AMA, 1988, Table 1), up from 119 in 1980. There are also 16 osteopathic medical schools. Allopathic medical school accreditation is carried out by the Liaison Committee on Medical Education, an agency jointly sponsored by the American Medical Association and the Association of American Medical Colleges. The osteopathic schools are accredited by the American Osteopathic Association.

The number of U.S. medical schools increased sharply between 1960 (85 schools) and 1980 (Schofield). Many schools also significantly enlarged their class size during that period. However, in the face of the oversupply of physicians and the increasing costs of medical education, growth in the number and class size of the allopathic medical schools came to a virtual halt in the mid-1980s. In 1988 a new osteopathic medical school was under development in California, and class size was still increasing in certain osteopathic schools.

In 1987 the allopathic medical schools had almost 64,000 full-time faculty and more than 66,000 students: a ratio of students to full-time faculty of 1.03:1 (AMA, 1988, Table 1). There were also more than 130,000 part-time faculty members, most of them volunteer. (The very low ratio is one of the reasons medical education is so expensive. However, medical school faculty are involved to at least some degree in the teaching of about 85,000 other health science students.) Teaching for medical students was done in more than 1,700 separate clinical facilities. For the 17,027 spaces allotted to medical students entering in the fall of 1987, there were 28,123 applicants, or 1.7 applicants for every space (AMA, 1988, Table 5). This ratio was down from its high of 2.8 in 1973–1975.

The average minimum curriculum time was 152 weeks, usually spread over 4 years. For 1986–1987 the total expenditures for the 127 allopathic schools was close to $12.6 billion, more than double the amount spent just 6 years before. Of that total, 42% came from various government sources (AMA, 1988, Table 3), down from 65% in 1976–1977.

Many of the schools that train health professionals have multiple functions. In medicine, for example, most schools are also centers of major biomedical research activities; they are responsible for training both doctors of medicine (M.D.s) and basic scientists (Ph.D.s) and are involved in the training of graduate physicians at the internship, resident, and fellowship (subspecialty) levels. Faculty of medical schools also instruct nursing, dental, and other students.

Historical Factors. Historically, several major trends influenced the current orientation of medical schools. The Flexner Report (1960), originally published in 1910, was very significant. Flexner is credited by some with initiating the modern medical education system (Cooper, 1979; Ebert). Banta (1971), among others, has pointed out that Flexner was not an initiator as much as he was a summarizer, catalyst, and publicizer of change. Nevertheless, it is the so-called Flexnerian model that is followed by most American medical schools today. This model has five principal features (Richmond, p. 3):

1. That a minimum of 2 years of undergraduate college work be required for admission to medical school.
2. That a 4-year curriculum be employed, with 2 years in the basic medical sciences followed by 2 years of supervised clinical work on both inpatient and outpatient hospital services.
3. That regular laboratory teaching exercises be included.
4. That a high level of quality in instruction be maintained through the use of full-time faculty.
5. That the medical schools be university-based.

These five elements reflect, however, only some of the many recommendations that Flexner made (Jonas, 1978, Chapter 8). They reflect in particular the model of medical education that has been developed at the Johns Hopkins University School of Medicine since its opening in 1893.

One result of the Flexner Report was a sharp decline in the number of proprietary medical schools, which had been very prominent until that time. Also disappearing was the preceptorship-apprenticeship orientation of clinical medical education. It is ironic that the popularity of medicine as a career, combined with modern air travel and electronic communications, in the late 1970s brought back the proprietary medical school—in the Caribbean.

Following World War II the federal government decided to provide financial support for biomedical research in the medical schools, rather than in the science departments of their parent universities. This decision was strongly influenced by the adamant opposition of the American Medical Association to direct federal aid to medical education. Supporting biomedical research in medical schools was one way that the federal government could indeed support medical education without appearing to do so directly. This approach had the effect of orienting the medical schools and their faculties toward research (Strickland, Chapters 3 and 4). The availability of research grants to support faculty salaries allowed the medical schools to expand the scope of faculty capabilities in the specialties and subspecialties. At the same time it focused the attention of medical school faculties heavily on research and away from teaching, among other things increasing the costliness of medical education. The problem of overspecialization in medicine only worsened.

In many states the legislatures expected their medical school hospitals to be the source of tertiary care and skilled care for large regions or the whole state. Both before and after the implementation of Medicare and Medicaid the states also expected the public medical school hospitals to care for their indigent populations. As populations shifted from the city to suburbs, the university-owned and university-associated hospitals of many private medical schools found that they were located in low-income areas. Thus, they also became the principal source of outpatient and inpatient care for large low-income populations (Freymann; Institute of Medicine, 1976).

Problems. The problems of medical education process and content are closely linked to the problems of physician distribution, supply, and costs and the role and functions of the physician in practice (Lewis & Sheps). The medical education community and the public have been engaged in a serious debate regarding the role of medical schools in producing physicians. Much of this debate can be found in the Health Manpower Hearings on legislation introduced in Congress in 1974 and 1975 (U.S. Senate). Testimony also can be found in the discussions between the professional associations and the (then) DHEW. As is true of many health policy debates, the positions and arguments of the various actors have changed little over time, although in the 1980s more attention is being paid to medical education process. The issues debated then, which are still being debated, include the following:

- Medical schools' responsibility for training primary care physicians.
- Appropriate curricula and training sites for the development of primary care physicians.
- Medical schools' responsibility for graduate medical education programs.
- Medical schools' possible role in improving the supply of physicians in underserved areas.
- Constraining the rise in health care costs.

It is notable that the debate on the content, role, and function of medical education has yet to make it onto the national political agenda. This is despite the fact that the state and federal governments play a major role in financing the system. The medical school, the orientation of its curriculum, the sites used for training, and the standards for evaluation are the critical components of health professional education. The training of the physician as generalist or specialist; the inpatient or outpatient orientation of the training; a curriculum emphasizing prevention and public health, and social and economic factors in health and disease; team teaching; and team practice all influence the way physicians practice, where they practice, and how they use other services (Jonas, 1978, 1982, 1984a).

Pleas made to government for understanding and flexibility (Cooper, 1978;

Rogers, 1980, 1982) were still being heeded in the late 1980s. It was unclear at that time how many schools were heeding the parallel pleas of Drs. Cooper and Rogers and others for creativity, resourcefulness, and responsiveness in the face of acknowledged problems.

In the 1980s the calls for major change in the content of medical education continued (Bok; Cooper, 1983; Jonas, 1984a; Kennedy; Petersdorf; Schweiker; Smith; Tarlov). Some new issues were introduced. They included the needs to (1) improve physicians' communication skills, (2) reintroduce "humanism" to medicine, (3) equip physicians to deal rationally with the increasingly complex ethical issues of the age of technological medicine, (4) provide physicians with computer literacy, and (5) create physicians who are truly creative, lifelong learners, and problem solvers.

A key issue is the place of health promotion/disease prevention in the medical school curriculum. As has been stated elsewhere (Jonas, 1988),

> . . . a significant portion of the deaths in the United States could have been prevented or postponed using known interventions. One reason this did not occur is because medical science and medical education are disease, not health, oriented. Since physicians are at the center of the health care delivery system, their disease orientation pervades the industry. Historically, there have been calls for physicians to focus more on disease prevention; however, medical education [by and large] does not teach disease prevention/health promotion.
>
> There are several reasons for this: conceptual discordance among medical school faculty between the "certainty" of curative medicine vs. the probability of risk factor reduction; gaps in the knowledge of effective interventions; the concept that health promotion/disease prevention are outside the province of physicians; the significant role of biomedical research grants in medical school funding; the close association of medical education and the acute care hospital; and the use of rote memory/lecture based teaching methods of traditional medicine vs. the problem-based learning necessary to teach disease prevention health promotion.
>
> Some medical schools have begun to use problem based learning and to introduce health promotion concepts [see below]. Widespread and long-lasting change requires support of the leadership in medical schools and the preventive medicine/public health community, and grant funding from state and federal sources to support research on medical education change.

The GPEP Report

Facing the many problems of medical education, in 1981 the Association of American Medical Colleges (AAMC) decided to undertake a comprehensive study. It was the first national study of medical education that the association had undertaken in 50 years. The AAMC established the Panel on the General Professional Education of the Physician and College Preparation for Medicine, commonly called GPEP. The panel's report, delivered in 1984, is a major contribution to the development of American medical education. In the introduction to its report (GPEP Panel, pp. xi–xiii) the group

- Affirmed "that all physicians, regardless of specialty, require a common foundation of knowledge, skills, values and attitudes."
- Affirmed "that the goal of the general professional education of physicians comprises both the acquisition of these attributes and the preparation for specialized education in medicine, and that these two purposes are not only compatible but also mutually supportive."
- Perceived a "continuing erosion of general education for physicians, an erosion that has not been arrested but is instead accelerating."
- Saw "continuing pressures (on the general education of the physician) to which we must accommodate with vigor and deliberate determination lest critical and irreversible damage is done." Among the pressures they observed were the following:

Chemical, mechanical, and electronic technologies available for prevention and treatment of disease will become even more complex, powerful, effective, and potentially dangerous. . . .

There will be an increasing recognition that many factors determining health and illness are not directly influenced by interventions of the health care system but are the consequences of life style, environmental factors, and poverty. . . .

Patients will increasingly need and demand advice and counsel from physicians and other health professionals about how to use special medical services to improve personal health. . . .

The principal providers of medical service in the near future are likely to be physicians employed by large corporations or by health service organizations covering specific population groups.

The panel was principally concerned with the direction to be taken in medical education to ensure that new physicians will be appropriately trained to practice medicine in the 21st century. It made 27 recommendations for change in medical education, grouped under five major conclusions:

Purposes of a general professional education
Baccalaureate education
Acquiring learning skills
Clinical education
Enhancing faculty involvement

Twenty-four of the recommendations concerned the process of medical education. The recommendations on content dealt with the three major substantive gaps in modern American medical education: understanding how the health care delivery system works; having the skills, knowledge, and attitudes necessary to integrate health promotion/disease prevention into medical practice; and being computer-literate. The recommendations on process focused on the conversion of medical education from its present approach—a teacher-centered, passive-learning mode without defined learning objectives—to a student-centered, problem-based, active-learning mode, with clearly defined, clinically relevant learning objectives.

The key is the introduction of problem-based learning. It uses clinical problems as a focus for student learning in all aspects of health sciences (Barrows; Barrows & Tamblyn). With problem-based learning as its focus, a new medical education system can be developed that will produce physicians equipped to solve the long-standing problems of the health care delivery system of the 20th century and meet the new challenges of the 21st century.

Making Changes in Medical Education

Change in any large institution is difficult. Change in medical education is particularly difficult. James B. Conant, a former president of Harvard University, has been quoted as saying that changing a medical school curriculum is like trying to move a graveyard. Steven Muller, president of Johns Hopkins University and chairman of the GPEP Panel, had this to say about change in medical education: "Change is already here, like it or not. More change is in view. Change breeds doubt. Doubt kindles choice. Choice is opportunity—the opportunity to do better or to do worse. We all will obviously seek to do our best" (Muller, p. 90). Change in the physician is the key to remedying many of the health services personnel problems that have been discussed in this chapter.

In the early 1970s a number of states established new medical schools (Fordham, 1979; Schofield). Several of these were described as community-based (Hunt & Weeks; Marder). They included the schools at Eastern Virginia, Center for the Health Sciences, the University of Illinois at Rockford, the University of South Alabama, and the University of Nevada. They rely more on decentralized community hospitals, outpatient settings, and use of preceptorships than do the older schools with strong tertiary-care hospital affiliations. A major interest of the state legislatures that established these schools was to increase the output of primary care physicians who would remain in the state to practice; many of these initiatives were successful (Marder).

Objectives-based curriculum design is a major element of the programs in the new medical schools at Southern Illinois University (Silber et al.), the University of Illinois at Urbana–Champaign (Sorlie), and the University of Missouri at Kansas City (1979). In the early 1980s the Texas College of Osteopathic Medicine (1980) at Fort Worth took the lead in attempting to develop a fundamentally health- and prevention-oriented curriculum along the lines proposed by Jonas in 1978. This was a major effort, aimed at making fundamental changes in both the process and the content of medical education in an existing school.

The effort was not successful, primarily because of a failure of administrative leadership at a critical moment in the change process. Although a majority of the faculty supported the change, a vociferous minority, which caught the attention of the administration, did not. Certain key compromises were made in the change program, especially in the area of substituting active for passive student learning. These compromises crippled the change movement, and it came to a halt. The school then drifted backward to a conventional program.

A different approach to making major changes in both process and content in an existing school was initiated at the University of New Mexico School of Medicine (Kaufman). The "parallel track" approach initiates change in only one portion the educational program. The experimental program is set up in tandem with the conventional program. It thus involves only a portion of the student body and faculty. Presumably, the program attracts students who want it and faculty who want to teach in the new way.

Parallel tracks, emphasizing problem-based learning and attention to previously ignored elements of medical practice, have been instituted in several other medical schools in the United States and other countries (Kantrowitz et al.) and generally have been successful. The parallel-track approach appears to hold the most promise for making effective change in other medical schools. Nevertheless, the disease-oriented, acute-care, passive-learning, teacher-centered approach to medical education is well entrenched and difficult to change.

Matching Education and Practice

In 1978 the Work Group on the Education of the Health Professions of the National Center for Health Services Research identified a series of policy issues in health professions education in general that, in their view, could be subjected profitably to research (Magraw et al.). They concluded that research should

- Address relationships between what is learned in health professions education and the effect of professional intervention on the care of individual patients and the health status of the American people.
- Examine health services and the health status of people in different regions and cultures in relation to variations in health professions education and practice.
- Address the lack of attention to preventive health measures in health professions education and professional practice and by the public.
- Address the effect of educational programs aimed at diminishing professional and disciplinary insularity on practice patterns and, subsequently, on the health status of the populations served.
- Identify contributions of education and practice to professional behavior and their effect on health services, health status, and relief from discomfort.

- Relate financing and reimbursement policies for education and practice to the educational system, practice patterns, and health status.
- Provide a better understanding of how health services research can influence changes in education, practice, health status, and relief from discomfort. [pp. 543–545]

Although the latter part of this chapter has focused on medical education and its problems, it is evident from the Magraw (1978) study conclusions that there are many similar problems at all levels of health professions education. It is also evident that the solutions to many of the problems in the functioning of health personnel will be found in the reform of health sciences education. In this regard, the most important task is to state clearly the goals and objectives of the health care delivery system. Then the knowledge, skills, and attitudes that health services personnel need in order to carry out their functions properly in the system can be clearly identified. Finally, the health sciences educational programs can be designed to teach students what they need and not teach them what they don't need. Easy to say; not easy to do.

References

American College of Surgeons and the American Surgical Association. *Surgery in the United States: A Summary Report of the Study on Surgical Services to the U.S.* Chicago: American College of Surgeons and the American Surgical Association, 1975.

American Medical Association. "84th Annual Report on Medical Education in the United States, 1983–84." *Journal of the American Medical Association, 252,* 1505, 1984.

American Medical Association. "Medical Education in the United States, 1987–1988" *Journal of the American Medical Association, 260,* 1033, 1988.

American Nurses Association. *Facts About Nursing 86–87.* Kansas City, MO: Author 1987.

American Nurses Association. *Fact Sheet* Kansas City, MO: Author.

Association of American Medical Colleges. "Graduates of Foreign Medical Schools in the United States: A Challenge to Medical Education." *Journal of Medical Education, 49,* 809, 1974.

Association of American Medical Colleges. *Weekly Report,* April 25, 1985.

Association of American Medical Colleges. "Declining Applicant Pool Conference." *Weekly Report,* June 23, 1988.

Bailey, B. J. "Manpower Issues for a Surgical Specialty: The Impact of Oversupply." *Journal of the American Medical Association, 253,* 1025, 1985.

Balinsky, W. L. "Distribution of Young Medical Specialists from Western New York." *Medical Care, 12,* 437, 1974.

Banta, H. D. "Medical Education: Abraham Flexner—a Reappraisal." *Social Science and Medicine, 5,* 655, 1971.

Barrows, H. S. *Problem-Based Learning in the Basic Science Years.* New York: Springer Publishing Co., 1985.

Barrows, H. S., & Tamblyn, R. *Problem-Based Learning*. New York: Springer Publishing Co., 1980.

Bloom, M. "The 'Other' Medical Schools: Coming Home." *Medical World News*, May, 28, 1979.

Blum, H. L. "*Health Planning: Lessons for the Future*, by Bonnie Lefkowitz" (book review). *Inquiry, 20*, 390, 1983.

Bok, D. *President's Report, 1982–83*. Cambridge, Mass.: Harvard University, 1984.

Bureau of Health Professions. *Diffusion and the Changing Geographic Distribution of Primary Care Physicians* (ODAM Rcport No. 4-83). Hyattsville, MD: U.S. Department of Health and Human Services, 1983.

Bureau of Health Professions. *Projections of Physician Supply in the U.S.* (ODAM Report No. 3-85). Rockville, MD: U.S. Department of Health and Human Services, 1985.

Bureau of Health Professions. *Fifth Report to the President and Congress on the Status of Health Personnel in the United States, March, 1986.* (DHHS Pub. HRS-P-OD-86-1). Rockville, MD: U.S. Department of Health and Human Services, 1986.

Butter, I. *Foreign Medical Graduates: A Comparative Study of State Licensure Policies* (DHEW Pub. No. HRA 77-3166). Rockville, MD: National Center for Health Services Research, 1976.

Carnegie Commission on Higher Education. *Higher Education and the Nation's Health*. New York: McGraw-Hill, 1970.

Castleton, K. B. "Are We Building Too Many Medical Schools?" *Journal of the American Medical Association, 216*, 1989, 1971.

Comptroller General. *Progress and Problems in Improving the Availability of Primary Care Providers in Underserved Areas* (USDHHS Pub. No. HRD 77-135). Washington, D.C.: General Accounting Office, 1978.

Cooper, J. A. D. "Academic Medical Centers and Government: An Indispensable Partnership." *Journal of Medical Education, 53*, 998, 1978.

Cooper, J. A. D. "Testimony Submitted by the Association of American Medical Colleges to the Subcommittee on Labor-Management Relations, Committee on Education and Labor, U.S. House of Representatives." Washington, D.C.: Association of American Medical Colleges, 1979.

Cooper, J. A. D. "President's Message." In Association of American Medical Colleges (Eds.), *Annual Report: 1982–83*. Washington, D.C.: AAMC, 1983.

Daniels, N. "Why Saying No to Patients in the United States Is So Hard." *New England Journal of Medicine, 314*, 1380, 1986.

"Doctor Surplus Breeds New Practice Forms." *Washington Report on Medicine and Health Perspectives*, April 25, 1983, pp. 1–4.

Dyckman, Z. Y. *A Study of Physician's Fees*. Washington, D.C.: U.S. Government Printing Office, 1978.

Ebert, R. H. "The Medical School." *Scientific American, 229*(3), 138, 1973.

Estes, E. H. "The Dispersion of Physicians." *Journal of the American Medical Association, 247*, 2406, 1982.

Engelhart, H. T. "Intensive Care Units, Scarce Resources, and Conflicting Principles of Justice." *Journal of the American Medical Association, 255*, 1159, 1986.

Fawcett, T. Analysis and Evaluation of Conceptual Models of Nursing, Philadelphia F. A. Davis, 1984.

Fein, R. *The Doctor Shortage*. Washington, D.C.: Brookings Institution, 1967.

Ferguson, R. P. "Declining Appeal of Foreign Medical Education for U.S. Students." *Journal of Medical Education, 62,* 719, 1987.

Flexner, A. *Medical Education in the United States and Canada*. New York: The Carnegie Foundation for the Advancement of Teaching, 1910. Reprinted, Washington, D.C.: Science and Health Publications, 1960.

Fordham, C. C. "Changing Medical Education—the New Schools." *New England Journal of Medicine, 301,* 719, 1979.

Fordham, C. C. "The *Bane Report* Revisited." *Journal of the American Medical Association, 244,* 354, 1980.

Freedman, S. A. "Megacorporate Health Care." *New England Journal of Medicine, 312,* 579, 1985.

Freidson, E. *Professional Dominance: The Social Structure of Medical Care*. New York: Atherton Press, 1970.

Freiman, M. P., & Marder, W. D. "Changes in the Hours Worked by Physicians, 1970–80." *American Journal of Public Health, 74,* 1348, 1984.

Freymann, J. G. *The American Health Care System: Its Genesis and Trajectory*. New York: Medcom Press, 1974.

Fuchs, V. *Who Shall Live? Health Economics and Social Change*. New York: Basic Books, 1974.

Fuchs, V. "The Rationing of Medical Care." *New England Journal of Medicine, 311,* 1572, 1984.

Fuchs, V., & Kramer, M. J. *Determinants of Expenditures for Physicians' Services in the United States, 1948–1968* (DHEW Pub. No. HSM 73-3013). Washington D.C.: U.S. Government Printing Office, 1972.

General Professional Education of the Physicians Panel. "Physicians for the Twenty-First Century." *Journal of Medical Education, 59*(11) (plus appendices), November 1984, Part 2.

Goldsmith, J. C. "The US Health Care System in the Year 2000." *Journal of the American Medical Association, 256,* 3371, 1986.

Gonzalez, M. L., & Emmons, D. W. *Socioeconomic Characteristics of Medical Practice, 1987*. Chicago: American Medical Association Center for Health Policy Research, 1987.

Graduate Medical Education National Advisory Committee (GMENAC). *Interim Report* (DHEW Pub. No. HRA 79-633). Washington D.C.: U.S. Government Printing Office, 1979.

Graettinger, J. S. "Results of the NRMP for 1988." *Journal of Medical Education, 63,* 491, 1988.

Green, R. "Health Care Rationing: Can It Happen Here?" *Medical World News,* November 12, 1984, p. 50.

Harris, J. E. "How Many Doctors Are Enough?" *Health Affairs, 5,* 73, 1986.

Hayward, R. A., et al. "Inequities in Health Services among Insured Americans." *New England Journal of Medicine, 318,* 1507, 1988.

Health Policy Agenda Steering Committee. "Health Policy Agenda for the American People." *Journal of the American Medical Association, 257,* 1199, 1987.

Health Resources Administration. *A Report to the President and Congress on the Status of Health Professions Personnel in the United States* (DHEW Pub. No. HRA 79-633). Washington, D.C.: U.S. Government Printing Office, 1979.

Health Resources and Services Administration. *Annual Report*. Rockville, MD: U.S. Government Printing Office, 1984.

Health Resources and Services Administration. *Annual Report*. Rockville, MD: U.S. Department of Health and Human Services, 1986.

Hemenway, D. "The Optimal Location of Doctors." *New England Journal of Medicine, 306*, 397, 1982.

Hunt, A. D., & Weeks, L. E. (Eds.). *Medical Education since 1960*. East Lansing, MI: Michigan State University, 1979.

Hudson, J. I., & Nourse, E. S. (Eds.). "Perspectives in Primary Care Education." *Journal of Medical Education, 50*, December 1975, Part 2.

Igelhart, J. K. "The Future Supply of Physicians." *New England Journal of Medicine, 314*, 860, 1986.

Imperato, P. J. (Ed.). "The Offshore Medical Schools." *New York State Journal of Medicine, 84*, 337, 1984. (a)

Imperato, P. J. "An Overview of New York State and the Offshore Medical Schools." *New York State Journal of Medicine, 84*, 337, 1984. (b)

Institute of Medicine. *Medicare-Medicaid Reimbursement Policies*. Washington, D.C.: National Academy of Sciences, 1976.

Institute of Medicine. *A Manpower Policy for Primary Health Care*. Washington, D.C.: National Academy of Sciences, 1978.

"JAMA 100 Years Ago: August 27, 1887." *Journal of the American Medical Association, 258*, 1123, 1987.

Jonas, S. *Medical Mystery: The Training of Doctors in the United States*. New York: W. W. Norton, 1978.

Jonas, S. "State Approval of Foreign Medical Schools." *New England Journal of Medicine, 305*, 45, 1981.

Jonas, S. "A Perspective on Educating Physicians for Prevention." *Public Health Reports, 97*, 199, 1982.

Jonas, S. "The Case for Change in Medical Education in the United States." *Lancet*, August 25, p. 452, 1984. (a)

Jonas, S. "The Historical and Theoretical Basis for the New York State Board of Regents' Policy Concerning Foreign Medical Students." *New York State Journal of Medicine, 84*, 345, 1984. (b)

Jonas, S. "A Modest Proposal for Controlling the Influx of United States Citizen Foreign Medical Graduates in the United States." *Federation Bulletin*, April 1985, p. 106.

Jonas, S. "Health Promotion in Medical Education." *American Journal of Health Promotion, 3*, 37, 1988.

Kantrowitz, M., et al. *Innovative Tracks at Established Institutions for the Education of Health Personnel*. Geneva: World Health Organization, 1987.

Kaufman, A. (Ed.). *Implementing Problem-Based Medical Education*. New York: Springer Publishing Co., 1985.

Kennedy, E. M. "Congressional Concerns about Physician Supply." *Journal of Medical Education, 63*, 117, 1988.

Kleinman, J. C., et al. "Physician Manpower Data: The Case of the Missing Foreign Medical Graduates." *Medical Care, 12*, 906, 1974.

Kleinman, J. C., et al. "Postgraduate Training and Work Experience of Non-ECFMG Certified Physicians in the U.S." *Medical Care, 13*, 445, 1975. (a)

Kleinman, J. C., et al. "A Reply to Stevens, Goodman and Mick." *Medical Care, 13,* 445, 1975. (b)

Lave, J. R., et al. "Medical Manpower Models: Need, Demand and Supply." *Inquiry, 12,* 97, June 1975.

Lewis, I. J., & Sheps, C. *The Sick Citadel.* Cambridge, MA: Oelgeschlager, Gunn and Hain, 1983.

Luft, H. S., & Arno, P. "Impact of Increasing Physician Supply." *Health Affairs, 5,* 31, 1986.

Magraw, R. M., et al. "Health Professions Education and Public Policy: A Research Agenda." *Journal of Medical Education, 53,* 539, 1978.

Maloney, J. V., & Reemtsma, K. "Cost Containment by a Naval Armada." *New England Journal of Medicine, 312,* 1713, 1985.

Marcus, S. A. "Trade Unionism for Doctors." *New England Journal of Medicine, 311,* 1508, 1984.

Marder, W. D. "Practice Patterns of Graduates of New Community-Based Medical Schools." *Journal of Medical Education, 59,* 345, 1984.

McClure, M. L. & Nelson, M. J. Trends in hospital nursing. In L. H. Aiken (Ed.) *Nursing in the 1980s:* Crisis, opportunities, challanges (pp. 59–73). Philadelphia: Lippincott, 1982.

McGuire, C. H., et al. *Handbook of Health Professions Education.* San Francisco: Jossey-Bass, 1983.

Mick, S. S. "Understanding the Persistence of Human Resource Problems in Health." *Health and Society, 56,* 463, 1978.

Miller, F. H., & Miller, G. A. H. "The Painful Prescription: A Procrustean Perspective?" *New England Journal of Medicine, 314,* 1383, 1986.

Mullan, F. S. M. "The National Health Service Corps." *Public Health Reports,* July–August (Suppl.) 1979.

Muller, S. "Medicine: A Learned Profession?" *Journal of Medical Education, 60,* 85, 1985.

Mulvihill, J. E., & Rosner, F. "Americans Studying Medicine Abroad." *New York State Journal of Medicine,* April 1979, p. 774.

National Advisory Commission on Health Manpower. *Report* (Vols. 1, 2). Washington, D.C.: U.S. Government Printing Office, 1967.

National Center for Health Services Research. *Financing Graduate Medical Education.* Hyattsville, Md.: U.S. Government Printing Office, 1979.

Navarro, V. "A Critique of the Present and Proposed Strategies for Redistributing Resources in the Health Sector and a Discussion of Alternatives." *Medical Care, 12,* 721, 1974.

Newhouse, J. P., et al. "Where Have All the Doctors Gone?" *Journal of the American Medical Association, 247,* 2392, 1982.

NY Ed. Law Article 139, Section 6902

New York State Department of Health. *Final Report of the New York State Labor-Health Industry Task Force on Health Personnel.* Albany, NY: Author.

New York State Education Department. *An Analysis of Current and Future Physician Supply and Requirements in New York State.* Albany, N.Y.: New York State Education Department, 1983.

"The Office Physician's Changing Patient Load." *Medical World News.* February 9, 1987, p. 58.

Petersdorf, R. G. "The Scylla and Charybdis of Medical Education." *Journal of Medical Education, 63,* 88, 1988.

Peterson, P. Q., & Pennell, M. Y. "Physician-Population Projections, 1961–1975: Their Causes and Implications." *American Journal of Public Health, 53,* 163, 1963.

Pierson, R. N. "Effects of Offshore Medical Students on Hospitals, Medical Schools and Physicians in New York State." *New York State Journal of Medicine, 84,* 352, 1984.

Record, J., et al. *Primary Care Staffing in 1990.* New York: Springer Publishing Co., 1981.

Reed, R. R., & Evans, D. "The Deprofessionalization of Medicine." *Journal of the American Medicine Association, 258,* 3279, 1987.

Reinhardt, U. E. *Physician Productivity and the Demand for Health Manpower.* Cambridge, MA: Ballinger, 1975.

Reinhardt, U. E. "The Health Professions' Collision Course." *Hospitals,* August 16, 1984, p. 86.

Relman, A. S. "Americans Studying Medicine Abroad." *New England Journal of Medicine, 299,* 887, 1978.

Richmond, J. *Currents in American Medicine: A Developmental View of Medical Care and Education.* Cambridge, MA: Harvard University Press, 1969.

Riddle, J. W. "Clinical Clerkships." *New York Journal of Medicine, 84,* 355, 1984.

Riehl, J. P., & Roy, C. *Conceptual Models for Nursing Practice.* New York: Appleton-Century-Crofts, 1980 2nd ed.

Riffer, J. "Physicians Trade Private Practice for Security." *Hospitals,* August 20, 1986, p. 66.

Rogers, D. E. "On Preparing Academic Health Centers for the Very Different 1980's." *Journal of Medical Education, 55,* 1, 1980.

Rogers, D. E. "Some Musings on Medical Education: Is It Going Astray?" *Pharos of Alpha Omega Alpha, 45,* 11, 1982.

Rosenberg, Charles E. *The Care of Strangers.* New York: Basic Books, 1987.

Rosenthal, M. M., & Frederick, D. "Physician Maldistribution in Cross Cultural Perspective: United States, United Kingdom, and Sweden." *Inquiry, 21,* 60, 1984.

Saywell, R. M., et al. "A Performance Comparison: USMG-FMG Attending Physicians." *American Journal of Public Health, 69,* 57, 1979.

Schloss, E. P. "Beyond GMENAC." *New England Journal of Medicine, 318,* 920, 1988.

Schofield, J. R. *New and Expanded Medical Schools, Mid-Century to the 1980's.* San Francisco: Jossey-Bass, 1984.

Schwartz, W. B., et al. "The Changing Geographic Distribution of Board-Certified Physicians." *New England Journal of Medicine, 303,* 1032, 1980.

Schwartz, W. B., et al. "Are We Training Too Many Medical Subspecialists?" *Journal of the American Medical Association, 259,* 233, 1988. (a)

Schwartz, W. B., et al. "Why There Will Be Little or No Physician Surplus Between Now and the Year 2000." *New England Journal of Medicine, 318,* 892, 1988. (b)

Schweiker, R. S. "Disease Prevention and Health Promotion." *Journal of Medical Education, 57,* 15, 1982.

Secretary's Commission on Nursing Final Report. Washington, D.C.: Department of Health and Human Services. December, 1988.

Secretary's Commission on Nursing Interim Report. Department of Health and Human Services: Washington, D.C. July, 1988.

Senior, B., & Smith, B. A. "The Number of Physicians as a Constraint on Delivery of Health Care." *Journal of the American Medical Association, 222,* 178, 1972.

Silber, D. L. et al. "The SIU Medical Curriculum: Systemwide Objectives-Based Instruction." *Journal of Medical Education, 53,* 473, 1978.

Smith, B. W. H., & Gerard, R. J. "A Federal Health Service Corps." *New England Journal of Medicine, 306,* 1045, 1982.

Smith, L. H. "Medical Education for the 21st Century." *Medical Education, 60,* 106, 1985.

Sorlie, W. E. *A Word about SBMS-UC*. Urbana-Champaign, IL: University of Illinois Press, 1979.

Stambler, H. V. "Health Manpower for the Nation—a Look Ahead at the Supply and Requirements." *Public Health Reports, 94,* 3, 1979.

Stamps, P. L., & Kuriger, F. H. "Location Decision on National Health Service Corps Physicians." *American Journal of Public Health, 73,* 906, 1983.

Steiber, S. R. "Physicians Who Move and Why They Move." *Journal of the American Medical Association, 248,* 1490, 1982.

Steinwald, B., & Steinwald, C. "The Effect of Preceptorship and Rural Training Programs on Physicians' Practice Location Decisions." *Medical Care, 13,* 219, 1975.

Stevens, R., et al. *The Alien Doctors*. New York: John Wiley, 1978.

Stillman, P. L., et al. "Students Transferring into an American Medical School." *Journal of the American Medical Association, 242,* 129, 1980.

Stimmel, B., & Benenson, T. F. "United States Citizens in Foreign Medical Schools and the Future Supply of Physicians." *New England Journal of Medicine, 300,* 1414, 1979.

Strauss, M. J., et al. "Rationing of Intensive Care Unit Services." *Journal of the American Medical Association, 255,* 1143, 1986.

Strickland, S. P. *Politics, Science and Dread Disease*. Cambridge, MA: Harvard University Press, 1972.

Surgeon General's Consultant Group on Medical Education. *Report: Physicians for a Growing America*. Washington, D.C.: Public Health Service, 1959.

Tarlov, A. R. "The Rising Supply of Physicians and the Pursuit of Better Health." *Journal of Medical Education, 63,* 94, 1988.

Texas College of Osteopathic Medicine. *Design of the Medical Curriculum in Relation to the Health Needs of the Nation*. Fort Worth, TX: Texas College of Osteopathic Medicine, 1980.

University of Missouri at Kansas City. *The Academic Plan for the School of Medicine*. Kansas City, MO: University of Missouri Press, 1979.

U.S. Bureau of the Census. *Statistical Abstract of the United States, 1987*. Washington, D.C.: U.S. Government Printing Office, 1987.

U.S. Department of Health and Human Services. *Health United States: 1987*. (DHHS Pub. No. PHS 88-1232). Hyattsville, MD: USDHHS 1988.

U.S. Senate, Subcommittee on Health and the Environment. *Current Health Manpower Issues* (Committee Print No. 96-IFC-34). Washington, DC.: U.S. Government Printing Office, 1979.

Weinberg, E., & Bell, A. I. "Performance of United States Citizens with Foreign Medical Education on Standardized Medical Examination." *New England Journal of Medicine, 299,* 917, 1979.

Wennberg, J. E. "Dealing with Medical Practice Variations: A Proposal for Action." *Health Affairs, 3,* 6, 1984.

Wennberg, J. E., & Lapenas, J. D. "On Choosing the Numbers of Needed Physicians." Report prepared for the GMENAC Panel on Geographic Variations. Washington, D.C.: Health Resources Administration, 1980.

Williams, A. P. "How Many Miles to the Doctor?" *New England Journal of Medicine, 309,* 958, 1983.

5

Nursing

Christine Kovner

This chapter presents an overview of the nursing profession. After a brief history of nursing, the chapter looks at how nursing is defined in law and by professional nurses. The various educational programs for nurses are described, as well as the levels of practice. Finally, current issues in nursing are analyzed within the context of the health care system. "Nursing" is a generic term that has been applied to a variety of practitioners from nurses' aides and assistants to nurse researchers with Ph.D.s. The focus of this chapter will be the professional registered nurse and the licensed practical nurse.

Historical Perspective

Aiken (1983, p. 408) points out four factors from nursing's history that influence nursing today:

1. Nursing developed as an occupation supportive of physicians.
2. Nurses work primarily in bureaucratic institutions.
3. Nurses are predominantly female.
4. Nursing's early educational history was linked to religious orders, with expectations of service, dedication, and charity.

Although English, Florence Nightingale (1820–1910) had a profound influence on American nursing. She advocated formal training for nurses and an administrative order for the hospital, with the matron (head nurse) as head (Rosenberg, 1987 pp. 122–141). After her success in decreasing the death rate of soldiers serving in the Crimean War, Nightingale opened a training school at St. Thomas's Hospital in England. The first training program in the United States was begun in 1872 at the New England Hospital for Women and Children in

Boston. Training schools increased from 15 in 1880 to 1,105 by 1909, all under the direction of hospitals (Kelly). Nursing students provided much of the care in these institutions. Married women and those over 30 were excluded, along with divorced women (Kelly, p. 32). Nurses were treated as subservient to both physicians and hospital administrators. According to Rosenberg (p. 236), until the 1920s the nurse's status was somewhat above that of domestic servant. However, Wilkerson (1985) suggests that public health nurses were "disciplined and well bred" (p. 1155) and "associate or co-worker of the physician" (p. 1157). In the early 1920s soul searching and reform were beginning. Prior to World War I, Presbyterian Hospital, in conjunction with Teachers College, Columbia University, developed a 5-year combined college-diploma program.

Early nursing leaders include Lillian Wald, public health nursing leader and founder of the Henry Street Settlement; Mary Mahoney, the first black nurse to graduate from a nurse training program; Annie Goodrich, the first dean of the U.S. Army School of Nursing; Adelaide Nutting, the first nurse to receive a professorship at Columbia Teacher's College; and Mary Breckenridge, founder of the Frontier Nursing Service. These early American leaders paved the way for today's nurses.

What Is Nursing?

Nursing includes caring for a newborn moments after birth and monitoring the blood pressure of a person brought into the emergency room following an auto accident. It is teaching the diabetic how to inject insulin and advising a senator on how to finance and organize home care services for the elderly. It is identifying the strengths of a family facing the knowledge that both mother and father have AIDS and convincing the illegal alien that being treated for tuberculosis at the government clinic will not jeopardize his status in this country. And it is adjusting the tubes and drips of the person in the ICU. But what is the legal definition of nursing? How do academic theoreticians define nursing? How do nurses themselves define it?

The American Nurses Association (ANA) (1980) suggests that authority for nursing is based on a social contract between society and the profession. It is further suggested that the legal authority for nursing (nurse practice acts) stems from this social contract, rather that the other way around (pp. 7–8).

Legal Definition

The ANA's (1981) suggested nursing practice legislation defines professional nursing as

> . . . services requiring substantial specialized knowledge of the biological, physical, behavioral, psychological, and sociological sciences and of nursing theory as the

basis for assessment, diagnosis, planning, intervention, and evaluation in the promotion and maintenance of health; the casefinding and management of illness, injury, or infirmity; the restoration of optimum function; or the achievement of a dignified death. Nursing practice includes but is not limited to administration, teaching, counseling, supervision, delegation, and evaluation of practice and execution of the medical regimen, including the administration of medications and treatments prescribed by any person authorized by state law to prescribe. [p. 6]

For example, in New York State a registered professional nurse is defined as

. . . diagnosing and treating human responses to actual or potential health problems through such services as casefinding, health teaching, health counseling, and provision of care supportive to or restorative of life and well-being, and executing medical regimens prescribed by a licensed or otherwise legally authorized physician or dentist. A nursing regimen shall be consistent with and shall not vary any existing medical regimen. (NY Education Law Article 139 Section 6902)

New York differentiates professional nursing from practical nursing, defining the later as "performing tasks and responsibilities . . . under the direction of a registered professional nurse or licensed or otherwise legally authorized physician or dentist." (NY Education Law Article 139 Section 6902) In some states nurses (or certain categories of nurses) may prescribe pharmacologic agents or deliver a baby; in other states they may not. In addition, some states require continuing education for license renewal.

Nursing is usually defined as diagnosis and treatment of human responses. However, each state has its own legal definition because regulation of the practice of nursing is a state responsibility. There are currently two legal categories of nurses in the United States: registered nurse and practical nurse. The registered nurse is sometimes called a registered professional nurse. The legal term for the practical nurse is sometimes licensed practical nurse or licensed vocational nurse. Under a state board of nursing each state licenses people to practice as registered nurses and defines what this practice is. As nursing developed in the United States, practitioners called themselves nurses. By 1923 legislation was enacted in all states for voluntary registration (Bullough). The first mandatory licensing law went into effect in New York State in 1947. It required that, with certain exceptions, only licensed professional nurses could legally use the title Registered Nurse. All states require that potential registered nurses attend an approved nursing program and take a national licensing exam, the National Council Exam for Registered Nurses (NCLEX-RN), developed by the National Council of State Boards of Nursing. In 1985, of the 81,519 first-time candidates educated in the United States and its territories taking the exam, 90% passed. This ranged from 23% passing in the U.S. Virgin Islands to 96% passing in Wyoming. New York had the largest number of examinees (6,804). In 33 states graduates of foreign schools of nursing must pass an examination prepared by the Commission on Graduates of Foreign Nursing

Schools prior to taking the NCLEX. Of the 47,420 nurses who took the test between 1978 and 1986 only 30% passed both the English and nursing components on the first examination (ANA, 1987, pp. 80–85).

Theoretical Definition

A classic definition of nursing is that of Virginia Henderson (1966), who states:

> The unique function of the nurse is to assist the individual (sick or well), in the performance of those activities contributing to health or its recovery (or peaceful death) that he would perform unaided if he had the necessary strength, will, or knowledge. And to do this in such a way as to help him gain independence as rapidly as possible. [p. 15]

The ANA (1980) proposes that nursing is concerned "with human responses to actual or potential health problems" (p. 8). Nurses do not treat the underlying health problems. The underlying health problems are usually diagnosed and treated by physicians. Some examples of human responses that are the concern of nurses are:

1. Self-care limitations.
2. Impaired functioning in areas such as rest, sleep, ventilation, circulation, activity, nutrition, elimination, skin, sexuality, and the like.
3. Pain and discomfort.
4. Emotional problems related to illness and treatment, life threatening events, or daily experiences, such as anxiety, loss, loneliness, and grief.
5. Distortion of symbolic functions, reflected in interpersonal and intellectual processes, such as hallucinations.
6. Deficiencies in decision making and ability to make personal choices.
7. Self-image changes required by health use.
8. Dysfunctional perceptual orientations to health.
9. Strains related to life processes, such as birth, growth and development, and death.
10. Problematic affiliative relationships. [ANA, 1980, p. 10]

Nursing care is based on theory that is both derived from other disciplines and developed by nurses. "The aims of nursing actions are to ameliorate, improve, or correct conditions to which those practices are directed, to prevent illness and to promote health" (ANA, 1980, p. 12). A distinguishing characteristic of nursing is that it includes nurturing to provide comfort—generative nurturing to develop new behaviors and protective nurturing involving surveillance. *Generative* implies newly developed, and *protective* implies monitoring (ANA, 1980, p. 18). Nurses encourage people to be responsible for their own health, and they work with patients to achieve mutually desirable outcomes.

There are many conceptual models and theories currently used and studied in nursing. Fawcett (1984) proposes that nursing is concerned with four concepts: patient, nurse, environment, and health. These four concepts are viewed differently in various models.

Orem (1980) proposes that nursing is helping the patient with self-care. When the patient is unable to provide self-care, this role is assumed by the nurse. She states five methods to help others:

1. Acting for or doing for another.
2. Guiding another.
3. Supporting another (physically or psychologically).
4. Providing an environment that promotes personal development in relation to becoming able to meet present or future demands for action.
5. Teaching another. [p. 61]

Rogers (1970), another popular nursing theorist, describes the person as an energy field, having no real boundaries. She proposes that the energy field of each person is in constant interaction with the environment, which is itself an energy field that is everything outside the human field (Riehl & Roy, p. 332). Wellness and illness are not differentiated within this model; rather, they are value judgments of society. Rogers differentiates nursing from other professions in that nursing's central concern is the unitary person. According to Rogers, "nursing aims to assist people in achieving their maximum health potential" (p. 86). The major premise of Rogers is that the person is a unitary whole and cannot be reduced to components such as organs or systems.

These two examples of nursing theory indicate what is either nursing's greatest strength or its greatest weakness—the diversity of opinion on what it is. It is a strength that nurses are open to new ideas and are not stagnant in a traditional view of nursing. Such an attitude will aid nurses in adapting to changes in the health care delivery system and creatively responding to clients' needs. But a problem with diversity is the lack of a cohesive voice for nursing. However, it can be said that nursing differs from medicine in its focus on the whole person. When a nurse takes a person's blood pressure, the focus is the entire person, whereas a physician's focus in the same situation would tend to be on the cardiovascular system.

Education of Nurses

One of the most confusing aspects of nursing is the variety of educational programs for educating nurses. Unlike medicine, which has consistent educational requirements, nursing offers the student a number of options. The practical nurse can attend programs in high schools, hospitals, junior colleges, or vocational schools.

Likewise, the registered nurse can attend a 2-year college program, a 3-year hospital-based (diploma) program, a 4-year college program, a 2-year master's degree program, or a nursing doctoral (N.D.) program, all of which enable the student to take the state licensing exam. State boards of nursing accept all of these programs as appropriate preparation for the licensing exam.

Licensed Practical Nursing (LPN/LVN)

The practical nurse provides direct patient care under the supervision of a registered nurse. The National League for Nursing (NLN) (1988) estimates the number of practical-nurse programs at 1,165. More than 50% of the programs are in technical or vocational schools. Others are in junior or community colleges (31.9%), hospitals (6.8%), secondary schools (6.7%), government agencies (1.4%), senior colleges or universities (1.1%), and independent agencies (0.8%). Enrollment in 1985 was 39,345, a decrease of 14% over 1984. Graduates in 1985 numbered 36,955, a decrease of 17% from 1984 (p. 177).

Registered Professional Nursing

During 1986 there were 1,469 educational programs for registered nurses in the United States, at the following educational levels: (1) associate degree, 776; (2) baccalaureate degree, 455; (3) diploma, 238; and (4) baccalaureate only for people already licensed as registered nurses, 161 (National League for Nursing). The NLN is the accreditation body for nursing programs. In 1986, 72.8% of R.N. programs were accredited (NLN, p. 13), with the North Atlantic region having the highest percentage (85.5%) and the West having the lowest (55.2%). Enrollments in professional nursing programs are dropping at an alarming rate. Total enrollments were 193,712 in 1986, an 11.1% decrease from 1985 (p. 28). Graduations from professional nursing programs dropped 6.2% (to 77,027) over the same period, with the largest drop (11.5%) for diploma programs (p. 38).

Accreditation standards do not specify specific course requirements. Consequently, curricula vary widely from school to school, and transfer of nursing course credits is extremely unlikely. The first associate degree program was begun in 1952 (Anastas). The typical associate degree program requires basic liberal arts courses such as English and sociology. In addition, science courses such as anatomy and physiology are required. Nursing courses usually include fundamentals of nursing (clinical skills), maternal and child health, and care of the acutely ill hospitalized adult patient. Practical experience is gained by practicing skills in the campus laboratory and care of patients in institutional settings such as hospitals. The nurses enrolled in associate degree programs are educated to be direct providers of care at the patient bedside. The programs are 2 academic years to 2 calendar years in length.

The typical diploma program is similar to the associate degree program, though usually under the auspices of a hospital. Often students are required to take liberal arts courses at a local college, and they receive college credit that can later be transferred to other colleges. The practical-experience sessions are usually longer than in the associate degree program, and the entire course takes about 3 years, with an emphasis on acute care (hospital-based) nursing. Diploma graduates who go to college often are not able to transfer the credits earned in the diploma program because until recently these have not been degree-granting institutions.

The curriculum of the baccalaureate program is similar to that of liberal arts programs in other fields. Because the program is at least 8 semesters long, the student takes more courses than in either the associate or the diploma program. Students take liberal arts courses such as English, math, and psychology and are required to take science courses such as microbiology, anatomy, and physiology. In addition, approximately half of the credits are usually in nursing courses. The organization of these courses varies from school to school. Some schools organize curricula developmentally and have courses devoted to care of infants, children, adults, and older people. Others base the curriculum on the relative health of populations and offer courses on prevention, episodic care, continuous care, and critical care. In addition, students learn to read and interpret research. Nurses are prepared to work in community settings and leadership positions as well as in acute-care settings. They are generalists who can provide care to individuals, groups, and families. Graduates are also prepared for advanced education in nursing.

Another opportunity for education in nursing is the external degree program, such as that offered by the Board of Regents of New York State. In 1971 an associate degree program was begun, followed by a baccalaureate degree program in 1976. Students obtain either degree by completing equivalency testing in liberal arts, sciences, and nursing. Students also must complete a practical exam. The program's philosophy is that what the person knows, rather than how the information was acquired, is what matters. California's state education system has a similar program. Graduates of these programs are eligible for state licensure (Anastas).

Graduate Education

Nursing degree programs at the master's and doctoral level concentrate on nursing courses, with the assumption that the baccalaureate graduate has had the basic liberal arts and science courses or will be required to make them up. Historically, specialists in nursing were educated in specialized hospitals or became specialists based on clinical practice with a particular type of patient. In the 1950s colleges and universities began offering programs for specialty education. By the 1960s postgraduate education for clinical practice specialization was in universities (ANA, 1980, pp. 21–22). The focus of these programs is expert competence. Functions of specialists include the following:

- Identification of populations or communities at risk.
- Direct care of selected patients or clients in any setting, including private practice.
- Intraprofessional consultation with nurse specialists in different clinical areas and with nurses in general practice.
- Interprofessional consultation and collaboration in planning total patient care for individual and groups of patients, and in planning and evaluating health programs for population groups at risk related to the specialty or the public in general.
- Contribution to the advancement of the profession as a whole and to the specialty field. [ANA, 1980, p. 26]

Master's Degree Programs. Registered nurses with baccalaureate degrees can earn master's degrees in advanced clinical practice, teaching, and nursing administration/management. Within these three broad areas students usually focus on a nursing content area such as adult health, maternal–child health, psychiatric–mental health, or community health. Specific programs include everything from nursing informatics (computers) to home health care management to geriatrics. Most students choose to focus on advanced clinical practice (56–72%) (NLN, pp. 79–81). For full-time students, maternal–child nursing is the most popular clinical area; for part-time students, medical-surgical nursing is.

In 1986 there were 189 programs offering a master's degree in nursing, an increase of 69 in the last decade (NLN, p. 73). In 1986 there were 19,958 students enrolled in master's degree programs. This was a dramatic increase over the 3,531 students enrolled in 1967. Only 28% were full-time, however (pp. 75–76), reflecting a steady decrease from the 78% full-time in 1967. This may relate to the decrease in federal funding for graduate education in nursing. The number of graduates per year has remained relatively stable, at about 5,200, over the 5-year period from 1982 to 1986 (p. 82).

Doctoral Programs. Nurses also earn doctoral degrees in nursing. There are three types of degrees offered. The N.D. (doctor of nursing) is similar to the M.D.; that is, it is the first professional degree, building on the earlier liberal arts or scientific education and preparing the student to take the state licensing exam to practice as a registered nurse. The D.N.S. and D.N.Sc. are professional doctorates that prepare the nurse for advanced clinical practice. The Ph.D. is a research degree, with requirements similar to the Ph.D. in other fields: extensive preparation in a narrow field and a dissertation. In 1986 there were 38 doctoral programs in nursing in the United States (NLN, p. 67), having grown from 5 programs in 1967. In 1986, 1,949 students were enrolled in these programs, and 249 graduated (p. 71), an increase in graduates of 322% over 10 years. In 1987 there were approximately 2,000 nurses with doctoral degrees in nursing, and in 1984 there were approximately 4,100 nurses with doctoral degrees in other fields, such as education, public health, law, and the social and biological sciences.

The NLN (1988) estimates that about 20,361 nurses work full-time in nursing education (p. 88). Ninety-eight percent of full-time faculty have graduate degrees, and 24% of those in baccalaureate and higher-degree programs have doctorates. Men continue to be underrepresented: only 3.3% of the full-time faculty are male (p. 89). Only 9% of full-time faculty were members of ethnic minority groups (p. 131).

Nurse Practitioners

Nurse practitioners are registered nurses with training beyond their basic education, usually prepared to provide primary care; they were first educated at the University of Colorado in 1965. They are prepared in areas such as care of children or the elderly, women's health, and the like. In 1980 there were 16,757 nurses who identified themselves as nurse practitioners (1.3% of R.N.s). Most (85%) had certificates; the remainder had master's degrees. As of 1984 there were about 208 nurse practitioner programs: approximately 60% master's programs and 40% certificate programs. In 1980 roughly 10% worked in rural areas and 47% in urban areas. Many practitioners are certified by professional organizations such as the National Board of Pediatric Nurse Practitioners, the ANA, and the American College of Nurse Midwives. Nurse practitioners are often viewed as a less costly alternative to medical care, although they practice nursing under the nurse practice act of their respective states (U.S. Department of Health and Human Services, 1984). As of 1983 Medicaid provided reimbursement for midwifery care in 32 states (Weston).

Government Aid for Nurse Education

During World War II, money was provided for nurse education. The Nurse Training Act of 1964 (P.L. 88-581) provided money for direct support of students to increase the supply of nurses. The Health Manpower Act of 1968, Title II, provided additional aid. The Nurse Training Act of 1971 provided money for categories of advanced practice. Federal aid for basic nursing education was at its peak of $102.5 million in 1976, declining to $60.3 million in 1979; it ended in 1983 (New York State Health Department, 1988). In 1988 Congress reauthorized the Nurse Education Act and included support for undergraduate education. Congress approved funding for fiscal year 1990 for undergraduate scholarships. As this book went to press, The President vetoed the funding measure. States provide substantial amounts of money for support of nursing programs, primarily in operational support of state colleges and universities (Institute of Medicine, 1983).

Careers in Nursing

There are approximately 2 million licensed registered nurses in the United States. About 1.6 million are employed, with an estimated 78.7% work-participation rate in 1984. These nurses work in settings that vary from hospital bedsides to occupational and industrial settings to elementary schools. About 68% of nurses work in hospitals, 8% in nursing homes, 7% in community health, 7% in ambulatory care, and 10% in other settings (ANA, 1987 p. 101). Unemployment is approximately 0.9% (Secretary's Commission).

About 34% of nurses actually employed in nursing work part-time, usually half-time. Of those licensed nurses not actively nursing, approximately 23% work in non-nursing jobs, and 69% are not looking for work. Many of those who were not working were over age 50 or had children living at home (Secretary's Commission).

Of the working nurses, about 67% work as staff nurses, 12% as supervisors or head nurses, 5% as administrators, and 0.2% as researchers. The remainder work as consultants, instructors, nurse specialists or clinicians, anesthetists, in private duty, or in other areas. Of the approximately 550,000 practical nurses (ANA, 1987, p. 104), 59% work in hospitals, 23% in nursing homes, 3% in community health, 9% in ambulatory care, and 7% in other settings.

Collective Bargaining

Nurses are organized in the work setting by professional organizations, under the auspices of state nurses associations, and by traditional trade unions. The ANA argues that it is appropriate for nurses to organize to improve both working conditions and the quality of care, although others argue that union membership is unprofessional. The issue of striking to improve conditions has long divided the nursing community: Some say that a strike is legitimate to attain improved conditions, and others argue that in a life-and-death profession such as nursing patient care should not be jeopardized under any circumstances. In 1974 the Taft-Hartley Act (P.L. 93-360) was amended to make nonprofit health facilities subject to National Labor Relations Board rulings. This means that nurses can join unions without fear of retribution. A continuing issue is whether the head nurse or supervisor is considered management and therefore not eligible to join the bargaining unit.

Registered nurses are organized into collective bargaining units in approximately 25% of private hospitals and 62% of government hospitals (ANA, 1987, p. 135). About 67% of the nurses were represented by state nurses' associations and the remainder by a variety of trade unions (p. 111).

Nursing Roles

Staff nurses typically work in direct patient care, where they provide nursing care to individuals who may be acutely ill, as in a hospital; chronically ill or recovering from illness, as in a home setting; or well but requiring preventive care, as in a health department or health maintenance organization (HMO). Supervisors or head nurses direct the care given by other nurses and nursing aides or other health workers. They may also provide direct care. Administrators manage a group of nurses. Nurse specialists or clinicians are generally experts in a narrow area of nursing, such as ostomy care or patients with pain. They provide care to patients, act as role models for nursing staff, and often serve as resource people for staff nurses. Consultants are often self-employed and provide a variety of services both to individual nurses and organizations. Instructors teach nursing in either health care settings or educational settings. They may teach in schools of nursing, provide orientation to new nurses, teach specialized classes, or conduct programs for nurse's aides. Researchers investigate nursing problems, such as how to decrease pain in patients following surgery. Private-duty nurses generally care for one patient for a large block of time (e.g., 8–12 hours a day) over several days to months. Nurses who work in public health plan and provide care for groups of patients, usually prevention and education.

Career Options

Historically, the major focus of nurses has been the care of the sick in institutions, particularly hospitals. Although most nurses still work in hospitals, the focus of nursing is moving away from that of dependent worker with a focus on illness to independent practitioner with a focus on health. Porter-O'Grady (1986) proposes that the role of the nurse will shift from one in which responsibility for the care and safety of the patient is defined by the institution to one that focuses on health, with responsibility determined by the client. She suggests that functions will move from direct care dominated by the physician to team interaction focused on prevention. For many nurses this transition has already occurred.

Nurses have flexible options for the nature of their work, the hours they work, and the settings in which they work. Most people think of the nurse as the person in white caring for a patient in the hospital; and although the majority of nurses have such jobs, many nurses work in other settings. Nurses work on a fee-for-service basis with clients who have mood disturbances, they deliver babies, and they work for government agencies developing policies for health care in certain geographic or political areas. Nurses teach schoolchildren about health, provide family planning services, administer intravenous nutritional therapy to people at home, and serve as patient advocates.

The typical staff nurse in a hospital spends her day caring for 6 to 10 patients. Nurses act as care integrators as well as caregivers (1982 McClure & Nelson). As care integrators, nurses manage communication and coordination of activities of other care providers. Nurses are the one type of health care provider who is with the patient 24 hours a day. Nurses provide direct care, which may include personal care such as bathing and help with toileting. Nurses administer medications and treatments, from intravenous fluids to dressing changes. Nurses teach the patient about his or her illness and about treatments that may be needed, and nurses assist patients to assume life-style changes that will improve their health. Nurses organize patient care across hospital departments, including radiology and laboratory. Nurses are usually the first persons to recognize an emergency and mobilize others to respond.

Another type of nurse manages a home care agency that provides nursing care to patients in their homes. She or he hires staff, assumes the financial responsibility for the agency, and serves as its manager. The nursing care must be coordinated so that the patient is getting the right care at the right time. In addition, nurses supervise the care provided by home health aides. They are responsible for the quality of care provided and for assuring that all government and accreditation regulations are met.

The nurse providing direct patient care in such an agency performs many of the same functions as those of the hospital nurse. There is, however, a greater focus on the patient (and/or family) assuming responsibility for the care. The nurse teaches the family along with providing the care. Nurses at home provide intravenous therapy, change dressings, administer medications, supervise respirators, and help families cope with the death of a loved one.

Another type of nurse is an attorney. She may work in the field of malpractice, either suing a hospital, doctor, and nurse or defending health providers against suits. She may work for a health agency in "risk management," advising on how to avoid lawsuits, or she may handle legal issues for a government agency. She understands the law and nursing. She is a lobbyist trying to get legislation passed. She is an advisor to government leaders at the city, state, and federal level. She may be a legislator or work for the executive branch of government to implement the law.

A nurse researcher spends her day reviewing journals, collecting and analyzing data, and writing reports on the research. She usually has a doctorate. Areas of research of interest to nurses include nursing practice, such as decision making and validating the efficacy of nursing practice; nursing education, such as learning strategies and methods to assess competence; and the administration, organization, and delivery of nursing services, such as the cost-effectiveness of nursing services and delivery models (Welch).

Public health nurses usually work for a government agency and typically see clients in a clinic setting, trace contacts of communicable disease patients, and provide community education. They may work in a school or an immunization clinic. They may design community education programs to prevent adolescent pregnancies or to decrease the spread of AIDS. Their focus is truly prevention and education to promote the health of a community.

Organized Nursing

The ANA is the national professional organization for nurses. Founded in 1897, its members are not nurses but state or territorial nurses associations. The so-called tri-level system is composed of individual nurses who may join local and/or district nurses associations. These in turn are usually organized by city or county into state associations. Delegates from the state associations meet annually at a national convention to set policy for the ANA. Approximately 20% of working nurses belong to the ANA (Kelly, p. 468).

The ANA also offers voluntary certification exams in a variety of nursing specialty areas, such as community health nursing, mental health nursing, and nursing administration. The ANA accredits programs for continuing education in nursing. It serves as a lobbying association for nursing and has a governmental affairs offices in Washington for this purpose.

The NLN, founded in 1893 and unrelated to the ANA, serves as the accreditation body for schools of nursing. Its subsidiary Community Health Accreditation Program (CHAP) accredits home health agencies. Membership is open to agencies, nurses, and non-nurses, although most members are in the nursing profession.

Sigma Theta Tau International is the honor society for nursing. An international organization located in St. Louis, its primary purpose is to foster scholarship in nursing. Membership is by election and restricted to those nurses who meet its academic and community service criteria.

Mason and Talbott (1985, p. 597) list 55 national nursing organizations. In addition to the general organizations described above, nurses belong to numerous specialty groups. The groups tend to have as a focus the specialty area or site of practice for nurses. The first such organization was the American Association of Nurse Anesthetists (Kelly, p. 462). Examples of other organizations include the American College of Nurse Midwives, the National Nurses Society of Addictions, the National Black Nurses Association, and the Society for Nursing History.

The National Center for Nursing Research is part of the National Institutes of Health (NIH) and was authorized under the Health Research Extension Act of 1985 (P.L. 99-158). Prior to its establishment, funding for nursing research was under the auspices of the Division of Nursing in the Health Resources and Services Administration. The purpose of the center is to conduct "a program of grants and awards supporting nursing research and research training related to patient care, the promotion of health, the prevention of disease and the mitigation of the effects of acute and chronic illnesses and disabilities" (Merritt). The initial budget for the center was approximately $16,200,000. The primary focus is support of extramural research. Organized nursing viewed authorization of the center as a milestone in the acceptance of nursing as a research-based profession.

Issues for the 1990s

The major issues for the 1990s are those of the health care industry in general: the cost and quality of health care. Nurses are being asked to provide high-quality care at a cost that society is willing to pay.

Diagnostic Related Groups (DRGs)

The federal government's attempt to control health care costs through a prospective payment system based on diagnostic related groups (DRGs) has had an impact on nurses. (See Chapter 12 for a detailed discussion of DRGs). Over time DRGs have decreased lengths of hospital stays and increased intensity of care required by patients, early patient discharge, and cost-consciousness (Mitchell & Dibbles). The introduction of DRGs forced nurses to analyze the cost of nursing care. Initially, there were fears that nurses would be fired as length of stay decreased along with patient census. Although there was some early evidence of a decreasing need for nurses, this situation quickly changed because the patients who remained in the hospital were sicker. In addition, the AIDS epidemic has countered some of the expected decrease in the need for nurses. Since hospitals are no longer reimbursed by Medicare on a cost basis, there is an increased push to isolate nursing costs so that attempts can be made to decrease them. Hospital nurses are the managers of patient care and play a vital role in allocating the hospital's resources. The nurse knows how the patient is progressing, where the patient should be at what time, and where the patient is going next. Under expert nursing care length of stay can be decreased and the patient discharged to well-organized care at home.

Many hospitals are now using acuity systems to measure the need for nursing care. Nurses use checklists to identify patient care needs. Results of the scoring are then translated into nursing hours required, and appropriate staffing is determined. Proprietary systems have been developed and sold, and many hospitals use systems developed for their special needs. Some have criticized the systems for their lack of validity, arguing that much of what nurses do cannot easily be quantified into mechanical tasks. These and other efforts are probably a result of the increased pressure on hospitals to use nursing resources efficiently.

Entry into Practice

In 1965 the ANA voted to (1) move toward the baccalaureate degree as the minimum educational requirement for licensure as a registered nurse and (2) require technical nurses to be prepared in 2-year college programs. In 1976 the New York State Nurses Association recommended that the state pass legislation to establish these two levels of nursing. This legislation has never been passed. In 1983, after years of debate, the NLN issued a statement of support for this proposal. As of 1988 only one state, North Dakota, requires the baccalaureate degree for professional nurses' licensure. This requirement was achieved by regulation of the North Dakota Board of Nursing rather than by legislation, as proposed in New York. This issue has divided the nursing community and pitted nursing against organized medicine and hospitals.

The argument for the proposal suggests that in the complex health care system 4 years of college is the minimal amount of education necessary to prepare nurses for practice. In addition, nursing is the only one of the major health professions (M.D., D.D.S., O.T., P.T.) that does not require at least a bachelor's degree. Proponents argue that nurses educated at the baccalaureate level provide better care. A recent study by Johnson (1988) that synthesized results of 139 studies found significant differences in communication skills, knowledge, problem-solving ability, teaching, and professional role between the baccalaureate-educated nurses and those educated in either a diploma or an associate degree program: baccalaureate nurses perform these functions at a higher level than graduates of either diploma or associate degree programs. The groups did not differ on autonomy and leadership behaviors.

Those who argue against the proposal suggest that graduates from both diploma and 2-year programs provide a fine level of care and may be even better at skills such as giving injections than those with baccalaureate education. They also argue that a 4-year education is more costly to society than a 2- or 3-year education and that requiring a baccalaureate degree further restricts entry into the nursing field. Intuitively, it seems to make sense that nurses who have a thorough grounding in the basic sciences, the social sciences, and the humanities will be better able to adapt to a changing health care environment and provide better care to patients than nurses with less education. But in view of the current nursing shortage it is unlikely that many states will require the baccalaureate as the minimum degree for licensure.

Independent Practice

Most working nurses are employees rather than independent practitioners. A phenomenon of the 1980s was a movement toward independent practice, defined as self-employment. Independent practice falls into three areas: private duty, individual fee-for-service practice, and group practice. It is interesting to note that in the late 19th century most nurses were independent practitioners employed by people to care for family members at home. The popularity of that type of practice waned, although there have always been nurses employed by families to care for sick members either at home or in the hospital. Such nurses contract with the patient to provide a set amount of care for a set fee.

Nurses in the mental health area are in the forefront of independent fee-for-service practice and, increasingly, nurses in other areas, such as geriatric care and cardiac patient care are providing nursing on a fee-for-service basis. For example, nurses provide care to patients who have cardiac problems, assisting the client to change life-style patterns and providing education and comfort. In this broad category are nurses who act as consultants to other nurses in areas such as setting up educational programs, organizing nursing services, or carrying out evaluation projects.

A major obstacle to independent practice is lack of benefit coverage or third-party reimbursement for nursing services. Since so much of health care is now reimbursed by third-party payers, consumers may be reluctant to purchase nursing services on a fee-for-service basis and not be reimbursed when they can receive a similar service from a physician and obtain reimbursement. For example, if a patient is recovering from surgery and has a wound that must be observed for signs of infection and healing, this can be done by either a nurse or a physician. If the patient sees the physician, the service is usually reimbursed by the third-party payer; if the patient sees a nurse for the service, it is not reimbursed.

If this same patient is homebound and has Medicare coverage, a visit by the nurse from a home health agency is reimbursed (as long as a physician orders the care), whereas the patient who is not homebound and visits the nurse in her office will not receive reimbursement. It is understandable that insurers do not want to increase the number of providers who are able to authorize service. There is also some sense to not encouraging another group of fee-for-service practitioners besides physicians. Nevertheless, the cost-benefit of reimbursement for more expensive medical care and not for nursing is difficult to appreciate.

In response to what some would argue is an irrational reimbursement system, community nursing centers have been proposed. Based on the HMO concept, a group of nurses would agree to provide nursing care for a defined population for a set reimbursable fee. Federal legislation has authorized the study of several such centers.

Many home care nurses work in a form of independent practice. They contract with an agency to provide patient care at a specific price per visit. Although these nurses are not directly paid by the patient or the insurer, they have many of the advantages of a fee-for-service practitioner. They are able to work as much as they like and earn more money by seeing more patients. If they are efficient and can complete their work quickly, they earn more money for fewer hours of work.

They generally do not have the advantages of institutional employment, such as health benefits, vacation days, and guaranteed work even when demand is slow.

Organized nursing and individual nurses are working to change the regulations for reimbursement. This is a slow and tedious process done on a state-by-state basis. For example, New York State now has "Third Party Reimbursement" requiring insurance companies to provide reimbursement for nursing care if requested by the insured group. This has had a nominal effect on reimbursement because most purchasers see payment to nurses as additive, not substitutive, so paying nurses as independent health practitioners would add to health costs and premiums. The ideal law, according to nurses, would require insurance companies to reimburse for any health care services currently covered that can be provided by a nurse.

Nursing Shortage

The most pressing issue as we enter the 1990s is the shortage of registered nurses, particularly in acute-care hospitals ("Federal Commission Finds Widespread Nursing Shortage,"; New York State Department of Health; Secretary's Commission on Nursing). The Secretary's Commission on Nursing (1988) concluded that "the reported shortage of RNs is real, widespread, and of significant magnitude" (p. iii). Examples cited include (1) the doubling of the hospital registered-nurse vacancy rate from 4.4% in 1983 to 11.3% in 1987, (2) 47% of community hospitals reporting use of agency nurses in 1987, and (3) the reported closing of hospital beds because vacant positions could not be filled. Available data suggest an increase in demand as the primary cause of the imbalance between supply and demand. Although the number of new graduates has declined, the supply of registered nurses has continued to grow. The Secretary's Commission reports an increase in the ratio between registered nurses and patients from 86:100 in 1984 to 96:100 in 1986. Nursing homes are employing more registered nurses possibly because of increased severity of illness related to earlier discharge from hospitals to nursing homes. It is likely that hospitals are using registered nurses where they previously used LPNs and nursing assistants. There has been a decrease in the use of both LPNs and nursing assistants in hospitals.

In addition, the Secretary's Commission (1988) Interim Report reports chronic problems of "low average salaries and compressed salary ranges, working conditions, problems with retention, and poor professional image" (p. vii). The most frequently cited factors influencing demand are, in order, patient acuity, number of patients, increased number of settings/services, and need for specialists and quality registered nurses. The most frequently cited factors affecting supply are decline in nursing students, increased options for women, poor working conditions, inadequate pay, out-of state migration, and poor image of nursing (ANA, April 1988; cited in New York State Department of Health).

Proposed solutions to the shortage include increasing the supply by recruiting more people into nursing and improving retention, thereby increasing supply; and decreasing the demand by having non-nurses perform activities currently performed by nurses and/or using technology to perform those activities. Specific solutions to increasing the supply have included raising starting salaries and increasing salary progression. As of 1986 the average maximum salary for a staff nurse was 136.4% of the average starting salary, whereas for an accountant that difference was 192.7% (ANA Fact Sheet). There is some evidence that hospitals are increasing the nursing salary progression.

Increasing the number of people entering the nursing field is a more elusive goal. Suggestions include improving the image and working conditions and increasing the amount of scholarship aid available. As the potential student pool decreases and women have more career choices, coupled with the reluctance of government to increase spending in health care, the likelihood that these proposals will provide long-term increases in entry into the field is not likely. As this chapter is being written, there is a major effort targeted at redefining the work of nurses. This includes efforts to have non-nurses do non-nursing tasks that nurses often do, such as transporting patients; redesigning the work setting, as in New England Medical Center's physician-nurse team approach, and using computers for communication. The shortage may be the major crisis of the 1990s and will require adjustment from everyone in the health care industry, not just nurses.

In many ways nursing exemplifies the cyclical or spiral nature of the world, with repeating patterns. In nursing's earliest days nurses were self-employed and responsible to the patients; today's nurses again want to be self-employed and responsible to their clients. In earlier times nursing care was primarily provided at home. Today there are many in nursing who think this is where nursing should take place. At times the nurse has been a team leader, coordinating and providing patient care and supervising LPNs and aides. Then, in the 1970s primary care—the nurse providing all of the care for a group of patients—was the vogue; and now there seems to be some movement toward hiring aides and assistants for the nurse. The nurse began as handmaiden to the physician; one circle that will surely not be redrawn is a return to that condition. Nurses will continue to work in an interdependent relationship with physicians in a variety of settings such as the acute-care hospital. Some nurses will also continue the dependent relationship when they work in a physician's office or in the operating room. But many nurses will move into areas of prevention and health promotion and work independently of physicians. Nursing has achieved independence; it remains to be seen how many nurses will choose this option.

References

Aiken, L. "Nurses." In D. Mechanic (Ed.), *Handbook of Health Professions* (pp. 407–431). New York: Free Press, 1983.

American Nurses Association. *Nursing Association Policy Statement.* Kansas City, MO: ANA, 1980.

American Nurses Association. *The Nursing Practice Act: Suggested State Legislation.* New York: ANA, 1981.

Anastas, L. *Your Career in Nursing.* New York: National League for Nursing, 1984.

Bullough, B. "Barriers to the Nurse Practitioner Movement: Problem of Women in a Women's Field." *International Journal of Health Services, 5,* 225, 1975.

Fawcett, J. *Analysis and evaluation of conceptual models of nursing.* Philadelphia: F. A. Davis, 1984.

"Federal Commission Finds Widespread Nursing Shortage." *The American Nurse, 20*(7), 10, 1988.

Henderson, V. *The Nature of Nursing.* New York: Macmillan, 1966.

Johnson, J. "Differences in the Performance of Baccalaureate, Associate Degree, and Diploma Nurses: A Meta-analysis. *Research in Nursing & Health, 11,* 183, 1988.

Kelly, L. Y. *The Nursing Experience.* New York: Macmillan, 1987.

Mason, D. J., & Talbott, S. W. *Political Action Handbook for Nurses.* Menlo Park, CA: Addison-Wesley, 1985.

McClure, M. L. and Nelson, M. J., Trends in Hospital Nursing in L. H. Aiken (ed.) *Nursing in the 1980's: Crisis, Opportunities, Challenges,* pp. 59–73, Philadelphia: Lippincott, 1982.

Merritt, D. "The National Center for Nursing Research." *Image, 18*(3), 84, 1986.

Mitchell, M., & Dibbles, S. "Acute Care Nursing: Impact of DRGs." In *Impact of DRGs on Nursing.* Washington, D.C.: Health Resources and Services Administration, 1988 pp. 5–31. (NTIS HRP-0907179).

National League for Nursing. *Nursing Data Review.* New York: NLN, 1988.

New York State Department of Health. *Final Report of the New York State Labor-Health Industry Task Force on Health Personnel.* Albany: Author.

Orem, D. E. *Nursing: Concepts of Practice.* New York: McGraw-Hill, 1980.

Porter-O'Grady, T. *Creative Nursing Administration: Participative Management into the 21st Century.* Rockville, MD: Aspen, 1986.

Secretary's Commission on Nursing. *Final Report. Secretary's Commission on Nursing Final Report.* Washington, D.C.: Department of Health and Human Services. December 1988.

U.S. Department of Health and Human Services. *Report to the President and Congress on the Status of Health Personnel in the United States* (Vol. 1). (DHHS Pub. No. HRS P-OD-84-4). Washington, D.C.: DHHS, 1984.

Welch, C. "Conference Report: Directions for Nursing Research in New York State." *The Journal of the New York State Nurses Association., 19*(3), 16, 1988.

Weston, G. *NPs and PAs: Changes—Where, Whether and Why.* Washington, D.C.: U.S. Department of Health and Human Services, National Center for Health Services Research, 1984.

Wilkerson, K. B. "Public Health Nursing: In Sickness or in Health." *American Journal of Public Health, 75,* 1155, 1985.

6

Ambulatory Care

Robert S. Lawrence and Steven Jonas

Ambulatory care is personal health care provided to an individual who is not a bed patient in a health care institution. It includes all health services, other than community or public health services, provided to noninstitutionalized patients. Once the almost exclusive domain of physicians and dentists, ambulatory care now includes the services of public health nurses, nurse-clinicians, physician assistants, social workers, optometrists, podiatrists, health assistants, and many others. Roemer (1981) provided the most comprehensive review of all features of this topic in *Ambulatory Health Services in America*. This chapter reviews the current organization of personal medical services provided in ambulatory settings but does not discuss mental health or rehabilitative services.

In 1986 the average person made 5.3 visits to a physician and spent 0.83 days in an acute-care hospital (833.1 short-stay hospital days per 1,000 population). Thus, 6.36 times more ambulatory care episodes than hospital days of care occurred (USDHHS, 1988, Tables 57, 64). This ratio is up from 4.3 in 1981 as the number of ambulatory visits increased from just under 5 per person and the number of hospital days declined sharply from 1,136.5 per 1,000 population in 1980. The unprecedented shifts away from inpatient care of the last decade have had enormous impact on the organization, staffing and financing of ambulatory services in the United States. The number of Americans who reported a visit to a physician increased from 66% in 1964 to 75.5% in 1986. A full 85.5% of the population had seen a physician in the past 2 years (USDHHS, 1988, Table 58). Meanwhile, the average length of stay in acute-care hospitals decreased from 8.1 in 1964 to 6.3 in 1986. Most patient-physician contacts now take place on an ambulatory basis.

Dr. Lawrence completed this chapter while a Fellow at the Center for Advanced Study in the Behavioral Sciences, where he was supported by a grant from the Henry J. Kaiser Family Foundation.

The rates of visits to physicians vary by age, gender, race, and socioeconomic status. About 91% of the very young (under 5 years) and 86.1% of the very old (75 years and over) have an annual visit with a physician; 70.3% of males and 80.3% of females report an annual physician visit; and 74.6% of whites and 73.0% of blacks saw a physician in 1986, compared with 67.3% and 57.0%, respectively, in 1964 (USDHHS, 1988, Table 58). The narrowing of the gap observed between the races also occurred for differences of physician use by the rich and the poor. In 1964, 57.5% of those with a family income less than $10,000 reported seeing a physician; 73.0% of persons living in families earning more than $35,000 did so. By 1986 these rates had increased to 75.0% and 79.3%, respectively. The enactment of Medicaid and Medicare accounts for much of the increased use of physicians by lower-income groups.

Somewhat paradoxically, the number of physician visits per person is actually higher among lower-income groups—those with less than $10,000 annual family income—than among those with annual family incomes above $35,000; the reported rates are 6.6 and 5.4, respectively. In part this reflects the marked differences in health status by income groups, with higher morbidity among those with low income (USDHHS, 1986, p. 84; Davis). Thus, access—as measured by the percentage seeing a physician yearly—has improved for the poor but still lags; whereas utilization—as measured by the number of physician visits per person per year—is higher because there is more sickness among the poor (Wilensky & Berk). For the elderly poor, ambulatory visits actually decreased by 20% between 1982 and 1986, when the federal government reduced support for health services (R. W. Johnson Foundation, 1987).

Whites report 5.4 visits per year and blacks, 4.8. Although a larger proportion of blacks live in poverty (a condition associated with higher utilization rates), they experience more problems with access to physician services than do whites, who constitute the majority of poor people. The percentage of visits occurring in hospital outpatient departments is almost double for blacks (24.2%) compared with those of whites (13.7%). Similar differences in hospital outpatient use exist by socioeconomic class. The inverse holds true for visits to doctors' offices and use of telephone contact with physicians when analyzed by race or socioeconomic status.

There are two major categories of ambulatory care. The dominant form is care provided by private physicians in solo, partnership, or private group practice on a fee-for-service basis. The other, growing dramatically in the last decade but still a distinct minority, is ambulatory care in organized settings that have an identity independent from that of the particular individual physicians practicing in it. This category contains hospital-based ambulatory services, including clinics, walk-in and emergency services, and the newer group practice and health promotion centers; freestanding "surgi-centers" and "emergi-centers"; health department clinics; neighborhood and community health centers (NHCs and CHCs); health maintenance organizations (HMOs); organized home care; community mental health centers; school and workplace health services; and prison health services.

Different ambulatory care settings provide service for diverse groups in the population. Results in utilization and quality of services provided also differ by demographic group. A decade ago Dutton analyzed the impact of the major forms of ambulatory care on patients in Washington, D.C., in terms that apply today:

> Sources used primarily by the poor—hospital outpatient departments, emergency rooms, and public clinics—contained important structural and financial barriers, and had the lowest rates of patient-initiated use. The prepaid system, in contrast, maximized patient's access to both preventive care and symptomatic care, and did not seem to inhibit physician-controlled follow-up care. The results suggest some perverse effects of fee-for-service payment: patients, especially poor patients, appeared to be deterred from seeking preventive and symptomatic care, while physicians were encouraged to expand follow-up services. Moreover, services in fee-for-service systems were distributed less equitably relative to both income and medical need than in the prepaid system. [p. 221]

Private Practice

Private practice remains the principal mode by which physicians provide services to patients in the United States. Only the licensure laws of the state limit the range of health care services that the physician can provide as an independent entrepreneur. The physician implicitly—and rarely in writing—contracts to provide these services to the patient in return for the payment of a fee, hence, the *fee-for-service* system.

Private practitioners care for patients on a fee-for-service basis in such settings as office space owned or leased by the physician, the patient's home (rare a few years ago but now increasing in frequency), or a bedded institution. When hospitalized under the care of his or her physician, the patient—or the patient's insurer—pays the hospital for all services other than physician care and pays the physician's fee directly. The physician remains a private contractor to the patient even in the hospital setting. Increasingly, physicians arrange for cross-coverage of ambulatory or hospitalized patients for nights, weekends, or holidays with other solo practitioners, or they form partnerships or group practices. Under these latter arrangements Medicare requires the covering physician to bill for services provided. Office billing arrangements follow the same pattern, although the distribution of practice income to the members of the group may use other systems to provide productivity incentives, reward longevity or partnership status, maintain the necessary specialty mix in the practice, or meet other goals set by the group.

As of 1985, 76% of the 426,000 nonfederal physicians in clinical practice were in office-based practice. Of these, just over 90% were in the fee-for-service system, compared with 95% a decade earlier (USDHHS, 1986, Table

73). Interns and residents in training comprised 16.7% of nonfederal practitioners. Full-time members of a hospital staff accounted for another 6.9%. Contrasting figures for the 19,976 federal physicians in 1985 are as follows: 6% office-based practitioners among the 15,877 physicians engaged in patient care, 19.8% interns and residents, and 74% full-time members of a hospital staff.

Data from the 1986 National Health Interview Survey show a continuing slow decline in the proportion of physician visits made to a doctor's office, from 55.9% of all contacts in 1983 to 55.5% in 1986 (USDHHS, 1988, Table 57). Visits to hospital outpatient departments increased slightly, from 14.9% to 15.0%, during the same period. The remaining 29.9% of physician contacts in 1986 were by telephone (13.2%), patient's home (about 1%), and laboratory or clinic facilities located outside the hospital. According to these patient interview data, just under 700 million visits to physicians in private offices or HMO practice occurred in 1986. The 25.7 million members of HMOs made about 115 million of these visits (Gruber). The growth of HMO membership from just under 7 million in 1976 to 29.3 million in 1987 accounted for the largest portion of the decrease in traditional private-practice office visits.

Other statistics capture some of the interesting dynamics of private practice during the past decade. The number of office visits lasting 10 minutes or less decreased from 47.3% in 1980 to 42.6% in 1985. Meanwhile, the proportion of visits generating a scheduled return visit increased modestly from 58.0% to 58.8% (USDHHS, 1988, Table 60). These changes held for both sexes and for all racial and age groups except those 75 years and over. The latter group had a slight increase in proportion of visits lasting 10 minutes or less from 35.1% to 36.9%. A corresponding increase in the proportion of visits identified as the patient's first visit occurred (from 15.3% to 17.7%) during the same period. Since first visits require more of the physician's time, it is possible that most or all of the decline in the number of short visits was the result of the concomitant rise in proportion of first visits. The data are not definitive on this matter. Alternative explanations include an ever more competitive health care market that encourages physicians to spend more time with their patients to increase patient satisfaction; the increase in the number of physicians relative to the patient population, which allows more time per visit with fewer visits per physician; and the proliferation of employee benefit options with annual enrollment periods, which raises the chance of the patient changing his or her physician because of changes in health insurance that increasingly emphasize managed care with closed panels of physicians.

Private practice is changing to compete with the HMOs and other forms of organized ambulatory care. One strategy is the development of women's health centers, special services marketed to women (Harrell; Wolinsky), or primary care centers staffed and run by women for women (Daily). Proponents of this strategy argue that women differ from men in the selection of health care services. Offering services designed to appeal to these differences will provide a competitive advantage.

Practitioners have become more aware of the role of practice organization in growth or maintenance of practice size. Attention to all of the types of encounters that patients have with the practice improves the patient's experience with office staff, the billing procedure, and the medical office environment. One practice found high patient satisfaction with all major elements of the practice after paying special attention to these various encounter points (Tulli).

Some practitioners have adapted to competitive pressures by contracting for part or all of their practice with an HMO, a preferred provider organization (PPO), or an independent practice association (IPA). These physicians must cope with a bewildering array of new organizational issues, including termination agreements, submission of data requirements, discipline procedures, no-solicitation covenants, arbitration clauses, rights to end treatment, use of consultants, compliance with state and federal laws, and exclusivity (Kucera & Warren).

With the arrival of freestanding emergency centers and surgi-centers some practices have responded with extended hours or increased walk-in services. One study compared two family practice groups using these adaptations with four freestanding emergency care centers (Chesteen, Warren, & Woolley). A total of 2,339 patient visits were examined, using data from both physicians and patients. Patient satisfaction with convenience and personal attention from the physicians and the cost of care were important in distinguishing the two forms of practice. The freestanding centers charged significantly more for their services ($45 vs. $27) but outperformed the family practices in convenience, time factors (waiting time, time spent with the physician, time to get an appointment, clinic location), and out-of-pocket costs. Patients judged the personal concern of the physician and the ability to see the same physician desirable attributes of the family practices.

Hospital-based Ambulatory Services

The hospital remains the institutional center of the U.S. health care system despite the enormous pressures in recent years to move the focus of care to the ambulatory setting. Inpatient services and revenues still drive the system. To a large extent the interest of hospital administrators in improving ambulatory services reflects a desire to expand the patient base on which the inpatient services draw. Thus, *outpatients* are treated in anticipation of their eventually attaining *inpatient* status.

Outpatients present with problems ranging from life-threatening, acute illnesses requiring emergency services to chronic conditions calling on rehabilitative and social services. Patients with routine medical problems closely resemble patients seeking care in private practitioners' offices. Most hospitals provide two levels of ambulatory care: emergency services and outpatient clinic care. In many inner-city areas the hospital ambulatory services may be the only source of health care, and patients frequently present to emergency departments with routine medical problems. In recent years hospitals have organized "walk-in" clinics to provide a middle ground between true emergency visits and scheduled outpatient clinic visits.

Insurers have traditionally paid hospitals more reliably for emergency services than for clinic services. As a result, hospitals have been more effective in organizing emergency services. In 1987, 95% of nonfederal, acute-care hospitals in the United States (5,273) had emergency units (AHA, 1988, Table 12A). Emergency services are intended to care for acutely ill or injured patients— particularly those with life-threatening or potentially life-threatening problems requiring immediate attention, or personnel and equipment not found in private practitioners' offices—and to offer prompt hospitalization if needed.

In contrast, clinic services are provided by only two kinds of hospitals: (1) those located in areas where patients cannot or will not attend private practitioner's offices for more routine care, usually for economic reasons (Roemer, 1981); and (2) those that have teaching programs. About 70% of community hospitals (3,671 in 1987) have organized outpatient departments (AHA, 1988, Table 12A), up sharply from 46% (2,451) in 1983 (AHA, 1984, Table 12A). These services for nonemergency problems compete with those offered by the private practitioner (economic considerations aside) whereas the emergency services that the office-based practitioner cannot provide do not. As hospitals expand their outpatient departments to increase their patient base, direct competition with private practitioners will continue to grow.

Hospital Clinics

Clinic services began growing in the voluntary hospitals in the latter part of the 19th century. By 1916, 495 hospitals had clinics, often serving both an educational and a charitable function (Roemer, 1975, 1981). Most were treated as the stepchild of the inpatient service, and physicians were often assigned to staff them as a duty in return for the privilege of hospitalizing their patients. From the beginning the clinics varied with the type of hospital (teaching vs. nonteaching, private voluntary vs. public). In community hospitals about 72% of emergency visits and 62% of clinic visits occur in hospitals not affiliated with medical schools (AHA, 1988, Tables 3, 8). Most of the literature on hospital ambulatory care in the United States describes teaching hospitals, so a true picture of the typical unaffiliated hospital is not available.

Most hospital clinics continue to fulfill their role of providing care for the poor, although little free care remains. Those patients not covered by Medicare, Medicaid, or commercial insurance must usually pay according to a means-tested, sliding fee scale. Municipal hospitals serve the uninsured living within their jurisdiction. In some states a "free care pool" exists to help offset the costs of providing unreimbursed care. As the pressure on hospitals from HMOs and PPOs increases, more teaching hospitals have reorganized their clinics to function as group practices (Block). Goldberg et al. (1987) conducted a controlled trial of the adoption of a group practice model within the medical clinic of a teaching hospital. Randomization produced similar groups of patients and residents, and the clinic activity of 2,299 patients and 28 residents was monitored for 11 months. The group-practice clinics had 20% more visits per month than the control clinics, primarily because there were twice as many overflow sessions (20.2 vs. 9.7 sessions per month). Patients spent 15% less time in completing scheduled visits in the group practice clinics. Regular users of the group-practice clinics had 7% more scheduled visits but 39% fewer walk-in visits. Continuity of care was not affected. The investigators concluded that the adoption of the group practice model for the medical clinic improved productivity, speeded up patient flow, and reduced unscheduled clinic visits.

The experiment also had important economic results. The hospital charges per patient were 26% lower in the group-practice clinics ($p = 0.003$). This difference was primarily the result of reduced inpatient charges that were 27% lower per hospitalized patient (Cohen et al.). The mean length of stay among group practice patients was 8.3, compared to 10.5 for the control group ($p = 0.011$).

Other hospitals have reorganized their clinics as components of an institution-wide HMO, some with satellite clinics set up to broaden the patient base (Nelson). The teaching hospital of the University of California at San Diego established an ambulatory clinic on the campus of its parent university several miles away to encourage faculty and students to seek care from medical school physicians and to use the teaching hospital for specialty and inpatient care (Selzer & Scholl). These and other strategies are becoming more widespread as teaching hospitals try to maintain, increase, and broaden the patient population necessary for medical education, clinical research, and fiscal viability. Insurers and payers are more dominant in the health care field (Goulet). Some health economists predict that 70% of the U.S. population will belong to HMOs and PPOs by the early 1990s and that at least 10% of the acute-care hospitals will have disappeared (Abramowitz; McManis & Hopkins; Sadowy & Wood).

Most hospital organizations now include participation in a PPO, HMO, or alternative delivery system to take advantage of these organizations' ability to direct groups of patients to the hospital (Merz). The PPOs appeared to have all of the necessary elements to guarantee success of new financing and service arrangements, but many did not live up to expectations. Merz (1986) argues that the four major participants in a PPO (providers, employers, employees or patients, and insurance carriers/administrators) must have an equal stake in the benefits gained from the risks taken. Patients, physicians, and policymakers appear to have accepted the constraints on public payments for medical services.

For employees the risks of rationed services and facilities appear inevitable (Mechanic) in return for affordable insurance premiums.

Ambitious strategies for expanding ambulatory care appear necessary for hospitals serving the inner city to survive. One example is the Lutheran Medical Center, serving a depressed Brooklyn neighborhood (Adams). The hospital, serving a population of 350,000 and providing more than 50,000 ambulatory visits per year, launched an aggressive program of community development that included the following:

1. Providing staff members to serve as resources and support staff for community groups.
2. Creating educational programs for the undereducated and underemployed residents of its service area.
3. Establishing a school health program.
4. Founding the country's largest federally supported neighborhood health center.
5. Contracting with the state of New York to provide health care for 10% less than the average cost for Medicaid patients.

New York City hospitals, with more than 10 million visits to outpatient clinics and emergency rooms each year, are under pressure to reduce the number of acute-care beds. Simultaneously, reduced Medicare reimbursement for graduate medical education squeezes them financially (Rogers, 1985). Hospital ambulatory services must expand and become more efficient if these institutions are to survive.

Clinic Organization and Staffing. The optimal organization of outpatient clinics to provide opportunities for teaching and research—especially in view of the current structure of medical education—is to have many disease-, organ-, or organ-system-specific clinics (Freymann, p. 255). The typical contemporary teaching hospital has three groups of clinics: medical, surgical, and others. The medical clinic group, which more and more commonly has a "general medical clinic" approximating the function of the general internist or a family practice unit, includes cardiology, neurology, dermatology, allergy, gastroenterology, and so on. Patients may stay in one or more specialty clinics for long periods if the general medical or family practice clinic is small or nonexistent; and specialty clinics admit patients directly, as walk-ins or on referral from the emergency room or inpatient service, rather than on referral from a general clinic. The surgical clinic group includes general surgery, orthopedics, urology, plastic surgery, and the like. Because surgical care is usually more episodic than is general medical care, patients are not as likely to remain in these clinics for long periods. The third group includes pediatrics and the pediatric subspecialties, obstetrics/gynecology and its subspecialties, and other specialties such as rehabilitation medicine.

Four groups of physicians staff teaching hospital clinics. Voluntary attending staff may draw clinic duty as part of their obligation to the hospital in return for receiving admitting privileges. In the 1980s many medical schools have become increasingly dependent on physician practice income, both to provide part of the support for medical staff doing the work, and, through "clinical practice plans," to gain some of that patient income for general support purposes. Thus, depending upon the particular arrangements, for some physicians the medical school hospitals have become more rather than less attractive places in which to work.

Full-time inpatient physicians, usually junior staff, may be assigned to teaching hospital clinics to carry out teaching, supervisory, and research functions. House officers, usually residents but occasionally interns, staff clinics on a rotating basis. Most teaching hospital clinics stress teaching and research (especially at the subspecialty-fellow level) rather than patient care. Because house officers usually rotate frequently among various subspecialty clinics for teaching purposes, patients with stable conditions coming to a subspecialty clinic, say, once every 3 months, may see a different physician each time. Finally, for very busy clinics, hospitals may hire outside physicians on a sessional or salaried basis to work exclusively in the clinic. They are usually not part of the regular hospital staff and do not participate in the educational programs.

Most hospital outpatient departments are open all day on weekdays, but many individual clinics, particularly highly subspecialized ones, meet once or twice a week. Some teaching hospitals have more than 100 different specialty and subspecialty clinics. Thus, hospital-based physicians working in the usual hospital clinic can concentrate on diabetes, peripheral vascular disease, or stroke in their teaching and research. This can be an advantage for the physician who has a focus confined to a particular disease or condition. It also may be helpful to the patient who has a single disease problem of a rather complex or unusual nature.

Three kinds of patients face difficulties in using such clinics. First is the patient with an ordinary problem for which no specialty clinic exists. Second is the patient with a disease like uncomplicated diabetes. Attending the diabetes clinic, such a patient is likely to have to defer to a diabetic patient who has complications. Third is the patient with multiple problems. These patients, often elderly, may end up attending a different specialty clinic each day of the week, causing multiple trips to the hospital and preventing one physician from looking at the patient as a person rather than as a collection of diseased organs and organ systems.

Thus, the basic conflict in hospital ambulatory services is established. The needs of specialty-oriented providers conflict with those of the patients with either ordinary problems or with several different problems requiring the care of specialists. Attempts to resolve this conflict by providing group practice arrangements within the clinic have all the advantages described earlier. By their success, however, they threaten the very existence of the subspecialty teaching/ research clinic. As hospitals become more responsive to community needs, in order to survive fiscally, the ambulatory clinics must provide more comprehensive services for most patients with common problems. As discussed below, educational reforms to improve the balance between generalists and specialists will also change the orientation of the physicians staffing these clinics (Jonas, 1978, Chapter 12). If teaching and research were oriented more toward an emphasis on the common rather than the uncommon and if hospitals defined their roles and responsibilities by community needs, the contradiction would resolve straightaway, and hospital clinics would be on the road to first-class status (Freymann, Chapter 18; Jonas, 1973).

The goal of organizing medical care in response to community needs is called community-oriented primary care, or COPC (Madison; Mullan; Mullan & Connor; Nutting et al.; Rogers, 1982). The major elements of COPC are

1. The clinical practice of comprehensive primary medical care.
2. The use of applied epidemiology in practice planning.
3. Community involvement in program planning.
4. The use of data gathered in practice planning and organization.
5. A continuing surveillance of community health status and needs.

All of these elements operate in a feedback loop. Any medical practice—solo, group, or hospital-based—can use the model. The principal problems are not conceptual; the ideas have been with us for many years. The problem is implementation.

Quality assurance requirements also influence the organization of ambulatory services. The University of Chicago Hospitals developed a system of clinic-based activity for all 60 of its clinics (Oswald & Winer). The staff developed indicators of quality of care to address both the servicewide and clinic-specific concerns. A single data collection and reporting instrument made it easier for hospital personnel to review and act on reports. The system appears to have improved care and encouraged better interdisciplinary cooperation in quality assurance activities. Other efforts to improve the quality of ambulatory services emphasize the medical record system (Barnett; Koster, Waterstraat, & Sondak). These include the advocacy of a standard outpatient medical summary to improve coordination among specialty clinics (Mak).

Because medical records are intended to assure continuity of care, with attention to applicable prior illness episodes, treatments, or laboratory data, some advocate the use of patient-carried records. Giglio and Papazian (1987) tested four types of patient-carried health records in a hospital outpatient department to determine the acceptability and use of the records. They estimated the costs and observed patient and physician reactions. A small record that fit in the patient's wallet was most acceptable, and the primary determinant of success was the physician's support of the process.

Hospital Emergency Services

Most U.S. hospitals provide emergency services, and over 97% of community hospitals with more than 200 beds have emergency departments (AHA, 1984, Table 12A). These units serve several functions, from caring for the acutely ill or injured patient to providing walk-in services to less acutely ill patients. Many physicians on the hospital staff also use the emergency room as a setting to assess a patient with a problem that either may lead to inpatient admission or requires equipment or diagnostic imaging facilities not available in the physician's office. Increasingly, extended-care facilities such as nursing homes or chronic-disease hospitals may use the emergency services of an acute-care facility for evaluation of a patient with a sudden change in medical status. Emergency services also continue to function as the primary source of unscheduled admissions to the hospital, accounting for most hospital admissions in many inner city institutions (Kessler & Wilson; Schroeder).

Two decades ago Weinerman et al. (1966, p. 1040) defined three categories of patients presenting themselves to emergency units:

1. *Nonurgent:* "Condition does not require the resources of an emergency service; referral for routine medical care may or may not be needed; disorder is nonacute or minor in severity."
2. *Urgent:* "Condition requires medical attention within the period of a few hours; there is a possible danger to the patient if medically unattended; disorder is acute but not necessarily severe."
3. *Emergent:* "Condition requires immediate medical attention; time delay is harmful to patient; disorder is acute and potentially threatening to life or function."

These terms derive from a professional perspective and are based on medical diagnoses. Most patients cannot make these distinctions and err in both over-intepreting and underinterpreting the gravity of symptoms. Most patients presenting to an emergency service feel that they need immediate attention, regardless of what the professional staff may think. Others know that they do not have an urgent or emergent problem. They simply use the emergency service because it is all that is available to them. A review done in the 1970s showed that the average distribution among patients using emergency services is about 5% emergent, 45% urgent, and 50% nonurgent (Jonas et al., 1976). The type and location of the hospital produce variations in these proportions (Torrens & Yedvab).

As discussed earlier, some hospitals have developed walk-in units to relieve the emergency services of the burden of the nonurgent patients and to respond to the competition from freestanding walk-in services or urgi-centers. With the organization of group practices in the outpatient clinics some hospitals have also provided "add-on" slots in the appointment schedule to accommodate the non-urgent patient demanding urgent attention. Financial incentives are forcing hospitals to make every effort to reduce the costly care of nonurgent patients in the emergency setting. These efforts include evening and weekend hours for walk-in units and after-hours telephone access for clinic patients. One study, however, found no difference in emergency service visits or hospitalizations between a group of patients randomized to telephone access to physicians, who in turn had access to computerized medical records, and control patients (Darnell et al.).

Managed systems of care often require subscribers to get prior approval before authorizing emergency services, and unauthorized use may not be covered. As the role of provider and insurer become commingled, it is easier to design (and enforce use of) more efficient and less expensive methods of providing non-urgent care. Published studies are not yet available reporting the effectiveness and safety of these interventions designed to contain costs.

Staffing for Hospital-based Emergency Services. Dramatic changes in the staffing of emergency rooms have occurred in the past two decades. Teaching hospitals once relied almost exclusively on junior house officers (interns and assistant residents) to staff their emergency services with backup supervision by more senior house officers or staff members. Nonteaching hospitals either had physicians with staff privileges cover the emergency services in rotation or relied on "moonlighters" from residency programs of nearby teaching hospitals. Most teaching hospitals now supplement the house officer staffing with full-time physicians, many board-certified emergency medicine specialists, and nurse-clinicians or physician assistants. At minimum, senior staff have responsibility for directing the emergency services. The debate has been intense at many institutions, as departments of medicine and surgery see their traditional domi-nance of emergency services erode. Some academic medical centers have accommodated by pragmatically using the emergency medicine specialists to manage the emergency department (providing direct patient care and supervising house officers in surgery and medicine) while adhering to their stated principles by denying the formation of emergency medicine residency programs.

The nonteaching hospitals have also shifted to full-time emergency medicine specialists, frequently contracting with a physician group serving several hospi-tals in the area (Gersonde; Hannas). The hospitals that contract for coverage from an emergency medicine group are willing to pay a premium in return for reliable staffing.

Changes in organization and staffing are linked with efforts to classify the levels of emergency services provided (American College of Emergency Physi-cians; Harvey). Hospitals now compete for classification as comprehensive or designation as a regional trauma center to assure the flow of patients with a higher chance of requiring admission to the inpatient service after being stabilized in the emergency department.

Freestanding Emergi-centers and Urgi-centers

First established in Delaware and Rhode Island in 1973, freestanding ambulatory care facilities providing emergency services and urgent care for nonurgent patients now operate throughout the United States. Some, such as the emergi-center, have the same 24-hours-a-day, 7-days-a-week access that hospital emergency services provide. Others, so-called urgi-centers or "Doc in the Box," provide less comprehensive emergency services and are commonly open 12 hours a day, 7 days a week. These centers do not serve truly emergent patients, and most do not receive ambulance cases.

Two groups of patients find these centers attractive: those seeking the convenience and access of emergency services without the delays and other forms of negative feedback associated with using hospital services for nonurgent problems and those whose insurance treats emergi-centers preferentially compared with physicians' offices (Chesteen et al.). Both hospitals and private practitioners feel the competitive pressures from these new centers. Hospitals have responded by sponsoring or buying emergi-centers and urgi-centers, and physicians have formed them. Several thousand of these facilities now exist. Precise data, however, are not available. There is no clear definition for the spectrum of services provided by an emergi-center. It can range from a group practice that has simply expanded hours and eased access for walk-in patients to hospitals with satellite services that are geographically separate but organizationally and administratively far from freestanding.

The National Health Interview Survey (USDHHS, 1988) does not report separately the use of emergi-centers. An estimated 200 million contacts with physicians in 1986 (16.3% of the total) occurred other than in doctor's offices, hospital outpatient departments and emergency rooms, or over the telephone. No data are available for the contacts with nurses, social workers, and other health professionals practicing in ambulatory settings. Lumped together with visits to emergi-centers are home visits and visits to "clinic or lab outside a hospital." An estimated 10%, or 20 million, of these "other" visits in 1986 were to freestanding emergi- and urgi-centers.

As these centers have increased in number and become familiar to more patients, many have evolved to offer a combination of walk-in and appointment services. The appointment services initially provided follow-up for the presenting complaint. They have evolved into more comprehensive routine ambulatory services, especially among the urgi-centers. Many now market their services as having all of the advantages of the personal relationship with a primary care physician plus the convenience of expanded hours and short waiting times. In many geographic areas the chain-sponsored urgi-center is a convenient and economic method for a newly trained primary care physician to enter practice without the expense of acquiring an office and equipment. The flexible hours of employment are attractive to nurses and other health workers.

Emergency Medical Services

Emergency medical services extend beyond the hospital emergency department or the freestanding emergi-center to include other services provided to accident victims or individuals suffering acute, life-threatening illnesses such as acute myocardial infarction or stroke. The goals of these services are to preserve life and reduce disability by providing prompt treatment and transportation to comprehensive treatment facilities. The intended recipients of care are patients with emergent or urgent problems.

The emergency prehospital care for these problems requires a functioning emergency medical services system with 15 parts (Hoffer): provision of labor force, training of personnel, communications, transportation, facilities, critical-care units, use of public-safety agencies, consumer participation, accessibility to care, transfer of patients, standard medical-record keeping, consumer information and education, independent review and evaluation, disaster linkage, and mutual-aid agreements. A principal goal has been to provide for the whole nation a set of coordinated emergency care dispatch centers, using the uniform emergency telephone number, 911.

The crucial first step in providing emergency prehospital care is the existence of a high-quality ambulance service to provide first aid on site and during transit to a hospital emergency department (Gibson, 1973). Ambulance services have evolved from their origins as for-profit services set up by funeral directors. No consistent pattern of responsibility for providing ambulance services exists across communities. In many large cities the department of health and hospitals is responsible for either providing the service or contracting with qualified ambulance services for coverage. In smaller communities volunteer fire departments or ambulance services struggle to provide adequate care, and many deficiencies persist.

Death from traumatic injury is the leading cause of death in the United States in years of potential life lost (McGinnis; Office of Disease Prevention), emphasizing the need to strengthen all links in the emergency services chain. In 1986 unintentional injuries among the population aged 1 to 64 cost over 2 million years of life (Morbidity and Mortality Weekly Report). Although improving ambulance services across the country would prevent only a small percentage of this loss, the size of the problem is such that small gains translate into a large number of lives saved (National Conference on Cardio-Pulmonary Resuscitation).

Ambulance services must have adequate staff and organization to respond quickly to calls, using vehicles appropriately designed and equipped, and then take the patient to the hospital emergency department most appropriate for the patient's problem. A successful intervention depends on a series of functioning communication links between the patient and the ambulance service, between the dispatcher and the ambulance and between the ambulance and the hospital (Gibson, 1973). Recently, the use of two-way radio and transmission of monitored data such as real-time electrocardiograms and vital signs has improved these links.

Gibson (1977) reviewed the policy issues in the development of emergency medical services that require adequate financing, personnel, equipment, and facilities—with strict standards for each—and the cooperation of professions, agencies, institutions, and local government units to work together and coordinate their resources. Federal legislation has been important in setting standards and in providing resources for local emergency medical services to achieve these standards. The National Highway Safety Act of 1966 set performance criteria and required the states to submit emergency medical services plans. The Emergency Medical Services System Act of 1973 (P.L. 93-154) authorized $185 million over 3 years to states, counties, and other nonprofit agencies to plan, expand, and modernize their emergency medical services. Additional laws passed in 1976 (P.L. 94-573) and 1979 (P.L. 96-142) extended the act and expanded its scope. The Robert Wood Johnson Foundation helped greatly to develop the national emergency medical services system (R. W. Johnson Foundation, 1977).

P.L. 93-154 had several important requirements: rural areas applying for assistance received special consideration; applications coordinating local systems with statewide systems received preferential treatment; the emergency medical services were to organize "in a manner that provides persons who reside in the system's service area and who have no professional training or financial interest in the provision of health care with an adequate opportunity to participate in the making of policy for the system"; and emergency services were to be provided without prior inquiry as to ability to pay.

The modernization of services included changing the ambulance design from a vehicle patterned after a hearse to a light van with space and equipment to provide cardiopulmonary resuscitation (CPR) by an ambulance attendant while en route to the hospital. Many attendants are now licensed emergency medical technicians, trained to provide life-support services and acute management of trauma. Training requirements for licensure vary from state to state. In 1978 a national standard course of 185 hours was established (National Training Course). Most ambulance personnel have a rating of EMT-A that requires at least 81 hours of training, and many are EMT-Paramedics with more than 1,000 hours of training. With improved equipment and staff training, emergency medical services have increased survival rates for victims of traumatic injuries and acute medical conditions (Hoffer; Jacobs et al.; Lewis et al.; Montgomery; Roth et al.; Sherman).

Other Hospital-related Ambulatory Services

Competition has stimulated the development of a range of hospital-related ambulatory and other services. Hospitals now operate satellite ambulatory care facilities, nursing homes, health promotion programs, alcohol and drug treatment centers, freestanding ambulatory surgery centers, emergi-centers, urgi-centers, ambulance services, HMOs or IPAs, PPOs, doctors' office buildings, hospital-supply purchasing plans, health care management consultancy, office building management, real estate development, progressive care retirement communities, insurance company management, and hotel/restaurant/resort management (Ermann & Gabel). A 1985 national survey of hospital chief executive officers asked about plans to expand or add services. Of the top 10 services in the list, 5 are exclusively ambulatory services, and the others each have a significant ambulatory part. They are (with percentages of hospitals planning to add or expand each) home health service (75.6%), in-house outpatient surgery (74%), PPO (62%), wellness and health promotion (57%), outpatient diagnosis (55.2%), HMO (41.1%), cardiac rehabilitation (40.3%), oncology (39.8%), general rehabilitation (37.5%) and substance-abuse control (31.5%) (Moore).

The freestanding ambulatory surgery center is an important new development. In 1984 more than 9 million males and 16 million females had surgical procedures in nonfederal short-stay hospitals (USDHHS, 1986). Approximately 40% of the procedures could be done in an ambulatory setting (Olson) without the patient staying overnight in a hospital bed, and each year the shift from inpatient to ambulatory surgery increases. Economic pressures, improved technology, and third-party payers contribute to this change (Berryman) as the patient base shifts to less costly settings. The acceptance of these changes by patients and surgeons has advanced the growth of outpatient surgery.

The facilities may be either in the hospital—in some instances using space from delicensed inpatient units—or freestanding. In 1983 approximately 370,000 procedures were performed in surgi-centers, and in 1984 there were about 300 such surgi-centers in the United States. Including ambulatory surgery done in hospitals themselves, about 5 million ambulatory procedures, or 24% of all surgical procedures, were done in 1983 (Shannon). Third-party payers now require that certain procedures be done on an ambulatory basis unless there is documented evidence that it would be unsafe for the patient. Patient satisfaction and quality of care seem to be good, and new centers continue to appear (Goodspeed & Earnhart). One study found that physician supply and insurance demand were more important than competition among hospitals in the development of ambulatory surgery centers and alternative forms of service delivery

(Chirikos & White). Another found that facility-fee reimbursement is adequate to maintain a high-quality surgical facility if the Accreditation Association for Ambulatory Health Care grants accreditation and Medicare approves licensure (McDonald).

Freestanding diagnostic imaging centers have experienced a parallel growth in recent years and present an economic challenge to hospitals offering outpatient imaging and radiology services. These new facilities require expensive equipment and must rely on referrals from other physicians to succeed. This creates complex relations among the hospitals, radiologists, referring physicians, and patients ("Meeting the Challenge"). Ethical, legal, and financial problems emerge when some of the referring physicians have financial interests in the success of the freestanding center. A variant is the hospital radiology department that offers mobile mammography services to the community (Krajewski & Gunn).

Patient convenience and cost-saving incentives stimulated the development of an outpatient intravenous antibiotic program in Minneapolis (Kind, Williams, & Gibson). Patients of all ages with bone, joint, skin, soft-tissue, and other infectious diseases, such as meningitis, received successful treatment. No significant morbidity and no mortality occurred, patient compliance was high, and cost savings were large. The necessary elements were an enthusiastic medical staff, a central admixture service in the hospital pharmacy, and a team of nurses for IV cannula care. The AIDS epidemic has prompted similar approaches to comprehensive ambulatory treatment of opportunistic infections and other complications of HIV infection (Pascarelli & Holtzworth). To support these ambulatory services many hospital pharmacies offer durable medical equipment (Smith & Popielarski), realizing net income while improving the continuity of patient care offered by the institution.

The number of hospitals that have developed health promotion/disease prevention (HP/DP) programs reflects the national interest in these areas. Growing professional awareness of the importance of preventive services and the positive image such services convey for the hospital account for the popularity of these programs. The American Hospital Association's Center for Health Promotion has been a major stimulus and guide for hospitals in developing HP/DP programs. The center has published several books on program development (Bader et al.; Kernaghan & Giloth; Longe & Wolfe), many pamphlets and patient-education materials, and audiovisual programs and audiocassettes. Several commercial companies provide HP/DP services, including some specifically designed for hospital employees.

Hospital-sponsored HP/DP programs have potential for improving the health of the American people. In 1986 those who died before the age of 65 suffered a loss of more than 12 million years of life (Morbidity and Mortality Weekly Report). More than 60% of all Americans who die each year do so prematurely (McGinnis) at a cost in medical care and lost productivity in the hundreds of billions of dollars. Successful application of primary prevention measures (immunizations, proper nutrition, exercise, avoidance of smoking and other substance abuse, use of seat belts and other accident prevention strategies, and moderate use of alcohol) and secondary prevention (screening for early detection and treatment of conditions before they become symptomatic) could postpone an estimated 45% of cardiovascular disease deaths, 23% of cancer deaths, and more than 50% of the disabling complications of diabetes.

The programs described above reflect the range of new ambulatory services developed by hospitals to broaden their patient base and strengthen their financial structure. New or expanded ambulatory services have emerged as dominant factors in marketing strategies (Anwar; Hellstern; Mashaw; Maurer; Phillips & Reeder; Stafstrom). This promises to change fundamentally the role of the hospital in U.S. health care.

Health Department Services

Nowhere is the diversity in the scope and variety of health care services provided in the United States more clear than at the level of the local health department. In most parts of the country the health department is responsible for some ambulatory services. These may range from immunization services only to comprehensive departments of health and hospitals offering the full range of acute and chronic health care services to inpatients, outpatients, schoolchildren, and the homebound. No consistent pattern exists for the allocation of responsibility for ambulatory services to municipal, county, or state governments; to health departments or voluntary agencies; or to private physicians under contract for part of their time versus full-time health department employees.

Typically, the local health departments avoid direct competition with private practitioners by restricting personal health services to those areas in which private physicians have little interest (routine well-baby examinations) or lack expertise (case finding, treatment, and contact investigation for venereal disease and tuberculosis). Where financial circumstances make an area unappealing to private practitioners, local health departments may expand the scope of their services to include ambulatory care of acute and chronic illnesses.

Roemer (1975) estimated that local health departments provided less than 3% of all ambulatory personal health services in 1975, excluding school health services. About half of local health departments provide school health services in their jurisdictions, and the remainder are about evenly divided between cooperative efforts of the school board and the local health department and the school board alone. School health programs focus on screening for vision and hearing problems, assuring that immunization levels are adequate, and case finding for contagious diseases. Students are referred for diagnosis and treatment. A few jurisdictions have integrated the school health program into the community or neighborhood health centers to provide comprehensive ambulatory services for preschool and school-age children.

The most frequently offered personal health services are well-baby care, tuberculosis and venereal disease control, prenatal and family planning services, adult chronic disease screening programs, mental health services, and home public health nursing and homemaker services. All are *categorical programs,* which care for categories of disease or persons. State or federal matching funds frequently stimulate the creation of these programs.

Efforts over the past 70 years to involve health departments in the delivery of comprehensive health services have usually been unsuccessful (Myers et al.; Rosen). Some have expressed optimism that this can change to improve services to the poor (Cashman; Miller & Moos; Miller et al.; Roemer, 1975). Miller (1985) envisioned local health departments as having major responsibility for the delivery of direct social *and* medical services to the poor. The history of local health departments, with their bureaucratic, categorically oriented administrative structure—plus close involvement with politically sensitive, financially pressed local governments—limits the chances for much progress in this direction (Jonas, 1977, Chapters 5, 7).

Because of the increasing concerns about environmental pollution—the safety of local water supplies, solid waste disposal—and the challenges of containing the AIDS epidemic, it is not surprising that most local health departments feel no desire to expand their role in providing personal health services.

Neighborhood and Community Health Centers

The contemporary community health center (CHC) represents the surviving heir of the Neighborhood Health Center (NHC) movement of the 1960s and early 1970s. Stimulated by funding from the federal Office of Economic Opportunity (OEO), part of the Johnson administration's "war on poverty," NHCs were set up to provide comprehensive ambulatory and social services to the poor living in inner cities and rural areas of the United States. They represented a new form of health care organized around full-time salaried physician staffing, multi-disciplinary team health care practice, and community involvement in both policymaking and facility operations (Davis & Schoen; Zwick). Although the NHCs never served more than 2 or 3% of the American people, they achieved symbolic importance. They demonstrated health services organized to meet community needs with a combination of clinical, preventive, and social services delivered by teams of professionals and community workers dedicated to the ideals of interdisciplinary practice.

Voluntary hospitals, local health departments, and other nonfederal entities sponsored similar NHCs (Schachter & Elliston; Stoeckle, Anderson, Page, & Brenner; Tennant & Day), although their numbers never matched those funded by OEO. All were influenced by the pioneering programs of the Gouverneur and Montefiore Hospitals (Lloyd & Wise) in New York City and the Tufts–Columbia Point NHC in Boston. The first medical director at Gouverneur, the late Dr. Howard Brown, brought with him the organizational experience of the Health Insurance Plan of Greater New York, one of the early prepaid group practices (Light & Brown), to build a comprehensive ambulatory care program that came to serve as a model for many later NHCs.

Although NHCs varied in size, program content, and methods of funding, they shared certain common features. Those established early usually cared for medically underserved inner-city minority groups. Later efforts by OEO stimulated the formation of rural NHCs, which more often served poor populations of mixed racial composition. The NHCs tried to use physicians, nurses, social workers, and community health workers in multidisciplinary team practice— with varying degrees of enthusiasm and success. The community health workers, hired from the service area, provided basic nursing and social service skills. NHCs pioneered in the training and employment of nurse practitioners and physician assistants. The professional staff members were salaried or paid on a sessional basis. The aim of the NHC was to provide comprehensive ambulatory services—preventive and rehabilitative as well as curative services—that were delivered sensitively and were affordable and of high quality, and to intervene in the cycle of poverty.

The typical NHC budget was large. Start-up costs for facilities and equipment were high, and most of the patients had no insurance. The NHCs usually related to a teaching hospital for inpatient services, specialty consultations, sophisticated laboratory and x-ray services, and supervision—if not the direct employment— of the medical staff.

The authorizing OEO legislation mandated "maximum feasible participation" in the operation and administration of the NHCs and the formation of Community Advisory Boards. The board members usually came from the area served by the NHC and previously served by the teaching hospital that now controlled the OEO grant. These hospitals were regarded with suspicion based on prior responsiveness to community needs. The boards frequently demanded the final word on major policy decisions. Eventually, the federal grants went directly to nonprofit corporations representing the served communities. These bodies, frequently called Community Boards, then contracted with the hospital for needed services. They often hired the professional staff directly.

The OEO view that the provision of job opportunities to service-area residents was at least as important as providing health care created additional tensions. The NHCs usually served minority groups living in extreme poverty who had few of the necessary health care skills and training, particularly in the professional and semiprofessional job categories. Control of the jobs for which the local residents might be eligible became a plum, for both positive and negative reasons.

Evaluation of the NHCs included general program evaluations (Orso; Resource Management Corporation), evaluations of quality of care (Morehead; Morehead & Donaldson), and cost analyses (Sparer & Anderson). By most accounts, in the mid-1970s NHCs were providing reasonable-quality care. A General Accounting Office report in 1978 noted that some programs were overstaffed, some centers were serving the nonpoor while there were many medically underserved areas with no programs at all, and there were some failures to collect third-party reimbursement (Comptroller General). The tendency toward expansion of service for the nonpoor may have represented an effort to resolve one of the basic contradictions of the original OEO NHC program. The NHCs' emphasis on the poverty population created a curious dilemma. In trying to develop an organization to enhance the health of the poor, the NHC was perpetuating a separate and distinct system of health care for the poor rather than integrating them into the mainstream of medical care.

At the peak of the original OEO NHC program in the early 1970s, an estimated 200 NHCs existed nationwide ("NENA"). By 1974, under the Nixon effort to dismantle OEO, the number had fallen to about 150 (Roemer, 1981). In the mid-1970s the program was renamed the Community Health Center program, and its scope was narrowed to concentrate on the delivery of medical care with less emphasis on the social roles of the NHC. The CHCs were encouraged to expand their services to the nonpoor (Davis & Schoen, p. 171). By the early 1980s more than 800 CHCs served more than 4.5 million people (Bureau of Community Health Services; Freeman et al.; Goldman & Grossman; Sardell). The program focused on urban and rural medically underserved populations. Support for the CHCs comes primarily from federal grant funds, third-party reimbursements, and fee-for-service on a sliding scale.

By the end of the Reagan presidency the number of CHCs had declined to 561, although 4.7 million people were still receiving care (D. Smith, personal communication, 1989). The strategy for the CHC program includes the following:

1. Work closely with state governments and medical societies.
2. Serve only high-need areas.
3. Support only well-managed projects.
4. Promote self-sufficiency in projects.
5. Help projects to adapt to changing conditions.

With the severe restrictions on federal funds available for discretionary programs imposed by pressures to reduce the deficit, the future of CHCs is uncertain. If, however, legislation is enacted providing health insurance for the 35 million Americans now lacking coverage (Himmelstein & Woolhandler), the CHCs have appropriate organization and staff to provide comprehensive ambulatory services.

Physician Supply and Specialty Distribution
for Ambulatory Services

Physician supply in the United States continues to grow. In 1950 there were 219,900 active physicians (14.1 per 10,000 population), by 1985 there were 534,800 (22.0 per 10,000 population), and by the year 2000 a projected 696,600 physicians will be in active practice (26.0 per 10,000 population) (USDHHS, 1986, Table 72). Despite the dramatic increase in the number of physicians, geographic maldistribution persists. New England continues to have the highest concentration, with 25.4 physicians per 10,000 population in 1983, followed by the Middle Atlantic states with 25.1 and the Pacific states with 22.2. The East South Central states lag far behind at 14.3, and the rest of the central areas of the country range from 15.8 to 18.6 (USDHHS, 1986, Table 71).

Specialty maldistribution also persists in ambulatory care in the United States. The dramatic post–World War II growth in specialization and biomedical research is responsible for the remarkable gains in understanding basic disease processes and in developing effective treatments for many of them. The price of this progress has been the failure to replenish the nation's supply of primary care practitioners. Recognizing the gravity of this problem, the American Medical Association (AMA) in 1966 appointed the Citizens Commission on Graduate Medical Education, usually referred to as the Millis Commission, to review the graduate education of physicians (Millis). The commission noted that since the Flexner Report a "process of specialization and consequent fragmentation has occurred so that responsibility is diffused and authority divided." [p. vi] The AMA took the position that the profession should discipline itself in establishing standards of practice and education to improve the balance between general and specialized postgraduate education. Citing the needs of the American people for ambulatory services that offer a balanced array of general and specialty services, the report stated that "medical schools and teaching hospitals should prepare many more physicians than now exist who will have the desire and the qualifications to render comprehensive, continuing health services, including preventive measures, early diagnosis, rehabilitation, and supportive therapy, as well as the diagnosis and treatment of acute and episodic disease states." [p. 30] The revolutionary changes in medical education needed to produce many more generalists did not, of course, take place.

Two decades later the Association of American Medical Colleges panel on the General Professional Education of the Physician presented its report, "Physicians for the Twenty-First Century," better known as the GPEP Report, describing the same problems of specialty maldistribution that had troubled the Millis Commission (Muller). The GPEP Report noted that any reform effort must accommodate the following pressures acting on the medical profession in the 1980s:

1. Rapid advances in biomedical knowledge and technology will continue.
2. Chemical, mechanical, and electronic technologies available for prevention and treatment of disease will become ever more complex, powerful, effective, and potentially dangerous.
3. Medical practice using these technologies will require an even higher degree of specialization.
4. There will be an increasing recognition that many factors that determine health and illness are not directly influenced by interventions of the health-care system but are the consequences of life-style, environmental factors, and poverty.
5. Patients will increasingly need and demand advice and counsel from physicians and other health care professionals about how to use special medical services to improve personal health.
6. The principal providers of medical service in the near future are likely to be physicians employed by large corporations or by health service organizations covering specific population groups.
7. The environment of medical education will be heavily influenced by the agencies that pay for medical services and that will shape the nature of these services. In a time of concern for containing medical costs, medical and financial incentives will be less and less congruent, complicating and intensifying ethical dilemmas in medicine. [Muller]

How the profession responds to these pressures will profoundly influence the organization and delivery of ambulatory care. This is especially true in the private sector, where the laws of supply and demand for specific services are less modulated by administrative planning than they are in organized settings. The past inertia of the medical education establishment and the nurturing and conservation of professional values conspire to resist the kind of changes called for by the Millis Commission and the GPEP Report (Jonas, 1978). Modern treatment successes have built on the growth of biomedical research and the training of specialists, clinical investigators, and basic researchers since World War II. During this same period the ranks of the primary care physicians in private practice thinned drastically. They reached a nadir about 1975, when only 16% of nonfederal physicians providing patient care in the United States described themselves as general or family practitioners (USDHHS, 1986, Table 73).

In 1975 there were 28,070 internists (9.8% of clinically active physicians) and 12,559 pediatricians (4.4% of active physicians). Even if all were functioning as primary care physicians—in fact, most of the internists practiced as consultants in 1975—only 30% of U.S. physicians were in primary care specialties. Experience with the National Health Service in the United Kingdom and with the Kaiser Health Plan had already shown that a proper mix for an industrialized country was 50 to 60% primary care and 40 to 50% specialty and subspecialty practitioners.

Policymakers in the 1960s interpreted the growing shortage of primary care physicians as a shortage of all physicians. New medical schools were built and existing ones expanded in response to capitation payments from the federal government (Hatch). The total number of professionally active physicians increased from 335,608 in 1975 to 490,410 in 1985. The proportion of primary care specialists, however, remained just under 30%. The overall growth in physician supply produced an actual decline in the proportion of family and general practitioners from 16 to 12.5% as newly trained generalists did not keep pace with losses from death and retirement. Rural areas were particularly hard hit as aging generalists died or retired and no primary care practitioners replaced them. With recent improvements in physician supply, rural residents are making more use of health services (Krishan et al.).

Despite the dramatic increase in the number of residency programs in family medicine that occurred after establishing this new specialty in 1969, the ranks of general and family practitioners increased only modestly from 45,863 in 1975 to 53,181 a decade later. Much faster growth rates for internal medicine and pediatrics almost doubled the total numbers in these disciplines while producing proportional gains of 9.8 to 12.2% and 4.4 to 5.2%, respectively (USDHHS, 1986, Table 73). Nonetheless, the Graduate Medical Education National Advisory Committee (GMENAC) projected continued specialty maldistribution into the 1990s, with excessive numbers of subspecialists and barely adequate numbers of primary care physicians (Report of GMENAC). The GMENAC used a needs-based requirement approach rather than an economic demand-based model. Weiner et al. (1987), using data from more than 10,000 children in three large HMOs, tested the validity of GMENAC for pediatrics. Delphi panels of pediatricians in the same sites provided normative data. If the HMO data rather than GMENAC's ideal projections were used, fewer pediatricians would be needed. Increased rates of delegation of pediatric care to nonphysicians (nurse-clinicians and physician assistants) in the HMOs made the Delphi panel projections still lower. There are some signs that the United States may have already moved from a position of physician shortage to one of patient shortage (Iglehart).

In 1974 the Robert Wood Johnson Foundation started a program to encourage academic medical centers to develop primary care training programs in internal medicine and pediatrics (Lawrence et al.). The Department of Health and Human Services funded a few pilot programs at the same time. In 1976 Congress passed Public Law 94-484, authorizing funding for postgraduate training in the three primary care disciplines: family medicine, internal medicine, and pediatrics. Guidelines for the new programs funded by the federal government required a minimum of 25% of training in ambulatory settings providing continuity of care.

For the first time educators made a concerted effort to plan the curriculum for the knowledge base of ambulatory care on the descriptive epidemiology of presenting problems. The planners hoped to avoid the problem described by Hodgkin (1966) in England: "A study of general practitioners . . . shows an inverse correlation between the frequency of disease and the emphasis given to instruction about diseases during medical training". The new training programs tried to capture the reality of the world of practice and prepare their trainees for satisfying and effective roles in ambulatory care. The emphasis was on learning how to manage "common problems uncommonly well" (Hatem, Lawrence, & Arky).

Rosenblatt et al. (1983), in their study of the content of ambulatory care, found that 50% of office visits to private doctors in the United States involved only 15 diagnostic clusters. For primary care internists and family practitioners only 11 diagnostic clusters accounted for 50% of visits. Some of these diagnostic clusters include conditions infrequently seen on the inpatient service of the typical teaching hospital. With family practice programs having pioneered a new and more balanced approach to ambulatory training, internal medicine and pediatrics programs incorporated more orthopedics, dermatology, office gynecology, and psychiatry in their curricula. The mismatch between training and practice finally began to disappear. The more rigorous 3-year residency training in family medicine that had replaced the 1-year rotating internship addressed lingering concerns about the competence of the general practitioner.

The changes taking place in hospital care reinforced the new interest in teaching students and house officers in ambulatory settings. Shorter lengths of stay under the DRG (diagnostic related groups) system of reimbursement and changes in case mix among hospitalized patients brought about by new technologies and day surgery programs have worked to reinforce the value of training in ambulatory settings (Perkoff, 1986). Other reasons for renewed interest in ambulatory training are the growing need for well-trained primary care physicians by organized medical groups and the increasing expectation among patients that their care will be more personal than it has been in the past. Paradoxically, some of the very organizations that need more primary care physicians are having a profound effect on the academic medical centers that train such physicians. Driven by strategies of cost containment, HMOs and similar provider systems both limit lengths of stay in hospital and restrict referrals to their own specialists, often at the expense of medical center faculty and specialty clinics (Vanselow & Kralewski).

A survey of all HMOs in the United States in 1986 (with a 44% response rate) showed a desire for the curricula of medical schools and residency programs to emphasize four topics:

1. Cost-effective use of diagnostic and treatment services.
2. Utilization review and quality assurance.
3. The role of the primary care "gate-keeper."
4. The financing of health services (Jacobs & Mott).

The HMOs identified the most important criteria for selecting physicians as board eligibility, motivation, bedside manner, ability to function as part of a team, adaptability to a changing health care environment, training in a U.S.

medical school, ability to relate to nonphysician staff members, and the reputation of the residency program in which the physician trained.

Including cost-effective use of diagnostic services in the curriculum addresses but one determinant of physician behavior. Epstein and McNeil (1985) reviewed physician characteristics and organizational factors that influenced the use of ambulatory tests. They found that specialty training, more recent physician graduation, and large group practice settings correlate with significantly higher test use. Data about other physician characteristics and organizational factors remain equivocal.

The United States is unique among industrialized countries in having no one dominant form of primary care practitioner. Excluded by the definitions used in P.L. 94-484, obstetrician-gynecologists continue to provide large amounts of primary care to their female patients. The AMA includes obstetricians in its definition of primary care physicians.

Despite the claims of organized internal medicine to be addressing the primary care manpower needs of the country, most internists continue to function as subspecialists (Steinberg & Lawrence). The landmark studies by Mendenhall et al. (1978, Mendenhall 1979) documented the phenomenon of "principal care." Subspecialists, such as those in nephrology or oncology, restrict their practices to patients having diseases in their subspecialty domain while accepting responsibility for management of most of the primary care needs of those patients (Mendenhall). Similarly, many surgeons function as part-time generalists when there is not enough demand for their surgical skills. They have neither the proper training nor, in many cases, the temperament to function effectively in this role.

Debate continues among those who favor the family practitioner model, those who favor separate care for adults and children by internists and pedicians, and those who favor family-oriented care provided by internist-pediatrician teams (Hudson & Nourse; McWhinney; Perkoff, 1978; Petersdorf). Academic units in family medicine have prospered in state-supported medical schools, but private universities have been inhospitable to the new specialty, preferring instead to develop primary care internal medicine and general pediatrics programs. Patients have accepted family practitioners well, especially in rural areas and physician-shortage areas.

Efforts to create a common primary care discipline have been sporadic and thus far unsuccessful. This is so despite the logic of shared goals, scarce resources for medical education, and a common desire for reform of reimbursement policies to establish parity between "cognitive" services provided by primary care physicians and "procedural" services delivered by specialists. The Primary Care Initiative at Brown University has established a pilot program of a common first year of postgraduate training for family practitioners, internists, and pediatricians, followed by disciplinary training in a shared ambulatory setting (D. S. Greer, personal communication, 1989). With growing signs of a physician surplus in the United States, it is hard to predict whether increasing competition for patients will encourage or discourage efforts to train a prototypical primary care physician.

Bertakis and Robbins (1987) studied patients randomly assigned to the care of family practice residents or primary care internal medicine residents in a teaching hospital ambulatory care setting. After 2 years, patients randomized to the internal medicine practice had a significantly higher frequency of visits to the primary care clinic, emergency room, and acute-care clinic and broken appointments. Internal medicine patients also had a significantly higher number of visits to all non–primary care clinics, especially dermatology, obstetrics-gynecology, and general surgery. Whether these differences in practice styles reflect basic characteristics of those trainees attracted to one form of primary care over another or the attitudes and behaviors of the supervising faculty was indeterminate.

Brook et al. (1987) evaluated 15 group practices in general internal medicine located in university hospitals and used data on the quality of residency education provided, access to and quality of care, and patients' satisfaction with that care to predict changes in ambulatory care programs. One-third of the patient population had no health insurance, the patients had twice the chronic illness rate of the general population, and 40% of the patients remained with the practice at least 2 years. Residents worked in the practice an average of 4 hours per week; few faculty members practiced more than 14 hours per week in the setting. Patient satisfaction was greater than in the general population despite waiting times that were regarded as excessive. Only 10% of eligible patients received an annual influenza vaccination. Most distressing was the finding that the residents did not value their educational experience in the practice.

During the most acute shortage of primary care physicians, training programs emerged to produce nurse practitioners (NPs) and physician assistants (PAs) to fill the gap. These "physician extenders" had knowledge and skills to care for families, adults or children, and some physician assistants were able to practice in medical or surgical subspecialties. The growth in physician supply is now threatening the role of these practitioners. Of 44 rural satellite health centers originally staffed by NPs and PAs in 1975, 12 practices had ceased functioning by 1984. Physician practices replaced eight of them. Of the remaining 32, 14 had physicians on the staff, and 18 remained NP or PA practices (Brooks & Johnson). The physician-staffed practices had higher patient use, charged more for office visits, and generated more of their income from fee-for-service. Similar shifts in staffing patterns are occurring in urban health centers, HMOs, and other organized forms of ambulatory practice.

The NP and PA penetration of private practice has been far less, in part because older, established private practitioners were more reluctant to delegate clinical responsibility than were younger physicians joining HMO and NHC staffs (Lawrence, 1977). If the freestanding health center staffed by NPs or PAs is passing from the scene, a new pattern of primary care practice is emerging in the Social HMO (SHMO). Combining clinical services with social and living-support services, these new organizations help the frail elderly remain in the community rather than become institutionalized when their health fails to the point at which they need help with activities of daily living (Greenberg, Leutz, & Abrahams; Harrington & Newcomer; Leutz et al.). McDonnell Douglas, persuaded of the opportunity for cost-effective health care for its retirees, was one of the first employers to offer SHMO coverage as a benefit (Ervin, Showe, & Mehta). If these demonstrations prove acceptable to purchasers, providers, and consumers, the SHMO will become an important source of primary care and other ambulatory services.

Conclusions

The health care system in the United States contains several paradoxes. We stand at the forefront of biomedical technology and are admired and emulated the world over for the sophistication of our specialty care, while millions of our citizens are denied access to these services by financial and social barriers. Our medical education institutions are preeminent yet seem unable to respond to the recommendations of the Millis Commission and GPEP for fundamental reform of their curricula. Specialty and geographic maldistribution persist despite two decades of federal and philanthropic efforts to stimulate programs in primary care service and education.

Ambulatory care is central to the resolution of these paradoxes. We need to pay more attention to the content of ambulatory services, to the potential for integration of preventive services with clinical care, and to the numbers and types of personnel needed to deliver these services to a population that is experiencing an unprecedented demographic shift. Failure to develop more effective, comprehensive ambulatory services by the end of this century will exact a heavy price in overburdened inpatient services filled with sick, elderly patients while younger adults die prematurely of preventable conditions.

References

Abramowitz, K. "Hospital Role on Decline." Physician Executive *12*(1), 2, 1986.

Adams, G. "Urban Hospital's Innovations Save Money, Win Support." *Health Progress,* *69*(1), 56–58, 62, 1988.

American College of Emergency Physicians. "Categorization of Emergency Services" (policy statement). *Annals of Emergency Medicine, 13,* 546, 1984.

American Hospital Association. *Hospital Statistics.* Chicago: AHA, 1984.

American Hospital Association. *Hospital Statistics.* Chicago: AHA, 1988.

Anwar, R. H. "Marketing the Ambulatory Care Physician." *Ambulatory Care, 7*(7), 29, 1987.

Bader, B. et al. *Planning Hospital Health Promotion Services for Business and Industry.* Chicago: American Hospital Publishing, 1979.

Barnett, G. O. "The Application of Computer-based Medical-Record Systems in Ambulatory Practice." *New England Journal of Medicine, 310*(25), 1643, 1984.

Berryman, J. M. "Development and Organization of Outpatient Surgery Units: The Hospital's Perspective." *Urologic Clinics of North America, 14*(1), 1, 1987.

Bertakis, K. D., & Robbins, J. A. "Gatekeeping in Primary Care: A Comparison of Internal Medicine and Family Practice." *Journal of Family Practice, 24*, 305, 1987.

Block, J. A. "Hospital Innovations in the Community: Ambulatory Care." *Bulletin of the New York Academy of Medicine, 55*, 104, 1979.

Brook, R. H., Fink, A., Kosecoff, J., Linn, L. S., et al. "Educating Physicians and Treating Patients in the Ambulatory Setting. Where Are We Going and How Will We Know When We Arrive?" *Annals of Internal Medicine, 107*, 392, 1987.

Brooks, E. F., & Johnson, S. L. "Nurse Practitioner and Physician Assistant Satellite Health Centers: The Pending Demise of an Organizational Form?" *Medical Care, 24*(10), 881, 1986.

Bureau of Community Health Services. *Community Health Centers.* Rockville, MD: U.S. Department of Health, Education and Welfare, 1979.

Cashman, J. *What Thirteen Local Health Departments Are Doing in Medical Care.* Washington, D.C.: Public Health Service, 1967.

Chesteen, S. A., Warren, S. E., & Woolley, F. R. "A Comparison of Family Practice Clinics and Free-standing Emergency Centers: Organization Characteristics, Process of Care, and Patient Satisfaction." *Journal of Family Practice, 23*(4), 377, 1986.

Chirikos, T. N., & White, S. L. "Competition in Health Care Markets and the Development of Alternative Forms of Service Delivery." *Health Policy, 8*(3), 325, 1987.

Cohen, D. I., Breslau, D., Porter, D. K., Goldberg, H. I., et al. "The Cost Implications of Academic Group Practice. A Randomized Controlled Trial. *New England Journal of Medicine, 314*(24), 1553, 1986.

Comptroller General. *Are Neighborhood Health Centers Providing Services Efficiently and to the Most Needy?* (Pub. No. HRD-77-124). Washington, D.C.: General Accounting Office, 1978.

Daily, M. C. "Women's Primary Care Clinics: Addressing the Women's Market." *Group Practice Journal, 35*(4), 22, 1986.

Darnell, J. C., Hiner, S. L., Neill, P. J., Mamlin, J. J., et al. "After-hours Telephone Access to Physicians with Access to Computerized Medical Records: Experience in an Inner-City General Medicine Clinic." *Medical Care, 23*(1), 20, 1985.

Davis, K., & Schoen, C. *Health and the War on Poverty: A Ten Year Appraisal.* Washington, D.C.: Brookings Institution, 1978.

Dutton, D. B. "Patterns of Ambulatory Health Care in Five Different Delivery Systems." *Medical Care, 17*, 221, 1979.

Epstein, A. M., & McNeil, B. J. "Physician Characteristics and Organizational Factors Influencing Use of Ambulatory Tests." *Medical Decision Making, 5*(4), 401, 1985.

Ermann, D., & Gabel, J. "The Changing Face of American Health Care: Multihospital Systems, Emergency Centers, and Surgery Centers." *Medical Care, 23*, 401, 1985.

Ervin, S. L., Showe, B. L., & Mehta, S. "Social HMOs and Employers: A Budding Relationship for Retiree Health Care." *Health Cost Management, 4*(4), 11, 1987.

Freeman, H. E. et al. "Community Health Centers: An Initiative of Enduring Utility." *Health and Society, 60,* 245, 1982.

Freymann, J. G. *The American Health Care System: Its Genesis and Trajectory.* New York: Medcom Press, 1974.

Gersonde, R. J. "Two Approaches to Providing Physician Coverage in E. R." *Hospital Topics, 49,* 50, 1971.

Gibson, G. "Evaluative Criteria for Emergency Ambulance Services." *Social Sciences and Medicine, 7,* 425, 1973.

Gibson, G. "Emergency Medical Services." *Proceedings of the Academy of Political Science, 32,* 121, 1977.

Giglio, R. J., & Papazian, B. "Acceptance and Use of Patient-carried Health Records." *Journal of the American Medical Record Association, 58*(5), 32, 1987.

Goldberg, H. I., Cohen, D. I., Hershey, C. O., Hsiue, I. L., et al. "A Randomized Controlled Trial of Academic Group Practice: Improving the Operation of the Medicine Clinic. *Journal of the American Medical Association, 257*(15), 2051, 1987.

Goldman, F., & Grossman, M. *The Production and Cost of Ambulatory Medical Care in Community Health Centers.* Cambridge, MA: National Bureau of Economic Research, 1982. (Working Paper No. 907)

Goodspeed, S. W., & Earnhart, S. W. "Planning, Developing, and Implementing a Freestanding Ambulatory Surgery Center." *Health Care Strategic Management, 4*(2), 18, 1986.

Goulet, C. R. "Blue Cross/Blue Shield Alternate Delivery System." *Health Matrix, 4*(4), 7, 1987.

Greenberg, J. N., Leutz, W. N., & Abrahams, R. "The National Social Health Maintenance Organization Demonstration." *Journal of Ambulatory Care Management, 8*(4), 32, 1985.

Gruber, L. R., Shadle, M., & Polich, C. L. "From Movement to Industry: The Growth of HMOs." *Health Affairs,* Summer 1988, p. 198.

Hannas, R. R. "Emergency Medicine—a Survey." *Southern Medical Bulletin,* December 1971, p. 11.

Harrell, G. D., & Fors, M. F. "Marketing Ambulatory Care to Women: A Segmentation Approach." *Journal of Health Care Marketing, 5*(2), 19, 1985.

Harrington, C., & Newcomer, R. J. "Social/Health Maintenance Organizations: New Policy Options for the Aged, Blind, and Disabled." *Journal of Public Health Policy, 6*(2), 204, 1985.

Harvey, J. C. "The Emergency Medical Services Systems Act of 1973." *New England Journal of Medicine, 292,* 529, 1975.

Hatch, T. D. "Health Human Resources in the United States of America." *Education Medica y Salud, 20*(3), 388, 1986.

Hatem, C. J., Lawrence, R. S., & Arky, R. A. *A Curriculum for the General Education and Training of Physicians in Primary Care Medicine.* Hartford, CT: National Fund for Medical Education, 1978.

Hellstern, R. A. "The Future of the ACC Industry and NAFAC (National Association for Ambulatory Care)." *Ambulatory Care, 7*(2), 18, 1987.

Himmelstein, D. U., & Woolhandler, S. "A National Health Program for the United States." *New England Journal of Medicine, 320,* 102, 1989.

Hodgkin, K. *Towards Earlier Diagnosis*. Edinburgh: Livingstone, 1966.

Hoffer, E. P. "Emergency Medical Services, 1979." *New England Journal of Medicine, 301,* 1118, 1979.

Hudson, J. I., & Nourse, E. S. "Perspectives in Primary Care Education. Part 2." *Journal of Medical Education, 50,* 23, 1975.

Iglehart, J. K. "From Physician Shortage to Patient Shortage: The Uncertain Future of Medical Practice." *Health Affairs (Millwood), 5*(3), 142, 1988.

Jacobs, I. M. et al. "Prehospital Advanced Life Support: Benefits in Trauma." *Journal of Trauma, 24,* 8, 1984.

Jacobs, M. O., & Mott, P. D. "Physician Characteristics and Training Emphasis Considered Desirable by Leaders of HMOs." *Journal of Medical Education, 62,* 725, 1987.

Jonas, S. "Some Thoughts on Primary Care: Problems in Implementation." *International Journal of Health Services, 3,* 177, 1973.

Jonas, S. *Quality Control of Ambulatory Care: A Task for Health Departments*. New York: Springer, 1977.

Jonas, S. *Medical Mystery: The Training of Doctors in the United States*. New York: W. W. Norton, 1978.

Jonas, S. et al. "Monitoring Utilization of a Municipal Hospital Emergency Department." *Hospital Topics, 54,* 43, 1976.

Kernaghan, S., & Giloth, B. E. *Working with Physicians in Health Promotion*. Chicago: American Hospital Publishing, 1983.

Kessler, M. S., & Wilson, K. C. "Emergency Department Key Factor in Hospital Admissions." *Hospitals,* Dec. 16, 1978, p. 87.

Kind, A. C., Williams, D. N., & Gibson, J. "Outpatient Intravenous Antibiotic Therapy: Ten Years' Experience." *Postgraduate Medicine, 77*(2), 105, 1985.

Koster, A., Waterstraat, F. L., Jr., & Sondak, N. "Automated and Ambulatory Record Systems: A Comparative Cost Analysis." *Journal of the American Medical Record Association, 58*(11), 26, 1987.

Krajewski, D., & Gunn, S. "Mobile Mammography Project." *Radiography, 53,* 69, 1987.

Krishan, I., Drummond, D. C., Naessens, J. M., Nobrega, F. T., & Smoldt, R. K. "Impact of Increased Physician Supply on Use of Health Services: A Longitudinal Analysis in Rural Minnesota." *Public Health Reports, 100*(4), 379, 1985.

Kucera, W. R., & Marren, J. P. "Guidelines for Physician Contracting with Alternative Delivery Systems." *Journal of Medical Practice Management, 2*(3), 200, 1987.

Lawrence, R. S. "Harvard Primary Care Program." Paper presented at the First Conference on Primary Care Delivery, Education and Research in Teaching Hospitals, September 28–30, 1977. *Journal of Ambulatory Care Management, 2,* 55, 1979.

Lawrence, R. S., DeFriese, G. H., Putnam, S. M., Pickard, C. G., Cyr, A. G., & Whiteside, S. W. "Physician Receptivity to Nurse Practitioners: A Study of the Correlates of the Delegation of Clinical Responsibility." *Medical Care, 15,* 289, 1977.

Leutz, W., Abrahams, R., Greenlick, M., Kane, R., & Prottas, J. "Targeting Expanded Care for the Aged: Early SHMO Experience." *Gerontologist, 28*(1), 4, 1988.

Lewis, R. P. et al. "Effectiveness of Advanced Paramedics in a Mobile Coronary Care System." *Journal of the American Medical Association, 241,* 1902, 1979.

Light, H. L., & Brown, H. J. "The Gouverneur Health Services Program: An Historical View." *Milbank Memorial Fund Quarterly, 45,* 375, 1967.

Lloyd, W. B., & Wise, H. B. "The Montefiore Experience." *Bulletin of the New York Academy of Medicine, 44,* 1353, 1968.

Longe, M. E., & Wolf, A. *Promoting Community Health through Innovative Hospital-based Programs.* Chicago: American Hospital Publishing, 1984.

Madison, D. L. "The Case for Community-Oriented Primary Care." *Journal of the American Medical Association, 249,* 1279, 1983.

Mak, H. K. "Hospital Outpatient Medical Summary." Medical Records and Health Care Information Journal *28*(1), 10, 1987.

Mashaw, R. "Marketing, Media and Medicine: Competing for ACC Patients." *Ambulatory Care, 7*(7), 31, 1987.

Maurer, M. P. "Marketing Planning for Ambulatory Care: Twelve Key Steps." *Journal of Ambulatory Care Marketing, 1*(1), 3, 1987.

McDonald, H. P., Jr. "Office Ambulatory Surgery in Urology. *Urology Clinics of North America, 14*(1), 27, 1987.

McGinnis, J. M. "National Priorities in Disease Prevention." *Issues in Science and Technology,* Winter 1988–89, p. 48.

McManis, G. L., & Hopkins, M. "Managed Care Plans: CFOs Weigh the Benefits." *Healthcare Financial Management, 41*(5), 52–54, 58, 1987.

McWhinney, I. R. "Family Medicine in Perspective." *New England Journal of Medicine, 293,* 175, 1975.

Mechanic, D. "Cost Containment and the Quality of Medical Care: Rationing Strategies in an Era of Constrained Resources." *Milbank Memorial Fund Quarterly: Health and Society, 63*(3), 453, 1985.

"Meeting the Challenge of Freestanding Imaging Centers: Options for Hospitals and Hospital-based Radiologists." *Journal of Health Care Technology, 1*(4), 257, 1985.

Mendenhall, R. C. "A National Study of Medical and Surgical Specialties: Part 3. An Empirical Approach to the Classification of Patient Care." *Journal of the American Medical Association, 241,* 2180, 1979.

Mendenhall, R. C., et al. "A National Study of Medical and Surgical Specialties: Part 1. Background, Purpose, and Methodology." *Journal of the American Medical Association, 240,* 848, 1978.

Merz, M. "Preferred Provider Organizations: The New Health Care Partnerships." *Hospital and Health Services Administration 31*(6), 32, 1986.

Miller, C. A. "An Agenda for Public Health Departments." *Journal of Public Health Policy, 6,* 158, 1985.

Miller, C. A., & Moos, M. K. *Local Health Departments: Fifteen Case Studies.* Washington, D.C.: American Public Health Association, 1981.

Miller, C. A. et al. "A Survey of Local Public Health Departments and Their Directors." *American Journal of Public Health, 67,* 931, 1977.

Millis, J. S. "The Graduate Education of Physicians. Report of the Citizens Commission on Graduate Medical Education." Chicago: American Medical Association, 1966.

Moore, W. B. "CEO's Plan to Expand Home Health Outpatient Services." *Hospitals,* January 1, 1985, p. 74.

Montgomery, B. J. "Emergency Medical Services—a New Phase of Development." *Journal of the American Medical Association, 243,* 1017, 1980.

Morbidity and Mortality Weekly Report. *37*(20), 319, 1988.

Morehead, M. A. "Evaluating Quality of Care in the Neighborhood Health Center Program of OEO." *Medical Care, 2,* 118, 1970.

Morehead, M. A., & Donaldson, R. "Quality of Clinical Management of Disease in Comprehensive Neighborhood Health Centers." *Medical Care, 12,* 301, 1974.

Mullan, F. "Community-Oriented Primary Care." *New England Journal of Medicine, 310,* 193, 1984.

Mullan, F., & Conner, E. (Eds.). *Community-Oriented Primary Care—Conference Proceedings.* Washington, D.C.: National Academy Press, 1982.

Muller, S. "Physicians for the Twenty-first Century. Report of the Panel on the General Professional Education of the Physician and College Preparation for Medicine." Washington, D.C.: Association of American Medical Colleges, 1984.

Myers, B. A. et al. "The Medical Care Activities of Local Health Units." *Public Health Reports, 83,* 757, 1968.

National Conference on Cardio-Pulmonary Resuscitation and Emergency Cardiac Care. "Standards for cardio-pulmonary resuscitation (CPR) and emergency cardiac care (ECC)." *Journal of the American Medical Association, 227* (Suppl.), 837–868, 1974.

National Training Course, Emergency Medical Technician/Paramedic, Course Guide. Washington, D.C.: U.S. Government Printing Office, 1978.

Nelson, S. R. "Hospital-Sponsored Group Practice." *Health Matrix, 2*(1), 7, 1984.

"NENA: Community Control in a Bind." *Health PAC Bulletin,* June 1972.

Nutting, P. A. et al. "Community-Oriented Primary Care in the United States." *Journal of the American Medical Association, 253,* 1763, 1985.

Office of Disease Prevention and Health Promotion, U.S. Department of Health and Human Services. *Disease Prevention/Health Promotion: The Facts.* Palo Alto, CA: Bull Publishing, 1988.

Olson, L. L. *Establishing Freestanding Ambulatory Surgery Centers: The Planning and Regulatory Process."* Chicago: American Medical Association, 1982.

Orso, C. L. "Delivering Ambulatory Health Care." *Medical Care, 17,* 111, 1979.

Oswald, E. M., & Winer, I. K. "A Simple Approach to Quality Assurance in a Complex Ambulatory Care Setting." *Quality Review Bulletin, 13*(2), 56, 1987.

Pascarelli, E. F., & Holtzworth, A. S. "Developing an Ambulatory Care Program for AIDS Patients." *Journal of Ambulatory Care Management, 10*(1), 44, 1987.

Perkoff, G. T. "General Internal Medicine, Family Practice or Something Better?" *New England Journal of Medicine, 299,* 654, 1978.

Perkoff, G. T. "Teaching Clinical Medicine in the Ambulatory Setting: An Idea Whose Time May Have Finally Come." *New England Journal of Medicine 314*(1), 27, 1986.

Petersdorf, R. G. "Internal Medicine and Family Practice." *New England Journal of Medicine, 293,* 326, 1975.

Phillips, J. H., & Reeder, C. E. "Ambulatory Care Centers: Structure, Services, and Marketing Techniques." *Journal of Health Care Marketing, 7*(4), 27, 1987.

Report of the Graduate Medical Education National Advisory Committee (GMENAC) to the Secretary (Pub. No. 81-651). Hyattsville, MD: U.S. Government Printing Office.

Resource Management Corporation. *Evaluation of the War on Poverty: Health Programs.* (Contract No. GA-654). Washington, D.C.: General Accounting Office, 1969.

Robert Woods Johnson Foundation. *Special Report.* Princeton, N.J.: Johnson Foundation, 1977.

Robert Wood Johnson Foundation. *Special Report: Access to Health Care in the United States: Results of a 1986 Survey.* Princeton, N.J.: Johnson Foundation, 1987.

Roemer, M. I. "From Poor Beginnings, the Growth of Primary Care." *Hospitals,* Mar. 1, 1975, p. 38.

Roemer, M. I. *Ambulatory Health Services in America.* Gaithersburg, Md.: Aspen Systems Corp., 1981.

Rogers, D. "Community-Oriented Primary Care." *Journal of the American Medical Association, 248,* 1622, 1982.

Rogers, D. "Policy Changes and Their Possible Impact on Hospital-Based Ambulatory Care." *Journal of Community Health, 10*(4), 226, 1985.

Rosen, G. "The First Neighborhood Health Center Movement—Its Rise and Fall." *American Journal of Public Health, 61,* 1620, 1971.

Rosenblatt, R. A., Cherkin, D. C., Schneeweiss, R., & Hart, L. G. "The Content of Ambulatory Medical Care in the United States: An Inter-Specialty Comparison. *New England Journal of Medicine, 309,* 892, 1983.

Roth, R. et al. "Out-of-Hospital Cardiac Arrest: Factors Associated with Survival." *Annals of Emergency Medicine, 13,* 237, 1984.

Sadowy, H. S., & Wood, S. C. "The Growth of Alternative Delivery Systems and the Implications for Hospitals." *Health Care Strategy Management 4*(7), 14, 1986.

Sardell, A. "Neighborhood Health Centers and Community-based Care: Federal Policy from 1965 to 1982." *Journal of Public Health Policy, 4,* 484, 1983.

Schachter, L. P., & Elliston, E. D. "Medical Care in a Free Community Clinic." *Journal of the American Medical Association, 237,* 11848, 1977.

Schroder, S. "The Increasing Use of Emergency Services." *Western Journal of Medicine, 130,* 67, 1979.

Selzer, S. R., & Sholl, J. G. "Development of a Campus-based Satellite Medicine Clinic." *Journal of Medical Education, 60*(6), 461, 1985.

Shannon, K. "Outpatient Surgery up 77 Percent: Data." *Hospitals,* May 16, 1985, p. 54.

Sherman, M. A. "Mobile Intensive Care Units: An Evaluation of Effectiveness." *Journal of the American Medical Association, 241,* 1899, 1979.

Smith, J. E., Popielarski, E. "Hospital Outpatient Pharmacies and Durable Medical Equipment." *American Journal of Hospital Pharmacy, 43*(4), 928, 1986.

Sparer, G., & Anderson, A. *Cost of Services at Neighborhood Health Centers: A Comparative Analysis.* Washington, D.C.: Office of Economic Opportunity, 1975.

Stafstrom, A. "The Right Staff—the Human Role in Financial Success." *Ambulatory Care, 7*(2), 8, 1987.

Steinberg, E. P., Lawrence, R. S. "Where Have All the Doctors Gone? Physician Choices between Specialty and Primary Care Practice." *Annals of Internal Medicine, 93,* 619, 1980.

Stoeckle, J. D., Anderson, W. H., Page, J., & Brenner, J. "The Free Medical Clinics." *Journal of the American Medical Association, 219,* 603, 1972.

Tennant, F. S., Jr., & Day, C. M. "Survival Potential and Quality of Care among Free Clinics." *Public Health Reports, 89,* 558, 1974.

Torrens, P., & Yedvab, D. "Variations among Emergency Room Populations: A Comparison of Four Hospitals in New York City." *Medical Care, 8,* 60, 1970.

Tulli, C. G., Jr. "One Key to Practice Growth: Improving Other Practice Encounters." *Group Practice Journal, 36*(6), 58, 1987.

U.S. Department of Health and Human Services. *Health United States, 1986* (DHHS Pub. No. PHS 87-1232). Washington, DC: U.S. Government Printing Office, 1986.

U.S. Department of Health and Human Services. *Health United States, 1987* (DHHS Pub. No. PHS 88-1232). Washington, DC: U.S. Government Printing Office, 1988.

Vanselow, N. A., & Kralewski, J. E. "The Impact of Competitive Health Care Systems on Professional Education." *Journal of Medical Education, 61,* 707, 1986.

Weiner, J. P., Steinwachs, D. M., Shapiro, S., Coltin, K. L., et al. "Assessing a Methodology for Physician Requirement Forecasting. Replication of GMENAC's Need-based Model for the Pediatric Specialty." *Medical Care, 25*(5), 426, 1987.

Weinerman, E. R. et al. "Yale Studies in Ambulatory Medical Care: V. Determinants of Use of Hospital Emergency Services." *American Journal of Public Health, 56,* 1037, 1966.

Wilensky, G. R., & Berk, M. L. "The Health Care of the Poor and the Role of Medicaid." *Health Affairs, 1*(4), 50, 1982.

Wolinsky, H. "New Trend in Patient Care: Women's Health Centers." *American College of Physicians Observer 6*(7), 1, 23, 1986.

Zwick, D. I. "Some Accomplishments and Findings of Neighborhood Health Centers." *Milbank Memorial Fund Quarterly,* October 1972. Reprinted in I. K. Zola and J. B. McKinlay (Eds.), *Organizational Issues in the Delivery of Health Services,* New York: Prodist, 1974.

7

Hospitals

Anthony R. Kovner

Smith and Kaluzny (1986) have characterized the health care system as a white labyrinth "so large, complex and subtle that it defies description." To many Americans, hospitals are just such white labyrinths. People often know little about how their local hospital works, and even those who work in hospitals often know little about departments or occupations other than their own. Yet hospitals, like other, more familiar local organizations, open, grow, merge, and even close.

This chapter surveys the following topics concerning hospitals: (1) historical development, (2) hospital statistics and characteristics, (3) factors affecting costs, (4) hospital structure, and (5) forces propelling and constraining change in hospitals. The primary focus is on the most common type of hospital—that which provides short-term, general, and acute care.

Historical Development

The development of American community hospitals can be divided into five periods:

1. The beginning, before 1870.
2. The first period of rapid growth, 1870–1910.
3. The period of consolidation, 1910–1945.
4. The second period of rapid growth, 1945–1980.
5. The present period of maturation and perhaps the end of growth in terms of the number and size of hospitals, 1980 and onward.

The section on Historical Development in this chapter remains in large part the same as in the first and second editions and was authored by Michael Enright and Steven Jonas.

The first hospitals were primarily of a religious and charitable nature, tending to provide care for the sick rather than providing for medical cure (Freymann, pp. 28–29; Starr, Chapter 4; Rosenberg). Hospitals began in the Middle Ages as places of refuge for the sick, the weary, and the poor. Beginning in the 17th century, several Western European countries, notably England, began to attempt to deal with the problem of the poor at the local level. Local governments were given the authority, and in some cases the responsibility, to build or provide institutions to house the poor. The "poor" included those who were unemployed, orphans or children whose parents could not care for them, the dependent elderly, and the mentally retarded, as well as poor ill persons. These institutions generally were called *almshouses* or *poorhouses*. In certain jurisdictions in England and the United States, some or all of these categories of poor people were housed together, from the first appearance of the poorhouses until well into the 20th century.

In the American colonies, the earliest hospitals were actually infirmaries in poorhouses. The first public institution designed solely for the care of the sick was the "pesthouse," built on the same grounds as the New York Workhouse. It was not until 1848 that the administrations of the two institutions were formally separated and an independent hospital was created (Freymann, pp. 28–29).

Private voluntary hospitals (those provided or supported by community leaders) in the United States go back to the 18th century (Freymann, pp. 22–24). These institutions also cared for the poor: Since hospitals could do little for their patients, there was no reason for the self-supporting sick to use them. The first voluntary hospital in the American colonies was Pennsylvania Hospital in Philadelphia (1751). New York Hospital was founded in 1769, followed by Massachusetts General Hospital in Boston in 1811 (Freymann, pp. 22–24). By 1873, however, there were an estimated 178 hospitals in the United States (Stevens, p. 52).

From 1870 to 1910, as biomedical science and technology developed effective means of intervention, hospitals evolved into local physicians' workshops for all types and classes of patients. More effective hospital care was achieved primarily through advances in general hospital hygiene, including the development of trained nurses and techniques for asepsis and surgical anesthesia. Between 1870 and 1910 there was a period of spectacular growth, the number of hospitals increasing from 178 in 1873 to more than 4,300 in 1909 (Stevens, p. 52). Medical care had become too complex for physicians to carry their entire armamentarium in their black bags; special equipment and consultation with other medical specialists became essential.

According to Starr (pp. 169–170), the period from 1750 to 1850 saw the formation of voluntary and public hospitals. From 1850 to 1890 there developed religious or ethnic institutions and specialized hospitals for certain diseases or categories of patients, such as children and women. The period from 1890 to

1920 saw the spread of for-profit hospitals owned by physicians. The period between 1910 and 1945 showed less growth than in the periods before and after.

The types of patients in the hospitals changed with each medical discovery. In 1923, the discovery of insulin drastically changed the character of treatment for diabetes. Liver extract reduced the incidence of pernicious anemia in 1929. Sulfonamides began to affect the treatment of pneumonia and some other infectious diseases in 1935, a trend that accelerated with the widespread use of antibiotics beginning in 1943, as well as the continuing development of immunization techniques. The development of rehabilitation services began to bring more disabled patients to the hospital. The 1950s saw chronic illness becoming progressively more important as a hospital problem. As infectious diseases generally have been conquered (with the notable exception of AIDS), hospitals are increasingly focusing on the pathology of trauma and degenerative and neoplastic disease.

The fourth period, 1945 to 1980, was a second major growth era for hospitals. It was marked by a tremendous increase in hospital services, costs, and technology and by a more modest expansion in the number of hospitals. Many small rural hospitals were built during this period, financed by federal monies under the Hill-Burton Act. A major factor influencing the increased breadth and intensity of inpatient hospital services was the rapid growth of hospital insurance. The Blue Cross system originally was developed during the Great Depression in order to help assure payment to hospitals. Hospital insurance developed rapidly through World War II as a result of collective bargaining agreements. In that period the federal government limited wage increases but not benefits. Finally, in 1965 the Medicare and Medicaid programs were created, the former providing health insurance for the elderly and the latter providing health benefits for the poor.

Since 1980, hospital occupancy rates have decreased, both with regard to the mean discharge rate (which is the ratio of total discharges in a year to number of beds) and average length of stay. In a study of 600 hospitals, Farley (1988) has calculated the average occupancy rate of community hospitals in the United States as declining nearly 20%—from 69.7 to 56.6%. At the same time that hospital occupancy has been decreasing, there are fewer independent hospitals. There has been an emergence in the industry of investor-owned and not-for-profit multihospital corporations (Starr, pp. 420–450). In 1986 multihospital systems owned, leased, or sponsored 1,953 hospitals and managed under contract 561 hospitals, putting more than one-third of U.S. hospitals under multihospital systems (AHA, 1987b).

Hospital care is big business. In 1986, hospital expenditures amounted to $179.6 billion, representing 40% of the nation's health expenditures and 4.4% of the nation's gross national product, or $720 per American (Ermann & Gabel). This compares with a 1972 expenditure level of $34.9 billion, which was 36.3%

of the nation's health expenditures and 3.0% of the nation's gross national product (Gibson et al.).

Hospital Statistics and Characteristics

There are two major agencies that count and classify hospitals in the United States: the American Hospital Association (AHA) and the National Center for Health Statistics (NCHS) of the U.S. Department of Health and Human Services. The AHA annually publishes the Hospital Guide issue of its journal *Hospitals*, followed by a companion publication, *Hospital Statistics*. These publications list each AHA-registered hospital, giving its basic characteristic as well as much summary data. The NCHS publishes the results of its Hospital Discharge Survey periodically in *Monthly Vital Statistics Report* and *Health and Vital Statistics*. The Hospital Discharge Survey gathers and analyzes data from a sample of hospitals on demographic characteristics of patients, descriptors of hospitals, morbidity and diagnoses, and surgical operations. Since 1976 a congressionally mandated annual report to the president, titled *Health: Unites States*, has appeared. It includes some data on hospitals, as well as health and financial data.

Hospital Statistics

Table 7.1 provides summary statistics on community hospitals. Community hospitals include general short-term hospitals under not-for-profit (voluntary), public (governmental), and investor-owned (proprietary) auspices. Other hospitals include federal hospitals and nonfederal, long-term mental and other hospitals.

Table 7.2 provides some additional key facts on community hospital size, utilization, employment, and expenditures. Community hospitals admitted more than 32 million patients in 1986, with an average stay of 7.1 days. Hospital occupancy, which is determined by dividing available bed days by patient days, was 64.3% in 1986 (AHA, 1987b). This is down dramatically (AHA, 1984b) from 1983 volume: by 4 million patients admitted, 1.5 days average stay, and 11% in hospital occupancy.

Although the number of community hospitals (see Table 7.1) has remained relatively the same—at about 5,800—since 1972, the average size of these hospitals has increased from 163 beds in 1976 to 172 beds in 1986 (AHA, 1987). Community hospitals employed 3,025,000 full-time equivalent staff in 1986. Community hospital expenditures totaled $140.6 billion in 1986, of which labor expenses were $75.8 billion of 54%.

Hospitals other than community (nonfederal, short-term general, and special) hospitals include federal, nonfederal psychiatric, tuberculosis and other respira-

Table 7.1 Community Hospital Facts: 1976 and 1986

	1976	1986
Total number of hospitals	5,857	5,678
Beds (thousands)	956	978
Patient admissions	33,979	32,379
Births (thousands)	2,962	3,584
Surgical operations (thousands)	16,832	20,469
Outpatients (thousands)	201,247	231,912
Hospital size, by number of beds		
6–24	290	211
25–49	1,124	993
50–99	1,446	1,376
100–199	1,370	1,382
200–299	711	752
300–399	376	437
400–499	234	216
500 or more	306	311
Community hospitals by type		
Nonprofit	3,368	3,338
Investor-owned	752	834
State and local government	1,836	1,556

Note: Community hospitals are nonfederal, short-term general and special hospitals (excluding psychiatric hospitals, tuberculosis and respiratory disease hospitals, and hospital units of institutions) whose facilities and services are available to the public.
Source: Adapted from American Hospital Association, *Hospital Statistics, 1987* (AHA, 1987b).

tory disease hospitals, long-term general, and other special institutions. In 1986 there were 1,163 of these hospitals, with 311,000 beds, 2.84 million admissions, and an average length of stay ranging from 20 to 119 days, as shown in Table 7.3.

Hospital Characteristics

Hospitals differ from one another with respect to size, mission, ownership, complexity, competitive environment, population served, endowment and financial situation, physical facilities, and costs per day of care or cost by patient diagnostic category.

As of 1986, 1,204 community hospitals had fewer than 50 beds apiece. Many of these hospitals were in areas with sparse populations, the nearest hospital being an hour's drive away from residents in the community. The 311 largest community hospitals of more than 500 beds (5.5% of the total) had about 22% of the nation's total community hospital admissions (AHA, 1987b).

Table 7.2 Community Hospital Key Facts: 1986

Average size	172 beds
Average length of stay[a]	7.1 days
Hospital occupancy	64.3%
FTEs (full-time equivalent employees) per 100 adjusted census	386
Expenditures (millions)	$140,654

Source: Adapted from *Hospital Statistics,* 1987 (AHA, 1987b).
[a]An aggregate figure including inpatient days plus an estimate of the volume of outpatient days, expressed in units equivalent to an inpatient day in terms of level of effort.

Hospitals differ with regard to the services they offer. For example, according to the 1986 AHA Hospital Guide, Nor-Lea General Hospital in Lovington County, New Mexico, had 28 beds and provided the following services: ambulatory surgery, health promotion, respiration therapy, physical therapy, family planning, ultrasonography, histopathological laboratory, blood bank, rehabilitation outpatient services, organized outpatient department, recreational therapy, day hospital, hospital auxiliary and volunteer services, patient representation, and geriatric services. New York University Medical Center in New York City had 878 beds and was listed as providing all of the services that Nor-Lea provided, other than an organized outpatient department and a day hospital. In addition, NYU Medical Center provided an intensive care unit, open heart surgery, x-ray radiation therapy, megavoltage radiation therapy, radioactive implants, diagnostic and therapeutic radioisotope facilities, magnetic resonance imaging, hemodialysis, occupational therapy, inpatient rehabilitation, psychiatric emergency services and consultation and education, clinical psychology, an emergency department, genetic counseling, lithotripsy, obstetrics, speech pathology, neonatal intensive care, pediatric inpatient care, CT scanning, and a cardiac catheterization laboratory.

Hospitals are similar to one another in that they provide inpatient care by nurses and physicians, the latter having a great deal of autonomy in deciding whom to admit and what services patients should receive. As organizations, hospitals have to be financially solvent. They all seek to survive and grow. Hospitals provide services every day and at every hour of the day. Some hospitals services are difficult to quantify and measure; for example, how can one measure the amount of health education services a patient receives? But all hospitals must be organized so that standby capacity is available to meet medical emergencies and to deal with critical and life-threatening situations. Hospitals are characterized by hierarchy and rules. There is little but increasing standardization of patient care. Nevertheless, there is overall agreement about the principal objectives of hospitals: curing and caring.

Table 7.3 Trends among Other Than Community Hospitals

	Hospitals		Beds (thousands)		Admissions		Average length of stay (days)	
	1976	1986	1976	1986	1976	1986	1976	1986
Federal hospitals	380	342	129	111	1,998	2,117	19	14
Nonfederal psychiatric hospitals	528	634	291	167	598	607	141	86
Nonfederal tuberculosis and other respiratory disease hospitals	21	4	4	0	12	4	64	27
Long-term general and other special	197	133	49	30	100	81	148	119
Short-term units of institutions	99	50	5	3	90	31	7	20

Source: Adapted from *Hospital Statistics, 1987* (AHA, 1987b).

Some Important Types of Hospitals

The American Hospital Association classifies hospitals in several ways. Those in which the average length of stay is 30 days or less are short-term hospitals. In long-term hospitals the average length of stay is more than 30 days. There are specialty hospitals—for example, ear, nose, and throat hospitals and those for women's diseases—and general hospitals. There are teaching and nonteaching hospitals, hospitals that are independent or are part of multihospital systems, public and private hospitals, and nonprofit or for-profit hospitals.

The following important types of short-term hospitals will be discussed: teaching, those in multihospital systems, public, and rural. These categories are not mutually exclusive. For example, Bellevue Hospital in New York City's Health and Hospital Corporation is a public teaching hospital that is part of a multihospital system.

Teaching Hospitals. In 1986, according to Fishman (personal communication, 1988), there were 358 nonfederal hospitals belonging to the Council of Teaching Hospitals (COTH) of the Association of American Medical Colleges. Relative to other hospitals, COTH hospitals are larger and are located in large urban areas. They offer more specialized services and provide more uncompensated care than non-COTH hospitals. In 1986, 53% of COTH hospitals averaged 5.9 times the volume of outpatient visits and performed an average of 4 times more surgical operations than did non-COTH hospitals. COTH hospitals averaged 5.9 times more employees than non-COTH hospitals.

Because of their commitment to the triad of teaching hospital missions— education, research, and patient care—COTH members also offer a large percentage of tertiary or highly complex services. For example, in 1986, 87% of COTH members reported having a cardiac catheterization lab (vs. 16% for non-COTH members); 74% reported a megavoltage radiation facility (only 13% for non-COTH hospitals), and 45% of COTH institutions reported the capability to perform organ transplants (only 3% of non-COTH hospitals reported having this service).

COTH members care for a disproportionate number of the poor. In 1985 nonfederal members of COTH had 20% of the nation's short-stay beds but 30% of the Medicaid bad debts and charity care; in 1984, COTH members comprised 6% of the nation's short-term nonfederal hospitals but claimed 49% of the total deductions for charity care ($1.2 billion) and 36% of the deductions for bad debt ($2.5 billion).

Multihospital Systems. Hospitals are part of a multihospital system when they are either leased under contract management or are legally incorporated by or under the direction of a board that determines the control of two or more hospitals (Ermann & Gabel). In 1986, there were 278 multihospital systems which included 2,514 hospitals and 429,837 beds. (AHA, 1987). In 1986, 44% of the nation's hospitals and beds were in multihospital systems.

Once the largest chain, Hospital Corporation of America (HCA), founded in 1968 with one hospital, sold 104 facilities to an employee group in 1987. HCA now owns 83 facilities and 18,700 beds which produced $2.9 billion in revenues in 1986–1987, 80 percent of HCA's total sales.

Large multihospital systems are not restricted to ownership and management of hospitals. National Medical Enterprises, another investor-owned system, is the fifth largest operator of domestic acute-care hospitals. Through a subsidiary, it is also the second largest nursing home operator. In addition, the company owns psychiatric hospitals, retirement centers, hospices, home health care agencies, durable medical equipment, and management contract businesses and entered the preferred provider organization business (Johnson. 1984.)

According to Ermann and Gabel (1984), investor-owned and nonprofit systems have different patterns of growth. Investor-owned systems average 23 hospitals per system and tend to be dispersed among many states. Individual nonprofit systems average 7 hospitals per system and tend to be regional, located in one or two states.

Large, public multihospital systems include those of the federal Veteran's Administration with over 160 hospitals, and the Health and Hospitals Corporation of New York City, whose 11 short-term hospitals have 7,778 beds. Large nonprofit hospital systems include the 28 Kaiser hospitals, which are part of the Kaiser-Permanente prepaid group practice system, (with revenues of over $4.8 billion in 1987) and the 28 hospitals owned by the Sisters of Mercy Health Corporation in three midwestern states.

Public Hospitals. Public hospitals are owned by agencies of federal, state, and local government. Federal hospitals typically have been designed for special beneficiaries: American Indians, merchant seamen, military personnel, and veterans. State hospitals typically have provided long-term psychiatric and chronic care, in the past especially for patients with tuberculosis. There are also state university or teaching hospitals that provide short-term general acute care.

There are two main types of local, short-term, general public hospitals. The first type has similar characteristics to smaller nonprofit hospitals, is located in small towns or cities of moderate size, is used by private attending physicians, and serves paying and indigent patients.

The second type is located in major urban areas. Physician staff is mostly salaried and mostly residents in training. The hospital's deficits are paid for from taxes. As of 1986, there were 1,556 state and local government general and other special hospitals with a total of 185,000 beds (AHA, 1987b). These 1,556 hospitals (27% of all community hospitals) provided 19% of the beds, 18% of the inpatient admissions, and 22% of the outpatient visits for all community hospitals (AHA, 1987b).

The urban public general hospitals usually provide care for poor persons, including an estimated 5 million undocumented aliens (Friedman). They often are the only institutions that will provide care for persons with special social problems: the "shopping bag lady," the poor prostitute, the poor drug addict or alcoholic, the disruptive psychiatric patient, the destitute aged person, and the prisoner. In certain areas, they are the only source of care for patients with special medical problems: the badly burned, the distressed neonate, the high-risk mother, and the victim of accidental or criminal life-threatening trauma (Friedman). In many areas they are also an important locus for health sciences education and for local employment.

Problems of public hospitals may include poor management, which can be due to a cumbersome civil service or patronage job system. Some public hospitals are saddled with the "pauper stigma," which has a long history and is deeply ingrained in the national psyche. Staffing by medical school specialty physicians, where it occurs, often impedes the development of comprehensive care. The location of hospitals in declining and poor urban areas results in more poor clients and more difficulty in recruiting staff.

Where municipal hospitals are the principal teaching institutions of medical schools—New York's Bellevue, Boston's City, New Orleans' Charity, Chicago's Cook County, and Los Angeles' General—the technical medical quality is probably superior to that of the average community hospital. However, with regard to surroundings, amenities, overall staffing, buildings, equipment, and budgeting, many local government hospitals are distinctly inferior.

Rural Hospitals. Rural areas are areas falling outside a metropolitan statistical area, which is defined as containing a city with a population of at least 50,000 or an urban area with a population of at least 50,000 and a total metropolitan population of at least 100,000 (AHA, 1988). In 1986, 2,638 of the nation's hospitals (46%) were rural. Seventy-one percent had fewer than 100 beds. Ten percent were investor-owned, 49% were private nonprofit institutions, and 41% were public facilities operated by state or local governments. The heaviest concentration of rural hospitals and hospital beds is in the West North Central United States, where three-quarters of the community hospitals and nearly 44% of staffed beds are in rural areas (AHA, 1988).

Between 1981 and 1986, admissions to rural hospitals dropped from 8.4 million to 6.4 million, a 24% decline. In 1986, rural hospital occupancy averaged 55%, and 37 rural hospitals closed. Key problems of rural hospitals include: threat of closure, thereby depriving local residents of access to care; the questionable financial viability of hospitals with fewer than 50 beds; difficulties in assuring quality of care in such hospitals when operated as independent units; and, difficulties in attracting skilled professionals to work in isolated rural localities. Rural American counties face different kinds of problems depending on economic structure. Although they are often thought to consist only of farm areas, rural counties can be classified as economically dependent on farming;

manufacturing; mining; oil and energy; large federal, state, or local government installations; federal lands; and retirement settlement communities or characterized by persistent poverty (AHA, 1988).

To survive in more competitive hospital markets, rural hospitals have undertaken a variety of innovative measures. According to the AHA rural hospital assessment (1988), these include seeking to increase patient volume by introducing or expanding ambulatory or long-term services. Many have sought to expand technological capabilities, increase referrals, or reduce costs through shared service or networking arrangements and consolidation activities.

Factors Affecting Costs

The determination of what should be appropriate hospital supply, utilization, and costs is a complicated subject about which the experts disagree.

Components of Hospital Costs

Bed supply is computed in terms of beds per 1,000 population. This bed-to-population ratio can be computed within age groups to avoid bias in interpreting use among populations. For example, the elderly use more hospital services than those in other age groups. Utilization is also computed in terms of admissions to the hospital per unit population and by length of hospital stay per admission.

Hospitals costs are composed of units of hospital service multiplied by cost per unit of service. For example, inpatient care in a 400-bed hospital may cost $300 per day if the hospital operates at 75% occupancy (300 occupied beds × 365 days per year), or $43,850,000 on an annual basis. Hospital costs can be lowered in many ways, such as by decreasing the cost per day or by reducing the cost per hospital stay for a particular diagnosis. Hospital costs can be decreased by shutting down hospitals or parts of hospitals, assuming the same number of days of hospitalization.

Hospital costs are composed of fixed and variable costs. *Fixed costs* stay the same as patient volume increases or decreases, within limits, while *variable costs* vary with higher and lower volume. If a wing of a hospital or an entire hospital is closed, this will eliminate certain fixed costs as well as variable costs, while if an existing wing or hospital is used less extensively without shutting down an entire unit, this only decreases variable costs and not fixed costs.

An Example[1]

Let us use a fictitious example to illustrate how decreasing the supply of beds and also decreasing the length of stay per admission will impact on hospital costs and

[1] I wish to acknowledge the assistance of Carol Noyes Marais in preparing this example.

Table 7.4 Hospital Supply, Utilization, and Costs in Years 1 and 2 in City X with Population of 1,000,000

Y1		
(1) Bed capacity (4.0 per 1,000)		4,000
(2) Patient days at 75% occupancy (4,000 beds × 365 days × 75%	=	1,095,000
(3) Cost at $300 per day (1,095,000 patient days × $300)	=	$328,500,000
(4) Admissions (1,095,000 patient days ÷ 7.6-day average length of stay)	=	144,079
Y2		
(1) Bed capacity (3.6 per 1,000) (decrease by 10%)		3,600
(2) Patient days (decrease length of stay by 10%) (144,079 admissions × 6.84-day average length of stay)	=	985,000
(3) Cost at $300 per day (985,500 patient days × $300)	=	$295,650,000
(4) Occupancy (985,500 actual patient days ÷ 1,314,000 available patient days)	=	75%

SAVINGS
$328,500,000 − $295,650,000 = $ 32,850,000 or 10%

capacity. Assume in year 1 (as shown in Table 7.4) a hospital per diem rate of $300 (or $2,280 per 7.6-day stay) in a city with a population of 1 million and a ratio of 4.0 beds per 1,000 people. Assume that in year 2 the same number of hospital admissions and the same resources per day are used to provide care. But now decrease hospital bed capacity by 10% and also decrease the average length of patient stay by 10%. Other things being equal, this would result in savings of $32.85 million, or 10%, and the same hospital occupancy rate of 75%. Other things are not equal, however. In reality, the effect on costs of decreasing capacity varies depending upon how many beds are taken out of service in how many hospitals. If hospital costs are similar in each of ten 400-bed hospitals, cost savings will be greater through closure of one hospital than through taking out of service one 40-bed wing in all 10 hospitals. This is because fixed costs eliminated by closure of an entire hospital are greater than fixed costs eliminated by closing 10 nursery units in 10 hospitals. Fixed costs include costs such as a proportion of the administrator's salary or of the salary of the security force or of the heating bill, which continue if one nursing unit is closed but not if one entire hospital is closed.

The purpose of this example is to begin to outline the factors that affect hospital costs and that policymakers and managers attempt therefore to influence. To illustrate the further complexity underlying the same example, costs per hospital day may actually increase in year 2 because of inflation and because more employees or more highly skilled employees and more nonlabor inputs of higher cost are used to provide the same days of service. This effect is called "increased intensity of service." Area hospital costs may rise even if one hospital is actually closed, for example, if it is a low-cost hospital and if other hospitals' costs per day of care do not fall because of higher volume. Even if area costs do not rise, access costs will increase for patients who live near a hospital that is closed.

Hospital Utilization

There are several measures of hospital utilization, including number of admissions; average daily census (average number of patients in the hospital); occupancy rate (percentage of beds occupied); average length of stay; total patient days (average daily census multiplied by number of days in time period considered); and discharges. These data can be modified and compared in various cross-tabulations: by geography (region, state); by hospital characteristics (bed, size, type, category of ownership); and by patient age, sex, and demographic modifiers. Analyses of hospital utilization data are vast; I shall cover only a portion of them.

In 1986 there were 35.2 million admissions to hospitals in the United States (AHA, 1987b). Of the admissions, 92% were to community hospitals, and 73% of the patient days were in such hospitals (AHA, 1987b). Although only 1.4% of admissions were to nonfederal short- and long-term psychiatric hospitals, these accounted for 16% of the total average daily census.

There are many determinants of hospital admission. Being separated or divorced, having comprehensive insurance, and having a long traveling time to a regular source of care all increase an individual's chance of being hospitalized (Andersen, et al., p. 13). Length of stay in a hospital varies by sex, age, and diagnosis, as well as family structure, degree of anxiety about health, beliefs about health care, and availability of alternatives to hospitalization, such as nursing homes and home health services (Andersen et al., p. 13).

Women are more likely to be hospitalized than are men (NCHS, 1983a p. 144). When obstetrical admissions are eliminated, the average length of stay (ALOS) is about the same for males and females. Length of stay in a hospital decreases as the patient's level of education and income rise, and it increases with age (Phelps, p. 112).

The use of community hospitals varies among age groups. In 1981, persons aged 65 years and over were discharged from the hospital at 2.7 times the rate of persons aged 15 to 44 and 5.4 times the rate of those under 15 years of age (NCHS, 1983b p. 148).

Diagnosis-specific length of stay has been declining with medical progress. In the 1950s physicians often recommended hospital stays of 4 to 8 weeks for a myocardial infarction. In the 1960s, for an uncomplicated myocardial infarction, this was shortened to 3 weeks, to 2 weeks in the 1970s, and then to 7 to 10 days in the 1980s. One study reports the theory that safe discharge can begin as early as day 3, and in the United Kingdom physicians have tried to take care of the patient exclusively at home, although neither of the latter two approaches is recommended in a recent *New England Journal of Medicine* editorial (Curfman).

In 1985 the most common DRGs (diagnosis related groups) accounted for 34.5% of all discharges in Farley's (1988) sample of 600 hospitals, as shown in Table 7.5. The percentage of total discharges associated with these 20 DRGs was quite stable between 1980 and 1985, increasing only 2.6%. However, there were large changes in individual case-mix proportions ranging from up by more than 84% for angina pectoris (DRG 140) to down by more than 72% for dilation and curettage (DRG 364). Changing coding practices to enhance hospital reimbursement explain part of this difference. Changing practice patterns or medical technology explain another part, such as knee procedures without complicating condition (DRG 222). For certain medical conditions, patients have moved from inpatient to outpatient settings (Farley).

The ALOS in community hospitals in 1986 was 7.1 days (AHA, 1987b). This compares with 7.7 days in 1976. There is wide variation in length of stay by age (AHA, 1985). In the third quarter of 1984, patients aged 65 and over stayed an average of about 8.8 days; those 65 and under stayed about 5.6 days per admission (AHA, 1985). There is variation in the ALOS by region and hospital bed size. For example, the ALOS in community hospitals ranged from 5.2 in Utah and 5.5 in Washington to 9.0 in Minnesota and 9.1 in New York (AHA, 1987b). In 1986 ALOS in community not-for-profit hospitals ranged from 4.6 days in hospitals with fewer than 25 beds to 7.9 days in hospitals with more than 500 beds. Variation in ALOS by hospital size may be explained in part by variation in severity of disease, but regional differences are difficult to explain on medical bases alone. In 1986 ALOS variance by type of short-term hospital was 6.1 days in investor-owned hospitals and 7.2 days in the nonprofits, with local government hospitals averaging 7.4 days (AHA, 1987b).

While cutting back on inpatient acute-care days, hospitals have increased services in the areas of long-term care and ambulatory care. The increases have not been great, if any at all, in the areas of emergency care and outpatient care, where there have been increases in visits to physicians' offices and freestanding ambulatory care and urgent care centers. The increases in hospital ambulatory care services have been in ambulatory surgery, health promotion, home care, hospice care, and chemical dependency (see Table 7.6).

With regard to long-term care, hospitals have increasingly converted acute-care beds to long-term care. This includes both skilled care and custodial care beds. From 1982 to 1986 the number of hospitals with SNF and other long-term-care beds increased as shown in Table 7.7.

Swing beds are hospital beds that can be used to provide either acute care long-term care (stays in swing beds average under 30 days). Medicare has approved payment for this kind of long-term care subject to specified requirements for hospitals of under 100 beds. From 1982 to 1986 the number of swing beds and reporting hospitals increased as shown in Table 7.8.

What Do Hospital Services Cost?

An article in *Harpers* in March 1984 details how high hospital costs can be (Hellerstein). Costs are presented for 25 days in the life of "Mrs. K.," whose hospital stay was in a New York City hospital. Costs are probably higher in this hospital, because of its location, age, and other factors, than in most other hospitals, and are certainly higher for this episode of illness because of the special services that Mrs. K. received. (Costs are higher in 1989 than in 1983.) Total costs for 25 days in the hospital, nearly all of this intensive care, were $47,311. This did not include the doctor's bills.

A breakdown of these charges by category of service is shown in Table 7.9. This is about $1,900 per day. During the 25-day stay, there were charges for 660 services, or an average of 26 per day. Billing for the fifth day of care is shown in Table 7.10; 42 services were billed on that day alone. Amounts ranged from $2.25 for a pharmacy item (14 pharmacy items are billed for, including $113.50 for IV solutions) to $500 for a room in the intensive care unit. Total charges for 1 day of care were $2,473.10, of which Blue Cross paid $2,259.10 (Blue Cross does not pay blood charges, which were $214).

Mrs. K. died on the 25th day. Questions can be raised as to whether all of these services were necessary, whether they could be provided more cheaply, and whether Mrs. K.'s admission was necessary. If she were going to die anyway within 25 days, should $47,311 have been spent on her care? How one might answer these questions may differ depending on whether one is Mrs. K's daughter, the hospital administrator, or Mrs. K's employer.

Economic Impact

The impact of hospitals on local economies can be very important. In small communities, hospital closure can remove a vital source of local employment and revenues to local hospital suppliers. Construction of a hospital means numerous jobs for construction workers and future hospital employees.

Ginzberg and Drennan (1985) have estimated the economic impact of hospitals in New York City to include the following: In 1983, the city's 102 hospitals spent $8.2 billion dollars. In 1981, these hospitals employed 127,676 workers. Also in 1981, 120,000 out-of-city patients (11% of discharges) received inpatient services in New York City hospitals. According to Ginzberg and Drennan, revenues from such patients are equal to those spent by 600,000 tourists on 4-day visits. Assuming a per diem inpatient average reimbursement rate of $360 and an average stay of 10.2 days, 120,000 nonlocal patients generated hospital revenues

Table 7.5 Casemix Proportions (Percent of Discharges) and ALOS (Days) for 20 Most Common DRGs, 1980 and 1985 Averages and 1980–85 Percent Change

Diagnosis related group (DRG)	Percent of discharges			DRG-specific ALOS (days)		
	1980 average	1985 average	1980–85 percent change	1980 average	1985 average	1980–85 percent change
391 Normal newborns	7.27	7.34	+ 1.0	3.44	2.90	–15.7
373 Vaginal delivery without complicating diagnosis	6.28	6.36	+ 1.3	3.24	2.63	–18.8
243 Medical back problems	2.33	2.21	– 5.2	8.33	5.90	–29.2
183 Esophagitis, gastroenteritis, and miscellaneous digestive diagnoses, age 18–69 without complicating condition	1.86	1.15	–38.2	4.65	3.60	–22.6
182 Esophagitis, gastroenteritis and miscellaneous digestive diagnoses, age greater than 69 or complicating condition	1.37	1.52	+10.9	6.95	5.51	–20.7
371 Cesarean section without complicating condition	1.31	1.90	+45.0	6.21	5.09	–18.0
39 Lens procedures	1.25	.55	–56.0	3.74	1.78	–52.4
355 Nonradical hysterectomy, age less than 70 without complicating condition	1.31	1.27	– 3.1	7.62	5.96	–21.8
127 Heart failure and shock	1.28	1.83	+43.0	10.67	8.22	–23.0
140 Angina pectoris	.86	1.59	+84.9	6.76	4.93	–27.1

14 Specific cardiovascular disorders, except transitory ischemia attacks	.97	1.24	+27.8	15.39	12.01	-22.0
430 Psychoses	.93	1.46	+57.0	16.74	15.06	-10.0
88 Chronic obstructive pulmonary disease	.91	.71	-22.0	10.35	8.50	-17.9
89 Simple pneumonia or pleurisy, age greater than 69 or complicating condition	.75	1.29	+72.0	11.24	8.83	-21.4
184 Esophagitis, gastroenteritis, and miscellaneous digestive diagnoses, age 0–17	.81	.73	– 9.9	3.67	2.94	-19.9
122 Circulatory disorders with acute myocardial infarction without cardiovascular complications, discharged alive	.84	.82	– 2.4	12.91	8.70	-32.6
364 Dilation and curettage with conization, except for malignancy	1.08	.30	-72.2	2.26	1.74	-23.0
390 Néonates with other significant problems	.68	1.10	+61.8	4.16	3.33	-20.0
294 Diabetes, age greater than 35	.80	.62	-22.5	9.29	7.43	-20.0
222 Knee procedures, age less than 70 without complicating condition	.74	.48	-35.1	5.03	2.77	-44.9
All patients in 20 most common DRGs, combined	33.61	34.48	+ 2.6	6.06	5.18	-14.6

Note: Calculations based on HCUP-2 patient records for 1980 and 1985. DRG rankings are based on 1982 HCUP-2 data.
Source: D. F. Farley, *Trends in Hospital Average Lengths of Stay, Casemix and Discharge Rates, 1980–1985.* (DHHS Publication No. (PHS) 88-3420), Hospital Studies Program, Research Note 11, National Center for Health Services Research and Health Care Technology Assessment. Rockville, MD: Public Health Services, p. 12.

Table 7.6 Selected Hospital-sponsored Ambulatory Care Utilization Trends, 1982–1987

	1982	1987[b]	% Change 1982–1987
Visits (in thousands)[a]			
Ambulatory surgery[c]	4,275	10,358	142.2
Emergency department	81,147	84,580	4.2
Organized outpatient Department[d]	313,666	309,364	–1.4
Programs (no. of hospitals)[e]			
Health promotion	2,324	4,583	97.2
Home care	784	2,018	157.4
Hospice	487	940	93.0
Rehabilitation	2,048	2,397	17.0
Psychiatry	1,227	1,437	17.1
Chemical dependency	1,009	1,448	43.5

[a]AHA annual survey.
[b]Projected figures, Division of Ambulatory Care, Health Promotion, and Women's and Children's Health.
[c]Surgical services provided to patients who do not remain in the hospital overnight.
[d]Visits by patients who are not lodged in the hospital while receiving medical, dental, or other services. Each appearance by an outpatient to each unit of the hospital counts as one outpatient visit.
[e]AHA Hospital Statistics; number of hospitals reporting for each year was approximately 90%.
Source: Division of Ambulatory Care, Health Promotion and Women's and Children's Health, American Hospital Association, 1987d.

Table 7.7 SNF Beds in Hospitals, 1982 and 1986

Year	No. of hospitals	% Hospitals	No. of beds
1982	797	12.8	56,336
1986	979	15.5	63,667
Other long-term-care beds			
1982	405	6.5	34,317
1986	559	8.9	38,478

Source: AHA Annual Survey, 1987e.

Table 7.8 Swing Beds in Hospitals 1982 and 1986[a]

Year	No. of hospitals reporting they have swing beds	No. of hospitals listing actual no. of beds	No. of swing beds
1982	63	60	824
1986	825	820	14,568

[a]This includes both Medicare-certified and noncertified beds.
Source: AHA Annual Survey, 1987e.

Table 7.9 Breakdown of Charges for Services Rendered to "Mrs. K." during 25-day Hospitalization

Intensive care	$12,000
Laboratory	11,201
Therapy	8,734
Drugs	6,365
Supplies	3,698
X-ray	2,870
Blood service	1,389
Operating room	521
EKG, EEG, etc.	366
Miscellaneous	167
Total	$47,311

of $440 million in 1 year. Applying an economic multiplier effect of about 2.0, as is done in analyzing tourist spending, the total economic impact of non-city-resident hospital stays is estimated at $888 million. Hospital expenditures, therefore, have an impact on the revenue side for hospital employees and suppliers as well as on the cost side for taxpayers and insurance purchasers.

Hospital Organizational Structure

The principal departments of the acute-care general hospital are the medical and , dental, nursing, other diagnostic and therapeutic support, financial, personnel, and hotel services. Most hospitals provide services both to inpatients who are admitted and assigned a bed and to outpatients who come to an emergency department, an outpatient clinic, or for a diagnostic or therapeutic service for a procedure not requiring admission.

Medical and Dental Departmental Organization

Physicians and dentists relate to hospitals in different ways. Attending physicians on the hospital staff who are not salaried often conduct much of their business in private offices that they own or rent. These physicians may admit patients to more than one hospital and may compete with the hospital for patients or customers. Other physicians may be salaried or paid by the hospital, relative to the amount of hospital work they do. These physicians often see patients or perform related activities in offices that are provided for them by the hospital. Some hospitals employ physicians to provide primary care in competition with other physicians who are attendings or local non-hospital-affiliated practitioners.

Table 7.10 Cost for One Day of Hospital Care for "Mrs. K."

Date	Description	Code	Total charges	First insurance charge	Due from patient
09/30	LAB AUTO BLOOD CT	1402101	$ 17.00	$ 17.00	
09/30	LAB CHEM—8	1401111	31.00	31.00	
09/30	LAB CHEM—8	1401111	31.00	31.00	
09/30	LAB DIFF	1402099	15.00	15.00	
09/30	SP HEM COAG STDY COM	1602007	$239.00	239.00	
09/30	SP HEMATOLOGY	1600000	49.00	49.00	
09/30	SP HEM RETIC CT	1602044	17.00	17.00	
09/30	SP HEM CBC	1602010	28.00	28.00	
09/30	LAB BACTERIA SM	1405011	16.00	16.00	
09/30	LAB ACT PAR THROM	1404001	27.00	27.00	
09/30	LAB PROTH DETER	1404011	17.00	17.00	
09/30	LAB FIBRIN QUAN	1404007	40.00	40.00	
09/30	LAB AUTO BLOOD CT	1402101	17.00	17.00	
09/30	LAB CHEM—20	1401104	31.00	31.00	
09/30	LAB TBC CULT	1405014	42.00	42.00	
09/30	LAB CHEM—20	1401104	31.00	31.00	
09/30	LAB RTN CULT	1405003	37.00	37.00	
09/30	LAB RTN CULT	1405003	37.00	37.00	
09/30	BLD BD ADMN FEE	1701028	207.00	207.00	
09/30	X-RAY CHEST—BED	1501128	74.00	74.00	
09/30	X-RAY CHEST—BED	1501128	74.00	74.00	
09/30	PHAR IV SOLUTIONS	2601003	16.00	16.00	
09/30	PHARMACY	2601000	39.00	39.00	
09/30	PHAR IV SOLUTIONS	2601003	21.00	21.00	
09/30	PHAR IV SOLUTIONS	2601003	16.00	16.00	
09/30	PHARMACY	2601000	3.70	3.70	
09/30	PHARMACY	2601000	13.50	13.50	
09/30	PHARMACY	2601000	11.00	11.00	
09/30	PHARMACY	2601000	2.40	2.40	
09/30	PHAR IV SOLUTIONS	2601003	21.00	21.00	
09/30	PHAR IV SOLUTIONS	2601003	21.00	21.00	
09/30	PHAR IV SOLUTIONS	2601003	18.50	18.50	
09/30	PHARMACY	2601000	2.25	2.25	
09/30	PHARMACY	2601000	2.25	2.25	
09/30	PHARMACY	2601000	2.50	2.50	
09/30	PLAT CONC PROC FEE	1701014	188.00		$188.00
09/30	FRSH FR PLA PROC FEE	1701019	26.00		26.00
09/30	INHAL RESPIRATOR	2102015	119.00	119.00	
09/30	DRESSING SET DISP	2708041	7.00	7.00	
09/30	VEST RESTRAINT	2709032	12.00	12.00	
09/30	INHAL BLOOD GAS MONT	2101034	354.00	354.00	
09/30	ROOM ICU		500.00	500.00	

Other hospitals contract with physician groups to provide emergency care or subspecialist services on hospital premises or in satellite centers. Some physicians are attendings who maintain their own practices distinct from the hospital but who also receive a part-time salary from the hospital for administrative work.

When physicians admit patients to the hospital, in most instances they are free to order whatever tests or treatments they deem necessary. Thus the physician basically determines the amount of services used and the consequent costs of patient care. Physicians have every reason to want the best possible hospital setting in which to practice medicine, especially when it is provided at little personal cost to them.

Although the physician is technically a guest in the hospital, the hospital is responsible for the care its staff renders patients on a physician's orders. Until relatively recently, hospitals could not be held liable for the wrongful conduct of a physician, but this principle has been significantly changed by a series of judicial decisions (Southwick, 1978b). Changing legal doctrines regarding negligence and the corporate liability of hospitals have established that hospitals are legally responsible and, to the extent that hospital negligence is involved, financially responsible for the care provided by their entire professional staff, including physicians.

Physicians are primarily organized along the lines of the medical specialties. The larger the hospital and the more specialized the medical services, the greater the number of separate medical departments. There is no universal logic to the way in which medical departments are categorized. Some are separated from the others by type of skill involved, some by the age or sex of their main patient group, and some by the organ or organ system that is their primary purview. Departments found in most hospitals include

1. *Internal medicine:* general diagnosis and therapy of adults for problems involving one or more internal organs or the skin, in which the principal tools do not involve a physical alteration of the patient's body by the physician.
2. *Surgery:* diagnosis and therapy in which the principal tools involve a physical alteration of a part of the patient's body by the physician.
3. *Pediatrics:* general diagnosis and therapy for children, primarily but not entirely with nonsurgical techniques.
4. *Obstetrics/gynecology:* diagnosis and therapy relating to the sexual and reproductive system of women, using both surgical and nonsurgical techniques.
5. *Psychiatry/neurology:* diagnosis and therapy for people of all ages with mental, emotional, and nervous system problems, using primarily nonsurgical techniques.
6. *Radiology/diagnostic imaging:* diagnosis and therapy, primarily through the use of x-ray and other internal imaging techniques.

7. *Pathology:* diagnosis, both before and after treatment.
8. *Anesthesiology:* principally concerned with preparing patients so that they may be surgically operated upon with no pain or discomfort during the procedure.

Other general medical departments include family and emergency medicine. Other, more subspecialized medical departments tend to be organized around organs and organ systems, for example, ophthalmology (eye); otolaryngology (ear, nose, and throat); urology (male sexual/reproductive system and the renal system for both males and females); orthopedics (bones and joints); and so on.

There are 23 medical specializations for which professional certification may be attained by passing a medical specialty board examination. Specialties other than the ones previously mentioned include allergy and immunology, proctology, dermatology, neurosurgery, nuclear medicine, physical medicine and rehabilitation, plastic surgery, preventive medicine, and thoracic surgery. There are clinicians other than physicians who also may be granted admitting privileges to a hospital; these include dentists and podiatrists.

Physicians and dentists practicing in hospitals have their own medical and dental staff organization, with bylaws, rules, and regulations that must be approved by the hospital's governing board. The medical staff bylaws specify procedures for election of medical staff officers by membership. The officers are given authority under the bylaws to enforce rules and regulations. The officers delineate privileges and recommend disciplinary action when necessary, through the committee structure. They enforce the bylaws and must oversee the committee structure and submit reports of medical staff activities to the governing board.

There are numerous medical staff committees in the hospital, some of which may include nonphysicians, particularly nurses, as members. The executive committee, if there is one, coordinates all activity, sets general policies for the medical staff, and accepts and acts upon recommendations from the other medical staff committees. The joint conference committee, if there is one, acts as a liaison between the medical staff and the governing board in deliberations over matters involving medical and nonmedical considerations. The credentials committee reviews applications by physicians to join the medical staff and considers the qualifications of education, experience, and interests before making recommendations to the executive committee, which will then make recommendations for appointment to the governing board. In some hospitals the joint conference committee is also involved in the process.

The infections control committee is responsible for preventing infections in the hospital, through routine preventive surveillance, tracking down of outbreaks of infection, and education of hospital personnel. The pharmacy and therapeutics committee reviews pharmacologic agents for inclusion in the list of drugs approved for use in the hospital. The tissue committee is responsible for ensuring quality control of surgery, principally by examining and evaluating bodily tissues removed during operations.

The medical records committee is responsible for certifying complete and clinically accurate documentation of the care given to patients. This committee also acts as a judge of clinical care, based on the written record. The utilization review committee evaluates the appropriateness of admissions and length of stay in the hospital and may review use of services and facilities for patients whose hospital care is being paid for by Medicare, Medicaid, and in certain cases by private insurers.

The tissue, quality assurance, and utilization review committees provide for review of each physician's professional work by other physicians. As the hospital has become more complicated and more critical of medical practice, the medical staff has been subjected to more scrutiny. In the hospital, the medical chain of authority exists side by side with an administrative chain. There are many areas of confused jurisdiction and overlapping or conflicting powers. Managers and physicians working together can attempt to integrate these hierarchies. Physicians are becoming more involved in hospital governing boards; boards of trustees are reviewing more closely the methods used to appoint physicians to hospital staff; and more full-time salaried physicians have been hired by hospitals, resulting in more direct physician-hospital reporting lines.

Because of the vested interests of various medical departments in a hospital, the addition of a full-time or part-time salaried chief of the medical staff and of medical departments can create latent or open conflict with trustees or management. To lessen controversy, in some hospitals appointments of chiefs are made for a specified period of time rather than for indefinite or lifetime tenure. As full-time chiefs of service become more common, many functions formerly handled by volunteer committees—such as quality-of-care review, medical records, and continuing medical education—have been taken over by full-time paid employees.

Many hospitals are now hiring salaried medical directors and quality-of-care review teams. As hospitals are made more accountable for alleged misconduct of attending physicians, much attention has been focused on the concept of due process. If a physician is to be deprived of his medical staff privileges, the process by which the decision is made must be capable of standing up to the scrutiny of the courts (Southwick, 1978a). Further, many hospitals now require physicians to have malpractice insurance as a condition of staff membership (Hollowell).

There were 73,171 resident physicians in training in American hospitals in 1986 (AMA). The number of hospital-salaried physicians other than resident physicians has more than quadrupled, from 10,000 in 1963 to 46,408 in 1986 AMA). Salaried physicians are employed in the hospital to supervise medical care in intensive care units, outpatient departments, and medical education. Attending physicians are affected by such hiring, as hospital-employed physicians may compete with them for patients, deny them medical staff privileges (particularly to physicians new to the community), more closely supervise their practices, and change a traditional patient-care orientation to more emphasis on teaching and research.

Models of Medical Services Organization

Shortell (1985) has conceptualized four different models of organization among physicians: traditional (departmental), divisional, independent-corporate, and parallel. Under the traditional model, while each department retains relevant medical specialists, it does not contain the support services required by the physicians to provide care. These include nursing, housekeeping, dietary, and clerical staff. Figure 7.1 illustrates a traditional hospital organizational chart, in which support services are organized separately from medical services. The medical staff's relationship to the hospital is indirect, as shown by the dotted line. Physicians are not a part of the hospital chain of command, as are nurses or assistant administrators. In hospitals, this is referred to as a *dual authority structure* (Smith, 1955). Most physicians are not hospital employees. Many physicians do not see themselves as obeying the hospital administration but rather as independent practitioners who must practice according to medical staff bylaws, rules, and regulations.

Shortell's second model of medical services organization, the divisional model, is characterized by the placement of functional support services within medical divisions, which are organized along departmental lines. Each division, such as medicine or physical medicine, includes many of the support services, such as nursing and clerical (and sometimes dietary and medical records and other services), it needs to do its tasks. Each medical division leaders is responsible for management, including financial management, of both medical and support services. The Johns Hopkins Hospital in Baltimore, Maryland, is organized along these lines (Heyssell et al.).

Under Shortell's third model, the independent-corporate model, the medical staff becomes a separate legal entity that negotiates with the hospital for its services in return for receiving support services. An independent group of physicians provides medical services to the hospital, under contract. A version of this type of model of organization is carried out by the Permanente medical groups, which have contractual relationships with the Kaiser Health Plan to form the Kaiser-Permanente medical care program, the nation's largest health maintenance organization.

Shortell's fourth model, the parallel model, involves the creation of a separate organization in order to conduct certain activities that are not handled well by the formal hospital organization. Certain physicians are selected to participate in a

Figure 7.1 Traditional (Departmental) Organizational Structure for Hospital Medical Services

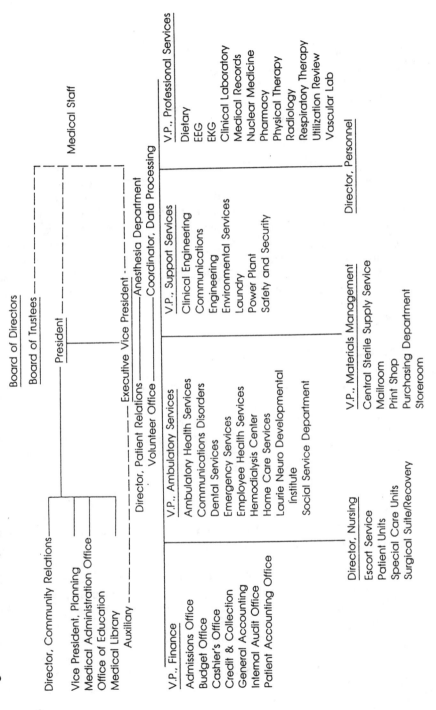

Board of Directors

Board of Trustees

President

Medical Staff

Executive Vice President

Director, Patient Relations
Anesthesia Department
Volunteer Office
Coordinator, Data Processing

Director, Community Relations

Vice President, Planning
Medical Administration Office
Office of Education
Medical Library
Auxiliary

V.P., Professional Services
Dietary
EEG
EKG
Clinical Laboratory
Medical Records
Nuclear Medicine
Pharmacy
Physical Therapy
Radiology
Respiratory Therapy
Utilization Review
Vascular Lab

V.P., Support Services
Clinical Engineering
Communications
Engineering
Environmental Services
Laundry
Power Plant
Safety and Security

Director, Personnel

V.P., Ambulatory Services
Ambulatory Health Services
Communications Disorders
Dental Services
Emergency Services
Employee Health Services
Hemodialysis Center
Home Care Services
Laurie Neuro Developmental Institute
Social Service Department

V.P., Materials Management
Central Sterile Supply Service
Mailroom
Print Shop
Purchasing Department
Storeroom

V.P., Finance
Admissions Office
Budget Office
Cashier's Office
Credit & Collection
General Accounting
Internal Audit Office
Patient Accounting Office

Director, Nursing
Escort Service
Patient Units
Special Care Units
Surgical Suite/Recovery

parallel organization for some percentage of their time, to work on important problems and report back to the formal structure. Some of these physicians would have positions in the formal structure as well. Shortell reports that parallel structures have been implemented at Saint Johns Hospital in Santa Monica, California, and at Fairfax Hospital in Virginia.

Other Patient Care Services

The functional divisions of the nursing service follow the patterns discussed in Chapter 5. Hospital diagnostic and therapeutic services, which may or may not be attached to one of the medical departments, include laboratory, usually under the direction of the department of pathology; electrocardiography, usually a part of internal medicine; electroencephalography, part of neurology; radiography, part of radiology; pharmacy; clinical psychology; social service; inhalation therapy, often part of anesthesiology or pulmonary medicine; nutrition as therapy; physical, occupational, and speech therapy, often attached to the department of rehabilitation medicince if there is one; home care; and medical records, among others.

Hospital Administrative Structure

The nonclinical services that the hospital provides can be categorized into four subsystems; finance, facilities and equipment, human resources, and management.

The financial subsystem includes capital, operating costs, and cash budgeting; pricing and cost allocation; long-range financial planning; and collection policies. In addition, some hospitals also have endowments to invest and grants to prepare and administer.

The facilities and equipment subsystem includes dietary, engineering, and environmental services; clinical engineering; power plant; grounds; housekeeping, communications, and purchasing services; and storeroom, among others.

The human resources system includes job analysis and description, job evaluation, wage and salary administration, recruitment, screening and selection, communication to employees, training and development, organizational development, collective bargaining, and labor contract administration.

The management subsystem includes planning and marketing; community, patient, and public relations; data processing and management information systems; legal services; and compliance with regulations, among others.

The organizational structure for a multihospital system is more complex and comprises a central headquarters, sometimes an intermediate divisional organization as well as the hospitals and other health care organizations, as shown in Figure 7.2.

Figure 7.2 Multihospital System Organizational Chart

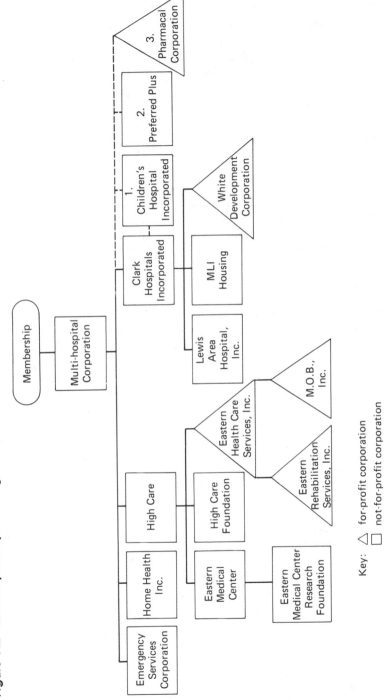

Key: △ for-profit corporation
      □ not-for-profit corporation

1. Participation Agreement with Multi-hospital; shared services with Clark Hospitals Incorporated

2. Management Contract

3. Joint Venture with Bliss Corporation (Multi-hospital owns ½ of the stock).

Forces Propelling and Constraining Change in Hospitals

As the 20-year period of expansion following passage of Medicare and Medicaid comes to an end, hospitals are changing rapidly. The forces that are constraining hospitals as they attempt to survive and grow include purchaser pressure for cost containment, competition from vertically integrated multihospital systems and local physicians, the conservatism of some traditionally oriented practicing physicians, the cost of rapidly changing new technology, slower growth of the national economy, and a changing philosophy of government toward hospital and health care expenditures.

The forces that are propelling hospitals to continued survival and growth include increased power of hospital managers, weakening power of physicians, new forms of hospital organizational structure, new markets for hospitals, the aging of the population, and changing customer expectations for service. These constraining and propelling forces are shown in Table 7.11.

Constraining Forces

Increasingly, limits are being placed on hospital reimbursement, at least for inpatient services. Revenues are being constrained in ways that they never have been previously. When costs run over the prospective reimbursable limits, this constrains future hospital investment and forces decision makers to make changes in the services they provide or in how they provide them. Furthermore, it is expected that the annual percentage increases allowed under the new reimbursement ceilings will increase more slowly than before, in relation to the historical ratio of medical to nonmedical price increases.

Large purchasers other than government, such as industrial corporations or coalitions of such corporations and their insurance carriers, are also pressing for

Table 7.11 Constraining and Propelling Forces Affecting Hospitals

Constraining	Propelling
1. Governmental and third party purchaser pressure for cost containment	1. New health markets other than inpatient care
2. Competition from multihospital systems and local physicians	2. Weakening power of physicians in the hospital
3. Conservatism of some traditionally oriented practicing physicians	3. New organizational structures
4. Cost of continuing technological advances	4. Increasing power of a more business-oriented management team
5. Slower growth of the economy	5. Aging of the population
6. Changing governmental philosophy toward health care	6. Changing customer expectations for service

cost containment. In exchange for "preferred provider" status and presumably increased or at least a guaranteed volume of business, hospitals are being required increasingly to offer discounted or guaranteed rates to large purchasers.

Hospitals in financial difficulty and lacking sophisticated managerial controls are increasingly merging with or being managed contractually by large multi-hospital systems, creating competition, a second external force constraining local hospitals. These systems, particularly those that are investor-owned, have greater access to capital markets as sources of money for expansion and renovation. As these systems lack local community ties, it is easier for them to close or sell local hospitals or particular services in geographical areas that are losing population or have increasing unemployment. There also is increased competition from local physicians. Hospitals are losing their monopoly in providing surgery, emergency care, diagnostic services, routine obstetrics, and rehabilitation. Such services are increasingly being provided locally by physicians and by new freestanding organizations, which are employing physicians who may be on a hospital's own attending staff.

A third constraining force is the continuing conservatism of older, more traditional attending physicians, who continue to view the hospital primarily as a doctors' workshop. From the perspective of these physicians, hospitals should be organized primarily to provide services to help physicians take care of their own patients. Physicians with these views lack interest in hospitals providing new services, which they may see as competitive with their own practices or as diluting allocation of resources away from the inpatient support services with which they are familiar and which they see as critical to their private practices.

The Medicare/Medicaid years have been marked by tremendous and costly technological changes in hospitals, the fourth constraining force. These include development and widespread implementation of computerized axial tomography (CAT) scanners, nuclear magnetic resonance (NMR) machines, radiation therapy, ultrasound, cardiac and intensive care, burn units, kidney dialysis, and organ transplants. It is difficult to forecast now what will be the high-technology innovations of the early 1990s, but they probably will be expensive. Fewer hospitals will be able to afford them or will wish to provide them because of the increased financial risks.

The same point applies to new technological advances in computers and information systems. Only certain hospitals, particularly those in multihospital systems, will be able to make the necessary investments and risk higher short-run costs now, in return for expected quicker response time, fewer recording errors, and eventual possible lower unit costs for greater volumes of information in the future.

The final two constraining forces on hospitals are the health of the economy and the philosophy of government officials toward hospital services. During the late 1970s and early 1980s, in contrast to the 40 years following World War II and including the last 20 years of Medicare and Medicaid expansion, the U.S.

economy has been growing at a much slower rate than it did previously. There is considerable feeling among federal and state government officials that not only must the rate of increase in hospital and health care expenditures be lowered but also that some competing areas of the economy require increased levels of investment relative to those required in health care. Such areas include defense; infrastructure, such as roads and bridges; criminal justice; and education.

Propelling Forces

Propelling forces are driving hospitals to respond to factors that threaten or constrain them and to take advantage of opportunities for enhanced survival and continuing growth. Our first propelling force is the identification and availability of new health care markets. Being constrained with regard to inpatient revenues, short-term hospitals are considering and implementing new services, such as home care and chronic care, which have been provided previously primarily by visiting nursing agencies, state mental hospitals, for-profit nursing homes, and other providers. Other newly organized services focus on ambulatory care. These include ambulatory surgery, freestanding emergency departments or urgent care centers, rehabilitation, day care, and health promotion/disease prevention programs. Some hospitals also are providing new support services in areas related to inpatient care, such as pharmacies, nurse registries, and parking lots, and even in areas not directly related to health care, such as motels and restaurants.

A second force propelling hospitals to move in new directions is the weakening organizational power of physicians in some hospitals, particularly those in multihospital systems. The accelerating development of a surplus supply of physicians diminishes physician leverage in opposing hospital responses to new market opportunities and enhances hospitals' negotiating positions with physicians for contractual relationships and joint ventures. It is becoming more difficult for physicians to gain hospital privileges or to admit patients to more than one primary hospital. Since multihospital systems operate in numerous markets rather than in a single geographical market, they tend to be less susceptible to local physician pressure than independent community hospitals.

Related to the weakening power of physicians in some hospitals are new organizational structures, a third propelling force and one that drives hospitals to focus effort in a few key directions. There may be separate organizations for different businesses, such as fundraising, research, or satellite health centers. Even within their main line of business—inpatient care—more hospitals are appointing medical directors and salaried chiefs of services to "administer" physician services. As physician leaders become more integrated into the hospital organizational structure, this streamlines the hospital decision-making process, thus enabling more options to be considered and implemented in a more timely way by hospital management.

A related, fourth propelling force is the increasing power, relative to that of the trustees and physicians, of a more business-oriented hospital management team. Medical services are being administered increasingly by salaried physician leaders who are being selected and rewarded for their management competence. Lay hospital managers are better trained and are being rewarded for taking more risks.

Partly as a result of improved medical care, life expectancy of Americans is increasing; hence, a fifth propelling force is the aging of the population. Those over 65 and those over 75 are making up an increasing proportion of the total population. The aged use more hospital services per capita than the rest of the population. They also use more of other types of health services, which hospitals also can provide and increasingly are providing. Such services range from retirement villages and congregate housing to nursing homes and include day-care, home care, and hospice care.

In a time of increasing competition among providers and of oversupply of providers, we can expect increased competition for hospitals in terms of quality of service as well as price. This is our sixth propelling force. In response to purchaser pressure, certain hospitals will compete primarily on price, while other hospitals will seek a niche in the marketplace by responding to the needs of those who are willing to pay more for customized services. For example, certain obstetrical hospitals can be marketed directly to women, more as a combination luxury hotel and beauty salon than as a workshop for physicians delivering babies for mothers. General hospitals may be preferred because, even though costs are higher, their food and nursing services are perceived to be better.

Summary

In this chapter we have reviewed the historical development of hospitals, key hospital characteristics, how hospitals differ from and are similar to each other, some of the key aspects of hospital costs, hospital organization, and some propelling and constraining forces for change in hospitals. Undaunted by the risks inherent in forecasting the future, I predict continuation of the following trends for hospitals in the early 1990s:

- Growth of larger multihospital systems that will become increasingly vertically integrated.
- Continuing high costs of hospital care.
- Increasingly differentiated hospitals or larger units within hospitals for patients of similar demographic characteristics and medical problems.
- Increasing standardization of treatment for patients of similar demographic characteristics and medical problems.

The reasons for these changes have to do with the increasing rationalization of the hospital industry. Larger hospital multiunit systems are formed for better response to competitive demands of large purchasers for adequate quality and lower cost. Such large systems can afford functional specialists in areas such as quality assurance and cost accounting and information systems so that treatment can be standardized and costs allocated for patients of similar age and sex and medical problems. New technology, information systems, and professional manpower is increasingly expensive, reimbursement is limited, and all hospitals cannot generate sufficient volume to provide a full range of services. So hospitals will increasingly specialize in the types of patients they can best take care of. This is less true in large areas of the country with dispersed populations, but even in those areas, hospitals will increasingly share services with other hospitals and partition services between periphery and central hospitals.

References

American Hospital Association. *Hospital Statistics,* Chicago: AHA, 1987 (b)

American Medical Association. *Physician Characteristics and Distribution in the U.S.* Chicago: AMA, 1987.

American Hospital Association. *Guide to the Health Care Field,* Chicago: AHA, 1987. (a)

American Hospital Association. *Hospital Statistics,* Chicago: AHA, 1987 (b)

American Hospital Association. *Environmental Assessment 1987.* Chicago: AHA, 1987. (c)

American Hospital Association. *Ambulatory Care, Health Promotion and Children's Health 1987.* Chicago: AHA 1987. (d)

American Hospital Association. *Annual Survey.* Chicago: AHA, 1987. (e)

American Hospital Association. *Environmental Assessment for Rural Hospitals 1988.* Chicago: AHA, 1988.

American Hospital Association. "Management Rounds: Business and Finance." *Hospitals, 59*(3), 36, 1985.

American Medical Association. *Physician Characteristics and Distribution in the U.S.* Chicago: AMA, 1987.

Andersen, R. et al. *Equity in Health Services: Empirical Analyses in Social Policy.* Cambridge, MA: Ballinger, 1975.

Applebaum, A. L. "Commission Report Addresses Future of Public General Hospitals." *Hospitals,* May 16, 1978, p. 95.

Association of American Medical Colleges. *A Description of Teaching Hospital Characteristics.* Washington, D.C.: AAMC, 1982.

Curfman, G. D. "Shorter Hospital Stay for Myocardial Infarction." *New England Journal of Medicine, 318*(17), 1123, 1988.

Ermann, D. & Gabel, J. "Multi-Hospital Systems: Issues and Empirical Findings." *Health Affairs, 3*(1), 50, 1984.

Farley, D. E. *Trends in Hospital Average Lengths of Stay, Casemix and Discharge Rates, 1980–1985* (Hospital Studies Program, Research Note 11). Washington D.C.: U.S. Department of Health and Human Services, 1988.

Freymann, J. G. *The American Health Care System: Its Genesis and Trajectory.* New York: Medcom Press, 1974.

Friedman, E. "Public Hospitals: Is 'Relevance' in the Eye of the Beholder?" *Hospitals,* May 1, 1980, p. 83.

Gibson, R. M., Lazanby, H., Levit, K., & Waldo, D. R. "National Health Expenditures, 1983." *Health Care Finacing Review, 6*(2), 1, 1984.

Ginzberg, E. & Drennan, M. P. "The Health Sector: Its Significance for the Economy of New York City." New York: Commonwealth Fund, 1985.

Hellerstein, D. "The Slow, Costly Death of Mrs. K." *Harpers,* March 1984, pp. 84–89.

Heyssell, R. M., Gaintner, R., Kues, I. W., Jones, A. A., & Lipstein, S. H. "Decentralized Management in a Teaching Hospital: Ten Years Later at Johns Hopkins." *New England Journal of Medicine, 310,* 1477, 1984.

Hollowell, E. "No Insurance—No Privileges," *Legal Aspects of Medical Practice,* April 1978.

Johnson, D. E. L. "Multi-Unit Providers: Survey Plots 475 Chain's Growth." *Modern Health Care,* May 15, 1984, pp. 65–84.

Kovner, A. R. *Really Trying: A Career Guide for the Health Services Manager.* Ann Arbor, Mich: AUPHA Press, 1984.

National Center for Health Statistics. Health & Prevention Profile. Washington D.C. U.S. Governmental Printing Office, 1983. (a)

National Center for Health Statistics. "Utilization of Short-Stay Hospital." *Vital and Health Statistics,* Series 13, No. 72, September 1983, p. 2. (b)

Pattison, R. V., & Katz, H. M. "Investor-Owned and Not-for-Profit Hospitals." *New England Journal of Medicine, 309*(6), 347, 1983.

Perrow, C. "Goals and Power Structures: A Historical Case Study." In E. Freidson (Ed.), *The Hospital in Modern Society.* New York: Free Press, 1963.

Phelps, C. E. "Effects of Insurance on Demand for Medical Care." In R. Anderson, J. Kravits, & O. Anderson (Eds.), *Equity in Health Services.* Cambridge, MA: Ballinger, 1975.

Relman, A. S. "The New Medical-Industrial Complex." *New England Journal of Medicine, 303,* 963, 1980.

Rosenberg, C. E. *The Care of Strangers,* New York: Basic Books, 1987.

Shortell, S. M. "The Medical Staff of the Future: Replanting the Garden." *Frontiers of Health Services Management, 1*(3) 3, 1985.

Smith, H. L. "Two Lines of Authority Are One Too Many." *Modern Hospital,* March 1955, pp. 59–64.

Smith, D. B., & Kaluzny, A. D. *The White Labyrinth,* (2nd ed.). Ann Arbor, MI: Health Administration Press, 1986.

Southwick, A. "Due Process: The Physician's Right to Due Process and Equal Protection." *Hospital Medical Staff,* June 1978. (a)

Southwick, A. *The Law of Hospital and Health Care Administration.* Ann Arbor, MI: Health Administration Press, 1978. (b)

Starkweather, D. B. "U.S. Hospitals: Corporate Concentration vs. Local Community Control." *Public Affairs Report Bulletin* (Institute of Governmental Studies, University of California, Berkeley), April 1981.

Starr, P. *The Social Transformation of American Medicine*. New York: Basic Books, 1982.

Stevens, R. *American Medicine and the Public Interest*. New Haven, CT: Yale University Press, 1971.

U.S. Department of Labor, Bureau of Labor Statistics. "The Employment Situation: January 1985." *Washington, D.C. News*, February 1, 1985, p. 2.

Wilensky, G. R. "Solving Uncompensated Hospital Care." *Health Affairs, 3*(4), 50, 1984.

8

Long-Term Care

Hila Richardson

The rapid growth of the elderly population and the increasing financial burden of long-term care on individuals and government have focused attention on the issues related to access, cost, and quality of long-term-care services. This chapter will discuss those issues, along with the current and future policy developments that are being suggested to address them.

Definition and Overview of Long-term Care

Long-term care is a range of health, personal care, social, and housing services provided to people who have lost or have never developed the capacity to care for themselves independently as a result of chronic illness or mental or physical disability. The level of assistance needed is on a continuum beginning with minimal help in performing basic activities in the home, such as bathing, dressing, using the toilet, ambulation, help with shopping, meal preparation, transportation, house cleaning, and other activities important for self-sufficiency. On the other end of the continuum is complete dependency on nursing services in a nursing home for all basic activities, plus care for such needs as ventilator-assisted breathing and tube feedings. The assistance provided can be continuous or intermittent, but it is assumed that most people will usually need it with increasing intensity for years, often for the remainder of their lives (Kane & Kane; Kutza).

The essential element in defining long-term care, therefore, is functional capacity. Because the level of mental and physical functioning varies enormously within age groups and chronic conditions (diabetes, arthritis, Alzheimer's disease), the amount of long-term care a person needs cannot be predicted solely by age or diagnosis. Further, neither the location of services nor the type of service can determine the amount of long-term care services needed because people of all levels of dependency use nursing homes or receive rehabilitation in their homes.

A fact often overlooked is that people of all ages need long-term-care services, although the elderly use them most frequently. Young people, including babies, can need long-term-care services because of mental and physical limitations at birth, spinal cord or brain injury resulting from traumatic accidents, and chronic debilitating conditions such as multiple sclerosis.

Over 70% of chronically disabled people receive long-term-care services in their homes from family members and friends (Soldo). When circumstances require more assistance than can be provided by this informal system, people can use the formal care system, which includes services such as home health, mental health programs, social services, transportation, and, finally, institutional services in nursing homes, rehabilitation facilities, and various housing arrangements. However, these services can be expensive is purchased privately, and publicly funded programs have eligibility requirements that exclude many elderly.

Given the uncertainty in predicting the levels and types of long-term-care services a person will need, the ability to plan for, budget for, or insure against the demand for the wide range of long-term-care services, health and social has become a major health policy and financing issue. In the last 10 years it has gained even more attention as projected growth in the aging population has raised increasing concern about future demand and expenditures.

The Elderly and the Need for Long-term Care

In evaluating the elderly population's need for long-term care, surveys use measures of functional capacity called activities of daily living (ADLs) and instrumental activities of daily living (IADLs). The ADLs are a measure of a person's dependence on others for assistance with personal care functions (i.e., preparing meals, shopping, housework, using the telephone, managing money). The 1984 National Health Interview Survey (NHIS) measured dependency of noninstitutionalized persons over 65 years of age in terms of their performance of both of these types of measures. The survey found that about 23% (6 million) of all noninstitutionalized persons 65 years or older were functionally dependent in performing one or more ADL and that the proportion of the elderly experiencing difficulty with each personal activity increased with age. For example, 17% of persons aged 65 to 74 years had difficulty with all ADLs, and nearly half of those over 85 years had difficulty with one or more activity (Dawson, Hendershot, & Fulton).

The same pattern existed for persons who have difficulty in performing IADLs. The percentage of persons having difficulty with these activities increased from 20% for those 65 to 74 years to 55% for those over 85 years. Similarly, the older the persons were, the more likely they were to receive assistance with home management activities, with over half of those 85 years and older receiving assistance with one or more activities.

Accompanying the increase in dependency, there is strong evidence that use of acute-care services, physician services, and nursing home services increases steadily with age, with a marked increase for hospital and nursing home services after 75 years. Those 85 and older have a threefold greater risk of losing their independence, seven times the chance of entering a nursing home, and 2 ½ times the risk of dying, compared to persons 65 to 75 years of age (Soldo & Manton).

Yet it should be noted that dependency increases gradually, over a period of 15 to 20 years. Further, these studies show that even in the oldest age group, about 50% of the elderly still do not have difficulty performing these daily activities. Other studies have shown that a small group of elderly persons account for most of the use of health services among the elderly (Kane & Kane).

However, the number of elderly people is expected to increase, so the number requiring high levels of assistance and health services is also expected to increase. This has been referred to as the demographic imperative for long-term care. It is based on the fact that for most of the 20th century the elderly have increased far more rapidly than the rest of the population. At the beginning of the century, fewer than 1 in 10 Americans was 55 or over, and 1 in 25 was age 65 or over. By 1986 one in five Americans was at least 55 years old, and one in eight was at least 65 (U.S. Senate Special Committee on Aging).

The most important projection in terms of estimating the need for long-term-care services is the number of people surviving into the oldest age ranges. As Figure 8.1 shows, the percentage of persons over 75 years of age is expected to represent nearly 50% of all persons 65 years or older by the year 2000. By 2050, 55% of persons over 65 years of age will be 75 years or older. The percentage of the oldest elderly, those over 85 years, is projected to increase from 10% of those over 65 years in 1990 to 24% in 2050.

Although these numbers are striking, there is no agreement on how to translate them into increased need for long-term-care services. There are many unknowns in predicting the influence of different life-styles and better medical management of chronic conditions such as arthritis, dementia, heart conditions, osteoporosis, and incontinence, all major contributors to dependency in the elderly. Nevertheless, there is agreement that the increase will occur.

Figure 8.1 Persons Age 75 and Over as a Percentage of Persons Age 65+, Actual and Projected, 1980–2050

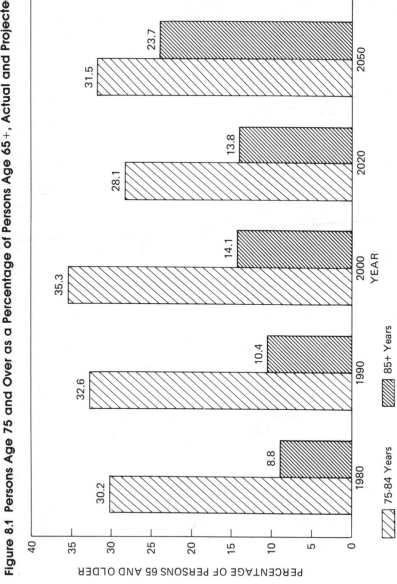

Source: U.S. Senate Special Committee on Aging, *Aging America: Trends and Projections, 1987–1988.*

Long-term Care Services: Delivery and Financing

Informal Care System

As stated earlier, Soldo (1984) estimated that over 70% of the care provided to elderly dependent persons in the community comes from relatives—especially spouses, daughters, and daughters-in law—friends, or neighbors; 16% also receive care from formal caregivers; and only 9% receive assistance exclusively from formal providers. Even though relatives are the main source of care for elderly people living alone, 18% have no one to rely on for even a few days, and 28% have no one they can depend on for a few weeks (Kasper).

Research has shown that, when possible, elderly people turn to the informal network for support first and most frequently. Only when the informal arrangements are not available or are inadequate do they seek help from formal organizations (Cantor). Moreover, when formal assistance is necessary, it does not substitute for informal care but provides additional services, particularly those requiring more technical and medical services beyond the ability of the informal caregivers (Soldo).

The dependent elderly living in the community is estimated to be 4.9 to 5.2 million people, two-thirds of whom are women. (General Accounting Office). Therefore, informal caregivers play an important role in controlling the amount of long-term-care services that would have to be purchased publicly or privately. As a result, programs to maintain the support from existing informal caregiver arrangements have been gaining interest. On both state and federal levels, programs have been funded to reduce the burden of family caregivers. These will be discussed later in the chapter.

Formal Care System

Nursing Homes. Although nursing home care is the service most closely associated with long-term care, only a small minority of the elderly are in nursing homes on any day. In 1985, of the 28.5 million persons over 65 years of age, 5%, or 1.3 million, lived in nursing homes (Hing). This proportion of the total elderly population residing in nursing homes has remained stable since 1973–1974, when the first National Nursing Home Survey (NNHS) was conducted (Hing).

However, 20% of the functionally dependent elderly people were in nursing homes in 1985. In fact, dependency in ADLs is one of the major predictors of nursing home admission. Other predictors include age, diagnostic condition, living alone, marital status, race, income, and lack of social support (Kane & Kane).

There were 19,100 nursing homes in the United States in 1985, more than three times the number of community hospitals. Their total of 1,624,200 beds was about double the number of community hospital beds. There has been a 22% increase in the number of nursing homes and a 38% increase in the number of beds since 1974 (Strahan). Nursing homes have remained mostly small, with an average of 85 beds.

Over 75% of nursing homes are owned by proprietary organizations. Only 20% are owned by voluntary groups or hospitals, and 5% are government-owned. Those owned by voluntary groups average 98 beds per facility, whereas the 1,000 public nursing homes had the largest average number of beds: 132 (Strahan).

Just over 50% of nursing homes are operated independently. There has been a significant increase in the number of nursing homes operated by what is referred to as a chain, usually a for-profit organization that operates a group of facilities. In 1977 nursing homes with chain affiliations were 28% of total homes, whereas in 1985 they were 41%.

Examples of the consolidation of chain ownership of nursing homes and beds are Beverly Enterprises, ARA, and Hillhaven, three of the largest chains. In 1973 they accounted for 2.2% of nursing home beds. Ten years later, they owned, managed, or leased 10% of the beds. Beverly alone controlled 40,000 beds in that year (Hawes & Phillips). This consolidation was largely accomplished by acquisition of existing homes. Since 1986, however, these major chains have begun to decrease their share of the nursing home market. For example, Beverly Enterprises announced plans to sell 170 facilities, or 15,000 to 20,000 beds, in 1988. Hillhaven also planned to sell about 30 homes (Mayer).

Until 1989 nursing homes were classified as either skilled nursing facilities (SNFs) for Medicare or Medicaid residents or intermediate care facilities (ICFs) for those covered by Medicaid. Each type of facility met distinct but overlapping conditions of participation to be certified to admit patients under the Medicare and Medicaid programs.

The SNFs were designated to provide a higher level of care to sicker patients and therefore required a licensed nurse on duty 24 hours a day and a registered nurse on day shifts. ICFs were considered to provide a lower level of care, more custodial than clinical, and were required to have a licensed nurse on duty only during the day. In practice, the distinctions between SNFs and ICFs always have been artificial because both types of facilities have served persons with a wide range of needs that often fluctuated between the definition of the two levels of care. The Nursing Home Reform Act, passed in 1987, ended the difference in staffing levels and mandated that ICFs provide the same range of services as SNFs. When the statute is fully implemented in 1990, all nursing homes will be referred to as nursing facilities (NFs).

The financial burden of nursing home care is shared almost equally between Medicaid (47.8%) and individuals (45%) (see Figure 8.2). Private insurers and Medicare paid only a small percentage of nursing home care in 1985 (General Accounting Office).

**Figure 8.2 Distribution of Nursing Home Expenditures
By Payer, 1985 (Total Expenditures = $36 Billion)**

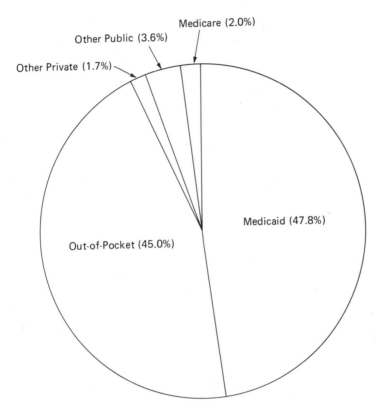

Source: U.S. General Accounting Office, *Long Term Care for the Elderly* (GAO/HRD-89-4)
Washington, D.C.: Author: 1988.

Medicaid covers both skilled and intermediate nursing home care. Because
Medicaid was enacted to cover health services for low-income people, it has
eligibility requirements, varying from state to state, that are based on income and
assets. Therefore, many elderly are not eligible for Medicaid coverage for costly
nursing home care unless they "spend down" their life savings to meet eligibility
requirements.

Given the expense of nursing home services (an average cost of at least
$22,000 per year), elderly people who require long nursing home stays often use
their income and assets to pay for nursing home service until they qualify for
Medicaid in their state. Nursing home residents are allowed to set aside a
monthly allowance from their own income and assets for personal needs. Also,

an allowance for the noninstitutionalized spouse can be set aside. However, these allowances have varied greatly among states, ranging from $30 to $70 per month for personal needs and $150 to $632 a month for maintenance (General Accounting Office). Recognizing the financial hardship this can mean for spouses, the Medicare Catastrophic Coverage Act of 1988 increased the amount of income and resources that an institutionalized person may retain for use by his or her spouse. Although Congress repealed this Act just 16 months after it was signed, this provision of the law was retained.

Medicare was not intended to cover nursing home care except for short-term care in a skilled nursing home after hospitalization. Regulations have strictly enforced the limitations on Medicare-covered skilled nursing care by limiting payment to care needed for recovery from an acute health condition rather than long-term care for a chronic condition. As a result, Medicare expenditures were less than 2% ($600 million) of total public and private expenditures in 1985 (Figure 8.2). The Medicare Catastrophic Act of 1988 expanded the skilled nursing care benefit, and, before its repeal in 1989, substantially increased Medicare's nursing home expenditures.

Hospital-Based Services. Because of the national decline in hospital occupancy, hospitals are looking for new services or conversions of existing facility space to more profitable uses than general acute care. The growing numbers of elderly in need of long-term care have become a primary target of hospital expansion. A 1985 survey found that 24% of hospitals owned SNFs, 12% owned intermediate care facilities, 33% provided home health services, and 14% provided homemaker services (Capitman et al.). A survey by the American Hospital Association of more than 3,000 hospitals found that 15% planned to add long-term-care beds in the future. Of this 15%, 61% planned to convert acute-care beds to skilled-nursing-care beds, and 29% planned to build new facilities (Pierce).

Another example of how hospitals provide long-term care is the swing-bed, a hospital bed that can be used interchangeably to provide acute, skilled, or intermediate care to patients. However, participation in swing-bed programs is currently limited to rural hospitals with fewer than 100 beds. To provide services, the hospitals must comply with most of the Medicare conditions of participation for nursing homes (Richardson & Kovner). In July 1986 there were 900 rural hospitals certified to provide swing-bed services (Shaughnessey, Schlenker, & Hittle).

Home Health Care. In the broadest sense, home health care encompasses the professional, paraprofessional, and supportive services provided in the home. It is generally classified as either medically related—skilled nursing, home health aide, rehabilitation, respiratory therapy services, emergency response systems—or as social or personal care such as homemaker, home-delivered meals, home companion services. Home care can be provided by a public agency (health department), private nonprofit organization (Visiting Nurse Association), proprietary organizations (private physician practices), and health facilities (hospitals and SNFs). These agencies serve people of all ages with extreme variation in needs. Most home care is provided to those over 65 years of age.

Advancements in technology for the home have made it possible to provide in-home therapies that previously could be provided only in the hospital (e.g., intravenous therapy, respirators, and parenteral nutrition). The home care sector now includes, in addition to direct service provider organizations, a wide range of medical equipment businesses and pharmacies.

It is estimated there are as many as 8,000 home health agencies in the nation (Kane & Kane). Of those, nearly 6,000 are Medicare-certified home health agencies (Lutz). To be certified to provide Medicare-covered services, the agencies have to meet conditions defining the care that can be provided, the personnel that must be employed, and the specific record documentation that is required. To provide home health services to Medicaid patients, regulations require that agencies meet the Medicare conditions of participants.

Table 8.1 shows the growth of Certified Home Health Agencies (CHHAs), by type of ownership, between 1972 and 1988. The number of CHHAs has more than doubled during those 16 years, with the greatest increase (65%) occurring between 1982 and 1986. Also of importance is the shift in the distribution of agencies by ownership. In 1972 Visiting Nurse Associations (VNAs) and official health agencies accounted for 80% of the CHHAs, representing 24% and 56.7% of those agencies, respectively. Ten years later these two types of CHHAs combined represented only 47.5% of all agencies. The shift had occurred as a result of the growth in proprietary and private nonprofit agencies. There were very few of these agencies in 1972. In 1982 they represented 35% of all CHHAs. Also, the number of hospital-based CHHAs nearly doubled during that 10-year span.

Since 1982 there has been a continuation and solificiation of this shift. By 1988 VNAs were less than 10% of CHHAs, official health agencies were 18%, and hospital-based CHHAs had continued to increase, representing 25%. The proprietary organizations had the largest proportion of agencies (32%), and the private nonprofit CHHAs represented 13%.

Medicare is the major public payer for home care, but as previously stated, it pays for only short-term SNF care. In 1985 Medicare accounted for just over half, or $2.3 billion of a total of $4.5 billion, of publicly funded home health care. Although still only 3% of total spending for home health, Medicare's share has been steadily increasing (Bishop & Karon).

In contrast to Medicare policies, Medicaid benefits for home health services can be extensive, depending on the state. They can include services by nurses, home health aides, social workers, housekeepers, and various therapists. Most states expanded their home health and community-based services under Section

Table 8.1 Medicare-Certified Home Health Agencies, by Ownership, 1972–1988

Type of ownership	1972		1983		1986		1988	
	No.	%	No.	%	No.	%	No.	%
VNA	531	24.0	517	14.2	510	8.5	498	8.7
Combination	55	2.5	59	1.6	62	1.0	53	0.9
Official health agency	1255	56.7	1211	33.3	1,192	19.9	1,066	18.4
Rehab-based	11	0.5	16	0.4	17	0.2	11	0.2
Hospital-based	231	10.4	507	13.9	1,350	22.5	1,458	25.2
SNF-based	7	0.3	32	0.9	117	1.9	101	1.7
Proprietary	43	1.9	628	17.3	1,918	32.0	1,840	31.8
Private nonprofit	N/A	N/A	632	17.4	824	13.7	760	13.1
Other	79	3.6	37	1.0	4	0.0	1	0.0
Total	2,212	100.0	3,639	100.0	5,994	100.0	5,788	100.0

Sources: Home Health Line, Vol. 9, February 6, 1984; and Home Health Line Vol. 13, May 16, 1988.

2176 waivers (Home and Community Based Waiver Program) in the 1981 Omnibus Reconciliation Act. In 1985, $1.1 billion of the $2.3 billion in public funds expended for home health were from the Medicaid program. Although home health programs have increased as a proportion of total Medicaid spending, from 0.02% in 1980 to 3% in 1985, they remain a small percentage of total Medicaid spending.

Community-based Services. Services based in the community are provided through voluntary, public, or proprietary organizations and include adult day care, hospice, respite, congregate meals, transportation, and case management programs. These services are supported by a combination of funds from Medicare, Medicaid, Title III of the Older Americans Act, and other federal, state, and local social services programs. The extent of the services provided and the eligibility requirements vary by funding source and by state and locality.

Through the social services block grant program, states may provide homemaker, home health aide, chore, adult day care, and adult foster care services. Under Title III of the Older Americans Act, established in 1965, available services include transportation, homemakers, and chore and home health aide services. In 1987 the Administration on Aging estimated that the number of client contacts for these services ranged from 6.3 million for transportation to almost 1 million for homemaker and home health aide services. Amendments to the Older Americans Act in 1987 authorized funds for nonmedical in-home services that included visiting and telephone reassurance, chore maintenance, and in-home respite and adult day care respite for families (General Accounting Office).

Adult Day Care Services. Adult day care is a program that offers a wide range of health and social services to the elderly during the day. Adult day care services are usually targeted to elderly in families where the caregivers work or to elderly living alone. Their goal is to delay or prevent institutionalization and provide respite for the caregiver. The services offered follow a medical or social model. The social model emphasizes social and recreational activities, crafts, discussion groups, and exercise. The medical model incorporates more rehabilitation, physical and mental assessment, nursing, and medical care.

Data on adult day care programs are still limited, but a survey done by the National Council on Aging found that there were about 1,200 adult day care centers in 1983. Programs were most commonly sponsored by nonprofit human services organizations, including government. Programs served an average of 19 clients per day, the typical participant being a 73-year-old female who lives with a spouse, relative, or friends (Von Behren).

Most adult day care programs surveyed offered social services, crafts, current events discussions, family counseling, reminiscence therapy, nursing assessment, physical exercise, ADL rehabilitation, psychiatric assessment, and medical care. The average daily fees charged were just over $20. Forty-three percent of the participants were Medicaid-eligible.

States finance adult day services with Medicaid funds and Social Security block grants. As of December 1985, 21 states had Medicaid waivers approved to offer such services (Pierce). Medicare does not cover adult day care. Most elderly people and their families pay for adult day care out of pocket.

There is conflicting evidence about the benefits of adult day care programs for clients. Some studies have shown improvement in mental and physical functioning of adult day care clients that delays nursing home admission, whereas others have concluded it does not have that effect (Kane & Kane). The conflicting evidence may be a result of the programs themselves, which tend not to be targeted to the highest-risk population groups or are not well integrated with rehabilitation services and medical supervision that might improve or maintain functioning. Adult day care programs may not appeal to the elderly unless they or their caregivers feel they are close to institutionalization. In such cases it may be a last attempt to forestall admission to a nursing home. Otherwise, the elderly may prefer other, less institutional sources of social and recreational activities, like senior centers and social clubs.

Respite Services. Respite services provide a temporary respite, or break, for the caregivers of the frail elderly or disabled chronically ill. There is no uniform definition of respite care. The services can be provided in or out of the person's home. In-home respite provides temporary homemaker, chore, or home health services. Out-of-home care includes adult day care and temporary stays in nursing homes, hospitals, group homes, or foster care homes. The type and scope of services and eligibility for services vary considerably among states (Kane & Kane; Meltzer). Since respites are in an early stage of development, there are no national data on the number and characteristics of such services.

States started using respite services for developmentally disabled and mentally retarded children in the 1960s. Research had shown that the ability to free the parents to care for nondisabled family members, including themselves, reduced their level of stress anxiety and isolation (Meltzer). The application of the concept to the elderly grew out of a combination of increasing interest in the role of the informal caregiver and the cost-containment effort to reduce expenditures of institutionalization.

Respite care may be paid for by Medicaid, a social services block grant, Older Americans Act funds, state general revenues, or privately. Medicaid rules require that respite care be provided only to elderly at risk of institutionalization. Some states require an assessment of functional limitations for admission to respite services (Pierce). With the passage of the Medicare Catastrophic Coverage Act in 1988, Medicare coverage was extended to respite services. The new benefit paid for the temporary services of a home health aide to provide respite for a spouse, relative, or friend caring for a Medicare beneficiary who cannot be left alone. This benefit was lost when the Act was repealed in 1989.

Few studies have been done to evaluate how respite care benefits the patient. One study of a group of Alzheimer's disease patients found that a 2-week in-hospital respite program had little effect on the patient's cognitive status and level of functioning. The changes, both positive and negative, that did occur depended on the patient's level of functioning on admission (Seltzer et al.)

An earlier study of a short-term respite program in nursing homes showed an unexpectedly high rate of institutionalization (12%) of the respite population within 1 month of use of respite services. Meltzer (1988) identified two possible explanations: (1) the use of respite might have been one last attempt to keep the patient with the family, suggesting that the institutionalization rate might have been even higher without respite; and (2) the respite experience reduced the family's resistance to institutional placement.

All in all, little is known about the respite concept. Research has not supported or refuted the hypothesis that respite care avoids institutionalization and reduces costs, nor has it demonstrated how services should be organized and provided to ensure a positive outcome for the patient and the caregiver.

Hospice Services. Hospice services are provided to the terminally ill and their families. Hospice is based on a philosophy of care, imported from England and Canada, that during the course of terminal illness the patient should be able to live life as fully and comfortably as possible. In the hospice approach, the family is the unit of treatment. An interdisciplinary team provides medical, nursing, psychological, therapeutic, pharmacological, and spiritual support during the final stages of illness, at the time of death, and during bereavement. The main goals are to control pain, maintain independence, and minimize the stress and trauma of death.

Most patients who need hospice care are elderly persons with cancer. More than 70% of hospice patients are Medicare-eligible (Tames). The pool of younger patients, however, is growing due to the needs of persons with acquired immune deficiency syndrome (AIDS). The palliative care and emotional support in a hospice, as well as less expensive care, have been accepted as a humane way to treat AIDS patients.

Increased federal and private insurance have spurred a boom in hospice care. In 1980 there were 269 programs. In 1986 that number had increased to 1500. Although there has been a similar growth in Medicare-certified hospices, they represent only a third of all hospices. In 1983 there were 119 Medicare-certified hospices, with 2,098 admissions. At the end of 1987 there were 417 Medicare-certified hospices, with 91,475 admissions (*Home Health Line,* 1988a).

Approximately 40% of the hospices were based in home health agencies, 30% were freestanding, 26% were hospital-based, and the remaining 3% were based in an SNF ((*Home Health Line,* 1988a).

The National Hospice Association has reported that the cost of hospice care is 30% lower than conventional care provided in the last month of life (Tames). The funding for hospice under Medicare strongly reinforces the intent to use ·

hospice as a cost-saving measure. For example, it is required that for at least 80% of the days in a hospice program, the patient is not in an inpatient setting like a hospital or nursing home. Also, the patient must waive other types of acute care, the patient's doctor must certify that life expectancy is 6 months or less, and 5% of services have to be furnished by volunteers in the patient's home with documentation of the cost savings from volunteers' services.

Despite these restrictions, the Medicare hospice benefits cover a comprehensive array of medical, nursing, and rehabilitation services in addition to medical appliances and supplies. There is a small coinsurance required for drugs. Inpatient respite care is provided for up to 5 consecutive days, and bereavement counseling is required but not reimbursed. To encourage the patient to remain in the home during crisis, Medicare will cover nurses, nurse's aides, and homemakers 24 hours per day. Reimbursement for hospice care was limited to a lifetime benefit of 210 days until 1989 coverage was allowed to continue if the beneficiary is recertified as terminally ill by an attending physician or hospice director. Total Medicare reimbursement for hospice care was 278 million in 1987 (*Home Health Line,* 1988a).

Hospice services have gained acceptance as an alternative to hospital care for the terminally ill. It is likely that hospices will continue to grow because of their philosophy toward caring for those at end of life and because services have been determined to be less expensive than those provided to patients in hospitals.

Case-Management Programs

Generically, case management refers to a method of linking, managing, or coordinating services to meet client needs and typically includes client assessment, service provision and follow-up (Zawadski & Eng). Case management demonstrations grew out of a concern about the cost of long-term-care services, particularly nursing home care. Most of the demonstrations (Coordinated Community-Oriented Long Term Care, the National Long Term Care Channeling Demonstration, the Medical Home and Community-Based Care Programs) had the goal of reducing public costs through substitution of community care for nursing home and hospital services.

In 1981, case management of community-based services was authorized for Medicaid reimbursement under Section 2176 of the Home and Community-Based Waiver Program of 1981. Today many states have assigned case management activities to agencies like the Department of Social Services, Areas Agencies on Aging, or Health Department special units. Also, case management for high-cost patients is offered by virtually all private insurers and many health management firms (Henderson, Sonder, Bergman, & Collard).

Zawadski and Eng (1988), in their review of eight demonstrations, differentiated the following three models of case management:

1. The prior authorization screening model, in which a health professional assesses the individuals considering institutional placement, determines whether alternative community services could be provided, and arranges for those services. Wisconsin has reported one of the most successful preadmission screening programs by assessing only those who were actually nursing home applicants, rather than all elderly at a high functional impairment level (Lindberg & Monson).

2. The brokerage model, wherein a health professional independently assesses an impaired individual, arranges services through other providers, and regular reassesses and follows the client. This is the model used by most private insurers.

3. The consolidated mode, in which a multidisciplinary team assesses needs and provides the services directly or under contract with other providers (e.g., hospitals, lab, home health agencies). The two most famous examples of this model are the Social Health Maintenance Organizations (SHMOs) and the On Lok Senior Health Services in San Francisco.

SHMOs are community-based programs that arrange for the provision of all primary-, acute-, and long-term-care services, including personal care and social services, for a fixed monthly prepaid fee. The sponsoring agency is therefore financially "at risk" and uses case management services to control the use of hospital and nursing home care while providing expanded home and support services. A federal demonstration of this concept is underway in four cities, serving about 15,000 elderly persons (Leutz et al.) The demonstrations are currently under evaluation, so it will be 1990 before their success at controlling costs be determined.

On Lok Senior Health Services is an extremely consolidated model of case management; the primary medical care, home health, and respite services are provided by On Lok multidisciplinary staff teams, which therefore maintain complete control over all of the services used. On Lok receives prospective monthly payments from Medicare, Medicaid, and individuals, for which it assumes full financial responsibility for the total health care of 300 physically and mentally frail elderly. A per diem fee is negotiated for hospital and nursing home services. A central feature of the program is a day health center linked to home health and in-home supports. Data from the program show a significant reduction in high-cost hospital and nursing home services and an increase in community services, particularly in-home personal care and support services (Zawadski & Eng).

Housing Services for Elderly People

Housing is increasingly recognized as playing a significant role in the continuum of long-term-care services. For example, the availability of affordable and appropriate housing for elderly people, particularly for those who are dependent, determines the need for institutional long-term-care services in the community. Housing programs and resources for the elderly can be at either end of the continuum. At one end are programs that are geared toward enhancing independent living and keeping elderly people in their homes (home equity conversion plans, home repair, shared housing). At the other end are semi-independent and sheltered arrangements (congregate housing, board and care) and nursing home care (Kane & Kane). A newer approach, Life Care Communities and continuing Care Retirement Communities (CCRCs), provide the full continuum of services from independent living to SNFs.

Following are the main housing programs and resources:

Federal housing: Federal subsidy has stimulated the building of approximately 1.5 million units of housing for elderly residents who meet income and age requirements. Recently, the issue of the elderly "aging in place" in subsidized housing has expanded support services for tenants to maintain them in their homes. These services include meals programs, homemakers, laundry service, on-site medical personnel, and transportation. The Robert Wood Johnson Foundation, for example, has awarded grants to 10 state housing financing agencies to develop programs to serve the needs of their elderly tenants ("Redefining Elderly Housing").

Home equity conversion: These programs allow elderly home owners to convert part of their home equity into cash without having to leave their homes and to be able to live in them until they die. The overall purpose is to provide cash for the 75% of the elderly who are homeowners to purchase long-term services, particularly in-home services and long-term-care insurance. However, Schole (1984) has identified the limitations of the concept: (1) the high cost of care relative to life expectancy and home value; (2) the reluctance of elderly people to sell their homes, their most valuable asset and one that represents their lifetime of labor and their independence; and (3) the complexity of the home equity conversion plans. As a result, the market is expected to be small and to develop slowly. By 1987, only 2,000 home equity conversions had been completed throughout the nation (Rivlin & Wiener).

ECHO housing: Elder Cottage Housing Opportunity (ECHO), often referred to as "granny flats," are small, freestanding, and removable units that can be located on the property of adult children to ensure accessibility of informal caregivers. There are no national data on the extent of their use. Thus far, their development seems to be hindered by zoning laws and concerns about loss in property values (Kane & Kane).

Home maintenance: These programs help poor elderly home owners with repairs (winterization, painting, plumbing, plastering, etc.) that will assist them in living independently in the homes. The programs are financed by both public (Community Development Block Grant, Title III of Older Americans Act, Title

XX of Social Security Act) and private community organizations. National data are not available on these programs.

Shared housing: This is a living arrangement in which two or more unrelated individuals share a house or an apartment. Examples of shared housing range from elderly people renting spare rooms to state agency–sponsored homes with 4 to 10 residents. In 1986, 670,000 elderly people shared housing with nonrelatives, a 35% increase in the last decade (Pierce).

Congregate living: This includes a variety of group-living and supportive service arrangements. Congregate housing generally occurs in multiunit apartment complexes. Residents usually can walk and eat independently. They may need assistance with housekeeping and personal care, and they have the option to have meal services. Congregate housing programs are operated by communities and public service agencies. Active state congregate housing programs operate in Arkansas, Connecticut Maine, Massachusetts, Minnesota, Mississippi, Ohio, and Oregon (Pierce).

Board-and-care homes: This is a broad category of housing that covers adult foster care homes, sheltered care facilities, halfway houses, and adult homes. They provide rooms, meals, help with ADLs, and some degree of protective oversight. Depending on the state, services may include supervising the use of medications by residents and linking residents to community services. A nationwide survey in 1987 reported approximately 41,000 licensed homes with about 563,000 beds (General Accounting Office). Data are not available on unlicensed homes. The residents pay for services themselves or receive Supplementary Security Income (SSI) to help pay for the facility (Kane & Kane). Board-and-care residents are both elderly people who need assistance with dressing and bathing due to physical and mental impairment and younger people who have mental impairment and cannot function without supervision.

Continuing Care Communities (CCRCs): As stated earlier, CCRCs combine independent living with access to nursing home care. As of 1986, 100,000 to 200,000 (less than 1%) of elderly people lived in about 700 CCRCs. There are predictions that by 1999 there will be 1,500 CCRCs with nearly 450,000 elderly residents. However, the high costs of these communities make them accessible to only a small proportion of the elderly. In 1989, only 13% of people over 75 years of age, the typical age for entering a community, had sufficient income and assets to pay the entrance fee and monthly charge (General Accounting Office). There is a large range in entrance fees and monthly charges, depending on the services contracted for. The median entry fee for a one-bedroom apartment was $49,927, and median monthly fees were $756 a person in 1987 dollars. The entry and monthly fees for a two-bedroom unit were $65,000 and $800, respectively, in the same year. Entry fees can range as high as $150,000. Two-thirds of the CCRCs provide some level of long-term-care services, including nursing home care. The others charge fees for these services (Cohen).

Issue in Long-Term Care

There is increasing concern that these existing long-term-care services will not be available, affordable, or of adequate quality to meet the needs of the growing number of elderly people. This section will discuss the basis for these concerns by describing the access, cost, and quality problems in long-term care.

Access: Problems in Supply and Eligibility

Access to long-term-care service depends on the supply of services relative to the need or demand for them and on the ability to reach services by overcoming financial, transportation or geographic barriers.

Supply. With respect to the supply of nursing home beds, there is an estimated national shortage of 250,000 such beds. For every person in a nursing home, there may be as many as two people not in nursing homes who are equally debilitated (USDHHS). Most states have restricted the supply of nursing home beds, to control Medicaid expenditures, by using the Certificate of Need (CON) regulations. By 1980, all but three states had CON laws for nursing home expansion (Kane & Kane). In addition, a number of states (10 in 1989) have established moratoria on the construction of new beds (American Health Care Association, personal communication, 1989). Nationally, the supply of nursing home beds has not kept pace with the growth in the elderly population (Harrington, Swan & Grant).

The availability of nursing home care is not equally distributed across the nation. The number of nursing home beds per 1,000 of the elderly population ranges from 22 in Florida to 96 in Wisconsin (USDHHS). There is no apparent correlation between the size of the elderly population and the supply of nursing home beds. Neither is there a correlation between the ratio of beds per 1,000 elderly population and the occupancy rate of nursing homes (USDHHS). For example, nursing home occupancy rates average 91% but can be as low as 70% and the nursing homes with low occupancy rates are not always in areas where there are more beds per elderly population unit. Such variation in supply affects the use of nursing homes even for elderly people with similar needs. A study of very dependent elderly—over 75 years of age, unmarried, and with low incomes—showed there was a greater likelihood they would be in nursing homes in the states with the largest number of nursing home beds per 1,000 elderly people (Scanlon, 1988). The findings of the study suggest that unmet needs may exists in those states with a low ratio of nursing home beds.

The access barriers created by the shortage of nursing home beds has made admission to nursing homes particularly difficult for the elderly poor who are very sick. Since nursing home administrators try to achieve a resident mix in their facility that optimizes their reimbursement (Institute of Medicine; Scanlon,

1980a,b), a shortage of nursing home beds allows them to be more selective in their admissions, accepting more profitable patients—those who are private-pay (and pay higher rates) or who are less sick and require less nursing care. Research has shown that patients who have labor-intensive needs such as tube feedings, those who require assistance with most ADLs, and those with mental and behavioral problems are the most likely to wait for nursing home placement (General Accounting Office).

There also is evidence to suggest that there are unmet needs for services in the community, including home health. A 1979 National Health Interview Survey found that a significant proportion of persons in the community who required assistance with ADLs were not receiving the help they needed (Scanlon, 1988). A similar survey, the 1982 National Long Term Care Survey, showed that the more dependent the elderly were, the greater the likelihood they had unmet needs (General Accounting Office).

Research is just emerging on how a prospective payment system (PPS) for hospitals will affect this demand for long-term care and increase concerns about access to services. In 1984 the implementation of prospective payment for Medicare patients using Diagnostic Related Groups (DRGs) created a reimbursement incentive to decrease the number of days the patient spends in the hospital by paying hospitals for each case rather than for the number of days. Claims have been made that since PPS has been instituted patients are discharged from the hospital "sicker and quicker."

One of the first studies on the effect of DRGs on the demand for long-term care was done by the National Association of Area Agencies on Aging. It found "a 365 percent increase in demand for case management, a 196 percent increase in demand for in-home skilled nursing, and a 63 percent increase in the demand for personal care services." (Pierce, p. 8) A survey of discharge planners by the U.S. General Accounting Office in 1987 revealed that the percentage of patients waiting in the hospital for posthospital care was greater in 1988 than 1982. About one-third said the supply of home care was a barrier to Medicare patients awaiting discharge (General Accounting Office).

Preliminary data indicate that in addition to an increase in the demand for nursing home services, there is also evidence to suggest that PPS has led to increasing severity of illness in nursing home patients. A study of changes in the location of death for the nation's elderly population before and after Medicare's PPS showed that although it was unchanged in 1981 and 1982, the percentage of deaths occurring in nursing homes increased from 18.9% in 1982 to 21.5% in 1985. The authors concluded that PPS had resulted in increased transfer of terminally ill patients from hospitals to nursing homes (Sager et al.). However, none of the studies has tried to evaluate the medical appropriateness of the increase in hospital discharges.

Finally, the inadequate supply of long-term-care services extends to housing. There is a widely recognized shortage of federally subsidized housing for elderly households. It is estimated that 2 million eligible families are not being served (U.S. Senate Special Committee on Aging). In addition, there are indicators that board-and-care homes are closing because the costs of operations are exceeding the SSI benefits and payments by the state social service agency (General Accounting Office).

Eligibility Barriers. In addition to access barriers created by shortages of resources, eligibility and service restrictions for Medicare and Medicaid programs, described earlier, prevent many elderly people from obtaining needed services that are available. Also, the social services block grants, Title III of the Older Americans Act, and Title XX of the Social Security Act, which fund community-based services, have limited funding and eligibility requirements. These eligibility restrictions not only create many "cracks" for people to fall through in qualifying for services, they also cause confusion about what services are available. For example, an elderly person may know there is a day care program available but may not know that it provides transportation. Lack of information about programs can also be a barrier to access. Because of these restrictions, available data show that few elderly people receive community-based services compared to the total number of dependent elderly in the community (General Accounting Office).

Financing Issues: Private and Public Responsibility

The major financing issue in long-term care is the distribution of public versus private responsibility in paying for services. On the public side, federal expenditures for health care and social programs for the elderly as a proportion of all spending on the elderly (retirement income, disability, housing programs, etc.) have increased from 6% in 1960, before Medicare and Medicaid, to close to 30% in 1986 (U.S. Senate Special Committee on Aging). As Figure 8.3 shows, expenditures for these programs represented about 53% of the $45 billion spent on long-term-care services for the elderly in 1985. However, the remaining 47% was paid for privately, leaving the elderly and their families paying out of pocket for almost half (44%) of all long-term-care expenditures (Figure 8.3). The Congressional Budget Office has projected that long-term-care expenditures could increase between 50% and 200% from 1985 to 2000 (General Accounting Office).

Expenditures for long-term care are mainly for nursing home care. In 1985, 80% ($36 million) of the $45 billion spent nationally for long-term care was for nursing home care. Medicaid spent $14.7 billion for nursing home care, representing more than one-third of total Medicaid spending and 42% of the nation's total nursing home bill (USDHHS). Payments to nursing homes accounted for more than 43% of state Medicaid budgets, with 19 states spending

Figure 8.3 Distribution of Total National Expenditures for Long-Term-Care Services by Payer, 1985 (Total Expenditures = $45 Billion)

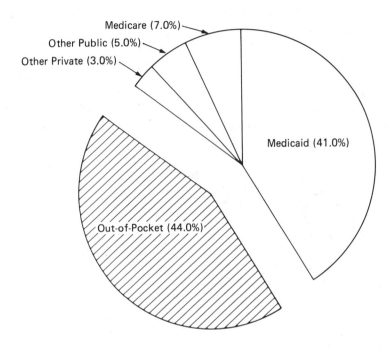

Source: U.S. General Accounting Office, *Long Term Care for the Elderly,* GAO/HRD-89-4, Washington, D.C.: Author, 1988, Table 4.1.

more than 50% of their Medicaid budgets on nursing home care in 1985 (Pierce). States have tried to reduce this burden on their budgets through cost-containment efforts primarily aimed at nursing homes.

The elderly and their families also have a major burden by paying out of pocket for about half of all long-term-care services. It is not surprising, therefore, that many elderly who need community or home-based services over years or who must enter a nursing home face impoverishment within only weeks. For example, those over 65 who are living alone and have an annual income between $9,700 and $15,000 would be impoverished after only 17 weeks in a nursing home with an annual average cost of $22,000. If their annual income is between $6,000 and $10,000, it would take only 6 weeks on average in a nursing home for an elderly person to become impoverished and dependent on Medicaid. These are elderly people who otherwise would not qualify for any form of public assistance (U.S. House Committee on Aging). As Vladeck (1983) has stated,

"Medicaid-reimbursed nursing home services have thus become the largest 'welfare' benefit available to formerly middle-class individuals and their families" (p. 360).

In order to defray this personal burden without increasing public expenditures, private long-term-care insurance has been proposed. The existing private policies covering long-term care, however, are both extremely limited in coverage and prohibitively expensive. A *Consumer Reports* survey ("Who Can Afford") found that only 70 insurance companies offer nursing home coverage. However, people who buy policies at age 65 may have to pay as much as $100 a month for adequate coverage. Another major drawback in private long-term-care insurance is that most policies pay a fixed benefit—ranging from $25 to $100—that is not adjusted for inflation. In each year after the purchase of the policy, the benefit will pay for a smaller part of the actual cost of care. Furthermore, there are major differences in the definition of covered nursing facilities, length of time benefits are paid, coverage, and eligibility for benefits ("Who Can Afford").

An analysis of long-term-care insurance options by Rivlin and Weiner (1988) found that only 1% of the elderly purchase long-term-care insurance. Moreover, the most optimistic projection is that only one-quarter to one-half of the elderly could purchase or would purchase policies by 2018. Thus, they conclude, there will continue to be a need for public financing to pay for most long-term care, particularly for the low- and middle-income elderly despite the increased availability of private policies (Rivlin & Weiner).

Other private financing approaches that have been suggested are the home equity conversions and the CCRCs discussed earlier. However, these approaches are also limited in the number of elderly they can reach. Therefore, it seems likely that most of the private sector responsibility for long-term-care expenses will continue to fall on individuals.

Quality of Long-Term-Care Services

Since most long-term care is provided by family and friends in the privacy of homes, concerns about quality of long-term-care services have historically centered on nursing homes. The nursing home sector has continually been plagued by scandals related to physical danger, filthy conditions, patient abuse, and negligence (Vladeck, 1980). Since 1974 the U.S. Senate Special Committee on Aging has issued two reports documenting the continued existence of these conditions. The most recent report, in 1986, charged that "thousands of our oldest, sickest citizens live in nursing homes which more closely resemble 19th century asylums than modern health care facilities." (U.S. Senate Special Committee on Aging). The committee found that almost one-third of the 8,852 SNFs failed to meet at least one basic federal health and safety standard in 1984. Almost 1,000 failed to meet three or more of these standards. The report also found that there had been an increase in violations of major conditions of participation, including a 75% increase in failure to provide physician supervision and a 61% increase in failure to provide 24-hour nursing care (U.S. Senate Special Committe on Aging).

The committee report and others have blamed the federal nursing home survey and certification regulations and enforcement mechanisms. A 2-year, $1.5 million study of the nursing home regulatory system by the Institute of Medicine (IOM) of the National Academy of Sciences (1986) found the major problem with the current survey and certification system was that it relied on a facility's ability to provide care, not whether the care is actually being delivered. A common example is that the survey process is mainly concerned about the facility having a dietitian, not how the food tastes or even if the patient is given the needed assistance to eat the food near the time it is served. The IOM report called for stronger regulations focused on patient outcomes determined through observation and direct contact with patients. As a result of this study, a number of nursing home reforms were passed in the Omnibus Reconciliation Act of 1987. These changes will require upgrading in staffing and nurse's aides' training, among other reforms related to patients' rights.

Defining and measuring quality of care in nursing homes is particularly difficult because a nursing home must be evaluated as an appropriate and sometimes final living situation for the residents. Quality of care over an extended period of time requires periodic and careful assessment of medical, functional, social, and psychological needs of the resident. Not all nursing homes have or can afford skilled professional staff able or motivated to do this.

Also, quality of care in a nursing home is closely related to quality of life—the resident's ability to have a sense of well being by making decisions about food, activites, and clothing; pursuing personal interests; having privacy; and being treated courteously and kindly by staff. These can be difficult and costly achievements for even the best nursing homes. Nursing home life must be institutional to some extent, particularly in large facilities. Nursing homes are built to look like hospitals, and the routine is geared to that of hospital staff. Although most nursing homes allow personal furniture and belongings, it is difficult to achieve a homelike atmosphere and privacy in an environment built with the main objectives of making it easy to clean and meeting fire and safety codes.

One of the critical elements of quality of life in nursing homes is the quality of the resident–staff relationship. Most of the care in nursing homes is provided by nurse's aides, who usually are low-paid, receive relatively little training in many states, and are inadequately supervised. They are often required to care for a large number of frail, very old residents, many of whom have mental impairments as well as physical disabilities. Not surprisingly, the turnover rate of nurse's aides ranges from 70% to over 100% a year (Institute of Medicine). Also, the nursing shortage has made it more difficult to recruit licensed and registered nurses for nursing homes, where the wages are lower than in acute-care facilities. This has intensified the problems with inadequate supervision and has put nurse's aides into the position of providing care they are untrained to provide.

According to the IOM report (1986), many of the quality problems can be handled by competent management and staff: "In most regions of the country, very good homes can be found—places that are well-managed, where competent, caring staff provide services in a conscientious, sensitive manner; where the dignity, privacy, and human needs of the residents are respected and provided for in thoughtful, and even imaginative ways" (Pill). However, it is acknowledged that these remedies increase costs. Reimbursement policies must recognize that maintaining the quality of patient care and life means higher costs.

The quality of home health services is particularly difficult to monitor because most of the time it cannot be observed. The patient contact occurs in the patient's home, often with only a paraprofessional home health aide or attendant and the patient present. Observation of the patient by a professional supervisor may occur only every 2 weeks and then may not include an observation of the care being provided.

Often quality problems in home care are also related to the difficulty CHHAs have in attracting and retaining experienced and reliable staff. Wages are so low that incomes of home health aides or attendants are near or below the federal poverty level. In Los Angeles home care workers made $3.72 per hour in 1987 and received no health insurance or fringe benefits. More than half of them depended on public assistance programs (Lutz). Until a recent contract settlement, home attendants working for the Medicaid program in New York City made $4.15 per hour, which gave them an annual income level of $7,000, less than the federal poverty level of $7,400 for two persons. Under the new contract, the hourly wages will be increased to $5.90 over a 3-year period, plus an enhanced health insurance benefit.

As with nursing homes, improving the quality of home care staff can also increase the costs of providing care. As Medicare and Medicaid develop more stringent limitations on eligibility for home health services, the agencies will be forced to cut their costs. It is already generally known that home health agencies cannot make a profit by providing only Medicare and Medicaid services. They also must provide privately paid nursing, personal care, and medical equipment services. This additional source of revenue serves to subsidize the publicly funded side of the agency's operation.

Proprietary and many voluntary home health agencies and necessary homes will continue to operate only as long as they can maintain sufficient profits. The choices for them will be either to resort to cost-saving measures, which may affect the quality of care, or to eliminate services to Medicare and Medicaid patients. Long-term-care providers will make the trade-offs between quality and cost if policies do not prevent them from doing so.

In summary, existing problems in access, financing, and quality of long-term-care services make obtaining appropriate, high-quality long-term care largely a matter of chance. The availability of services depends on the state and locality in which one lives. It also depends on whether one has just the right amount of income and assets to qualify for Medicare, Medicaid, or other public programs or so much income that any amount of services can be purchased. Those who are unlucky enough to fall between those two extremes, will be forced to use most of what income and assets they have until they are poor enough to obtain Medicaid. Once services have been obtained, their quality will largely depend on luck in getting personnel who, despite poor wages and little status, will be competent, considerate, and remain on the job.

Although these problems and inequities have existed for decades, the policies and programs to address them have been slow in developing because of resistance at both state and federal levels to increased spending. The next section will describe the current, and what appears will be the future, approaches to these problems by the federal and state governments.

Strategies for Change: Federal and State Approaches

Federal Approach

Since the early 1980s the federal government has limited its role in long-term care to research aimed at demonstrating whether long-term-care costs could be reduced by (1) substituting home- and community-based services for nursing home care and (2) using a combination of case management and capitated funding as incentives to control the use of services. The results of the demonstrations intended to substitute community services for nursing home care showed that expanded community services led to only a small reduction in nursing home use and, in fact, actually increased aggregate costs of services. However, the demonstrations did show that the increased services benefited patients and their families and were most successful in improving their quality of life (Kemper; Weissert, Cready, & Parvelak). One additional but unexpected finding from the evaluation of these demonstrations was that informal caregivers did not stop giving care when formal care was added—an argument often used against expanding community-based services (Christianson).

The SHMOs are the federally supported demonstration on capitation and case management. The SHMO demonstrations have placed limits on long-term-care benefits ranging from $6,500 to $12,000 (Pierce). This has raised concern about unrealistic restrictions on access to these services because this amount would cover only about 6 months in a nursing home. The four demonstration sites are expected to save $3 million to $6 million over 3 years in decreased use of hospitals and nursing homes (Pierce). As stated earlier, the impact of the SHMOs will not be known until the evaluation is completed in 1990.

To successfully address the issues in financing of long-term care, more systemwide federal reforms have been suggested. For example, adding a Medicare Part C for long-term care has been advocated to get long-term care disentangled from the state welfare system and make it an entitlement program like the other services under Medicare. Also, establishing federal and minimum standards for Medicaid coverage of long-term-care services has been discussed. So far, there has been no significant attempt at the federal level to develop policies or programs that would address these more fundamental changes.

The federal government has been more aggressive in the area of quality in nursing home care than in financing reforms. The 1987 Omnibus Reconciliation Act (OBRA) included a nursing home reform package with the following major features:

1. Upgrade nurse's aides by setting minimum hour and content standards for training programs and requiring testing of knowledge and clinical skills.
2. Preadmission screening to prevent admission to nursing homes of people whose only need is for services related to mental illness or mental retardation.
3. Minimal nurse staffing requirements for 24-hour licensed nursing services and a full-time registered nurse 7 days a week.

Although these measures are needed, they will cost money to implement. If the increased costs associated with these improvements are not recognized through increases in reimbursement, the nursing homes will have to find other ways to cut costs. Ironically, these cost reductions might undermine any improvements in quality gained from the implementation of the legislation. Also, since there is no provision for increasing the wages of the nurse's aides, their positions will be upgraded without a commensurate increase in salary. Without better nurse's aide salaries, the nursing homes will still be faced with turnover and burnout in this labor force.

State Approaches

Without policy direction at the federal level, states have been undertaking their own programs to reduce their Medicaid budgets. The programs have focused on decreasing costs of nursing homes and home- and community-based services. More recently, states have become more active in encouraging the development of private long-term-care insurance through removing regulatory barriers and developing tax incentives.

The approaches to reducing Medicaid spending fall into three general areas: (1) targeting access, (2) limiting payment, and (3) encouraging private responsibility.

Targeting Access. The most widely used method for targeting access is case management, particularly preadmission screening. Preadmission screening is currently used by 45 states (Pierce). The programs range from a broad screening of applicants who are likely to become Medicaid-eligible within a certain time to screening only those who have decided to enter a nursing home. Wisconsin and South Carolina have been so successful in the latter approach that it is likely to become more widespread. However, savings from keeping less sick patients in the community ultimately may be offset by limiting nursing homes to heavier-care patients whose care is more costly.

Case management as a targeting function ranges from coordination and monitoring of service delivery to state organizational structure that has a total gatekeeping function. Oregon provides a good example of the latter and represents the direction in which most states are likely to move.

Major components of the Oregon system include relocation planning, risk intervention, and preadmission screening. All functions are performed by case managers, who assess client needs and develop a care plan authorizing the provision of Medicaid services. They also identify services available through other resources for those not eligible for Medicaid. Other case managers assigned to relocation planning help institutionalized older people return to the community. Since 1982, more than 5,000 nursing home patients have been relocated to community settings (Justice). This case management function is part of the Senior Services Division (SSD), which has centralized control over all major state funds for the elderly, including Medicaid, social services block grants, Older Americans Act funds, and SSI. The state estimated that in 1986 the combined nursing home and community-based services cost the state $13 million less than if the reorganization had not occurred. This represented an 11% reduction in state expenditures for these services (Justice). Also, the Oregon model that relocates and arranges for other services can indirectly improve access. Case management without these features is more likely to result in limiting access only.

Limiting Payment. States have been experimenting with ways to avoid the open-ended health insurance reimbursement model that pays retrospectively for services that are prescribed and provided by providers of nursing home care, home health, and other community-based services. The approaches range from tinkering with the nursing home reimbursement system to placing a cap on the total value of services that can be provided. States may be experimenting with more than one approach.

Prospective payment is the most popular reimbursement reform (Pierce). A specific form of prospective payment, case-mix payment, is gaining in use. Seven states (Illinois, Maryland, Minnesota, Montana, New York, Ohio, and West Virginia) have adopted a case-mix approach to establishing nursing home reimbursement rates (Swan, Harrington, & Grant). Case-mix reimbursement is based on an asessment of each resident's condition and an estimate of the actual amount of nursing time and other resources that patient will need (Schlenker). The assessment usually measures ADLs, mental status, medical conditions, and behavioral problems. After the assessment, residents can be grouped according to the level of resources they require. Although case-mix systems help prevent facilities from losing money when accepting Medicaid residents with heavier care needs, they are mainly intended to restrict cost by setting ceilings for average costs of different case-mix groups. The Health Care Financing Administration is sponsoring a national study on the use of case-mix reimbursement for nursing homes.

There are two concerns about case-mix reimbursement. One is that paying nursing homes less money as residents improve creates the potential for nursing homes to increase the residents' dependency and care requirements to maximize reimbursement. (Kane & Kane; Swan et al.). The second concern is that the increase in reimbursement will not necessarily mean an increase in services. Patient case-mix reimbursement formulas can be targets for "gaming" to increase reimbursement. To control this potential, New York State has implemented a new, more stringent quality assurance system that will be looking more closely at how care is provided and the outcome of the care to determine if the patient has received the needed services. Also, the New York State program has a quality-of-life component that will assess such areas as resident participation in activities as an indicator of their progress.

Half of the state Medicaid programs still use retrospective cost-based reimbursement for home care, but it is expected most states will change to prospective payment. (Pierce). Of those who have already changed, 29 states have established prospective maximum payment rates for home health care services adjusted by type of provider (nurse, nurse's aide, physical therapist, etc.). Development of case-mix reimbursement for home health services is difficult because there is not a sufficient data base on home health recipients. Also, it is difficult to assess the population with multiple and changing health problems, differing home and family situations, variation in travel time and the time required to perform the same unit of service

In setting maximum payable amounts for home and community services under the Section 2176 waiver programs, most states have used a percentage of the average cost of nursing home care as the limit above which services may not be authorized. The range is usually between 75 and 90% (Pierce). Maine has a per-client cap equal to the state's potential expense of providing ICF care for that person. This maximum amount is programmed into the state's Medicaid computer so that spending cannot exceed the limit (Justice). Arkansas currently limits its personal care services to a maximum of 72 hours per client per month ($442/month). Although Wisconsin does not set maximums for individuals, it sets an average payment level for counties, and the counties are not reimbursed if the average cost for all recipients exceeds the contract level (Justice).

As states become more restrictive in payment for long-term care, providers are forced to reduce their costs in order to keep operating. To balance the negative effect these reductions might have on quality, Illinois has been using an outcome base reimbursement, a concept originated by Robert Kane at the University of Minnesota. The Illinois scheme uses incentive payments for reaching goals in the resident's condition and in the environment.

Despite the potential of this scheme to protect quality of care, it is naive to assume that continually reducing nursing home or home health payments to make them more efficient will not affect quality and access. As Scanlon (1988) has pointed out with respect to nursing homes; "Because of virtually guaranteed high occupancy, nursing homes have little need to compete. A likely response to lower Medicaid reimbursement is therefore a reduction in staff and other resources devoted to providing care" (Pill).

Encouraging Private Responsibility. Because the insurance industry is regulated by states, the states must remove legal and regulatory barriers that increase the industry's financial risk in developing private long-term-care insurance. States also can take steps to encourage the sale of policies. One of these steps is sponsoring educational campaigns to inform elderly citizens of the limitations of Medicare in covering long-term-care services. The Washington State insurance commissioner, for example, runs a program that uses trained senior volunteers to conduct public meetings and assist individuals in assessing insurance policies (Pierce). Colorado has enacted a tax reduction for purchasing long-term-care policies. Other state proposals include waiving Medicaid asset eligibility requirements for those who have used up benefits through long-term-care insurance policies and making long-term-care insurance available to state employees (Pierce).

These initiatives are still in experimental stages, but it is likely that will spread over the next 5 to 10 years as insurance companies develop more attractive service and financing packages. Nevertheless, the ability of long-term-care insurance to lead to Medicaid savings will not be known for at least 10 to 15 years, when those purchasing policies now will actually need to use the services covered.

The other major area in which states are able to encourage private responsibility is the use of tax incentives to support family and informal caregiving. States provides tax incentives through use of exemptions, deductions, and tax credits. Only five states (Arizona, Idaho, Iowa, North Carolina, and Oregon) have tax incentive programs. Iowa's program allows informal caregivers to claim a deduction of up to $5,000 for eligble expenses. The disabled relative must be eligible for Medicaid and have a statement from a physician stating the person cannot live independently. The combination of these two requirements means the program is targeting those at higher risks for institutionalization (Pierce).

In contrast, Oregon has a very limited program that allows a credit of up to 8% of eligible expenses, to a maximum of $250. Oregon also is the only state of the five to limit income eligibility of the caregivers to $17,500 (Pierce).

Thirteen states make direct payments to family members who provide services to dependent persons. Average monthly payments range from $119 a month in Florida to $400 a month in Minnesota. States have various guidelines for payments, including requirements that the caregivers demonstrate financial hardship and that the dependent person live in the same household (Pierce).

Tax incentive programs have the advantage of keeping the dependent elderly person in the family home, where it is assumed that he or she will get the best care. However, the few programs that exist have been so small, it is unlikely that they will be sufficient incentive for daughters and daughters-in-law to leave the labor force for caregiving responsibilities. As a result, they have limited ability to create more direct care.

Conclusion and Future Direction

The development of a national strategy to address the need for long-term care is one of the most necessary and challenging areas in health policy. Variations in level of need and demand among individuals, localities, and states and the range of needed services that crosses the boundaries between health, social services, and housing make it difficult to imagine that the problems of equity and quality can be addressed without a strong federal role.

That federal role can confront the problems with a comprehensive reform of the health system or address them incrementally, with changes in existing programs. However, the goals of any national approach should be the same:

- To achieve equity in the distribution of resources and the distribution of financial responsibility.
- To ensure access for functionally impaired persons of all ages based on their need for services, including personal care services, homemaker assistance, and housing.
- To expand support for informal caregivers.
- To fund education, training, and decent salaries to attract health personnel into long-term care.

A social insurance model, where those of all ages pay a small amount to receive benefits when needed, may be the only federal approach that can provide universal access to long-term-care services while offering protection against financial disaster to all. The fears of exorbitant cost and insurmountable administrative problems have made a social insurance approach seem out of the question during this era of fiscal constraint. However, the future social and political environment may provide a different perspective. The financial and emotional devastation that often accompanies the need for long-term-care services may no longer be socially acceptable. The private sector approaches may provide unacceptably limited solutions. Major financing reforms that, for example, shift resources from acute to chronic care may become options for increasing publicly funded long-term-care services without increasing public expenditures. The expected demands for long-term services from persons with AIDS, combined with increased demand by the elderly, may force choices that shift resources to long-term care.

These changes cannot be predicted with certainty. Neither can the actual need for services be identified. The need will depend on the social and economic trends that determine the availability of informal caregivers in the home and the purchasing power of the elderly in the future. Also, changes in medical science and technology will influence the prevalence and treatment of the major disabling chronic conditions (arthritis, osteoporosis, heart conditions) and the conditions that lead to dependence (incontinence and dementia).

This uncertainty, however, does not excuse inaction; it makes action essential. Taking the opportunity to develop a national policy that can be the basis for planning and financing adequate long-term-care services before they are needed can prevent a future with an ever-widening gap between the health needs of elderly people and the health resources available to help them and their caregivers.

This uncertainty, however, should not prevent action. It is essential that a national policy for the planning and financing of long-term-care services be developed now. Without it, the future does hold one certainty: an ever-widening gap between the need for long-term-care services and the resources available to meet that need.

References

Bishop, C. E., & Karon, S. L. *Composition of Home Health Care Expenditure Growth.* Waltham, Mass: Bigel Institute for Health Policy, 1987.

Cantor, M. "The Family: The Basic Source of Long Term Care for the Elderly." In P. H. Feinstein, M. Gornick, & J. N. Greenberg (Eds.), *Long Term Care Financing and Delivery Systems: Exploring Some Alternatives.* Washington, D.C.: Health Care Financing Administration, 1984.

Captiman, J. A., Prottas, J., MacAdam, M., Leutz, W., Westwater, D., Yee, D. L. "A Descriptive Framework for New Hospital Roles in Geriatric Care." *Health Care Financing Review,* Annual Supplement, 17–25, December 1988.

Christianson, J. B. "The Effect of Channeling on Informal Caregiving." *Health Services Research, 23*(1), 99, 1988.

Cohen, M. A. "Life Care: New Options for Financing and Delivering Long Term Care." *Health Care Financing Review,* Annual Supplement, 139, December 1988.

Dawson, D., Hendershot, G., Fulton, J. "Aging in the Eighties: Functional Limitations of Individuals Age 65 years and Over." *Advance Data from Vital and Health Statistics,* No. 133 (DHHS Pub. No. PHS 87-1250 Hyattsville, MD: National Center for Health Statistics, 1987.

General Accounting Office. *Long Term Care for the Elderly* (HRD-89-4). Washington, D.C.: Author, 1988.

Harrington, C., Swan, J. H., & Grant, L. A. "Nursing Home Bed Capacity in the States, 1978–86." *Health Care Financing Review,* 9(1), 33, 1988.

Hawes, C. & Phillips, C. D. "The Changing Structure of the Nursing Home Industry and the Impact of Ownership on Quality, Cost, and Access." In B. H. Gray (Ed.), *For-Profit Enterprise in Health Care.* Washington, D.C.: National Academy Press, 1986.

Henderson, M. G., Sonder, B. A., Bergman, A., & Collard, A. F. "Private Sector Initiatives in Case Management." *Health Care Financing Review,* Annual Supplement, 89–95, December 1988.

Hing, E. "Use of Nursing Homes by the Elderly: Preliminary Data from the 1985 National Nursing Home Survey." (DHHS Pub. No. PHS 87-1250). Hyattsville, MD: National Center for Health Statistics, 1987.

Home Health Line, 13, 177, May 9, 1988. (a)

Home Health Line, 13, 194, May 23, 1988. (b)

Institute of Medicine. *Improving the Quality of Care in Nursing Homes.* Washington, D.C.: National Academy Press, 1986.

Isaacs, J. C., & Tames, S. *Long-Term Care: In search of National Policy.* Washington, D.C.: National Health Council, 1986.

Justice, D. *State Long Term Care Reform.* Washington, D.C.: Center for Policy Research, National Governor's Association, 1988.

Kane, R. A., & Kane, R. L. *Long-Term Care: Principles, Programs and Policies.* New York: Springer Publishing Co., 1987.

Kasper, D. *Aging Alone: Profiles and Projections* New York: The Commonwealth Fund, 1988.

Kemper, P. "Overview of the Findings." *Health Services Research, 23*(1), 161, 1988.

Kutza, E. A., "Allocating Long-Term-Care Services." In J. Meltzer, F. Farrow, & H. Richmond (Eds.), *Policy Options in Long-Term Care.* Chicago: University of Chicago Press, 1981.

Leutz, W., Abrahams, R., Greenlick, M., Kane, R., & Prottas, J. "Targeting Expanded Care to the Aged: Early SHMO Experience." *The Gerontologist, 28*(1), 4, 1988.

Lindberg, G., & Monson T. "Long Term Care Initiatives in Hennepin County, Minnesota." Notes from the Field. *American Journal of Public Health,* 79(4), 519, 1989.

Lutz, S. "Despite Pitfalls, Home Care keeps Growing." *Modern Health Care,* June 24, 1988, pp. 24–37.

Mayer, D. "Nursing Home Market Reaches All-Time High." *Health Week,* August 8, 1988.

Meltzer, W. *Respite Care: An Emerging Family Support Service.* Washington, D.C.: The Center for the Study of Social Policy, 1982.

Pierce, R. M. *Long Term Care for the Elderly: A Legislator's Guide.* Washington, D.C.: National Conference of State Legislatures and the American Association of Retired Persons, 1987.

"Redefining Elderly Housing." *Long Term Care Management, 18*(3), 4, 1989.

Richardson, H., & Kovner, A. R. "Swing-Beds: Experience and Future Directions." *Health Affairs, 6*(3), 61, 1987.

Rivlin, A. M., & Wiener, J. M. *Caring for the Disabled Elderly: Who Will Pay?* Washington, D.C.: The Brookings Institution, 1988.

Sager, M. A., Easterling, D. V., Kindig, D. A., & Anderson, O. W. "Changes in the Location of Death after Passage of Medicare's Prospective Payment System: A National Study." *New England Journal of Medicine, 320*(7), 433, 1989.

Scanlon, W. J. "Nursing Home Utilization Patterns: Implications for Policy." *Journal of Health Politics, Policy and Law, 4*(4), 619, 1980. (a)

Scanlon, W. J. "A Theory of Nursing Home Market." *Inquiry, 17*(1), 25, 1980. (b)

Scanlon, W. J. "A Perspective on Long Term Care for the Elderly." *Health Care Financing Review,* Annual Supplement, 7–15, December 1988.

Schlenker, R. E. "Case Mix Reimbursement for Nursing Homes." *Journal of Health Politics, Policy and Law, 11*(3), 445, 1986.

Scholen, K. "An Overview of Home Equity Conversion." In P. H. Feinstein, M. Gornick, & J. N. Greenberg (Eds.), *Long Term Care Financing and Delivery Systems: Exploring Some Alternatives.* Washington, D.C.: Health Care Financing Administration, 1984.

Seltzer, B., Rheaume, Y., Volicer, L., Fabiszewski, K. J., Lyon, P., Brown, J. E., & Volicer, B. "The Short-Term Effects of In-Hospital Respite on the Patient with Alzheimer's Disease." *The Gerontologist, 28*(1), 121, 1988.

Shapiro, E., & Tate, R. "Who Is Really at Risk of Institutionalization?" *The Gerontologist, 28*(2), 237, 1988.

Shaughnessy, P. W., Schlenker, R. E., & Hittle, D. F. *An Evaluation Study of the National Swing-Bed Program in the 1980's.* Denver: Center for Health Services Research, University of Colorado Health Sciences Center, 1987.

Soldo, B. "Supply of Informal Care Services: Variations and Effects on Service Utilization Patterns." In W. Scanlon (Ed.), *Project to Analyze Long-Term Care Data* (Vol. 3). Washington, D.C.: The Urban Institute, 1984.

Soldo, B., & Manton, B. "Dynamics of Health Changes in the Oldest Old: New Perspectives and Evidence." *Milbank Memorial Fund Quarterly, 63*(2), 286, 1985.

Strahan, G. "Nursing Home Characteristics: Preliminary Data for the 1985 National Nursing Home Survey." *Advance Data from Vital and Health Statistics,* No. 131, (DHHS Pub. No. PHS 87-1250). Hyattsville, MD: Public Health Service, 1987.

Swan, J. H., Harrington, C., & Grant, L. A. "State Medicaid Reimbursement for Nursing Homes, 1978–86." *Health Care Financing Review, 9*(1), 33, 1988.

Tames, S. "The Booming Hospice Industry." *Medicine and Health Perspectives, 41*(16), 1987.

U.S. Department of Health and Human Services, Health Care Financing Administration. *Long-Term Health Care Policies* (HCFA Pub. No. 87-02170). Washington, D.C.: U.S. Government Printing Office, 1987.

U.S. House of Representatives, Select Committee on Aging. *Long-Term Care and Personal Impoverishment: Seven in Ten Elderly Living Alone Are at Risk* (Comm. Pub. No. 100-631). Washington, D.C.: U.S. Government Printing Office, 1987.

U.S. Senate Special Committee on Aging. *Aging in America.* Washington, D.C.: U.S. Department of Health and Human Services, 1988.

U.S. Senate Special Committee on Aging, *Nursing Home Care: The Unfinished Agenda,*
    Staff Report, May 21, 1986.
Vladeck, B. *Unloving Care: The Nursing Home Tragedy.* New York: Basic Books, 1980.
Vladeck, B. "Nursing Homes." In D. Mechanic (Ed.), *Handbook of Health, Health Care
    and Health Professions.* New York: The Free Press, 1983.
Von Behren, R. *Adult Day Care in America: Summary of a National Survey.* Washington
    D.C.: National Council on the Aging, 1986.
Weissert, W. G. "Hard Choices: Targeting Long Term Care to the 'At Risk' Aged."
    Journal of Health Politics, Policy and Law, 11(3) 463, 1986.
Weissert, W. G., Cready, M. C., & Parvelak, J. E. "The Past and Future of Home and
    Community-Based Long Term Care." *Milbank Memorial Fund Quarterly, 66*(2),
    1988.
"Who Can Afford a Nursing Home?" *Consumer Reports,* May 1988, pp. 300–311.
Zawadski, R. T., & Eng, C. "Case Management in Capitated Long Term Care." *Health
    Care Financing Review,* Annual Supplement, 75–81, December 1988.

9

Mental Health Services

Steven S. Sharfstein and Lorrin M. Koran

Who is mentally ill? The precise boundaries for the concept of "mental disorder" are not clear and are influenced by philosophic, social, and cultural considerations. This is also true for the concepts of physical disorder and notions of health versus disease. Every society includes individuals who present behavioral or psychological deviancy significant enough to qualify for a definition of mental illness. These syndromes are associated with painful emotional symptoms or significant impairment in important areas of social or occupational functioning or present as an inability to think, remember, or concentrate. Such syndromes also significantly increase the potential for general medical illness, pain, disability, and even death. The cause of mental disorder may be biological, developmental, psychological, environmental, or a combination of these. The important boundary line is the person's level of distress and dysfunction that is expressed primarily through a behavioral syndrome.

Mental health services are expensive. In 1980 it was estimated that 8% of the nation's health expenditures, or $20 billion, went for the direct treatment of individuals with mental disorders. The specialty mental health sector accounted for about half of this expenditure, the general medical sector one-third, and the human services and nonhealth sector one-sixth (Frank & Kamlet). If one adds alcohol and drug abuse services to mental care, approximately 14% of the health dollar goes for direct treatment costs. The indirect costs—that is, those due to lost productivity, disability, and death—are approximately double the direct costs (President's Commission, vol. 2, p. 530). These dollar estimates can only begin to suggest the magnitude of human suffering caused by mental disorder.

The delivery of mental health care is beset by many difficulties. It is a pluralistic delivery system with inequitable access, variable quality, and high costs. There is a major public health problem in the delivery of continuous care for the chronically ill, many of whom have been deinstitutionalized from psychiatric institutions over the past two decades. The public health problem of homeless people, especially wandering schizophrenic individuals and substance abusers, rivals other major medical crises today, such as the AIDS epidemic. This is partly because of a fragmentation of services, including general medical and social welfare services, and an uneven approach by state government toward the direct care needs of these individuals. Stigma issues remain (Rabkin), and public apathy toward the suffering of the mentally ill also hampers care.

Forms of Mental Disorders: DSM-III-R

In 1980, after 5 years of intensive work, the American Psychiatric Association published the third edition of its *Diagnostic and Statistical Manual of Mental Disorders* (DSM-III). The manual included more than 200 mental disorders, grouped in 17 categories, and it improved upon earlier editions in several ways. The term "mental disorder" was carefully defined. Diagnostic criteria were given for each disorder in order to increase the reliability of diagnoses. New diagnostic entities were created to take account of discoveries in the last 20 years regarding the causes, natural history, and treatment responsiveness of many forms of mental disorder. In 1984–1985 work commenced on a revision of DSM-III, and changes were made on the basis of empirical support from well-conducted research studies, increased clinical experience with DSM-III, and, in the case of a new diagnosis under consideration, the extent of research support for the category as contrasted to its perceived potential for abuse. There were three national field trials on the development of diagnostic criteria for disruptive behavior disorders, pervasive developmental disorders, and generalized anxiety disorder and agoraphobia. DSM-III-R was approved by the American Psychiatric Association board of trustees at the end of 1986 and published in 1987. The major diagnostic classes in DSM-III-R are as follows:

1. Disorders usually first evident in infancy, childhood, or adolescence (including developmental disorders, disruptive behavior disorders, anxiety disorders of childhood or adolescence, eating disorders, gender identity disorders, tic disorders, elimination disorders).
2. Organic mental disorders (disorders caused by or associated with impaired brain tissue function).
3. Psychoactive substance use disorders (including alcohol, drugs, and tobacco).
4. Schizophrenia.
5. Delusional (paranoid) disorders.
6. Mood disorders (bipolar disorders and depressive disorders distinquished).
7. Anxiety disorders (including panic disorder with or without agoraphobia and agoraphobia without a history of panic disorder, social phobia,

obsessive-compulsive disorder, post-traumatic stress disorders, and generalized anxiety disorders).

8. Somatoform disorders (physical symptoms suggesting physical disorders without organic findings).
9. Dissociative dirorders.
10. Sexual disorders (including the pedophilias and sexual dysfunctions).
11. Sleep disorders (a new category, including various insomnia and hypersomnia disorders, sleep–wake schedule disorders and parasomnias).
12. Factitious disorders.
13. Impulse control disorders not otherwise classified.
14. Adjustment disorders.
15. Psychological factors affecting a physical conditions.
16. Impulse control disorders (including pathological gambling and kleptomania).
17. Personality disorders (enduring maladaptive patterns of relating to, perceiving, and thinking about the environment and oneself).
18. Conditions not attributable to a mental disorder.

This last category is an attempt in DSM-III and DSM-III-R to avoid labeling all socially deviant behavior as symptomatic of a mental disorder; it includes antisocial behavior, malingering, and various marital problems.

The Prevalence of Mental Disorders

Recent findings from the National Institute of Mental Health (NIMH) Collaborative Epidemiology Catchment Area (ECA) program, a five-site community and institutional sample of the adult population of the United States, suggest new and more reliable prevalence rates for specific mental disorders. These prevalence rates are for 6-month periods and are based on the 1980 census. It is estimated that 29.4 million Americans aged 18 and over suffer from mental disorders, which represents 18.7% of the adult U.S. population (Locke & Regier). The prevalence rates for specific mental disorders are as follows:

1. Anxiety disorders—estimated to affect 8.3% of the adult population, or 13.1 million adults, in any 6-month period. Anxiety disorders are the most prevalent mental disorders.
2. Substance abuse disorders—affecting 7% of the population, with 5%, or 7.9 million adults, suffering from alcohol abuse or dependence and another 2% of the population, or 3.1 million people, suffering from other substance abuse or dependence.
3. Affective disorders—estimated to affect 6% of the population, or 9.4 million adults.

4. Schizophrenic disorders—although affecting only 1% of the adult population, approximately 1.5 million people, schizophrenia creates the highest social disability, accounting for about half of all public mental health dollars spent in the United States. It is the most common condition found among the mentally ill homeless.

In addition, there are estimates that approximately 2 million children have severe mental disorders, and only 500,000 of them receive any kind of treatment (NIMH, 1987). Especially troubling is the rate of teenage suicide. Although suicide was the eighth leading cause of death in the United States in 1982 for all ages combined, it was the third leading cause of death for age groups under 35. Teen suicides have increased dramatically over the last 25 years, increasing from 444 in 1958 ot 1,764 in 1975 (Weed).

Another important mental disorder is senile dementia, which affects approximately 3 million elderly and will continue to increase as the population ages. More than 20% of those over age 80 have symptoms of senile dementia. One form of dementia, Alzheimer's disease, affects approximately 1 million to 1.5 million people in the United States and is a major cause of nursing home placement (Goldman, Cohen, & Davis).

Of the 15 to 23% of the population afflicted by a mental disorder, only one in five receives any treatment from a mental health professional. The majority (57%) are evaluated and treated (with varying degrees of appropriateness) in the primary care/outpatient medical sector of the health care system. A small proportion (3%) are treated as inpatients in the general hospital or nursing home sectors. Twenty percent either receive no treatment or are seen by other human service providers such as clergymen or social welfare agencies (Regier et al).

The data that follow focus on the mental health sector of the U.S. health care delivery system. One must remember, however, that only one-fifth of mentally disordered people receive care in this sector. Training primary care physicians to recognize and treat mental disorders and establishing better linkages between the general health sector and the mental health sector are vital to improving the major portion of mental health care (Browskowski et al.; Goldman et al.; NIMH, 1983a, Series DN, No. 2).

Treatments and Services for the Mentally Ill

The term "mental health care" encompasses diverse preventive, therapeutic, and rehabilitative activities. Preventive mental health care aims at promoting mental health and preventing specific mental disorders. The first objective is difficult to attain because it is vague: Few people agree on exactly what promotion of mental health is. The second preventive aim has met with some success: Disorders such as syphilitic dementia and pellagrinous psychoses, for example, now rarely occur. Efforts to prevent childhood mental disorders through prenatal care, neonatal screening, childhood immunizations, adequate nutrition, and preschool education are receiving increased study. But primary prevention of schizophrenia, mania, depression, and other mental disorders of adult life remains beyond our powers (Langsley).

Therapeutic mental health services include individual, family, and group psychotherapies; hypnosis; psychodrama; expressive therapies such as art therapy; milieu therapy; medications; electroconvulsive therapy; and psychosurgery. Psychotherapies rely primarily on structured conversation and understanding aimed at changing a patient's attitudes, feelings, beliefs, defenses, personality, and/or behavior. The therapist's procedures vary across schools of psychotherapy and with the nature of the patient's problem. Psychoanalysis, for example, employs techniques such as free association and interpretations based on psychoanalytic theory to bring about personality restructuring. Most forms of psychotherapy, however, have much in common (Frank). Psychotherapy, hypnosis, and psychodrama are generally used to treat mental disorders other than psychoses and organic brain syndromes. Milieu therapy involves arranging the physical setting and social organization of an inpatient treatment setting to encourage socially acceptable and responsible behavior.

Most drugs effective in treating mental disorders have been available for less than 30 years. These include phenothiazines and other drugs for treating schizophrenia; tricyclic and other antidepressants for depression, panic attack, and obsessive-compulsive disorders; lithium and carbamazepine for manic-depressive disorders; and benzodiazapines for anxiety states (Barchas et al.). Amphetamines have been used to treat hyperactive children since the 1930s. Electroconvulsive therapy, which is effective for certain forms of depression, schizophrenia, and mania, was introduced in 1938 (Fink). Psychosurgery (neurosurgery used to treat a mental disorder) was widely used to treat schizophrenia in the late 1940s and early 1950s but is rarely used today for any mental disorder, usually as a treatment of last resort (Bernstein et al.; National Commission).

Rehabilitative mental health care includes occupational therapy, social skills training, and reeducation aimed at helping the patient return to normal living patterns. It may begin in an inpatient setting with patient self-government activities and social activities and can progress through transitional settings such as halfway houses, group homes, or supervised apartments. Rehabilitative care is employed primarily with patients suffering from chronic psychoses, drug addiction, or alcoholism.

Brief History of Mental Health Care in the United States

The mentally disordered in colonial America were treated slightly better than their European counterparts: Fewer were tortured, burned, hanged, or drowned as witches. The Salem witch trials of 1691–1692, during which 250 persons were tried and 19 executed, were an exception, not the rule. Throughout the colonial period, most mentally ill people were kept at home or wandered from town to town and often were lodged in jails or almshouses (workhouses). This remained the general pattern until the 1840s (Shryock).

As early as 1756, however, mentally ill patients were admitted to the newly established Pennsylvania Hospital, and in 1773 the first American mental asylum was established under government auspices in Williamsburg, Virginia. These two institutions marked the beginnings of humanitarian treatment of mentally disordered patients in America, although some treatments administered within their walls until the 1800s were primitive, including bloodletting, purges, and administration of emetics.

In the early 1800s the Quakers and American physicians exposed to European psychiatry encouraged the view that mental illness was treatable and espoused kind and sympathetic methods. Partly as a result, a few mental hospitals were opened where "moral treatment" (combining work, recreation, education, and kind but firm management) was predominant (Bockoven). Violent patients, however, were segregated in separate wards, and in most of the country mentally disordered paupers and blacks were sent to workhouses and jails (Mora). In 1841 an alliance of professionals and reformers began lobbying legislatures for improved care. Members of the first specialty medical society, the Association of Medical Superintendents of American Institutions for the Insane (now named the American Psychiatric Association) developed program information and statistics.

In 1854, Dorothea Dix, a citizen reformer, and many of the physicians who were part of this new specialty society managed after 4 years of intense lobbying to get Congress to pass the "12,225,000 Acres Act," a large federal land grant sale to provide federal funds to build mental hospitals. It represented the culminating effort of a group of farsighted and idealistic social reformers and physicians who believed that mental illness could be cured through kind and firm moral reeducation and circumstances far from the chaos of cities and the corrupting influences of modern life. President Franklin Pierce vetoed this bill with the following message:

> If the Congress has power to make provision for the indigent insane . . . the whole field of public beneficence is thrown open to the care and culture of the Federal Government. . . . I readily . . . acknowledge the duty incumbent on us all . . . to provide for those who in the mysterious order of providence are subject to want and to disease of body or mind, but I cannot find any authority in the Constitution that makes the Federal Government the great almoner of public charity throughout the United States. To do so would, in my judgement, be contrary to the letter and spirit of the Constitution . . . and be prejudicial rather than beneficial to the noble offices of charity.

Dorothea Dix, exhausted and dispirited, took 6 months off, then reorganized her allies and began the pursuit, state by state, of asylum care for the mentally ill.

She personally led to the founding of some 32 state mental hospitals, an extraordinary accomplishment (Foley & Sharfstein).

Despite the reformers' successes, the quality of care in state mental hospitals rapidly declined. Outright neglect and custodial care were fostered by the overcrowding of hospitals with criminals, alcoholics, vagrants, and state paupers; by a tendency to build larger institutions to keep per capita expenditures down; and by an increasing pessimism regarding the curability of mental disorders. Since mental hospitals were located away from population centers, the dismal conditions within them were easily ignored for a time. In the 1870s and 1880s a new wave of reform began, with criticisms of commitment procedures, the use of restraints, and the low level of staff training (Deutsch). Between 1890 and 1990 New York State reformed its mental institutions, but few states followed its example.

In 1908 Clifford Beers, a former mental patient, exposed the cruel conditions in public and private asylums with his autobiography, *A Mind That Found Itself.* Together with William James, Adolf Meyer, and others, Beers helped launch the National Committee for Mental Hygiene (NCMH), which lobbied on behalf of the mentally disordered and carried out a national census of institutionalized mental patients until the Bureau of the Census took this over in 1923. During World War I, the U.S. Army Surgeon General's office asked the NCMH to organize the psychiatric branch of the Army Medical Corps. For many years the NCMH surveyed conditions in mental hospitals. Inspection and accreditation of mental hospitals was not undertaken by the Joint Commission on the Accreditation of Hospitals until 1958.

At the beginning of this century, mental health care was primarily hospital-based, and biological approaches dominated etiological theories and applied treatments. During World War I, however, psychological and social contributions to cause and treatment were forcibly brought home to professionals and the public alike. Thousands of men were rejected for military service because of psychoneuroses. War neuroses ("shell shock") accounted for a large proportion of psychiatric casualties. Psychiatrists saw that situational stress could precipitate a mental disorder in "normal" individuals as well as in those with "psychopathic constitutions." Psychological and social techniques were soon employed widely by military psychiatrists to treat war neuroses and return soldiers to the front (Strecker). Early intervention prevented chronic disability. These lessons were lost on the military until World War II, but psychiatrists carried them back into civilian life.

In the 1920s the mental hygiene movement, nurtured by the National Committee for Mental Hygiene and strengthened by Freud's psychological theories and the experience gained in World War I, captured the popular imagination. As Deutsch (1947) writes,

Enthusiasm for mental hygiene swept the social work field. . . .[There was an] accelerated trend toward organizing mental hygiene clinics in the community. Most of them were connected with mental hospitals; some were attached to outpatient departments of general hospitals or to social agencies, courts and correctional institutions; some were independently created. . . . The movement was oversold by overenthusiastic converts who advanced mental hygiene as a sure cure for practically every ill that beset the world. (pp. 362–363)

In the 1930s the advance of the mental hygiene movement was slowed by the weight of the Depression, limited scientific knowledge regarding the prevention of mental disorders, and conflicts among various schools of psychiatric theory.

Between 1910 and World War II, psychoanalysis gradually came to dominate psychiatric training, outpatient care, and popular views of the nature of humanity. It did little, however, for severely disturbed individuals who, for the most part, remained in poorly funded, sparsely staffed, biologically oriented, custodial state institutions. In the 1930s new hope for these severely disturbed patients was raised by the discovery of new biological treatments: insulin coma, drug-induced convulsive treatments, electroconvulsive therapy, and psychosurgery. The Federal Public Works Administration added more than 60,000 beds to state the local mental institutions.

World War II again focused public attention on mental disorders: 1.75 million men were rejected for service because of mental or emotional disturbance, and a large number of veterans returned with emotional problems. In 1946 Congress passed the National Mental Health Act, which established the NIMH and gave new federal support for mental health services, training, and research. The Veterans Administration estabished psychiatric hospitals and outpatient clinics. Most inpatient treatment, however, still took place in state institutions, whose deplorable conditions were graphically described by two journalists, Mike Gorman and Albert Deutsch. Partly to compensate for limited professional personnel, institutions and outpatient clinics began to use group psychotherapy, which allowed one professional to treat many patients at once.

By the mid-1950s the number of persons hospitalized in state and county mental hospitals reached its peak: 558,900. At the same time, however, effective drugs for treating schizophrenia and mania were discovered (reserpine and chlorpromazine). These drugs replaced insulin coma and psychosurgery and allowed many patients to behave more rationally in institutions, to leave them, or to avoid hospitalization entirely. Effective drug treatment stimulated the introduction of milieu therapy, halfway houses, and aftercare.

In 1955 Congress established the Joint Commission on Mental Illness and Health, representing 36 organizations, to examine the nation's mental health care. The commission's 1961 report, *Action for Mental Health,* concluded that half of the patients in the state mental hospitals were not receiving active treatment. The commission's recommendations set the stage for the emphasis on community mental health care that marked the 1960s. They recommended establishing one fully staffed community mental health clinic per 50,000 citizens, limiting the bed complement of large psychiatric hospitals to a maximum of 1,000, and encouraging the use of community-based, short-term inpatient care.

Many of the commission's recommendations were incorporated in a 1963 Message to Congress by President Kennedy, the first presidential message Congress had ever received on behalf of the mentally ill and the mentally retarded. Congress responded with the Mental Retardation Facilities and Community Mental Health Centers Construction Act, which, in part, created federal support for community-based mental health services delivered by community mental health centers (Foley & Sharfstein). The 1960s also saw the introduction of additional effective drug treatments for mental disorders: benzodiazepines for anxiety disorders, tricyclic and monoamine oxidase-inhibiting drugs for depressions, and lithium for manic-depressive psychosis. Behavior therapy became popular for treating certain neuroses and behavior disorders, and research began to demonstrate the effectiveness of various psychotherapies (Bergin; Malan; Smith & Glass).

Congress continued to expand NIMH financial support for psychiatric and behavioral science research, psychiatric education in medical schools, residency training of psychiatrists, and community mental health centers. The creation of Medicare and Medicaid (Titles VIII and XIX of the Social Security Act) helped transfer some of the costs of caring for the chronically mentally ill to the federal treasury. Federal welfare support (Social Security Disability Income) and food stamps provided a minimal level of economic support for chronically mentally ill patients discharged from state hospitals. Unfortunately, the necessary networks of community medical, mental health, and human services agencies were inadequately organized and underfunded.

The 1970s saw a decline in federal support for mental health research and training and slow growth in funding for community mental health centers. The Carter administration renewed presidential interest in mental health. In 1977 President Carter appointed a President's Commission on Mental Health, with Mrs. Carter as honorary chairperson. The Commission's 1978 report included an extensive review of the magnitude of the nation's mental health problems and of the resources available to meet them. The problems inherent in transferring the care of chronically mentally ill patients from state hospitals to community agencies began to be recognized. Detailed recommendations were made for increasing community services for chronic mental patients; improving access to care for underserved groups (children, minorities, rural citizens, and the aged); improving insurance coverage for mental health services; encouraging federal support for training personnel for underserved areas and population groups; increasing public understanding of mental disorders; protecting patients' rights; and expanding the knowledge base through increased federal support of research (President's Commission).

The 1980s have been a period of fiscal retrenchment, with increasing numbers of Americans on the poverty rolls, cutbacks in programs for the poor, an increase in the number of homeless, and a new public health menace—the AIDS epidemic. During this time NIMH service programs, along with programs aimed at chemical dependency treatment, were block-granted to states, but the NIMH continued a major leadership role through its community support program and demonstration projects aimed at the homeless mentally ill. Indeed, the major public mental health problem in this country is the sight of the homeless mentally ill wandering the streets, often hallucinating, rummaging through garbage and sleeping on grates. This issue more than others has received attention through legislative hearings, the media, and public outcry. It is symptomatic of the release of thousands of patients from state facilities and the imperfect psychiatric technology that can help patients in the acute phase of a psychosis but does not provide a long-term cure. Patients then find themselves in underfunded community mental health programs, and when they discontinue treatment, they are readmitted to hospitals for short-term stays.

Legal advocacy for mental patients also received a strong federal push with the passage of legislation in the mid-1980s, and in 1987 the Medicare program was expanded to include additional outpatient care as well as day treatment. The NIMH mission has expanded in the area of research and neuroscience. Our knowledge of the brain is rapidly increasing, making the field of mental disorders one of the most exciting areas in medicine today.

Mental Health Personnel

Many types of professionals and nonprofessionals serve the mentally ill, including psychiatrists, nonpsychiatric physicians, psychologists, social workers, nurses, vocational rehabilitation counselors, occupational therapists, expressive art therapists, and teachers. In 1982 NIMH surveys identified 390,000 filled staff positions in 4,200 mental health facilities in the United States, excluding the Veterans Administration (NIMH, 1985). Slightly more than one-third of the total staff were professional, another third were other patient-care staff with less than a baccalaureate degree, and about a third were administrative, clerical, and maintenance staff. In this chapter we will describe the core mental health professions: psychiatrists, psychologists, social workers, and nurses.

Psychiatrists

The number of psychiatrists per 100,000 population doubled between 1955 and 1980 from 6.4% per 100,000 to 13.2% per 100,000 (Beigel & Sharfstein, 1984). Psychiatrists account for approximately 2 to 4% of staff positions in state and county mental hospitals, private psychiatric hospitals, and freestanding outpatient clinics and multiservice outpatient facilities. In nonfederal general hospitals, however, psychiatrists account for 8.5% of full-time equivalent (FTE) staff positions (NIMH, 1985).

Psychiatrists are physicians with postgraduate training of 4 years duration. The first year after medical school requires at least 6 months of general medicine and neurology; three years of psychiatric residency training follow. Psychoanalysts undergo additional years of education and training, including a personal psychoanalysis and supervision of their treatment cases. About 10% of all psychiatrists are psychoanalysts.

The American Psychiatric Association (APA) surveyed psychiatrists in 1982 and 1983. The APA study showed that there were approximately 37,000 psychiatrists in the United States in 1982. Survey responses of almost 20,000 were analyzed in a major report, *The Nation's Psychiatrists* (Koran).

The major findings of the study were as follows:

1. The proportion of women among active psychiatrists increased from 11% in 1965 to 17% in 1982. Psychiatry ranks first among medical specialties in the proportion of women practitioners.
2. Representation of ethnic minorities among active psychiatrists has increased to about 20%, but blacks and Native Americans remain underrepresented in comparison with their proportions in the general population.
3. The proportion of active responding psychiatrists certified by the American Board of Psychiatry and Neurology had increased since 1965 from less than 50% to 69%.
4. All states experienced increases since 1970 in their ratios of psychiatrists to population. However, the relative geographic distribution of psychiatrists has changed little.
5. The mean number of hours worked per week by psychiatrists in 48.7, and the most commonly reported primary work setting is private practice, accounting for 57.7% of active psychiatrists. This proportion is smaller for psychiatrists than for other physicians.
6. Seventy percent of active psychiatrists work in two or more settings.
7. Psychiatrists' medical training is directly utilized in the care of almost two-thirds of the patients seen in a typical work week. Medical diagnostic and treatment skills are applied indirectly in the care of all patients.
8. The mean number of patients seen by active psychiatrists in a typical week is 36.5.
9. The national adjusted gross professional annual income of active psychiatrists in 1982, adjusted for regional differences in the cost of living, was $82,200.

The largest proportions of patients treated by psychiatrists suffer from affective disorders (23%), schizophrenia (17%), anxiety disorders (13%), or personality disorders (11%). About 45% of psychiatrists' patients are seen for individual psychotherapy, half with medication and half without. An additional 20% are seen primarily for medication management, 18% for evaluation or consultation, and 0.5% for electroconvulsive therapy. The remaining patients are treated by means of psychoanalysis (2.2%) or other psychotherapies (12.5%). Thus, about two-thirds of psychiatrists' patients receive evaluation or treatments that depend on medical skills.

Even as the number of psychiatrists has grown steadily, a shortfall during the 1970s is only recently being made up by an increase of psychiatrists in residency positions. Whether there is an oversupply or undersupply of psychiatrists continues to be disputed. On the east and west coasts, many private practitioners complain of oversupply, but many areas of the country continue to experience an extremely short supply of psychiatrists in public, administrative, and rural settings. In 1982 there were 4 psychiatrists per 100,000 population in Idaho, compared to 31 per 100,000 in New York (Koran).

About 50% of medical mental health services, including medical management and counseling is provided by nonpsychiatric physicians (Talbott, 1985), such as general practitioners, family physicians, emergency physicians, neurologists, internists, and others. Psychiatrists are important teachers of these specialists, both in medical school and in postgraduate training.

Psychologists

The number of psychologists per 100,000 population tripled from 1955 to 1980, from 8.2 to 25 per 100,000. In 1984 psychologists accounted for 3.5% of FTE staff positions in specialty and mental health organizations (NIMH, 1987).

Psychologists are nonmedical professionals who may have either a master's or doctoral degree in one of many kinds of psychology, including experimental, social, general, and clinical (Rodnick). Only psychologists trained in clinical psychology programs must have supervised clinical experience. About 28,000 psychologists, of whom 90% held doctoral degrees, were providing mental health services in 1982 in mental health facilities, schools, community agencies, and private practices (Van den Bos & Stapp). Private practice is the primary professional setting of about 25% of all psychologists; 40% practice primarily in organized care settings, and 23% in academic settings. Psychologists working in mental health facilities carry out psychotherapy, diagnostic testing, research, teaching, and administrative duties and offer consultation to other human services agencies.

Psychologists have been extremely successful in lobbying the federal and state government to allow direct third-party payments without requiring physician referral or supervision (Meltzer). Psychologists have also been pressing for hospital admitting privileges, and they debate with psychiatrists the qualifications necessary for practicing psychotherapy. On the one hand, a medical education is not needed to be a skilled psychotherapist or to counsel or treat physically well individuals whose mental disorders do not require medications. On the other hand, only psychiatric physicians can prescribe indicated psychotherapeutic drugs, knowledgeably treat the large proportion of mentally disordered patients who suffer from both physical disease and mental disorder (Hall et al.; Koranyi; Tsuang & Simpson), and be relied on to recognize organic diseases masquerading behind mental symptoms (Hoffman & Koran; Lishman). Psychologists working in organizational settings are also finding themselves in competition with social workers and marriage and family counselors, who claim to offer the same psychotherapeutic services at even lower cost to the organization.

Social Workers

The number of social workers per 100,000 population tripled between 1955 and 1980, from 12.6 to 36.5 (Beigel & Sharfstein, 1984). In 1984 social workers accounted for 5.2% of FTE staff positions in mental health specialty facilities (NIMH, 1987).

Social workers may have a bachelor's, master's, or doctoral degree in social work, although a master's or doctoral degree is encouraged for those doing clinical work. Three-quarters of social workers in mental health facilities have a master's or doctoral degree (NIMH, 1983b). Most social workers practice in organized settings. Primary practice is the primary work setting for 12% and the secondary work setting for 8%.

Psychiatric social work received great impetus from the mental hygiene movement and child guidance clinics of the 1920s and 1930s. The social worker obtained diagnostic information from the child's parents concerning the child, the parents, and the environment, pooled this information with that gathered by the psychologist and psychiatrist, and then carried out therapy with the child's parents (Modlin). Today social workers like to practice with individuals and also be uniquely skilled to bring resources of community, health, and welfare agencies to bear on patients' problems. They also offer consultation to human services agencies and to a lesser degree engage in research and teaching. Most recently, social workers have become quite active in a variety of administrative roles, especially in the public sector.

Registered Nurses

In 1982 psychiatric nurses amounted to 11.1% of FTE staff positions in specialty settings. Registered nurses accounted for almost 30% of staff positions in nonfederal general hospitals and 50% of full-time staff positions in private psychiatric hospitals, compared to only 8.2% of such positions in state and county mental hospitals (NIMH, 1985).

Some training in psychiatric nursing is part of all general nursing education programs. A small percentage of registered nurses pursue specialized training in psychiatric nursing and pursue master's or doctoral degrees. Registered nurses are the largest group providing professional care in mental health facilities.

The role of the psychiatric nurse includes supervising patients' interactions on the inpatient unit, administering medications, assisting in other somatic treatments, helping patients with activities of daily living, and in some instances engaging in individual, group, or family therapy. Psychiatric nurses with advanced training participate in research, teaching, and administration and offer consultation to nurses and other workers in medical units and public health agencies (O'Toole).

Recently, nurses, following the lead of social workers and psychologists, have been lobbying state legislatures to permit increased autonomous practice; that is, being able to see patients without a prior referral or without supervision. However, the scope of practice for nurses has remained quite circumscribed (Carter).

Delivery of Mental Health Services

From the mid-19th century to the mid-20th century, psychiatric services in this country were primarily based in long-stay institutions supported by state government, and patterns of practice were relatively stable. In the past 35 years, remarkable changes have occurred. These changes include a reversal of the balance between institutional and community care, inpatient and outpatient services, and individual and group practice. Meanwhile, the rate of patient care episodes per 100,000 population has nearly tripled. Today, of the approximately 35 million Americans with mental disorders, almost 55% are seen entirely in the primary care sector or only in general health care settings. Fifteen percent are seen in the specialty mental health sector, and approximately 20% are not in treatment at all (Regier et al.).

Deinstitutionalization, or the departure of thousands of individuals from the large state hospital system, has occurred over the last three decades and has had a significant impact on the mental health care delivery system. At the peak of public asylum psychiatry in 1955, 559,000 Americans were hospitalized in state and county mental hospitals. Now only 75,000 to 100,000 people are long-stay residents in state mental hospitals, and total beds number around 120,000. In 1955, three of four patient care episodes took place in state hospitals, one of four in community settings. Today three of four patient care episodes occur in community settings, only one of four in institutional-type settings (Manderscheid & Witkin).

These changes occurred as a result of a number of forces, not the least of which was a change in the legal environment in the 1960s, when patient rights suits established the principle of treatment in "the least restrictive setting."

Further, social psychiatrists had established the deleterious effects of long-term institutional care, that is, the so-called social breakdown syndrome. The arrival of effective psychiatric medications ameliorated patients' behavioral symptoms and allowed discharge into the community. The increased proportion of the population with private insurance coverage for psychiatric services has also stimulated utilization. Probably the most significant factor in spurring the discharge of patients from state hospitals, however, was financing. With the federal Social Security titles—Medicare, Medicaid, supplemental Social Security—it became advantageous for states to discharge patients into a variety of nursing homes or board-and-care-type settings and utilize new federal dollars to deal with state fiscal concerns. As long as patients remained in state institutions, they were not eligible for federal funds. With the passage of Medicaid (Title XIX) in 1965, patients who moved into the community and into long-term-care institutions that were not institutions for mental diseases could be supported through that program, which provided a 50% federal subsidy. In 1972, with the passage of Supplemental Social Security (Title XVI), patients discharged from hospitals could pick up federal payments for board-and-care homes and other group living arrangements and for their daily support and also Medicaid for their treatment cost. This cost shifting strongly encouraged the emptying of state facilities because of the fiscal pressure on state budgets.

Admissions to state mental hospitals and the number of psychiatric beds in general hospitals increased dramatically during this same period. Most admissions, however, were actually readmissions, as hospitals experienced a "revolving door," with patients admitted for multiple acute stays. Further, nursing homes have become a substitute for state mental hospitals and have assumed the long-term-care function. One estimate places three-quarters of a million Americans with chronic mental illness in nursing homes (Goldman & Manderscheid). Most often, the mental disorders are of an organic nature, although nearly 100,000 patients have another psychiatric diagnosis, not a dementia nor other organic mental disorder, that requires long stay.

Decline in the use of state hospitals has had negative effects. Many patients—perhaps a million—have been discharged into communities that are ill-prepared to provide the therapeutic and rehabilitative services they need, such as halfway houses, aftercare programs, sheltered workshops, and psychosocial rehabilitation (Borus; Talbott 1980). Some have become homeless wanderers, shifted from the back wards to living on the streets. Many patients now reside in unlicensed and uninspected board-and-care homes that do not offer or arrange for active treatment (Lamb).

Since 1978 the NIMH, through its Community-Support Program, has provided leadership to states and local communities to help them build systems of coordinated and cooperative mental health, health, and human services agencies to meet the needs of the chronically mentally ill (Morrissey & Goldman).

In the past quarter-century, outpatient services have exhibited dramatic growth. The rate of additions to outpatient care doubled between 1969 and 1983, from 576 to 1,148 per 100,000 population. Most of this growth occurred in freestanding psychiatric clinics and community mental health centers, but non-federal general hospitals also registered large increases in patient volume (NIMH, 1987).

Although more than triple their 1969 number, patient additions to partial care in 1983 (177, 332) still represented less than 5% of patient additions to all mental health service organizations (NIMH, 1987).

The Settings for Mental Health Services

The number of organizations providing specialized mental health services rose nearly 50% between 1970 and 1984, from 3,005 to 4,438. Most of the increase is attributed to the growth in general hospitals with psychiatric units and in private psychiatric hospitals, which grew from 150 in 1970 to 220 in 1984, the great majority being part of investor-owned, for-profit medical chains. In 1970 there were 797 psychiatric units in general hospitals; there were 1,347 in 1984. In contrast, the number of VA medical centers and state and county mental hospitals have decreased during the same period. Indeed, nearly all of the decrease in inpatient beds during this period can be attributed to reductions in state and county mental hospitals, which decreased their bed count from 413,000 beds in 1970 to 130,000 in 1984, a decrease of 68%. Nonetheless, state and county mental hospitals still accounted for about 50% of all psychiatric beds in 1984, compared to 79% in 1970. Between 1982 and 1984, the number of beds in private psychiatric hospitals and in psychiatric units of general hospials increased more than the number decreased in state and county mental hospitals, resulting in an increase in the number of psychiatric beds for all organizations.

The number of organizations providing outpatient psychiatric services also increased between 1970 and 1984 and at a much greater rate than inpatient additions, rising 32% between 1969 and 1983. Partial hospitalization services also have grown considerably, from 778 in 1970 to 1,817 in 1984. These data are all abstracted from organizational information collected by the Survey and Reports Branch of the Division of Biometry and Applied Sciences at the NIMH (Witkin et al.).

If one adds the growth characteristics enumerated above to the growth of the mental health personnel, one can see that the mental health system, in the words of our modern corporate managers, "has expanded and diversified its portfolio." Indeed, expenditures by mental health organizations rose from $3.29 billion in 1969 to $14.4 billion in 1983, an increase of approximately 340%. Measured in constant (that is, noninflated) dollars, the increase was only 39%. State mental health agency funds account for 41% of the total, followed by federal funds with

13%. Funding sources, however, vary considerably by type of organization and location across the country (Witkin et al.).

In 1963 the federal government initiated a new type of mental health organization: community mental health centers (CMHCs). The CMHC program was an effort to provide access to an integrated set of services to residents of a specific geographic area (catchment are) containing from 70,000 to 200,000 persons. By 1980 there were 798 federally initiated CMHCs providing services in about half the country. Centers had to provide inpatient, outpatient, 24-hour emergency, partial hospitalization, and consultation/education services directly or through affiliative arrangements and had to treat individuals regardless of ability to pay. Later, centers were required to develop additional services, including rehabilitative aftercare services; specialized services for substance abusers, for children and adolescents, and for the elderly; and research and evaluation programs.

By 1980, 46% of the admissions to outpatient care in mental health facilities occurred in federally funded CMHCs, compared to 31% in freestanding psychiatric clinics. In addition, CMHCs accounted for 14% of all inpatient episodes (NIMH, 1983b, pp. 27, 88). Although federal grants to CMHCs totaled $314 million in 1980, this represented less than 5% of public funding for mental health services. In launching this program, the federal government bypassed state mental health agencies, which until that time had been slow to establish community-based programs. An unfortunate result was that CMHCs failed to focus on providing services to chronically mentally ill patients discharged from state mental hospitals (Morrissey & Goldman). Patients with diagnoses of neuroses and personality disorders were the largest group admitted to care (21%), with substance abusers (13%), and depressed patients (13%) next (President's Commission, Vol. 2, p. 319).

Between 1963 and 1982, successive administrations held varying views of the appropriate federal role in funding mental health services through the CMHC program. Republican administrations tried to limit it to a demonstration program, whereas Democratic administrations sought to expand the program gradually nationwide (Ochberg). With Public Law 97-35 (the 1981 Omnibus Budget Reconciliation Act), the Reagan administration repealed the legislation authorizing the CMHC program and consolidated all federal funds for mental health and alcohol and drug abuse services into a block grant program for the states, funded at 21% less (30% with inflation) than the previous year's appropriation (Estes & Wood). In addition, many states took steps to decrease their Medicaid expenditures, which had been an important source of funds for CMHCs. CMHCs ceased to be a federally recognized reporting category for mental health statistics. Depending on the services they operated and controlled directly, they were reclassified as multiservice mental health organizations, freestanding psychiatric outpatient clinics, or psychiatric units of nonfederal general hospitals. A 1983 survey of a sample of former CMHCs revealed that the cutbacks in federal and state funding had caused more than one-third of the centers to reduce staffing and services (Estes & Wood).

CMHCs were designed to remedy some of the deficiencies long recognized in the U.S. mental health care delivery system; however, the achievement of this laudable aim was blocked by various obstacles. Growth of nonfederal sources of funding was slower than expected. Insurance coverage for some services (day treatment, consultation and education, home visits) was quite limited. Some CMHCs had difficulty in obtaining provider status under state Medicaid plans, and some states limited CMHC participation in Medicaid. Local governments often allocated very little money to CMHCs, particularly in poverty areas. Nonetheless, older CMHCs depended less on federal funds than younger ones did (NIMH, 1974). The declining participation of psychiatrists in providing services and in administering CMHCs, together with the small percentage of CMHC caseloads represented by patients with severe mental disorders, led some to ask whether CMHCs were evolving into social agencies rather than providers of mental health care (Fink & Weinstein). Some CMHCs aroused local opposition when, because of their attempts at preventing mental disorders, they plunged into local political conflicts about resource allocation. CMHCs were not able to cure social inequities and injustices rooted in economics, politics, and racism (Musto).

The long-term effect of the CMHC experiment on the pattern of mental health service delivery is yet to be determined. Nonetheless, the experiences of CMHCs with catchment area responsibility; multigency agreements; the integration of different levels of care; consumer participation; and local, state, and federal politics provide a rich record to be consulted by those interested in planning improvements is general health care service delivery.

Insurance Coverage for Mental Disorders

Insurance coverage for mental health care has always lagged behind coverage for other medical care. Only 13% of the payment for mental illness treatment comes from private insurance dollars, compared with 28% for general medical care. States pay almost 50% of the cost of mental health care, while paying less than 15% of the cost of other medical treatments (Sharfstein et al.).

An analysis of data from the Bureau of Labor Statistics from 1979 to 1984 revealed changes in the level of insurance benefits for mental and nervous disorders in the private sector. Virtually all individuals with private health coverage have some inpatient psychiatric treatment included in the benefit package. Fewer than half of all individuals, however, have coverage for inpatient psychiatric treatment that is equal to the coverage for other illnesses, and this proportion is falling. In 1984, 48% had equal mental and general health coverages, compared to 58% in 1981. The limitations on psychiatric benefits include limitations on days of care and separate dollar limits, including fixed dollar caps on an annual or lifetime basis.

For outpatient care, although the vast majority (96%) has some coverage, this coverage is often quite restricted. In 1984 a total of 89% of all participants—up from 82% in 1981—had some outpatient coverage, subject to limitations such as additional copayment charges, higher deductibles, and specific dollar limitations. In this survey, the percentage of participants with any coverage for the treatment of alcohol abuse increased from 38 to 61% between 1981 and 1984 (Brady, Sharfstein, & Muszynski).

Differences in insurance for psychiatric versus other conditions arose in the 1920s and 1930s when hospital insurance was first written. Inpatient treatment for mental disorders then occurred largely in state-funded mental hospitals or in private mental hospitals used primarily by the wealthy. Although treatments and treatment settings have changed, rising health care costs, the absence of strong consumer demand for mental health coverage, and insurers' continuing fear of the potential cost of this coverage have kept these restrictions in place.

Today psychiatrists treat approximately twice the proportion of patients with no health insurance as do other physicians. Mental health coverage has been curtailed in a number of plans, including those under the Federal Employees Health Benefits Program (FEHBP). The Blue Cross/Blue Shield FEHBP, for example, in 1982 imposed a 50-visit limit on outpatient mental health treatment and a 60-day annual limit on inpatient care, whereas in the past treatment was limited only by medical necessity (Sharfstein & Taube).

Psychiatric care will not be adequately covered by insurance until the surrounding economic myths are addressed. The first myth is that costs of psychiatric treatment are uncontrollable and unpredictable, but experience contradicts this. For example, the Blue Cross/Blue Shield FEHBP had no limits on mental health coverage from 1967 to 1981, aside from the same deductibles and copayments as for general medical care. After the initial jump in costs immediately following the introduction of broader psychiatric benefits between 1967 and 1969, mental health care accounted for 7.2 to 7.7% of the total benefits paid from 1970 to 1981 (Sharfstein et al.), indicating that mental health costs are stable over time.

In 1971 the Rand Corporation began a health insurance study that enrolled 7,500 persons at six sites across the country in 14 different insurance plans. Patient copayments ranged up to 95%, with a maximum dollar expenditure of $1,000 per family (Brook et al.). The study found that expenditures for mental health care constituted only about 5% of the total health care costs for all insurance plan enrollees. Depending on copayment levels, between 7.1 and 9.6% of the population studied used mental health benefits, including visits to general practitioners and internists. Recall that the NIMH Epidemiological Catchment Area study recently reported mental illness prevalence rates of 15 to 23% of the population (and included only a portion of all mental disorders)

(Myers et al.). Only a small percentage of the Rand study population (0.4) saw clinicians more than 40 times a year (Brook et al.). This study and others underscore the stability over time of costs for mental health care under insurance (Krizay; Wells et al.).

Many of the restrictions on insurance coverage for psychiatric care appear to stem largely from concern about the costs of long-term custodial care or intensive psychotherapy. The standard treatment regimen for intensive psychotherapies involves a minimum of three therapy sessions a week. Within the FEHBP, which placed no restriction on the annual number of outpatient visits for more than a decade, the number of persons receiving intensive psychotherapeutic treatment ranged from 0.9% of all psychiatric outpatients treated in 1971 to 1.1% of those treated in 1973. The cost for treatment for this population during the same period ranged from 8.7% to 10.3% of the total cost of physicians' treatment of mental disorders (Sharfstein & Magnas).

Another myth is that mental health care costs are unstable because liberal coverage encourages unnecessary and excessive use. Supporters of this view cite data such as these: 9% of outpatient users of mental health care in the Blue Cross/Blue Shield FEHBP accounted for 45% of the total cost (Sharfstein & Taube). That someone with insurance may be more likely to initiate medical care and, once under care, be more likely to opt for more extensive treatment is not a phenomenon limited to mental health care. Insurance encourages utilization of all physician services. The Rand study, for example, reported that 1% of utilizers of medical care in their 7,500-person sample accounted for 28% of the total expenditures (Wells et al.).

A third myth is that mental health care is not cost-effective. However, a body of evidence suggests that expenditures for psychotherapy produce savings elsewhere in the economy through increased employee productivity, reduced absenteeism, and lower costs for other medical care (Jones & Vischi; Mumford et al.). For example, beneficiaries covered by the Blue Cross/Blue Shield FEHBP who began outpatient psychotherapy following diagnosis of chronic medical disease used 56% fewer medical services during the third year after diagnosis than did beneficiaries with the same diseases who received no outpatient psychotherapy (Schlesinger et al.). Considering costs and benefits from a broad societal perspective, the introduction of lithium for the treatment of manic-depressive psychoses produced a conservatively estimated 10-year savings of $4.2 billion ($2.9 billion in unexpended treatment costs plus $1.3 billion in productivity gains) (Reifman & Wyatt).

A final myth is that psychiatric treatment is not accountable to insurance carriers. Utilization review in the form of peer review has become the cornerstone of organized psychiatry's accountability to payers and consumers. Many insurance carriers have chosen to put strict limits on psychiatric care rather than implement peer review procedures. The APA developed peer review services in the early 1970s to give insurers the option of providing psychiatric care limited only by medical necessity, thereby enhancing their opportunity to achieve savings through cost avoidance in other areas of medical care. More than 400 psychiatrists nationwide now review mental health benefits claims for 24 national and local insurers. Three psychiatrists review each case, basing their evaluations on guidelines in the APA's *Manual of Psychiatric Peer Review,* which is regularly revised by the APA. In 1982 the APA conducted 5,000 reviews for Civilian Health Medical Program of the Uniformed Services (CHAMPUS) and 965 reviews for other third-party payers.

The cost savings reported from the APA program are impressive. Aetna Life and Casualty's peer review costs in 1981 were about $20,000; its estimated savings were $2.4 million. Mutual of Omaha Insurance Company estimated a savings of about $300,000 during its first year of participation in the program. CHAMPUS reports that peer review has led to "outright savings" of $5 million a year since it began participating 3 years ago. Additional savings in costs of medical care avoided as a result of peer review may be three to four times greater than the direct savings. Peer review has been effective in assuring that necessary and appropriate care is delivered (Sharfstein et al.).

Medicare

The general benefits and costs of Medicare, a federal program that insures through the Social Security system some health care costs of individuals aged 65 and over and disabled individuals regardless of age, are described in Chapter 12. About 29 million people are insured under Medicare. Under Part A (hospital insurance), benefits for inpatient treatment in a psychiatric hospital are limited to 190 days in a lifetime. Only 150 of these days (90 benefit-period days plus 60 lifetime-reserve days) can be used in any one benefit period. Benefits for psychiatric care in a certified general hospital or extended-care facility are the same as for any other form of medical care. This provision has increased the use of general hospitals to provide psychiatric care for the elderly. Medicare was the principal expected payment source for 78% of elderly patients admitted to psychiatric inpatient units in general hospitals in 1980 (NIMH, 1985).

Under Part B (supplementary medical insurance), benefits for physicians' outpatient care for mental illness was limited to 50% of the charges or $250, whichever is less (see below). Benefits for physicians' inpatient care for mental illness are the same as for other illnesses; that is, they are not limited. One hundred home visits are also covered and may be provided by mental health agencies.

A relatively small part of Medicare payments are for psychiatric services. In fiscal year 1981, about 2.4% of Medicare interim payments ($995 million of the approximately $41 billion in total interim reimbursements) was expended for psychiatric services. The breakdown of psychiatric payments was as follows:

Psychiatric hospitals (private & state)	$190,000,000
General hospitals	630,000,000
Psychiatrists and psychologists	115,000,000
Hospital outpatient services	45,000,000
Other institutions (SNFs, HHAs)	15,000,000
Total	$995,000,000

Thus, inpatient hospital services for psychiatric care (psychiatric hospitals plus general hospitals) accounted for 82% of Medicare reimbursements for psychiatric care. This represents approximately 2% of all Medicare reimbursements. Considered alongside the prevalence of mental disorders among the elderly, these percentages are strikingly low. After reviewing these and other data, the President's Commission on Mental Health recommended increased mental health benefits under Medicare as well as national standards for minimum mental health benefits and other service expansions and improvements under Medicaid (President's Commission, vol. 2, pp. 517–526).

In December 1987 Congress expanded the outpatient psychiatric benefit in Medicare as part of the Budget Deficit Reduction Act of 1987. Outpatient benefits were increased in two stages over a 2-year period to $2,200 annually, with a 50% copayment. This quadrupling in benefits basically keeps the out-patient psychiatric benefit on par with inflation since 1965. Benefits were expanded for partial hospitalization, which was established as a reimbursable service. Perhaps most significantly, all limits and special copayments were removed for "the medical management of psychopharmacologic agents" for Medicare beneficiaries. This type of "medical management" will be covered on a par with outpatient treatment for other medical illnesses, that is, with an 80–20 copayment and no visit or dollar limits. The definition of medical management is yet to be worked out in regulations.

Medicaid

Medicaid is a combined federal and state program that covers certain health care costs for eligible persons with incomes falling below stated levels. Eligibility standards and covered health care services vary from state to state; however, in no state is care of patients under age 65 in mental institutions included. The federal government views this as a responsibility long borne by the states through their own mental hospitals. Although no other restrictions by diagnosis are permitted, states can and have limited the amounts of covered mental health care. An APA survey revealed a typical set of limits in most states:

> For inpatient hospital care most states limit the number of days allowable to 30 or less per year. Inpatient physician visits are generally provided for but allowed

charges are usually set unrealistically low. Outpatient physician visits for psychiatric care are typically limited to 20 to 30 visits per year with maximum fees per visit usually set will below prevailing charges. (Muszynski et al., p. 865)

Few utilization data are available because states are not required to keep records by diagnosis. It has been estimated, however, that $2 billion in Medicaid funds was expended in fiscal year 1979 for care of the chronically mentally ill (Health Care Financing Administration). This sum represented about 9% of all 1979 Medicaid expenditures. Medicaid was the principal expected payment source for 23% of patients admitted to psychiatric inpatient units in general hospitals in 1980; private insurance was the principal expected payment source for 43%, Medicare for 15% and personal resources for 7%. Eight percent used "other" resources, and 4% made no payment (NIMH, 1985).

Legal Issues

Laws and their interpretations change with the times, and laws regulating the delivery of mental health services are no exception. Legal issues receiving substantial judicial attention in the past two decades have included commitment procedures, the right to treatment, the right to refuse treatment, and the insanity defense in criminal proceedings (Stone).

Civil commitment to a mental institution deprives a mentally disordered person of liberty, in exchange for treatment. The grounds for civil commitment vary in different states but include judgments that the person is dangerous to self or others, is unable to care for physical needs, or needs care or treatment. Recent rulings show a movement toward restricting the grounds for civil commitment, reducing the length of time a person can be committed by physicians without judicial review, abolishing indeterminate stays during which the patient cannot initiate discharge or release, and requiring commitment through the courts, with due process guarantees for longer-term commitments (Appelbaum, 1984a). In a 1978 case, *Addington v. Texas*, the U.S. Supreme Court determined that the standard of evidence for civil commitment should be "clear and convincing evidence," rather than the standard of "beyond a reasonable doubt" that applies in criminal proceedings. Applebaum has argued that the general principle behind these and other decisions of the Burger Court in the mental health arena was the desire to limit judicial intrusiveness into the operation of state-level institutions, such as hospitals, prisons, and schools (Applebaum, 1984b).

The civil and personal rights of committed and voluntary mental patients have been given increasing statutory recognition. These rights include the right to communicate with persons outside the institution; to keep clothing and personal effects; to practice religion freely; to receive independent psychiatric examination; to manage or dispose of property; to retain licenses, permits, or privileges established by law; to enter into contracts; to marry; and to sue and be sued (McGarry & Kaplan).

The Mental Health Law Project, sponsored by the American Civil Liberties Union Foundation, the American Orthopsychiatric Association, and the Center for Law and Social Policy, has been engaging in litigation and consulting with legislatures and mental health organizations to help secure these and other patient rights. Because of this attention to procedures and rights, seriously disturbed individuals are being given more humane care. But the conflicts, involving patients' rights to liberty, their need for care or treatment, and the state's interests in protecting their welfare and in preventing harm to others, remain (Roth).

A constitutional right to treatment for involuntarily committed patients was first recognized by a court in *Wyatt v. Stickney* in 1972. Guardians of involuntarily committed patients sued the Alabama mental health commissioner, charging that inadequate care was rendered in a state mental hospital. A federal district court judge agreed that patients had a right to treatment that included the right to certain standards of care. With the aid of medical and psychiatric consultants, he defined these standards to include individual evaluation, active treatment, minimum staffing ratios, detailed nutritional and physical standards, and compensation for work performed. But the judgment had certain limitations: It did not apply to voluntary patients, and it set no penalty for noncompliance. The mental health commissioner, a psychiatrist, did not contest the inadequacy of care at the state's institutions. He was fired and replaced by a finance officer.

Although lower courts have recognized a right to treatment on the part of involuntarily committed patients, the U.S. Supreme Court has not. The right to treatment recognized in 1974 by the Fifth Circuit Federal Court of Appeals in *O'Connor v. Donaldson* was rejected in 1975 by the U.S. Supreme Court (Weiner). The court held in this case, however, that states have no right to confine "a nondangerous individual who is capable of surviving safely in freedom by himself or with the help of willing and responsible family members and friends" (Weiner, p. 462).

The federal district court that decided *Wyatt v. Stickney* has remained active in working for improved levels of care in Alabama's state mental hospitals. Similar cases may therefore force state legislatures to allocate more resources to institutional care of the mentally disordered and to community-based care (Kaufman). Right-to-treatment cases on behalf of the mentally retarded have had some success in this regard (McGarry & Kaplan). Right-to-treatment litigation does raise the dangerous possibility that lawyers and judges rather than mental health professionals may begin determining the details of hospital administrative practices and the adequacy of individual treatment plans. If courts intrude too far on the decision-making prerogative of mental health professionals working in state institutions and departments of mental health, even fewer will work there than do now (Robitscher).

The right of committed patients to refuse treatment is not widely recognized.

Since committed patients are deprived of their liberty in exchange for treatment that is presumably in their best interests, to allow them to refuse it would seem contradictory. On the other hand, the state's coercive power must be restrained to prevent capricious application. Committed patients usually are regarded as legally incompetent to decide whether to accept particular treatments, although exceptions are made for electroconvulsive therapy and psychosurgery in a few states on the grounds that these treatments may harm patients or change them irrevocably. Electroconvulsive therapy, however, is much safer than many common surgical procedures; it is not known to cause permanent brain damage, and it brings about well-documented benefits (Avery & Winokur; "Electroconvulsive Therapy"; Fink; Janicak et al.). In most states, a committed patient's only grounds for refusing medications is religious principle, recognized by the Second Circuit Federal Court of Appeals in *Winters v. Miller* in 1971. These grounds for refusing were then recognized by the U.S. Supreme Court in the same year.

In Massachusetts, Colorado, and Oklahoma, however, committed mental patients can refuse treatment, except in narrowly defined emergencies, unless they are found incompetent by a judge. If a patient is found incompetent, the judge will decide "whether the patient, if competent, would have consented to the administration of antipsychotic drugs" (Gutheil, p. 213). Gutheil (1985) believes that the failure in Massachusetts "to defer in the average case to medical judgment may have introduced significant delays and impediments to the good treatment of patients in the name of protecting their rights" (p. 216). He plans an empirical study of this question.

In California the 1983 decision by the Federal District Court for the Northern District of California in *Jamison v. Farabee* established a review process when a treating psychiatrist wishes to use neuroleptic (antipsychotic) medication to treat an involuntary patient who has refused medication or who cannot give informed consent. Rather than resorting to judicial review, as in Massachusetts, the California decision requires an outside psychiatrist to examine the patient and the clinical records and then to approve or deny the medication's use. NIMH has funded a study of the implementation of *Jamison v. Farabee,* to identify costs, effects, and problems and their probable causes (Hargreaves). Because all laws and judicial policy decisions are social experiments, more frequent empirical investigations of their effects are desirable.

That involuntary treatment is not limited to psychiatric settings is often forgotten. Nonpsychiatric physicians on medical and surgical units of general hospitals use or prescribe restraints, psychoactive and other medications, intravenous fluids, and nursing care for patients who have refused these treatments (Applebaum & Roth).

The invocation of an insanity defense during John Hinckley's trial for the attempted assassination of President Reagan stimulated great public and professional interest in this difficult area of law. The Insanity Defense Work Group of the APA subsequently issued a review of the legal history of this concept and an exploration of potential changes in its application. The American Medical Association (1984) and the American Bar Association (Riley & George) also issued position statements. Whereas the APA and the ABA argued for the preservation in criminal trials of a more constrained insanity defense "based on inability to appreciate the wrongfulness of one's conduct at the time of the offense" (Glass, p. 399), the AMA argued for the abolition of the insanity defense and the enactment of laws "providing for acquittal when the defendant, as a result of mental disease or defect, lacked the state of mind (mens rea) required as an element of the offense charged" (AMA, p. 2967).

The APA group noted that most insanity acquittals are not awarded by juries; they result from concurrence between the prosecution and the defense. Among other issues, the group discussed (1) abolishing the insanity defense, (2) allowing a "guilty but mentally ill" verdict, (3) changing current standards employed in defining the legal concept of insanity, and (4) the appropriateness of current dispositions for defendents found "not guilty by reason of insanity" (Insanity Defense Work Group). Although this point of intersection between psychiatry and the law episodically receives great public attention, the intersection points discussed earlier affect far greater numbers of citizens.

"Mental health" encompasses the entire adaptation of the individual. Legal issues closely interrelate with psychiatric ones. Psychiatrists are often expected to perform a social control role in the process of hospitalizing and treating potentially dangerous patients. At the same time, the legal system is concerned with punishment for wrongdoing and not for illness. Patients have individual legal rights, but when their judgment is impaired, what is their right to treatment? When their judgment is impaired by a mental disorder, who decides what is more important—freedom or health? These questions will continue to be debated within our democracy, within the medical and legal professions as well as between them.

Conclusion: Progress in Understanding Mental Illness and the Promotion of Mental Health

Mental health care has grown, diversified, and prospered, especially over the last 35 years. Large state hospitals have been supplemented and supplanted by psychiatric units in general hospitals, new outpatient clinics, community mental health centers, day treatment, halfway houses, and private practitioners. Treatment has become more effective and specific, based on our growing understanding of the brain and behavior. Psychopharmacologic treatment has made possible the shift out of long-term custodial institutions, and psychosocial treatments continue the process of care and rehabilitation in community settings. Recent advances in the biological and behavioral sciences will continue to create improved opportunities for diagnosing, treating, and preventing mental disorders (Institute of Medicine).

Problems remain. Financing mental health care is difficult, and insurance coverage is inadequate. More extensive education of general physicians regarding mental disorders and their treatment is needed. Most mental health care takes place in the general physician's office, and the integration of mental health with general health services is a task that must continue well into the 1990s. This requires an integration of the financing streams, an end to discrimination under private health insurance, and a greater awareness on the part of general physicians of the mental and emotional problems of their patients.

The diversity of settings and treatments and of professionals who deliver mental health care is both a strength and a weakness of the overall system. The extent to which various settings and professionals are substitutable is a hotly debated subject and in need of studies of outcome and efficacy. Whereas there is a great deal of choice for the consumer of mental health care, being an informed consumer and making choices based on scientific evidence is difficult. The growth in our knowledge base and the opportunities for new discoveries give one optimism and hope. But governmental and nongovernmental support for research and service innovation is necessary. We hope that our readers will help provide the necessary political support for these continuing efforts.

References

American Medical Association. "Report of the Board of Trustees: Insanity Defense in Criminal Trials and Limitation of Psychiatric Testimony." *Journal of the American Medical Association, 251,* 2967, 1984.

Appelbaum, P. S. "Standards for Civil Commitment: A Critical Review of Empirical Research." *International Journal of Law and Psychiatry, 7,* 133, 1984. (a)

Appelbaum, P. S. "The Supreme Court Looks at Psychiatry." *American Journal of Psychiatry, 141,* 827, 1984. (b)

Appelbaum, P. S., & Roth, L. H. "Involuntary Treatment in Medicine and Psychiatry." *American Journal of Psychiatry, 141,* 202, 1984.

Avery, D., & Winokur, G. "Mortality in Depressed Patients Treated with Electroconvulsive Therapy and Antidepressants." *Archives of General Psychiatry, 33,* 1029, 1976.

Barchas, J. D., et al. (Eds.). *Psychopharmacology: From Theory to Practice.* New York: Oxford University Press, 1977.

Beers, C. W. A. *A Mind That Found Itself.* New York: Doubleday, 1939.

Beigel, A., & Sharfstein, S. S. "Mental Health Care Providers: Not the Only Cause or the Only Cure for Rising Costs." *American Journal of Psychiatry, 141* (5), 668–672 1984.

Beigel, A., & Sharfstein, S. S. (Eds.). *The New Economics and Psychiatric Care.* Washington, D.C.: American Psychiatric Press, 1985.

Bergin, A. E. "The Evaluation of Therapeutic Outcomes." In A. E. Bergin et al. (Eds.), *Handbook of Psychotherapy and Behavior Change.* New York: John Wiley, 1971.

Bernstein, I. C., et al. "Lobotomy in Private Practice: Long Term Follow Up." *Archives of General Psychiatry, 12*, 10, 1975

Bockoven, J. S. *Moral Treatment in Community Mental Health.* New York: Springer Publishing Co., 1972.

Borus, J. F. "Deinstitutionalization of the Chronically Mentally Ill." *New England Journal of Medicine, 305,* 339, 1981.

Brady, J., Sharfstein S. S., & Muszynski I. L. "Trends in Private Insurance Coverage for Mental Illness." *American Journal of Psychiatry, 143,* 10, 1986.

Brook, R. H ., et al. "Does Free Care Improve Adults' Health?" *New England Journal of Medicine, 309,* 1426, 1983.

Broskowski, A., et al. (Eds.). "Linking Health and Mental Health." In *SAGE Annual Reviews of Community Mental Health* (Vol. 2). Beverly Hills, CA and London: Sage Publications, 1978.

Carter, E. W. "Psychiatric Nursing." In H. I. Kaplan & B. J. Sadock (Eds.), *Comprehensive Textbook of Psychiatry* (Vol. 1, 4th ed.). Baltimore and London: Williams and Wilkins, 1985.

Deutsch, A. "The History of Mental Hygiene." In J. K. Hall et al. (Eds.), *One Hundred Years of American Psychiatry.* New York: Columbia University Press, 1947.

"Electroconvulsive Therapy: Consensus Conference." *Journal of the American Medical Association, 254* (15), 2103, 1985.

Estes, C. L., & Wood, J. B. "A Preliminary Assessment of the Impact of Block Grants on Community Mental Health Centers." *Hospital and Community Psychiatry, 35,* 1125, 1984.

Fink, M. *Convulsive Therapy: Theory and Practice.* New York: Raven Press, 1979.

Fink, P. J., & Weinstein, S. P. "Whatever Happened to Psychiatry? The Deprofessionalization of Community Mental Health Centers." *American Journal of Psychiatry, 136,* 406, 1979.

Foley, H. A., & Sharfstein, S. S. *Madness and Government: Who Care for the Mentally Ill.* Washington, D.C.: American Psychiatric Press, 1983.

Frank, G. F., & Kamlet, M. S. "Direct Costs and Expenditures for Mental Health Care in the United States in 1980." *Hospital and Community Psychiatry, 36,* 165, 1985.

Frank, J. D. "Common Features of Psychotherapy." *Australian and New Zealand Journal of Psychiatry, 6,* 34, 1972.

Glass, R. M. "Realities Not Myths." *Journal of the American Medical Association, 253,* 399, 1985.

Goldman, H. H., Cohen, G. D., & Davis, M. "Expanded Medicare Outpatient Coverage for Alzheimer's Disease and Related Disorders." *Hospital and Community Psychiatry, 36*(9), 939, 1985.

Goldman, H. H., & Manderscheid, R. W. "Chronic Mental Disorder in the United States." In R. W. Manderscheid & S. A. Barrett (Eds.), *Mental Health, United States, 1987* (DHHS Pub. No. ADM 87-1518). Washington, D.C.: U.S. Government Printing Office, 1987.

Gutheil, T. G. "Rogers v. Commissioner: Denouement of an Important Right-to-Refuse-Treatment Case." *American Journal of Psychiatry, 142,* 213, 1985.

Hall, R. C. W., et al. "Physical Illness Presenting as Psychiatric Disease." *Archives of General Psychiatry, 35,* 1315, 1978.

Hargreaves, W. A. *Jamison versus Farabee Implementation: The External Investigator.* Paper presented at the American Psychiatric Association Annual Meeting, Dallas, Texas, May 1985.

Hoffman, R. S., & Koran, L. M. "Detecting Physical Illness in Patients with Mental Disorders." *Psychosomatics, 25,* 654, 1984.

Insanity Defense Work Group. "American Psychiatric Association Statement on the Insanity Defense." *American Journal of Psychiatry, 140,* 681, 1983.

Institute of Medicine. *Research on Mental Illness and Addictive Disorders: Progress and Prospects.* Washington, D.C.: National Academy Press, 1984

Janicak, P. G., et al. "Efficacy of ECT: A Meta-Analysis." *American Journal of Pschiatry, 142,* 297, 1985.

Jones, K. R., & Vischi, T. R. "Impact of Alcohol, Drug Abuse and Mental Health Treatment on Medical Care Utilization." *Medical Care, 17,* ii–82 1979.

Kaufman, E. "The Right of Treatment Suite as an Agent of Change." *American Journal of Psychiatry, 136,* 1428, 1979.

Koran, L. M. (Ed.). *The Nation's Psychiatrists.* Washington, D.C.: American Psychiatric Association, 1987.

Koranyi, E. K. "Morbidity and Rate of Undiagnosed Physical Illnesses in a Psychiatric Clinic Population." *Archives of General Psychiatry, 36,* 414, 1979.

Krizay, J. "Federal Employees' Experience as a Guide to the Cost of Insuring Psychiatric Services in the Various States." *American Journal of Psychiatry, 139,* 866, 1982.

Lamb, H. R. "The New Asylums in the Community." *Archives of General Psychiatry, 36,* 129, 1979.

Langsley, D. G. "Prevention in Psychiatry: Primary, Secondary, and Tertiary." In H. I. Kaplan & B. J. Sadock (Eds.), *Comprehensive Textbook of Psychiatry* (Vol. 1, 4th ed.). Baltimore and London: Williams and Wilkins, 1985.

Lishman, W. A. *Organic Psychiatry.* London: Blackwell Scientific Publications, 1978.

Locke, B. Z., & Regier, D. A. "Prevalence of Selected Menal Disorders." In C. A. Taube & S. A. Barrett (Eds.), *Mental Health, United States, 1985* (DHHS Pub. No. ADM 85-1378). Washington, D.C.: U.S. Government Printing Office, 1985.

Malan, D. H. "The Outcome Problem in Psychotherapy Research." *Archives of General Psychiatry, 29,* 719, 1973.

Manderscheid, R. W., & Witkin, M. J., et al. "Specialty Mental Health Services: System and Patient Characteristics-United States." In C. A. Taube & S. A. Barrett (Eds.), *Mental Health, United States, 1985* (DHHS Pub. No. ADM 85-1378). Washington, D.C.: U.S. Government Printing Office, 1985.

McGarry, A. L., & Kaplan, H. A. "Overview: Current Trends in Mental Health Law." *American Journal of Psychiatry, 130,* 621, 1973.

Meltzer, M. L. "Insurance Reimbursement, a Mixed Blessing." *American Psychologist, 30,* 1150, 1975.

Modlin, H. C. "Psychiatric Social Service Information." In A. M. Freedman et al. (Eds.), *Comprehensive Textbook of Psychiatry* (Vol. 2). Baltimore: Williams and Wilkins, 1975.

Mora, G. "Historical and Theoretical Trends in Psychiatry." In A. M. Freedman et al. (Eds.), *Comprehensive Textbook of Psychiatry* (Vol. 2). Baltimore: Williams and Wilkins, 1975.

Morrissey, J. P., & Goldman, H. H. "Cycles of Reform in the Care of the Chronically Mentally Ill." *Hospital & Community Psychiatry, 35,* 785, 1984.

Mumford, E., et al. "A New Look at Evidence about Reduced Cost of Medical Utilization Following Mental Health Treatment. *American Journal of Psychiatry, 141,* 1145, 1984.

Musto, D. A. "Whatever Happened to 'Community Mental Health'?" *Public Interest, 39,* 53, 1975.

Muszynski, S., et al. "Paying for Psychiatric Care." *Psychiatric Annals, 14,* 861, 1984.

Myers, J. K., et al. "Six-Month Prevalence of Psychiatric Disorders in Three Communities." *Archives of General Psychiatry, 41,* 959, 1984.

National Commission for the Protection of Human Subjects of Biomedical and Behavioral Research. *Psychosurgery* (DHEW Pub. No. OS 77-0001). Washington, D.C.: U.S. Government Printing Office, 1977.

National Institute of Mental Health. *Patterns in Use of Nursing Homes by the Aged Mentally Ill* (DHEW Pub. No. ADM 74-69). Washington, D.C.: U.S. Government Printing Office, 1974.

National Institute of Mental Health. *Mental Health Services in Primary Care Settings: Report of a Conference, April 2–3, 1979.* (DHHS Pub. No. ADM 83-995.) Rockville, Md.: U.S. Government Printing Office, 1983. (a)

National Institute of Mental Health. *Mental Health, United States: 1983* (DHHS Pub. No. ADM 83-1275). Rockville, Md.: U.S. Government Printing Office. 1983. (b)

National Institute of Mental Health. *Mental Health, United States: 1985* (DHHS Pub. No. ADM 85-0000). Rockville, Md.: U.S. Government Printing Office, 1985.

National Institute of Mental Health. *Mental Health, United States, 1987* (DHHS Pub. No. ADM 87-1518). Washington, D.C.: U.S. Government Printing Office, 1987.

Ochberg, F. M. "Community Mental Health Center Legislation: Flight of the Phoenix." *American Journal of Psychiatry, 133,* 56, 1976.

O'Toole, A. W. "Psychiatric Nursing." In A. M. Freedman et al. (Eds.), *Comphrehensive Textbook of Psychiatry* (Vol. 2). Baltimore: Williams and Wilkins, 1975.

President's Commission on Mental Health. *Report to the President—1978* (Vols. 1–6). Washington, D.C.: U.S. Government Printing Office, 1978.

Rabkin, J. "Public Attitudes toward Mental Illness: A Review of the Literature." *Schizophrenia Bulletin, 10,* 9, 1974.

Regier, D. A., et al. "The DeFacto U.S. Mental Health Services System." *Archives of General Psychiatry, 35,* 685, 1978.

Reifman, A., & Wyatt, R. J. "Lithium: A Brake in the Rising Cost of Mental Illness." *Archives of General Psychiatry 37,* 288, 1980.

Riley, W. D., & George, B. J., Jr. "Reform, Not Abolition." *Journal of the American Medical Association, 251,* 2947, 1984.

Robitscher, J. "Implementing the Rights of the Mentally Disabled: Judicial Legislative and Psychiatry Action." In F. J. Ayd, Jr., et al. (Eds.), *Medical, Moral and Legal Issues in Mental Health Care.* Baltimore: Williams and Wilkins, 1974.

Rodnick, E. H. "Clinical Psychology." In H. I. Kaplan & B. J. Sadock (Eds.), *Comprehensive Textbook of Psychiatry* (Vol. 1, 4th ed.). Baltimore and London: Williams and Wilkins, 1985.

Roth, L. H. "A Commitment Law for Patients, Doctors and Lawyers." *American Journal of Psychiatry, 136,* 1121, 1979.

Schlesinger HJ, Mumford E, Glass GV, Patrick C, Sharfstein SS: Mental health treatment and medical care utilization in a fee-for-service system: outpatient mental health treatment following the onset of a chronic disease. American Journal of Public Health. 73:422–428, 1983.

Sharfstein, S. S. et al. *Health Insurance and Psychiatric Care: Update and Appraisal.* Washington, D.C.: American Psychiatric Press, 1984.

Sharfstein, S. S., & Magnas, H. L. "Insuring Intensive Psychotherapy." *American Journal of Psychiatry, 132,* 70, 1975.

Sharfstein, S. S., & Taube, C. A. "Reductions in Insurance for Mental Disorders: Adverse Selection, Moral Hazard, and Consumer Demand." *American Journal of Psychiatry, 139,* 1425, 1982.

Shryock, R. H. "The Beginnings: From Colonial Days to the Foundation of the American Psychiatric Association." In J. K. Hall et al. (Eds.), *One Hundred Years of American Psychiatry.* New York: Columbia University Press, 1947.

Smith, M. L., & Glass, G. V. "Meta-Analysis of Psychotherapy Outcome Studies." *American Psychologist, 32,* 752, 1977. Rockville, MD: Dept of Health, Education, and Welfare.

Stone, A. A. *Mental Health and Law: A System in Transition.* National Institute of Mental Health (DHEW Pub. 75-176). 1975.

Strecker, E. A. "Military Psychiatry: World War I, 1917–1918." In J. K. Hall et al. (Eds.), *One Hundred Years of American Psychiatry.* New York: Columbia University Press, 1947.

Talbott, J. A. *Contemporary Social Issues and Decisions That Will Affect the Future Practice of Psychiatry.* Unpublished manuscript 1985.

Talbott, J. A. (Ed.). *State Mental Hospitals: Problems and Potentials.* New York: Human Sciences Press, 1980.

Tsuang, M. T., & Simpson, J. C. "Mortality Studies in Psychiatry." *Archives of General Psychiatry, 42,* 98, 1985.

VandenBos, G. R., & Stapp, J. "Service Providers in Psychology: Results of the 1982 APA Human Resources Survey." *American Psychologist, 38,* 1330, 1983.

Weed, J. A. "Suicide in the United States: 1952–1982." In C. A. Taube & S. A. Barrett (Eds.), *Mental Health, United States, 1985* (DHHS Pub. No. ADM 85-1378). Washington, D.C.: U.S. Government Printing Office, 1985.

Weiner, B. A. "Supreme Court Decisions on Mental Health: A Review." *Hospital and Community Psychiatry, 33,* 1982.

Wells, K. B., et al. *Cost Sharing and the Demand for Ambulatory Mental Health Services.* Santa Monica, CA: Rand Corporation, 1982.

Witkin, M. J. et al. "Specialty Mental Health System Characteristics." In R. W. Manderscheid & S. A. Barrett (Eds.), *Mental Health, United States, 1987* (DHHS Pub. No. ADM 87-1518). Washington, D.C.: U.S. Government Printing Office, 1987.

10

Financing for Health Care

James R. Knickman and Kenneth E. Thorpe

A key factor that shapes the delivery of health care in the United States is the evolving system for financing services. The types of services delivered and the organizational approaches to delivering services are heavily influenced by how health care is paid for and the aggregate resources available for health care.

The financing system that has evolved over the past 25 years in the United States involves a complex blend of public and private responsibilities. This system varies substantially from the largely public financing systems that exist in many European countries. An understanding of how health care is paid for is useful for developing an understanding of the general organization of health care in America.

Payment approaches for health care have been undergoing tremendous changes since the early 1980s. The basic approach for reimbursing hospital care has been completely restructured by many payers for care, and payment approaches for physicians and long-term-care providers also are being restructured. As emphasized here, financing approaches vary from provider to provider and from payer to payer, and financing approaches will continue to evolve over time. Thus, this chapter attempts to explain not only the current structure of financing approaches but also the principles behind the financing system.

In explaining how the American health care financing system operates, this chapter focuses on

- What health care resources buy.
- Where resources come from.
- How health care providers are paid.
- Why health care expenditures have been increasing.

As displayed in Table 10.1, $500 billion, or just over 11% of the gross national product (GNP), was spent for health purposes in 1987. These expenditures represent $1,987 per year for each person. Thus, the health care sector represents a major element of the American economy. As a component of the economy, health care has been growing at a fast rate over the past 25 years. As a point of comparison, health expenditures totaled only $43 billion in 1965, or 6.2% of the GNP. From 1965 onward, outlays for health rose, on the average, 10.6% each year. Although the rate of increase in costs between 1986 and 1987 was 9.8%, which was much lower than the peak inflation rate of 15.3%, growth in health care expenditures continues to exceed by a wide margin the overall inflation rates prevalent in the American economy. An important element of the study of health care finance, therefore, is analysis to understand the dynamics of spending in the United States and to understand what is being achieved by the ever-increasing health care expenditure levels.

What the Money Buys

National health care expenditures, as measured by the federal Health Care Financing Administration (HCFA), are grouped into two categories: (1) research and medical facilities construction and (2) payments for health services and supplies (see Table 10.2). Personal health care expenses constitute the bulk of the latter, $442.6 billion in 1987. Five types of personal health care expenditures account for over 80% of the 1987 total: 38.9% went to hospitals, 20.5% to physicians, 8.1% for nursing home care, 6.8% for drugs and drug sundries, and 6.6% for dentists' services. The other categories of expenditures are "other professional services," such as podiatry and private speech thereapy, 3.2%; "other health services," 2.4%; administrative expenses, 5.2%; government public health activities, 2.9%; and construction, 1.7%. The costs of medical education are not included in these HCFA figures, except insofar as they are inseparable from hospital expenditures and biomedical research.

Where the Money Comes From

Ultimately, the people pay all health care costs. Thus, when we say health care monies come from different sources, we really mean that dollars take different routes on their way from consumers to providers: through government, private insurance companies, and independent plans, in addition to out-of-pocket payments. In 1987 close to 28% of personal health care expenditures were directly out-of-pocket ($123.0 billion). At the same time, the government share exceeded 39% (about $175.3 billion), with the federal government bearing nearly three-fourths of that. Finally, almost 32% was paid through insurance companies ($139.1 billion) (Letsch et al.).

Table 10.1 Aggregate and Per Capita National Health Expenditures, by Source of Funds and Percentage of Gross National Product, Selected Calendar Years, 1929–1983

Calendar year	Total GNP[a]	Total health expenditures			Private health expenditures			Public health expenditures		
		Amount[a]	Per capita	% of GNP	Amount[a]	Per capita	% of Total	Amount[a]	Per capita	% of Total
1929	$ 103.3	$ 3.6	$ 29	3.5	$ 3.2	$ 25	86.4	$ 0.5	$ 4	13.6
1935	72.2	2.9	23	4.0	2.4	18	80.8	0.6	4	19.2
1940	99.7	4.0	30	4.0	3.2	24	79.7	0.8	6	20.3
1950	284.8	12.7	82	4.5	9.2	60	72.8	3.4	22	27.2
1955	398.0	17.7	105	4.4	13.2	78	74.3	4.6	27	25.7
1960	503.7	26.9	146	5.3	20.3	110	75.3	6.6	36	24.7
1965	688.1	43.0	217	6.2	32.3	163	75.1	10.7	54	24.9
1966	753.0	47.3	236	6.3	34.0	170	71.8	13.3	67	28.2
1967	796.3	52.7	260	6.6	33.9	168	64.4	18.8	93	35.6
1968	868.0	58.9	288	6.8	37.1	181	63.0	21.8	107	37.0
1969	935.5	66.2	321	7.1	41.6	202	62.9	24.5	119	37.1
1970	982.4	74.7	359	7.6	47.5	228	63.5	27.3	131	36.5

1971	1,063.4	82.8	393	7.8	51.4	244	62.1	31.4	149	37.9
1972	1,185.9	93.6	429	7.9	58.5	268	62.3	35.4	162	37.7
1973	1,326.4	103.4	468	7.8	64.0	290	61.9	39.4	178	38.1
1974	1,434.2	116.3	522	8.1	68.8	309	59.1	47.6	214	40.9
1975	1,549.2	132.7	590	8.6	76.3	340	57.5	56.4	251	42.5
1976	1,718.0	150.8	665	8.8	87.9	388	58.3	62.8	277	41.7
1977	1,918.3	170.2	743	8.9	100.1	437	58.8	70.1	306	41.2
1978	2,163.9	190.0	822	8.8	110.1	476	57.9	79.9	346	42.1
1979	2,417.8	215.1	920	8.9	124.2	531	57.7	90.9	389	842.3
1980	2,631.7	248.0	1,049	9.4	142.2	601	57.3	105.8	448	42.7
1981	2,957.8	285.8	1,197	9.7	164.2	688	57.4	121.7	510	42.6
1982	3,069.2	322.3	1,337	10.5	186.5	774	57.9	135.8	564	42.1
1983	3,406.0	357.2	1,473	10.5	209.7	865	58.7	147.5	609	41.3
1984	3,772.0	388.5	1,587	10.3	228.8	935	58.9	159.6	652	41.1
1985	4,015.0	419.0	1,696	10.4	244.0	987	58.2	175.0	708	41.8
1986	4,240.0	455.7	1,827	10.7	266.8	1,069	58.5	188.9	757	41.5
1987	4,527.0	500.3	1,987	11.1	293.0	1,164	58.6	207.3	824	41.4

aIn billions of dollars.

Source: Adapted from R. M. Gibson et al., "National Health Expenditures, 1983," *Health Care Financing Review, 6,* Winter 1984; and R. M. Gibson, "National Health Expenditures, 1978," *Health Care Financing Review, 1,* Summer 1979, Table 1.

Table 10.2 Aggregate and Per Capita Amount and Percentage Distribution of National Health Expenditures, Selected Calendar Years, 1970–1983

Type of expenditure	Aggregate amount ($ millions)									(Aggregate amount ($ billions)			
	1970	1975	1977	1978	1979	1980	1981	1982	1983	1984	1985	1986	1987
Total	$74,740	$131,465	$169,994	$192,448	$215,100	$248,000	$285,800	$322,300	$355,400	$388.5	$419.0	$455.7	$500.3
Health services and supplies	69,449	123,211	161,247	183,007	204,600	236,100	272,700	308,100	340,100	372.7	403.4	439.3	483.2
Personal health care expenses	65,723	116,297	149,139	167,911	189,600	219,100	253,400	284,700	313,300	340.1	368.3	401.6	442.6
Hospital Care	27,799	52,138	67,914	76,025	87,000	101,300	117,900	134,900	147,200	156.1	166.7	178.4	194.7
Physicians' services	14,340	24,932	31,242	35,250	40,200	46,800	54,800	61,800	69,000	74.4	81.4	91.6	102.7
Dentists' services	4,750	8,237	11,650	11,800	13,300	15,400	17,300	19,500	21,800	24.6	27.1	29.6	32.8
Other professional services	1,595	2,619	3,700	4,275	4,700	5,600	6,400	7,100	8,000	10.8	12.4	14.1	16.2
Drugs and drug sundries	8,406	11,812	13,810	15,098	17,100	18,500	20,500	21,800	23,700	26.5	28.5	31.3	34.0
Eyeglasses and appliances	2,100	2,981	3,455	3,879	4,700	5,100	5,600	5,500	6,200	7.0	7.8	8.7	9.5
Nursing home care	4,677	9,886	13,364	15,751	17,400	20,400	23,900	26,500	28,800	31.6	34.7	37.4	40.6
Other health services	2,058	3,691	4,005	4,333	5,100	5,900	7,000	7,600	8,500	9.0	9.8	10.7	12.0

Expenses for prepayment and administration	2,286	3,717	7,844	7,500	8,600	9,200	10,600	13,400	15,600	21.7	22.6	23.9	25.9
Government public health activities	1,440	3,198	4,264	5,073	6,400	7,700	8,600	10,000	11,200	11.0	12.5	13.8	14.7
Research and medical facilities construction	5,291	8,254	8,746	9,441	10,400	11,900	13,200	14,200	15,300	15.8	15.6	16.4	17.1
Research	1,862	3,186	3,714	4,287	4,700	5,400	5,600	5,900	6,200	6.9	7.5	8.3	8.8
Construction	3,429	5,068	5,032	5,154	5,700	6,500	7,600	8,300	9,100	8.9	8.1	8.0	8.3
Per capita amount													
Total	$358.63	$604.57	$768.77	$863.01	$920.01	$1,049.07	$1,197.32	$1,336.79	$1,458.90	$1,587.01	$1,695.67	$1,826.45	$1,986.89
Health services and supplies	333.25	566.61	729.22	820.68	875.11	998.73	1,142.44	1,277.89	1,396.10	1,522.47	1,632.54	1,760.72	1,918.98
Personal health care expenses	315.25	534.82	674.46	752.98	810.95	937.13	1,061.58	1,180.84	1,286.10	1,389.30	1,490.49	1,609.62	1,757.74
Hospital Care	133.39	239.77	307.13	340.93	372.11	428.51	493.93	559.52	604.20	637.66	674.62	715.03	733.23
Physicians' services	68.81	114.66	141.26	158.08	171.94	197.97	229.58	256.33	283.20	303.92	329.42	367.13	407.86
Dentists' services	22.79	37.88	52.69	59.64	56.89	65.14	72.48	80.88	89.40	100.49	109.67	118.64	130.26
Other professional services	7.65	12.04	16.73	19.17	20.10	23.69	26.81	29.45	32.80	44.12	50.18	56.51	64.34
Drugs and drug sundries	40.33	54.32	62.45	67.70	73.14	78.26	85.88	90.42	97.20	108.25	115.34	125.45	135.03

Table 10.2 (continued)

Type of expenditure	Aggregate amount ($ millions)									(Aggregate amount ($ billions)			
	1970	1975	1977	1978	1979	1980	1981	1982	1983	1984	1985	1986	1987
Eyeglasses and appliances	10.07	13.71	15.62	17.40	20.10	21.57	23.46	22.81	25.20	28.59	31.57	34.87	37.73
Nursing-home care	22.44	45.46	60.44	70.64	74.42	86.29	100.13	109.91	118.20	129.08	140.43	149.90	161.24
Other health services	9.87	16.97	18.11	19.43	21.81	24.96	29.33	31.52	34.80	36.76	39.66	42.88	47.66
Expenses for prepayment and administration	10.93	17.09	35.47	44.94	36.78	38.92	44.41	55.58	64.00	88.64	91.46	95.79	102.86
Government public health activities	6.91	14.71	19.28	22.75	27.37	32.57	36.03	41.48	45.90	44.93	50.59	55.31	58.38
Research and medical facilities construction	25.39	37.96	39.55	42.34	44.48	50.34	55.30	58.90	62.80	64.54	63.13	65.73	67.91
Research	8.93	14.65	16.80	19.23	20.10	22.84	23.46	24.47	25.40	28.19	30.35	32.27	34.95
Construction	16.45	23.31	22.76	23.11	24.38	27.50	31.84	34.42	37.30	36.36	32.78	32.06	32.96

Source: R. M. Gibson, "National Health Expenditures, 1983," Health Care Financing Review, 6, Winter 1984, Table 2.

Public Outlays

The 39% of personal health care expenditures transferred by the public sector in 1987 ($175.3 billion) compares with 39% in 1980, 22% in 1965, 22% in 1950, and 9% in 1929. The increase, especially since 1965, is largely a result of greater federal expenditures. Proportionately, state and local government outlays have remained rather constant over time, in the 10 to 13% range. The significant rise in federal spending is accounted for by the Medicare and Medicaid programs, Title XVIII and XIX, respectively, of the Social Security Act.

Medicare. Medicare was inaugurated on July 1, 1966. It provides a range of medical care benefits for persons aged 65 and over who are covered by the Social Security system. The 1972 amendments to the Social Security Act extended benefits to persons aged 65 and older who do not meet the criteria for the regular Social Security program but who are willing to pay a premium for coverage. In July 1973 benefits were further extended to the disabled and their dependents and those suffering from chronic kidney disease (Russell et al.).

Part A of the program, financed by payroll taxes collected under the Social Security system, provides coverage for care rendered in a hospital, an extended-care facility, or the patients home. Part B, a voluntary supplemental program that pays certain costs of physicians' services and other medical expenses, is supported in part by general tax revenues and in part by contributions paid by the elderly (Somers & Somers). Neither Part A nor Part B of Medicare, however, offers comprehensive coverage. Built into the program are deductibles (set amounts the patient must pay for each type of service each year before Medicare begins to pay) and co-insurance (a percentage of charges paid by the patient). Limitations on the amount of coverage exist as well. Hospital benefits cease after 90 days if the patient has exhausted his lifetime reserve pool of 60 additional days; extended-care facility benefits end after 100 days. Home health care visits are limited in number to 100 (Russell et al., p. 51).

In 1988, Congress passed a bill to substantially expand Medicare coverage. This legislation, the Medicare Catastrophic Act of 1988, set limits on the maximum out-of-pocket costs that beneficiaries are responsible for in the case of hospital care, physician services, and pharmaceuticals.

The Medicare Catastrophic Program, however, was greeted unenthusiastically by many elderly, and at the time this chapter was written, Congress was coming to a decision to abandon the program. The program's unpopularity is caused by its financing approach which passes along the costs of the program to the elderly in the form of new premiums and income-related surcharges to the elderly's federal income tax. The elderly particularly objected to the added income tax, in part because many of the wealthy elderly who were required to pay the maximum tax already had arranged for similar supplementary insurance coverage through private insurance companies.

Quality and cost of care delivered by public programs have been long-standing issues. Medicare amendments passed in 1972 established professional standards review organizations (PSROs) to monitor the quality and quantity of institutional services delivered to Medicare and Medicaid recipients. The 1982 Tax Equity and Fiscal Responsibility Act (TEFRA), discussed below, replaced the PSROs with a "utilization and quality control peer review organization" (PRO). Subsequent legislation (P.L. 98-21) required that hospitals covered under Medicare's new case payment system contract with a PRO by 1984. The new PROs differ substantially from the old PSROs: PROs are to be statewide organizations unless exceptional circumstances pertain; they may be for-profit as well as nonprofit operations; they require participation of only a small segment of area physicians; and they operate under contract with the Health Care Financing Administration, with performance judged against preestablished and quantifiable contract objectives.

As with quality and cost reviews, recent changes in Medicare provisions have changed radically the way Medicare pays for hospital care. The TEFRA legislation of 1982 was designed to provide incentives for cost containment. Most important, TEFRA established a case-based reimbursement system (DRGs, or diagnosis related groups) while also placing limits on the rates of increase in hospital revenues. TEFRA was followed in 1983 by Title VI of P.L. 98–21, which established a prospective payment system. Discussion of the principles of these 1983 amendments is provided later in this chapter.

Medicaid. Unlike Medicare, Medicaid is a program run jointly by federal and state governments; the name is more or less a blanket label for 50 different state programs designed specifically to serve the poor. Beginning in January 1967, Medicaid provided federal funds to states on a cost-sharing basis (according to each state's per capita income) so that welfare recipients could be guaranteed medical services. Payment in full was to be afforded to the aged poor, the blind, the disabled, and families with dependent children if one parent was absent, unemployed, or unable to work. Four types of care were covered: (1) inpatient and outpatient hospital care, (2) other laboratory and x-ray services, (3) physician services, and (4) skilled nursing care for persons over age 21. By July 1970 home health services and early and periodic detection and treatment of disease for persons under age 21 also were covered.

The 1972 Social Security Act amendments added family planning to the list of "musts." Prescriptions, dental services, eyeglasses, and care in an "intermediate facility" (institutions that do not qualify as skilled nursing homes or those serving the mentally retarded) are allowable "optionals," as is coverage of the medically indigent (those who are self-supporting except for medical care costs). Under the 1972 amendments, coverage of the medically indigent is, by law, tied to their payment of monthly premiums, the amount graduated by income. Deductibles and co-payments also are allowed on all services for the medically indigent and on optional services for welfare recipients (Russell et al.).

Eligibility for Medicaid is determined by the states but must include cash assistance recipients and, with the passage of the Deficit Reduction Act of 1984 (P.L. 98-368), three other groups: poor children up to age 5, pregnant women who are poor and who will qualify for cash assistance programs when their children are born, and pregnant women in two-parent families with an unemployed principal wage earner. States also may expand coverage to special groups such as individuals who become poor or due to expenditures on health care.

State flexibility in determining eligibility standards for cash assistance has created wide variation in Medicaid coverage. Some states set income thresholds below the federal poverty level. Others expand coverage to a categorically or medically needy group. As a result, many poor individuals are not eligible for Medicaid. For example, in 1979 the ratio of Medicaid recipients to individuals living below the poverty line ranged from 115% in Massachusetts to 24% in several states (Muse & Sawyer). Moreover, of those with incomes below 125% of the poverty level, more than 25% have no health insurance, and another 20% of the "near poor" are uninsured (Davis & Rowland).

Because of the gaps in insurance coverage for the poor and near poor that are not taken care of by the Medicaid programs, much recent debate and analysis has focused on how to pay for services to individuals uncovered by Medicare, private insurance, or Medicaid. Five states (New York, New Jersey, Massachusetts, South Carolina, and Florida) have established bad-debt and charity-care pools to pay for hospital services and, in some cases, physician services for individuals who have no source of payment for their medical care. These programs have developed, in part, to spread the burden of the costs of care to indigents across the hospital system. The pools are generally funded through some form of tax or surcharge on hospital revenues from third parties (Lewin & Lewin).

Some states, as well as the federal government, are exploring mandatory insurance coverage by employers and also methods for extending insurance on an individual basis to the near poor (Wilensky, 1988). Other states have established "risk pools" to make insurance coverage more accessible to individuals who historically are "medically uninsurable" because of chronic medical problems (Laudicina).

Other Public Expenditures. In 1987 Medicare and Medicaid accounted for 74.5% of public outlays for personal health care services. The next-largest expenditure category, state and local government outlays (excluding the state share of Medicaid), accounted for 7.4% of the $175.3 billion spent on public programs (Letsch et al.). Included here are funds used to operate psychiatric hospitals and other long-term-care facilities, as well as acute-care general hospitals at the county and municipal levels.

There are four remaining significant personal health care categories for which government monies are spent: (1) federal outlays for hospital and medical services for veterans ($9.6 billion in 1987, 5.5% of public personal health care expenditures); (2) provision of care by the Department of Defense for the armed forces and military dependents (in 1987, $9.7 billion; 5.5%); (3) worker's compensation medical benefits ($8.9 billion; 5.1%); and (4) other federal, state, and local outlays for personal health care ($3.6 billion; 2.1%), including support for maternal and child health programs, vocational rehabilitation, Public Health Service and other federal hospitals, the Indian Health Service, temporary disability insurance, and the Alcohol, Drug Abuse, and Mental Health Administration. In contrast, all government public health activities are recorded as costing only $14.7 billion in 1987. It must be noted, however, that while federal prevention and control operations are included in this figure, excluded are funds expended by other than health departments at the state and local levels for air and water pollution control, sanitation, and sewage treatment (Letsch et al.). The relatively low level of government funding for public health activities deserves special attention in view of the growing recognition of the relationship between the environment and health and the importance of preventive care and health promotion.

Worker's compensation is an insurance system operated by the states, each with its own law and program, that provides covered workers with some protection against the costs of medical care and loss of income resulting from work-related injury and, in some cases, sickness (Congressional Research Service; Price, 1979a, b; U.S. National Commission on State Workmen's Compensation Laws. The first worker's compensation law was enacted in New York in 1910; by 1948 all states had enacted such laws). The theory underlying worker's compensation is that all accidents, irrespective of fault, must be regarded as risks of industry and that the employer and employee shall share the burden of loss.

Finally, public spending for research and facilities construction totaled approximately $10.8 billion in 1987. Public outlays for research totaled $8.2 billion in 1987, with the federal government the source for the vast majority (see Table 10.2).

Private Health Care Expenditures

The bulk of private health care expenditures comes from two sources: individuals receiving treatment and private insurers making payments on the behalf of patients. In 1987 private expenditures totaled $262.1 billion, 59.2% of all personal health care expenditures. In 1965, prior to the advent of Medicare and Medicaid, private expenditures accounted for 76.9% of all personal health care expenditures; in 1935, 82.4%; in 1929, 88.4% (Gibson). This recent decline in the private share of total expenditures is due primarily to the sharp drop in out-of-pocket payments associated with increased federal spending. In 1965, 53% of personal health care expenditures was paid directly by the patient; in 1987, it was only 28%. Yet because of inflation and other factors, the per capita dollar amount paid directly in 1983 was four times what it was in 1965 (Gibson; Letsch et al.)

Private insurers have paid between 20 and 32% of personal health care costs since 1965. Their share was $45.3 billion in 1978, 27% of the total; compared to $139.1 billion, or some 31.4% of the total, by 1987 (Gibson; Letsch et al.).

Before considering private health insurance in any depth, the manner in which the term "insurance" is used in the health care industry should be clarified. "Insurance" originally meant, and still usually refers to, the contribution by individuals to a fund for the purpose of providing protection against financial losses following relatively unlikely but damaging events. Thus, there is insurance against fire, theft, and death at an early age. All of those events occur within a group of people at a predictable rate but are rare occurrences for any one individual in the group.

When medical insurance began, it was in this tradition. From 1847, when the first commercial insurance plan designed to defray the costs of medical care was organized, to the 1930s, health insurance consisted essentially of cash payments by commercial carriers to offset income losses resulting from disability attributable to accidents. Sickness benefits (cash payments during sickness) began as an extra, a "frill" on accident insurance policies. As with accident insurance, emphasis was on the replacement of income lost, in this instance as a result of contracting certain specified and catastrophic communicable diseases, such as typhoid, scarlet fever, and smallpox (Health Insurance Institute). With the organization of Blue Cross and Blue Shield, a new policy developed: reimbursing health care costs in general.

Health care utilization is not a rare occurrence. On the average, each person in the United States visits a physician five times a year. One of every six Americans is admitted to a hospital at least once a year. Other than coverage for catastrophic illness, a fairly rare event, health insurance has become a mechanism for offsetting expected rather than unexpected costs. The experience of the many is pooled in an effort to reduce outlays for any one individual to manageable prepayment size. Perhaps the term *assurance* more appropriately describes the health care payment system that has evolved. In Britain *assurance* is used to denote coverage for contingencies that must eventually happen (life assurance), whereas *insurance* is reserved for coverage of those contingencies, like fire and theft, that may never occur.

Structure of the Private Insurance Industry. The organization of private insurance in the United States is undergoing dramatic changes. Before 1980 virtually all private insurance was provided by either the national system of Blue

Table 10.3 Enrollment in Managed and Unmanaged Group Health Plans, 1988

Group Plan	% Enrollment
Managed FFS[a]	43
Unmanaged FFS	28
HMO	18
PPO	11

[a]FFS, fee-for-service insurance.
Source: Health Insurance Association of America, *Employer Survey,* Washington: Health Insurance Association of America: 1988.

Cross and Blue Shield plans or by commercial insurance companies, which offered health care insurance as one of many types of insurance products available to employers. These insurance companies charged employers or individuals annual premiums and generally paid health care providers on what is termed a fee-for-service basis. A set amount, often prescribed by the insurance plan or negotiated between the insurer and the provider, was paid by the insurance company to a provider each time a beneficiary used a covered service.

In the 1980s, however, a range of new insurance approaches and a range of new relationships between insurers and providers have emerged. Health maintenance organizations (HMOs), which deliver services on a capitated basis rather than a fee-for-service basis, have been expanding rapidly; they accounted for 18% of all private insurance in 1988 (Gabel et al.). Preferred provider organizations (PPOs), which either limit beneficiaries to a set list of physicians and other providers or provide economic incentives to use physicians who have offered discounts to the insurer, also are expanding rapidly; they accounted for 11% of all private insurance in 1988 (see Table 10.3).

Table 10.3 indicates that fee-for-service insurance still accounts for 71% of the health insurance market. However, 43% of private insurance policies are fee-for-service but use some "managed" care approaches to limit utilization. These approaches include second surgical opinion requirements, preadmission certification review, and length-of-stay reviews.

The growth of insurance plans that do not rely on unmanaged fee-for-service coverage has been a response to the rapid rise in insurance premiums that has faced both employers and individuals. Insurance premiums have been increasing at a rate that far exceeds general inflation rates, and employers have been seeking alternative insurance approaches that can reduce employer costs.

A second major change in the structure of the insurance industry is the growth of self-insured or self-funded health plans. Self-insurance refers to the assumption of claims risk by an employer, union, or other group, whereas self-funding refers to the payment of insurance claims from an established bank or trust account (Arnett & Trapnell). Self-insurance offers potential advantages to employers: They are exempt from most premium taxes and are able to retain interest on reserves (Arnett & Trapnell). Moreover, they have generally been exempt from state laws mandating minimum benefits under the Employee Retirement Income Security Act of 1974 (ERISA). Recently, however, a U.S. Supreme Court decision ruled that a Massachusetts mandated-benefit law is not preempted by ERISA because it applies to insurance contracts purchased for plans subject to ERISA.

The growth in self-insurance has been significant, accounting for over 17% of all private health insurance benefit payments in 1983, compared to less than 10% in 1975 (Arnett & Trapnell). One common operational mode of self-insured plans is the administrative services only (ASO) plan. Under an ASO plan, the insurance carrier handles the claims and benefits paperwork for the self-insured group. Insurance claims are normally paid from an employer bank account.

Blue Cross and Blue Shield. The establishment of payment mechanisms to defray the costs of illness can be traced to the Great Depression. Previously hospitals had sought to assure reimbursement for their services through public education campaigns directed at encouraging their users, middle-income Americans, to put money aside for unpredictable medical expenses (Law). When hard times proved the inadequacy of the savings approach, attention turned to the development of a stable income mechanism. A model was at hand in the independent prepayment plan pioneered in 1929 at Baylor University Hospital in Texas to assure certain area schoolteachers of some hospital coverage. Under the plan, 1,250 teachers prepaid 50 cents a month to provide themselves with up to 21 days of semiprivate hospitalization annually.

In the early 1930s nonprofit prepayment programs offering care at a number of hospitals were organized in several cities. The American Hospital Association (AHA) vigorously supported the growth and development of these plans, soon to be named Blue Cross, and the special insurance legislation that was required for their establishment in each state (Law). The AHA set standards for plans and then offered its seal of approval to plans meeting the standards. A provider–insurer partnership was firmly established; indeed, not until 1972 did national Bule Cross formally separate from the AHA.

Whereas Blue Cross developed as a hospital insurance system, Blue Shield developed independently, beginning in 1939 as an insurer for physician services. These two insurers tend to be financially and organizationally distinct, but they have many similarities and most often work together to provide hospital and physician coverage. Blue Cross and Blue Shield both are local or statewide undertakings organized for the most part under special state enabling acts. In most states a department or commissioner of insurance supervises the "Blues," issuing or approving their certificates of incorporation, reviewing their annual income and expenditure reports, and monitoring the rates subscribers pay into the program and the rates the programs pay to the providers (Law).

In line with their nonprofit status, both programs, at least initially, were committed to "community rating." Under such a policy a set of benefits is offered at a single rate to all individuals and groups within a community, regardless of age, sex, health status, or occupation of community members. In essence, the rate represents an averaging out of high- and low-cost individuals and groups so that the community as a whole can be served with adequate benefits at reasonable cost (Somers & Somers). When commercial for-profit insurance companies entered the field, however, they did so with a policy of "experience rating," charging different individuals and population subgroups different premiums, based on their use of services. Low-risk groups could secure benefits at lower premiums. As a result, the Blues began to offer a multiplicity of policies with differing rate and benefit structures, and they generally have adopted experience rating. Had they not, their health insurance portfolios would have been heavily composed of adverse risks (Krizay & Wilson).

Commercial Insurance. Commercial insurance companies (Aetna, Metropolitan Life, etc.) entered the general health insurance market cautiously. They had realized losses on income-replacement policies during the Depression and were leery of the Blues' initial emphasis on comprehensive benefits. However, a Supreme Court decision recognizing fringe benefits as a legitimate part of the collective bargaining process, following as it did the freezing of industrial wages during World War II, proved too much of a temptation. Business was shopping for insurance carriers, and the commercials responded (Somers & Somers).

In the main, Blue Cross offers hospitalization insurance; Blue Shield, coverage of in-hospital physician services and a limited amount of office-based care. The commercials offer both. As in the case of the Blues, commercial insurance is primarily provided to groups through employee fringe-benefit packages negotiated through collective bargaining. Individual coverage can be purchased, but it is usually quite expensive or has limited coverage. The commercials also sell major-medical and cash payment policies. The former, directed primarily at catastrophic illness, pay all or part of the treatment costs beyond those covered by basic plans. They are sold on both a group and an individual basis.[1] Cash-payment policies pay the insured a flat sum of money per day of hospitalization and are usually sold directly to individuals, often through mass advertising campaigns. Although the daily cash-payment sum is usually small, it can help defray costs left uncovered by other insurance.

Like the Blues, the commercials are subject to supervision by state insurance

---

[1] Blue Cross and Blue Shield also sell group major-medical policies. In 1983 they had more than 40% of such coverage (Arnett & Trapnell).

Table 10.4 Number of HMO Members, (in Millions), 1976–1987

Year	As of June	As of December
1976	6.0	na
1977	6.3	na
1978	7.5	na
1979	8.2	na
1980	9.1	na
1981	10.2	na
1982	10.8	na
1983	12.5	na
1984	15.1	na
1985	18.9	na
1986	23.7	25.7
1987	28.6	29.3

na, data not available.
Source: Adapted from Gruber, R., Shadle, M., & Polich, C. L. "From Movement to Industry: The Growth of HMOs," *Health Affairs, 7*(3), p. 198.

commissioners, although such supervision does not include rate regulation. One general requirement is that commercials establish premium rates high enough to cover claims made under the insurance they provide. Solvency of the insurer is the principal aim of insurance commission surveillance in this instance (Krizay & Wilson).

HMOs. The form of health insurance that is reshaping the way many Americans relate to the health sector is the HMO. HMOs integrate the delivery of health care and insurance for health care. Although there are many different types of HMOs, the essential idea is that an annual payment is made by or for beneficiaries and then a group of providers delivers all covered services for this "capitated" payment. The HMO concept fundamentally changes the traditional approach of paying physicians and other providers on a fee-for-service, "piecework" basis. An HMO is paid a capitated amount to "maintain" (and when necessary, to restore) the health of an enrollee.

Table 10.4 displays the growth in HMO members between 1976 and 1987, when 29.3 million Americans received care through HMOs. The 1987 membership is five times that of 1976. The number of HMOs has grown from 176 in 1976 to 650 in 1987 (Gruber, Shadle, & Polich).

There are four distinct types of HMOs, which vary in how the fiscal agent relates to the providers of care (Group Health Association of America). The traditional type of HMO is a "staff" model in which the fiscal agent employs salaried physicians who generally spend all of their time delivering services to the HMO's enrollees. A "group" model is a slight variant of this in that the physicians as a single group contract with the fiscal agent to deliver services. In a "network" type of HMO the fiscal agent has contracts with multiple physician groups to provide services to enrollees; often the physician groups deliver services to non-HMO patients also. The fourth HMO type is the "independent practice association" (IPA) model, in which the fiscal agent contracts with a range of physicians, who work in independent practices or multispeciality group practices to provide services to HMO enrollees. Again, IPA physicians generally provide services to both HMO enrollees and patients with other forms of insurance.

HMOs vary in how they relate to hospitals. Some HMOs own their own hospitals, and others have varying forms of fiscal arrangements with community hospitals. The fiscal arrangements can include some version of a capitation payment or some form of discounted per diem or per case reimbursement mechanism.

The reason for increased enrollment in HMOs in recent years is principally the expectation and claim that HMOs reduce health care costs while providing coverage that has fewer co-payment features and uncovered services. Many studies have found that HMOs, particularly group and staff models, reduce hospital use and total costs (Arnould et al.; Luft, 1978, 1981; Manning; Roemer & Shonick; Wolinsky). Physicians working in HMOs generally have a strong incentive to use resources efficiently because of the capitated payment approach. Most important, HMO providers have strong incentives to avoid hospitalizations. Studies consistently indicate that even after adjusting for demographic differences, HMO patients are hospitalized 15 to 40% less often than fee-for-service patients (Luft, 1981).

PPOs. In addition to HMOs, the other growing form of insurance coverage is that which uses PPOs. As with HMOs, there are many different types of PPOs. However, the general concept involves beneficiaries using physicians who have agreed to give price discounts to the insurer. The beneficiary usually is provided some incentive to use a preferred provider, in the form of either lower insurance premiums or waiver of cost-sharing requirements.

As indicated in Table 10.3, PPOs accounted for 11% of the private insurance market in 1988. PPOs have been growing, especially in areas where there is significant competition for patients among physicians and other health care providers. In competitive markets insurers are best able to persuade providers to offer price discounts in return for a chance to increase patient volume. A recent survey found that PPOs are often established not by insurers but by groups of physicians interested in maintaining patients in the face of competition from HMOs (de Lissovoy et al.).

Extent of Private Health Insurance Coverage in the United States. Private health insurance coverage for Americans is extensive but far from complete. As of 1987, all but 37.1 million, some 17.6% of the nonelderly population, had some form of health insurance. These latest figures show the continuation of a reversal in the long-time trend toward reductions in the number of the individuals without health insurance (Swartz).

Although large numbers of individuals have some health insurance, the breadth of their coverage is uneven. In 1962 the proportion of the population having some coverage for hospitalization and physicians' services was 70% and 65%, respectively (Gibson et al.). The same was not true, however, of the proportions of the population covered for other services. In 1962, for example, some nursing home coverage was held by only 3% of the population; for dental care the figure was 0.5%. These proportions have increased throughout the past two decades. By 1981 the proportion of the population having some hospital insurance had increased from 70% to over 83%, and the proportion having some coverage for physicians' services increased to over 72%. Further, from 1960 to 1981 the number of Americans with some major-medical coverage increased from 33 to 156 million (Health Insurance Association of America).

An examination of the proportion of total consumer expenditures met by private insurance for various types of care indicates variations in coverage (see Table 10.5). As noted earlier, in 1987 expenditures made through private health insurance amounted to about 31.4% of the total. Table 10.5 translates that percentage for 1987 and prior years into the proportions of expenditures met for the several categories of health care covered by such insurance. It is clear that many individuals have some coverage for drugs, physicians' office visits, and dental care, although the coverage often does not go very far.

One type of service that has very poor insurance coverage is long-term care that is custodial in nature. In discussing Medicare, it was noted that coverage for long-term care that involves rehabilitation has recently been expanded. However, very few long-term-care services are for rehabilitation; most are custodial, involving chronic care of the frail elderly. Medicare pays less than 3% of all long-term-care costs, and private insurance pays less than 1%.

The current system of financing long-term care relies on out-of-pocket expenditures by the elderly who can afford such expenditures. In most states, after an elderly person becomes impoverished by the costs of services, the state Medicaid program will cover services.

Although private insurance has played a very small role in insuring long-term-care services, in recent years a market for private insurance has been emerging, and the number of policies has been expanding. In addition, numerous proposals have been made for developing an integrated public–private insurance system for long-term-care services that would combine private insurance and some public resources now devoted to Medicaid long-term-care services (Knickman).

Table 10.5 Percentage of Consumer Health Expenditures Met by Private Health Insurance, 1950–1987

Year	Total	Hospital care	Physicians' services	Prescribed drugs (out-of-hospital)	Dental care
1950	12.2%	37.1%	12.0%	a	a
1960	27.8	64.7	30.0	a	a
1965	30.5	70.1	34.0	2.4%	1.6%
1966	30.4	71.0	34.0	2.7	2.0
1967	31.8	76.7	36.7	3.5	2.5
1968	34.5	78.8	40.5	3.6	3.1
1969	35.5	77.7	41.1	4.0	3.9
1970	37.2	77.7	43.7	3.9	5.3
1971	39.1	80.9	43.7	4.9	6.3
1972	39.0	76.5	45.8	5.0	7.2
1973	39.0	75.4	46.0	5.6	8.1
1974	41.4	77.3	49.8	6.2	11.0
1975	45.0	82.6	51.3	6.7	15.8
1976	47.0	84.6	53.1	7.9	19.6
1977	45.5	79.3	52.9	7.9	20.2
1981	54.5	82.9	58.9	13.4	34.9
1982	56.2	83.2	60.4	14.6	34.4
1983	56.5	83.5	60.6	14.8	34.9
1984	56.0	80.0	62.6	14.6	35.7
1985	55.5	79.4	62.2	14.8	36.5
1986	55.8	79.4	62.9	15.1	37.4
1987	56.2	79.5	62.9	15.6	37.6

aCoverage insignificant.
Source: Adapted from M. S. Carroll & R. H. Arnett III, "Private Health Insurance Plans in 1977: Coverage, Enrollment and Financial Experience," *Health Care Financing Reviews, 1,* Fall 1979, p. 14; R. M. Gibson, K. R. Levitt, H. Lazenby, & D. Waldo, "National Health Expenditures, 1983," *Health Care Financing Review, 6,* Winter 1984, Table 3; S. Letsch et al., "National Health Expenditures, 1987," *Health Care Financing Review, 10,* Winter 1988, Table 1.

How the Money Is Paid Out

Paying Physicians

As indicated in Table 10.2, physican services account for approximately 20% of all health care expenditures. However, the method used to pay physicians influences not only this 20% of the health care bill but also the large share of health care costs that are controlled largely by physicians' decisions. It is important to emphasize the role of physicians in deciding when a patient uses hospital resources and in prescribing drugs and medical tests.

As already mentioned, methods used by insurers to reimburse physicians are undergoing substantial change. The growth of HMOs and PPOs is changing the ability of physicians to set prices freely. Increased regulation of fees by Medicare also is affecting the way physicians are reimbursed.

Fee for Service. The dominant approach to paying physicians continues to be some variation of a fee-for-service approach. A traditional fee-for-service approach is a simple system in which a physician sets a price for each type of service delivered, and then the patient or the insurer pays this price.

For individuals who have no insurance for physician services, traditional fee-for-service generally is used. Even when an individual has private insurance, fee-for-service rates are generally charged, with the patient paying any share of the rate the insurer judges to be above a stated payment scale. Insurers use a wide range of methods for establishing payment scales for covered services.

The Medicare program has used a complicated system for establishing what fees it will pay physicians. This system is based in part on a comparison of each doctor's fee schedule for a given type of service with those of other physicians in a community. Medicare will never pay an individual physician an amount that exceeds the 75th percentile of charges by all physicians in a community (this is termed the "prevailing" fee). However, the Medicare program also has used a cost of living index, termed the Medicare Economic Index, to constrain the growth in the maximum payment it will pay in a community for each type of physician service (Congressional Budget Office).

The Physician Payment Review Commission has recommended extensive revisions in the method Medicare uses to set fee-for-service rates. One proposal is based on the use of what are termed "relative value scales" (RVS) to set rates for different types of physician services. The RVS system is devised by comparing the relative resources required to deliver different types of services, including physicians' time and training requirements (Hsiao & Stason).

Implementation of an RVS approach to reimbursement would, over time, lead to relative increases in reimbursements for cognitive services (i.e., physicals and diagnostic visits) and relative decreases in rates for physician services that involve procedures. This rebalancing would occur because current reimbursement systems have led to higher rates for procedures than makes sense based on objective input measures involving time, training, or relative expertise.

Preferred Provider Approaches. An alternative to traditional fee-for-service payment approaches is the use of negotiated discounts by physicians or groups of physicians. PPOs use this discounting approach to set reimbursement rates for patients covered by a participating insurer. In many ways, however, the discounting approaches inherent to PPOs are not distinct from fee-for-service approaches but rather a variation on the fee-for-service idea. Physicians continue to be paid on a service-by-service basis but at a somewhat lower rate than is charged for non-PPO patients.

Capitation and Salary. The alternative forms of provider reimbursement are capitation and salary. The latter approach is self-explanatory; its use as a payment mechanism for health professionals is widespread. Certainly, from the employer's point of view, a salary system has the merit of administrative simplicity. When the employer is the government, there is the added benefit of flexibility: The movement of providers into areas of medical scarcity and unpopular jobs is more easily accomplished under a salary system than under other payment mechanisms. From the provider's point of view, he or she has an income protected from sudden fluctuations in supply and demand, has no bill collection problems, and usually receives extensive fringe benefits (Roemer, 1962).

Various types of capitation approaches are used by individual practice associations to compensate physicians. There were more than 400 IPAs across the country in 1987 (Gruber et al.), and the payment approaches used by these organizations vary substantially. Some pay individual physicians using discounted fee-for-service plans, but most put physicians at some financial risk for the costs of their patient's care. Often a physician receives a capitated annual payment for each patient who uses that physician as a primary provider. The capitated payment is meant to cover certain forms of primary care and, depending on the arrangement, some share of specialty care, ancillary services, and hospital care. The physician thus has strong incentives to manage resources efficiently.

Another form of capitation is to have a group of IPA physicians receive some percentage of a fee-for-service rate, with the remaining percentage held in escrow to assure that aggregate health care costs across the group do not exceed targets. The escrow amounts are distributed to the physicians at the end of the year if utilization targets are met.

Paying Hospitals

There are two major approaches to hospital reimbursement: retrospective and prospective; although there are numerous modes of payment within these two categories (Glaser, 1984).

Retrospective Payment. Retrospective rates for payment to hospitals by third-party payers and individuals are set after services are provided. There are two major modes of retrospective payment: charges and cost. Most commercial insurers and some Blue Cross plans reimburse hospitals on the basis of submitted charges. Charges are simply prices set by hospitals. Most hospitals set charges for basic and intensive-care room and board, as well as for each service provided. These prices may or may not reflect the true economic costs of the particular service. Often the variation above cost is a function of patient mix. Charges will exceed actual costs to the extent that a hospital serves a large number of nonpaying patients and to the extent that "cost-based" insurers actually pay amounts that are less than actual costs.

The more sophisticated retrospective payment mode is based on cost. The determination of cost never involves individual patients; rather, it is a matter of negotiation between hospitals and third-party payers such as Blue Cross and Medicaid. Cost reimbursement is used when insured patients receive their benefits as services rather than as dollar indemnities. Almost all group health insurance policies in the United States now provide service benefits rather than dollar indemnities. To determine reimbursable costs, third-party payers sumtotal hospital costs, decide which costs are "allowable," then, using a formula, reimburse hospitals on a per-patient-day basis.

Prospective Payment. The most significant change in hospital payment methodologies in the last 5 years has been recent expansion in prospective payment systems. Of special importance were the changes in the method used by Medicare to pay hospitals. In the Tax Equity and Fiscal Responsibility Act (TEFRA) of 1982, Congress established a cost-per-case basis for hospital payment. TEFRA also placed a ceiling on the rate of increase in hospital revenues that would be supported by the Medicare program.

The 1983 amendments to the Social Security Act further defined the case payment system. These amendments created a revolutionary method of paying hospitals for inpatient care to Medicare patients, one that is based on DRGs. Under this system, hospitals are paid a preestablished amount per case treated, with payment rates varying by type of case. The DRGs measure hospital output by originally classifying patients into 23 major diagnostic categories (MDCs), based on major body systems. The MDCs are divided further into 47 diagnostic groups based on the patient's diagnosis or the surgical procedure used and on age, sex, and other clinical information. One additional group is also used for cases in which diagnosis and surgical procedure do not match (Grimaldi & Micheletti).

Not all hospitals are included in Medicare's case payment system. Certain specialty hospitals, such as children's, long-term-care, rehabilitation, and psychiatric hospitals are exempt. So are certain states, such as New Jersey and Maryland, that have approved alternative payment systems. Moreover, certain hospital costs, such as direct medical education and capital-related costs, continue to be reimbursed on a cost basis and are excluded from costs used to calculate case payment rates. There is continuing debate, however, about how to include capital costs in the case payment system.

Payment that an individual hospital receives for treating Medicare patients in a given DRG depends on the DRG's "cost" weight multiplied by a "standardized" average cost for all Medicare patients. The standardization process includes adjustments for differences in wages and teaching intensity. Also, different rates are set for urban and rural hospitals. Payment amounts to hospitals are also adjusted each year by an "update factor," consisting of a measure of the price of goods and services purchased by hospitals. In addition, a discretionary adjustment factor (DAF) accounts for changes in new technology and productivity. Although Congress originally set the DAF at 1 percentage point each year, the Deficit Reduction Act of 1984 capped these adjustments at 0.25%.

Two aspects of this payment system depart significantly from previous methods used to pay for Medicare patients. First, the DRG concept holds that the "best" measure of hospital output is the diagnosis treated rather than individual services provided or length of stay. That is, the *basis* of payment is the case treated rather than ancillary or routine inputs to hospital care.

Second, unlike retrospective payment methodologies, DRG payments are determined prospectively and are fixed. Although a portion of the initial rates for fiscal year 1984 were determined by historical costs, subsequent rates of increase in the payments are controlled before payment is made. Hence, Medicare now has the ability to control the per-case rate of increase for Medicare patients.

The use of DRGs as a basis for hospital payment transcends Medicare and is spreading rapidly to other payers. As of 1985, at least 12 states had adopted case-based systems to pay for hospital care (Hellinger). New Jersey and New York, for example, use a DRG system as the basis of payment for all third-party payers. Other states, such as Pennsylvania, Utah, Ohio, Michigan, and Washington, employ a DRG system to pay hospitals for Medicaid. Finally, other states, such as Arizona, Oklahoma, and Kansas, employ a DRG system to pay for Blue Cross patients.

Use of classification schemes as the basis for hospital payment assumes that the classifications are clinically meaningful and "reasonably" homogeneous with respect to resource consumption. There is, however, mounting evidence that some of the DRG categories do not satisfy either requirement (Prospective Payment Assessment Commission). Perhaps the most common criticism of the DRG categories is that they include patients with dissimilar resource needs because they often do not account adequately for differences in patient complexity or severity of illness (Horn et al.). Variation in severity within each DRG category is cause for concern if patient complexity can be assessed before admission to the hospital: this can create an incentive to divert more complex patients to other hospitals. Longer-run consequences may include shedding unprofitable DRG "products" and expanding the volume of "profitable" services to ensure hospital financial viability. Changes in hospital service mix may not be entirely undesirable, however, if increased patient volume allows hospitals to eliminate facility duplication and exploit economies of scale. On the other hand, narrowing the scope of services may adversely affect access to care in some cases.

Research concerning the impacts of the new Medicare DRG payment system indicates that that approach is significantly changing hospital utilization patterns. Medicare hospital admissions decreased 15.9% during the first 3 years of the new reimbursement system, and average length of stay decreased 17% (Guterman et al.). Although it is difficult to determine exactly how much of these dramatic reductions in utilization are attributable to DRGs, research studies do document that utilization rates fell much more quickly in states where the DRG system was implemented compared to the states that received waivers to delay or avoid implementation.

The reduction in hospital use has not been without side effects, however. In particular, evidence consistently indicates sharp increases in posthospital use of services, including home health care, and nursing home care, as well as increased readmissions (Guterman et al.). The tighter regulation of Medicare payment rates also may be responsible for part of the rapid growth in cost of private insurance as hospitals shift some of their costs from Medicare to private insurance. That is, higher rates may be charged for individuals with private insurance to compensate for any operating losses associated with care delivered to Medicare patients.

The Rising Costs of Health Care

National spending for health care grew an average of 12.7% per year from 1970 to 1987. In addition, the rate of increase in health care costs has consistently far exceeded the rate of inflation in the general economy. Thus, health care expenses each year account for an increasing share of the nation's GNP.

Several factors have contributed to the rise in medical costs: general inflation in the economy, population growth, the development of new medical technology, and an increased "intensity" of services provided to all patients. Rapid development of medical technology and intensity of medical care services have been encouraged by growth in the extent of health insurance coverage and previous retrospective, cost-based payment systems that rewarded higher reported costs with higher payments (Feldstein). As insurance coverage increases, the out-of-pocket cost to the patient is reduced, leading to increases in demand for higher-quality medical care and hence to rising prices. The growth in the comprehensiveness of third-party insurance coverage is stimulated in part through federal government tax subsidies (Phelps). Under current tax law, employer payments to employees for health insurance are not considered taxable income. Because these tax subsidies reduce the price of health insurance, they provide incentives to purchase more health insurance.

Despite the theoretical connection between the extent of health insurance and costs, until recently there was little persuasive empirical evidence that increased health insurance coverage led to greater use of health care services. Some even argued that more comprehensive insurance, especially for ambulatory care, would *reduce* total spending by encouraging preventive health care and more "appropriate" hospital use (Roemer et al.).

Recent data from the Rand Corporations's Health Insurance Experiment (Newhouse et al.) provide considerable insight into the connection between insurance coverage and utilization. The experiment ran from late 1974 through January 1982 and enrolled 7,706 individuals between the ages of 14 and 61 who belonged to 2,756 families. Families were assigned randomly to one of four major types of experimental plans.

1. A "free-care" plan, in which all care was received without charge (i.e., there were no co-insurance or deductible requirements).
2. An individual deductible plan, which imposed a 95% co-insurance rate on outpatient care, up to a maximum out-of-pocket expenditure of $450 per family, with all care beyond that amount (either inpatient or outpatient) free at time of service.
3. A series of intermediate co-insurance plans with cost-sharing requirements of either 25% or 50%.
4. "Income-related catastrophic" plans that included a 95% co-insurance requirement with income-related maximum dollar spending caps.

The results of the experiment were quite robust. Health care spending was almost 50% lower in plans with 95% cost-sharing, compared to those in the free-care plans. Perhaps of more interest was the finding that any cost sharing—even just for ambulatory care services—reduced costs, compared to the free-care plans.

Another important finding from the experiment was that, in general, the reduced utilization of health care due to cost sharing did not affect most measures of health status. However, two exceptions to these findings were slight increases in blood pressure for individuals with high blood pressure at the start of the study and for individuals who had low incomes (Brook et al.).

The system of third-party reimbursement also has been implicated as a primary factor spurring the recent growth in new medical technology. Although in certain instances new technology has increased the length and quality of life, it is often very costly. As one observer of the system has noted, "with some important exceptions, the norm for hospital care in the United States approximates the maxim, 'if you think it will help, do it' " (Aaron & Schwartz, p. 7). Since most patients are insulated from the true social costs of medical care, our present system encourages the uses of services that may yield only slight, if any, positive diagnostic information, often regardless of cost. The HCFA, for example, found that the increased per-admission intensity of care accounted for over 20% of the growth in expenditures for community hospital inpatient care over the past 10 years (Freedland & Schendler).

Although the spread of new technology undoubtedly offers unprecedented medical benefits, some innovations are of marginal value. Further, facilities and services unavailable in the late 1970s or found only in medical centers are now offered in a substantial number of community hospitals. The increase in diagnostic imaging by computerized axial tomography (CAT) has been impressive, more than doubling since 1980 (Office of Technology Assessment). Similarly, rapid diffusion of magnetic resonance imaging (MRI) has occurred. The medical benfits of CAT scanning are well known; for instance, it has reduced the need for exploratory surgery. Yet growth in new technology has expanded the potential pool of recipients as well as symptoms diagnosed. Thus, although it is true that new technology provides unprecedented medical benefits, the downside is that new technology increases expenditures.

The battle over medical efficacy, new technology, and health care expenditures has escalated with the advent of Medicare's DRG payment system. Under the DRG system, hospitals may become more reluctant to purchase new technologies that add significantly to their operating costs because reimbursement rates will not automatically increase with an expenditure for technology. Moreover, the rate of technological diffusion in the industry will be sensitive to the method ultimately chosen by the HCFA to reimburse hospitals for capital expenditures. Yet, to date, the tremendous growth in new medical technology shows no perceptible signs of abating. Each year new, more expensive technologies with the potential for saving and improving the quality of life appear. Many consider cost increases resulting from advances in and greater use of medical technology as the necessary price of improvements in health care, if not health. Opponents suggest that a substantial portion of the utilization of technology is generally unnecessary. They link a proportion of the increase in ancillary service to physician fear of exposure to malpractice claims. Indeed, small increases in diagnostic accuracy often require substantial increases in the health care bill. This concern has increased interest in redirecting resources into programs—especially public health interventions—with more favorable cost–benefit implications.

Some observe that any appreciable reduction in spending can be accomplished only by denying medical benefits (Aaron & Schwartz). Others note that increased cost sharing may reduce spending and utilization, often without deleterious effects on health status (Brook et al.). Thus, the debate continues surrounding the health implications of recent attempts, such as the expansion of the DRG system, to reduce the rate of growth of health care costs. At the very least, the debate over efficiency, access, and quality will heighten in the coming years.

Conclusion

Money funds the health care delivery system, but the routes dollars take from consumers to providers can be labyrinthine. Some dollars go directly, some via the government, and some through insurance companies. Most health care providers are paid by salary, but some are paid on a piecework basis. Hospitals are paid for services provided in numerous ways. Some insurers base payments on what the hospital charges, whereas others pay on the basis of allowable average costs. Still others, notably Medicare and some Medicaid and Blue Cross plans, pay hospitals on a "case" basis, with the payment rate set in advance.

In the United States in the 1960s and 1970s a health insurance system that emphasized coverage for hospital care, with physician service in hospitals generally being more lucrative than in the office setting, "tilted" the system in the direction of utilization of the most expensive component of the system. Technological change, a significant factor in rising health care costs, was often poorly planned and evaluated, with decisions frequently made on the basis of universal access rather than cost-effectiveness.

The 1980s, however, have seen a virtual revolution in the financing and structure of medical care delivery. Fundamental changes in the methods used to pay health care providers, growing involvement by employers and employees in direct negotiation with providers, and a projected aggregate surplus of physicians have led to the changes in the structure of the delivery system. Perhaps most notable has been the move from retrospective to prospective modes of payment. Although prospective per-case payment systems are generally restricted to in-patient hospital care, considerable research and development efforts—aimed at designing prospective case payment systems for long-term care, home health care, outpatient care, and payments to physicians—are currently underway. In some quarters, across-the-board capitation payments may prove feasible.

The 1980s also saw the beginning of dramatic changes in the organization of medical practice. The growth in prepaid group practices, ambulatory surgery, and the "unbundling" of hospital services are indicative of the magnitude of recent changes in the delivery system. New alignments between providers, employers, and employees—in the form of HMOs, PPOs, and self-insurance ventures—also reflect the recent entrance of the consumer into direct financial negotiation with health care providers.

References

Aaron, H., & Schwartz, W. *The Painful Prescription: Rationing Hospital Care*. Washington, D.C.: The Brookings Institution, 1984.

Arnett, R., III, & Trappell, G. "Private Health Insurance: New Measures of a Complex and Changing Industry." *Health Care Financing Review, 6,* 2, Winter 1984.

Arnould, R., et. al. "Do HMOs Produce Services More Efficiently?" *Inquiry, 21,* 3, Fall 1984.

Brook, R., et al. "Does Free Care Improve Adults' Health? Results from a Randomized Controlled Trial." *New England Journal of Medicine, 319,* 1426, 1983.

Carroll, M. S., & Arnett, R. H., III. "Private Health Insurance Plans in 1977: Coverage, Enrollment and Financial Experience." *Health Care Financing Review, 1,* 3, Fall 1979.

Christensen, S., & Kasten, R. "Covering Catastrophic Expenses under Medicare." *Health Affairs, 3,* 5, 79, 1988.

Congressional Budget Office, U.S. Congress. *Physician Reimbursement under Medicare: Options for Change.* Washington, D.C.: U.S. Government Printing Office, 1986.

Congressional Research Service. *Workmen's Compensation: Role of the Federal Government.* (1B75054). Washington, D.C.: Library of Congress, 1976.

Davis, K., & Rowland, D. "Uninsured and Undeserved: Inequities in Health Care in the United States." *Milbank Memorial Fund Quarterly: Health and Society, 61,* 149, 1983.

de Lissovoy, G., T. Rice, D. Ermann, & J. Gabel. "Preferred Provider Organizations: Today's Models and Tomorrow's Prospect." *Inquiry, 23,* 7, Spring 1986.

Feldstein, M. S. *The Rising Cost of Hospital Care.* Washington, D.C.: Information Resources Press, 1971.

Freeland, M. S., & Schendler, C. E. "National Health Expenditure Growth in the 1980's: An Aging Population, New Technologies, and Increasing Competition." *Health Care Financing Review, 4,* 3, 1983.

Gabel, J., DiCarlo, S., Fink, S., & de Lissovoy, G. "Employer-sponsored Health Insurance in America: Preliminary Results from the 1988 Survey." *Research Bulletin.* Washington, D.C.: Health Insurance Association of America, January 1989.

Gibson, R. M. "National Health Expenditures, 1978." *Health Care Financing Review, 1,* 1, Summer 1979.

Gibson, R. M., Levitt, K., Lazenby, H., & Waldo, D. "National Health Expenditures, 1983." *Social Security Bulletin, 6,* 2, Winter 1984.

Grimaldi, P., & Micheletti, J. *Diagnosis Related Groups: A Practitioner's Guide.* Chicago: Pluribus Press, 1982.

Group Health Association of America. *HMO Industry Profile: Trends, 1985–1986* (Vol. 4) Washington, D.C.: Group Health Association of America, 1986

Gruber, L. R., Shadle, M., & Polich, C. L. "From Movement to Industry: The Growth of HMOs." *Health Affairs, 7*(3), 197, 1988.

Guterman, S., P. W. Eggers, Riley, G., Greene, T. F., & Terrell, S. A. "The First 3 Years of Medicare Prospective Payment: An Overview." *Health Care Financing Review, 9*(1), 67, 1987.

Health Insurance Association of America. *Sourcebook of Health Insurance Data, 1984 Update.* New York: Health Insurance Association of America, 1985.

Health Insurance Institute. *Source Book of Health Insurance Data, 1974–75.* New York: Health Insurance Institute, 1975.

Hellinger, F. "Recent Evidence on Case-Based Systems for Setting Hospital Rates." *Inquiry, 22,* 1, Spring 1985.

Horn, S., et al. "The Severity of Illness Index as a Severity Adjustment to Diagnosis-Related Groups." *Health Care Financing Review, 5* (Suppl.), 1984.

Hsiao, W., & Stason, W. "Toward Developing a Relative Value Scale for Medical and Surgical Services." *Health Care Financing Review, 1,* 23, 1979.

Knickman, J. "Private Long-term Care Insurance: Alleviating Market Problems with Public-Private Partnership." *Health Economics and Health Service Research, 9,* 135, 1988.

Krizay, J., & Wilson, A. *The Patient as Consumer*. Lexington, MA: D. C. Heath, 1974.

Laudicina, S. "State Health Risk Pools: Insuring the 'Uninsurable'." *Health Affairs, 7*(4), 97, 1988.

Law, S. A. *Blue Cross: What Went Wrong?* New Haven, CT: Yale University Press, 1974.

Lewin, L., & Lewin, M. "Financing Charity Care in an Era of Competition." *Health Affairs, 6*(1), 47, 1988.

Letsch, S., et al. "National Health Expenditures, 1987." *Health Care Financing Review, 10*, 109, Winter 1988.

Luft, H. "How Do Health Maintenance Organizations Achieve Their Savings?" *New England Journal of Medicine, 298*, 1336, 1978.

Luft, H. *Health Maintenance Organization: Dimensions of Performance*. New York: John Wiley, 1981.

Manning, W. "A Controlled Trial of the Effects of a Prepaid Group Practice on Use of Services." *The New England Journal of Medicine, 310*, 23, June 1984.

McCarthy, C. M. "Incentive Reimbursement as an Impetus to Cost Containment." *Inquiry, 12*, 320, 1975.

Muse, D. N., & Sawyer, D. *The Medicare and Medicaid Data Book, 1981* (HCFA Pub. No. 03128). Washington, D.C.: U.S. Department of Health and Human Services, 1982.

Newhouse, J. P., et al. "Some Interim Results from a Controlled Trial of Cost Sharing in Health Insurance." *New England Journal of Medicine, 305*, 1501, 1981.

Office of Technology Assessment. *Policy Implications of the CT Scanner: An Update*. Washington, D.C.: U.S. Office of Technology Assessment, 1981.

Phelps, C. E. "Taxing Health Insurance: How Much Is Enough?" *Contemporary Policy Issues, 3*, 2, Winter 1984.

Price, D. N. "Workers' Compensation Programs in the 1970s." *Social Security Bulletin, 42*(5), 3, 1979a.

Price, D. N. "Workers' Compensation Coverage, Payments and Costs, 1977." *Social Security Bulletin, 42*(10), 18, 1979b.

Prospective Payment Assessment Commission. *Report and Recommendation to the Secretary, U.S. Department of Health and Human Services*. Washington, D.C.: U.S. Government Printing Office, 1985.

Roemer, M. I. "On Paying the Doctor and the Implications of Different Methods." *Journal of Health and Human Behavior, 3*, 4, Spring 1962.

Roemer, M. I., et al. "Copayments for Ambulatory Care: Penny-wise and Pound-Foolish." *Medical Care, 13*, 457, 1975.

Roemer, M., & Shonick, W. "HMO Performance: The Recent Evidence." *Health and Society, 51*, 271, 1973.

Russell, L., et al. *Federal Health Spending, 1969–74*. Washington, D.C.: National Planning Association, 1974.

Somers, H., & Somers, A. R. *Doctors, Patients and Health Insurance*, Washington, D.C.: The Brookings Institution, 1961.

Swartz, K. *The Uninsured with a Special Focus on Workers*. Unpublished report, The Urban Institute, 1989.

U.S. National Commission on State Workmen's Compensation Laws, *Report*. Washington, D.C.: U.S. Government Printing Office, 1973.

Wilensky, G. "Filling the Gaps in Health Insurance." *Health Affairs, 7*(3), 133, 1988.

Wolinsky, F. "The Performance of Health Maintenance Organizations: An Analytic Review." *Milbank Memorial Fund Quarterly, 58*(4), 4, 1980.

11

Health Care Cost Containment: Reflections and Future Directions

Kenneth E. Thorpe

Despite vigorous efforts to control health care costs, health care expenditures continue to rise at rates exceeding general inflation. In 1987 health care accounted for 11.1% of our gross national product (GNP), compared to 9.8% just 5 years earlier (Health Care Financing Administration). The sustained rise in health care expenditures has raised a number of concerns. First, public expenditures for health care account for a substantial portion of the federal budget. Thus, recent efforts to reduce the size of the federal budget deficit (estimated at approximately $140 billion in 1989) have focused attention on publicly financed health care programs. Second, recent increases in premiums paid by employers have skyrocketed. Health care benefits account for a growing percentage of employers' total compensation to employees, as costs per employee have risen 43% between 1984 and 1988. Rates for the 77 Blue Cross and Blue Shield plans nationally will increase between 15 and 25% during 1989 (Mullen). Third, the sustained premium increases are not limited to traditional forms of insurance coverage. Employers deciding to "self-insure" also faced large increases during 1988, averaging approximately 20% (Mullen). Perhaps even more distressing is the 16.9% projected rise in rates by health maintenance organizations (HMOs), medical supermarkets widely touted as the consummate cost-containment mechanism, during 1989.

The continued escalation in health care costs suggests that efforts by third-party payers to lower cost growth have largely failed to achieve their goal. Although some payers have reduced their expenditures over time, spending by others has increased, leaving the overall rate of growth largely unaffected. The factors accounting for the sustained increase in health care costs, the effects of recent public and private sector attempts to control this growth, and an assessment of the future direction of health care cost containment serves as the focus of this chapter.

270

Factors Accounting for Health Care Expenditure Growth

The United States currently spends over $600 billion, some $2,000 per capita, on health care (Health Care Financing Administration). This represents a 9.8% rise between 1986 and 1987 alone, a $45 billion jump. Four major factors generally account for these large yearly increments: general economy-wide inflation, inflation specific to the health care industry (over and above general rates of inflation), population growth, and changes in the nature and intensity of health care delivery. The relative contributions of these factors to yearly changes in health care costs are discussed below.

Approximately 32% of the yearly rise in health care spending is traced to general inflation (Freeland & Schendler). This includes inflation in the price of inputs used in the delivery of medical care (e.g., electricity, material, etc.). Another 11% of the yearly increase is traced to population growth. Thus, approximately 43% of the yearly rise in health care costs stem from general trends in the economy.

Fifty-seven percent, or $25.6 billion, of the most recent increase in health care spending is traced to the health care "marketplace." Of this portion, some 22%, or $10 billion, of the most recent increase is the result of "real" (as opposed to the general level of inflation noted above) changes in health care prices. This includes rapid growth in wages paid to health care workers, as well as rising interest rates for capital expansion. Finally, the remaining 35%, or $15.6 billion, stems from continued changes in the "intensity" of a health care visit. The intensity of care refers to the volume of medical care inputs used by physicians to treat patients (e.g., ancillary tests, procedures) per visit. Thus, among those factors specific to the health care industry, changes in the intensity of care account for over 60% of the yearly change in expenditure growth.

Two factors commonly thought responsible for the rise in health care costs are the rapid spread of comprehensive health insurance (traced to demand-side distortions) and technological change (a supply-side issue). These factors and their interrelationships are explored below.

Demand Side Distortions

Economists have traditionally identified the spread of health insurance as a primary cause for health care cost growth (Pauly). The rapid spread of health insurance has generated continued increases in demand for health care, in terms of both volume and perceived quality. The rapid increase in the scope (type of health care insured) and comprehensiveness (the proportion of a health care bill paid by a third party) of health insurance during the 1960s and 1970s has been traced to the tax treatment of health benefits (Manning et al., 1987). In particular, employer contributions for health insurance benefits are exempt from federal and state income taxation. With employer health benefit contributions exceeding $130 billion, this exemption translates into a $41 billion revenue loss (Pauly). The tax treatment subsidizes the marginal dollar of fringe benefits employees receive from employers relative to other forms of compensation (e.g., wages), therefore increasing the demand for health insurance relative to other goods.

The tax treatment of health insurance benefits has two consequences. First, individuals purchase more insurance than they would without the tax subsidy. Second, more extensive health insurance results in higher health care spending. With respect to insurance, the tax laws encourage individuals to purchase less preventive care and insure against marginal risks. More comprehensive policies with few cost-sharing obligations also lead to higher spending. The magnitude of the additional expenditures is substantial. One recent experimental study, conducted by the Rand Corporation, examined the impact of insurance on health care spending. Their results indicate the use of services respond to the level of cost sharing. In short, per capita expenditures in plans with no cost sharing were approximately 33% greater than in plans with a 95% co-insurance obligation (Manning et al., 1987). Moreover, relative to a free-care plan, per capita spending among those enrolled in plans with 25% co-insurance was approximately 15% lower. Lower expenditures did not result in measurable reductions in patient health status. For example, for an average individual enrolled in the plan, the Rand study did not detect significant differences in health status across insurance plans during the 3-year tracking period. These findings suggest that low co-insurance obligations result in higher rates of utilization with few measurable short-run health benefits.

Supply Side Factors

Imperfect information and cost-increasing technological changes represent two supply side factors that distinguish the health care industry from more "competitive" markets. These factors, in conjunction with the demand side distortions noted above, also have contributed to the real changes in medical care prices as well as intensity of medical care over time.

Imperfection Information. Potential consumers of medical care have imperfect information concerning its price and quality. High search costs and extensive health insurance coverage reduce the potential net benefits of searching for lower-cost providers. The importance of search costs and their impact on medical care prices have received much attention. The "increasing monopoly" thesis, outlined by Pauly and Satterthwaite (1981), consists of two observations. First, consumer information concerning physicians and other providers decreases with higher numbers of providers. Second, if search for providers is more difficult, consumers are less price-sensitive, and physicians have more discretion in increasing fees. Thus, according to this thesis, growth in the per capita number of physicians would result in higher prices.

Even with extensive price shopping by consumers, comprehensive health insurance coverage reduces any potential savings resulting from identifying low-cost providers. Thus, both high search costs and extensive health insurance coverage dilute the incentives for consumers to engage in vigorous price shopping.

Further complicating the consumer's task is the lack of information concerning provider quality. Measuring the quality of care provided by individual physicians or hospitals has traditionally been very difficult. Although we have witnessed an explosion of medical outcomes research over the past 5 years, outcome-based measures remain in their infancy. Instead, consumers often have used proxies such as the physician's board certification or a hospital's teaching affiliation as a signal for higher quality. As a result, higher perceived quality is also associated with higher fees and costs. At issue is whether these higher fees and prices reflect unobserved quality differences. Thus, price competition among providers will continue to be limited until consumers are able to compare both price and quality differences accurately.

Despite the informational problems facing consumers, hospitals and physicians do compete. However, the features of the health care delivery system noted above have encouraged competition in perceptions of quality rather than price. This includes both inadequate information on price and quality differences as well as the pervasiveness of first-dollar health insurance coverage. Thus, instead of competing on a price basis to attract patients, hospitals have competed to attract physicians (and through them patients). Hospitals in more concentrated (competitive) markets attempt to attract physicians through specific capital investments. These capital investments include the latest technologies, a broad range of clinical services, and other amenities. Since new technology increases service intensity, quality competition is quite costly. Whether the additional service intensity translates into better health outcomes remains at issue.

That hospitals have traditionally pursued competition in quality, rather than in price, has been the subject of numerous empirical investigations. The results generally conclude that, other factors held constant, hospitals in more competitive markets produce more services and have significantly higher costs (Robinson & Luft, 1985, 1987). Although these results generally held through the mid-1980s, efforts by state governments and other payers to encourage price competition have altered the behavior of hospitals. The more recent role of competition and market structure are discussed below.

Technological Change. The demand side distortions noted above, combined with traditional "non-price" competition among providers, have created an environment for rapid adoption and diffusion of new technologies. These technologies generally fall into three categories: replacing accepted medical practices (e.g., hip replacement techniques and coronary artery bypass surgery), new therapies (e.g., liver, heart, and other organ transplants), and new imaging devices (e.g., magnetic resonance imaging). Without question, many of these new technologies clearly extend years of active life to many who would have died even 20 years ago. The down side is that many of the new technologies have large price tags.

Although international comparisons of health care delivery systems often raise more questions than they answer, one recent study has attempted to document the role of technology in increasing health care costs (Aaron & Schwartz). Based on their analysis of the U.S. and British health care systems, Aaron and Schwartz conclude that per capita health care costs would fall 10% if U.S. physicians used 10 key technologies (e.g., hip replacement, computed tomography, intensive care units) and intensive care at (population adjusted) rates similar to their British counterparts. Their analysis did not detect significant differences in health status resulting from the less intensive use of these technologies.

The critical role assumed by technological change (discussed above as increased service intensity) in rising health care costs has generated a growing volume of research focused on practice patterns and the appropriateness of medical procedures. This research has been spurred by international comparisons as well as by large variations in practice patterns documented domestically. One early pioneer, John Wennberg, noted magnitude differences in rates of specific procedures completed by physicians. Fourfold differences in hysterectomy rates, prostatectomies, tonsillectomies, and other common surgical procedures were discovered within and between states (Wennberg, 1984). Subsequent research indicates that these variations are not related to underlying differences in patient characteristics but rather to physician's practice patterns. These large variations among common procedures have resulted in a significant body of research aimed at examining the "appropriateness" of these differences.

Researchers at the Rand Corporation also have been active in examining the appropriateness of various practice patterns. Their studies of four surgical procedures—coronary artery bypass surgery (CABG), carotid endarterectomy, coronary angioplasty, and upper gastrointestinal endoscopy—examined the magnitude of unnecessary procedures and hospitalizations. With respect to CABG, the Rand researchers judged that 44% of the procedures examined were performed for inappropriate reasons (Chassin). Some 17% of coronary angiographies, used to diagnose blockages in heart arteries, were deemed inappropriate, as were a similar volume of gastrointestinal endoscopies. Eliminating inappropriate surgery would result in continued savings of billions of dollars per year. Although the precise magnitude of the savings remains speculative, if the rates of inappropriate use found in these procedures are extrapolated, reducing unnecessary use could reduce health care spending by $50 billion per year.

Efforts to Control Rising Health Care Costs: The Early Experience

This section summarizes previous and current efforts by third-party payers to control health care costs. We focus specifically on hospital cost containment, an area attracting most of our cost-control efforts.

Historically, third-party payers have implemented four distinct methods of cost control: control over the inputs used by hospitals, control over hospital admitting practices, limits on hospital payment, and the development of alternative (i.e., competitive) delivery systems. During the 1970s, public payers most actively pursued these cost-containment activities. By the mid-1980s, however, private payers adopted many of the cost-control techniques discussed below.

Limits on Hospital Inputs

Historically, efforts to control the use of inputs by hospitals have focused on capital expenditure decisions. Government has assumed a major role in initially financing and subsequently limiting hospital capital expansion for more than 40 years. The initial role of the government in health planning was to facilitate expansion of the hospital industry. In this capacity, the Hospital Survey and Construction Act (Hill–Burton bill) of 1946 supplied federal funds to underwrite new hospital construction. These funds were allocated to states according to population and state per capita income levels to redress a perceived shortage and maldistribution of hospital beds. Using some simple bed-to-population guidelines, local health planners allocated the funds to expand the nation's hospital bed supply.

In light of the rapid growth in the capacity of the hospital sector, health planning efforts have recently focused on limiting future hospital capital expansions. Although some voluntary efforts preceded, the most comprehensive planning efforts commenced in 1974 with the National Health Planning and Resource Development Act. This act provided federal funding for local health systems agencies (HSAs) and state health planning and development agencies. The health planning act developed because of growing concern over rising hospital costs increasingly linked to facility (both physical plant and technology) duplication. Thus, a primary role of the HSAs was to develop planning recommendations for specific hospital investments exceeding some dollar threshold (often $100,000). Based on the work of the local HSAs, a certificate of need (CON) was usually issued at the state level granting the capital spending. Although health planning agencies reached their peak during the 1970s, HSAs have generally been phased out during the mid-1980s.

In practice, state CON programs differed both in structure and organizational goal. They varied according to four characteristics thought to be related to their potential effectiveness (i.e., their stringency): (1) the program's orientation (i.e., planning/redistribution or cost containment), (2) locus of decision making (state or local), (3) the scope of formalized review standards, and (4) extent of an appeals process exemptions.

Early evaluations of the ability of the CON process to control were quick to question the cost-containment capabilities of the program. Although the CON process appeared initially to reduce the growth rate in hospital beds, it was accompanied by a larger rise in total assets per bed (Salkever & Bice). Moreover, even those CON programs that, *ex ante,* appeared more restrictive had little impact on total capital expenditures (Joskow). These results suggest that hospitals merely substituted one form of "unconstrained" capital investment for beds.

Other studies examining the effectiveness of the CON process focused on the diffusion of specific technologies. Those examining the role of the planning process in slowing the diffusion of potentially "duplicative" technologies (e.g., computerized tomography [CT]) and expensive new technologies (e.g., new surgical techniques) into hospitals were also negative (Sloan, Valvona, & Perrin). Although the CON process may have achieved other objectives, containing capital expenditures and total health care spending was not among them. Although the growing interest in competition among health plans and hospitals contributed, the inability of the CON process to achieve its fundamental goal— slower rates of capital expansion and overall cost growth—ultimately led to its decline.

Regulating the Utilization of Medical Care

This section focuses on public sector efforts to limit the utilization of hospital services. More recent attempts by the private sector to manage the course of a patient's treatment are addressed below.

Efforts to prevent unnecessary and low-quality care delivered to publicly insured patients commenced in 1972 with the advent of professional standard review organizations (PSROs). The goals of the PSRO program, albeit quite broadly defined, were to "promote the effective, efficient, and economical delivery of health care services of proper quality." Thus, the language in the enacting legislation included both cost-containment and quality-enhancement goals. The lack of clear direction in the program's goals likely contributed to the inability of most PSROs to focus their efforts effectively. In practice, PSROs focused primarily on Medicare and Medicaid beneficiaries, although some anticipated a broader spillover to privately insured patients. Despite the broad range of goals articulated under the original act, most PSROs attempted to reduce the length of stay among the Medicare population.

Evaluations of the PSRO program have produced mixed results. On average, the PSROs appeared to reduce total days of hospitalization among Medicare patients by 1.5% (Congressional Budget Office). PSROs appear to have reduced total days through reductions in length of stay rather than by preventing admissions. Although some studies suggest the PSRO program produced some public sector savings, these costs appear to have been shifted to other payers (Congressional Budget Office). The impact of the program on the Medicaid population remains unknown. When considering the administrative costs of the program, Medicare savings (through reduced utilization) were nearly offset by the costs of the program. Viewed more broadly, the Congressional Budget Office researchers found that savings to the Medicare program were offset by increases in charges (and expenditures) by private payers. Hence, when administrative costs and charges in total health care expenditures were examined, the PSROs appeared less effective.

The PSROs were replaced with peer review organizations (PROs) in 1984. The PROs differ from their predecessor, the PSROs, in that PROs are awarded on a competitive bidding process, based in part on their ability to achieve specific utilization goals. These goals are developed through negotiations with the Health Care Financing Administration (HCFA) and relate to five objectives (Office of Technology Assessment, Appendix G): (1) to reduce unnecessary hospital readmissions; (2) to assure the provision of adequate care, which, if not given, would cause serious complications; (3) to reduce the risk of mortality associated with specific procedures and conditions; (4) to reduce unnecessary surgery; and (5) to reduce avoidable postoperative or other complications. Negotiations between a PRO and the HCFA define specific performance markers (e.g., reduce readmissions resulting from substandard care by 20% used to evaluate the effectiveness of each PRO).

Beginning in 1989, PROs will assume an extended set of responsibilities beyond hospital care, including review of outpatient procedures, home health care, and care provided to military personnel and their families.

Although the jury is still out on the effectiveness of the PRO program, specific programs specified in the contracts appear to have been beneficial. In contrast to the PSRO program, PROs have influenced (albeit slightly) the rate of hospitalization among Medicare beneficiaries. The percentage of admissions denied by the PROs range from a high of 4.79% in Florida to 0.32% in Vermont (Health Care Financing Administration). Whether these reductions warrant the program's expense (estimated at $300 million in 1990) and administrative costs imposed on hospitals remains at issue.

Hospital Rate Setting (1969–1980)

Attempts to limit payment rates to hospitals represents a third cost-containment strategy. Between 1969 and 1974, 15 states introduced some form of hospital rate-setting program (Coelen & Sullivan). Although similar in their objectives, these programs differed with respect to a number of key design features, including the unit of payment, the scope of revenue covered (i.e., the number of payers and proportion of total revenue included), and a variety of design issues defining the actual prospectivity of the payments. These technical design features largely determined the restrictiveness of the rate-setting rules and ultimately their effectiveness. A brief description of these programs and their impact on reducing hospital expenditures follows.

Hospital rate setting generally refers to some form of prospective payment (i.e., the determination of payment rates prior to services rendered) by third-party payers. Methods actually used to define the payment rates are, in practice, quite complex. The essential elements include a base year and a trend factor. For example, Medicaid and Blue Cross payments to New York hospitals during 1989 were calculated by using a 1981 base year increased each year by an allowable trend factor. In this case, actual payment rates to hospitals are effectively divorced from individual hospital spending decisions. Thus, the degree of prospectivity built into the rate-setting system depends on the frequency in which the base year is moved. More stringent or restrictive rate-setting programs (such as the New York State program) move the base year infrequently. The trend factor used to define allowable revenue increases is also critical in determining the ability of rate-setting programs to control cost growth. The allowable trend factor could differ by multiple percentage points depending on key design decisions. For instance, trend factors may or may not include allowances for technological change. Moreover, allowed increases in wages may reflect more general wage trends or focus specifically on changes in the health care sector. Beyond these basic elements, most rate-setting programs differ with respect to the unit of payment (e.g., per diem, per case), who sets the rates (e.g., a separate rate-setting authority), and the extent to which historic (base year) costs are subjected to efficiency screens. These efficiency screens often compare each hospital's inpatient costs (after a variety of adjustments) to the mean or median within the state. In more restrictive programs, costs above the mean are "disallowed" and not recognized in developing the base year for subsequent payment. In contrast, less restrictive programs effectively pass-through all historic costs into the base.

Although state rate-setting programs differed with respect to a variety of important design issues, they also shared some common characteristics. First, rate-setting programs generally determined rates of payment prospectively. Second, the prospective rates generally applied only to inpatient operating expenses, leaving physician fees, direct medical education spending, capital, and outpatient expenses unregulated. In addition to the features noted above, state rate-setting programs varied in other respects. Three states—New Jersey, Maryland, and New York—established regulated per diem rates of payment. Elsewhere, rate setting focused on department revenue or total revenue caps. The number of payers within each state participating in the rate-setting program also varied. Prior to 1980 the rate-setting program in one state, Maryland, included all third-party payers. Programs in other states were more limited. Most programs included Medicaid and Blue Cross plans, although some, such as Indiana and Kentucky, covered only Blue Cross plans.

An impressive volume of research has examined the impact of state rate setting on hospital costs (Eby & Cohodes). The research generally concludes that state rate-setting programs reduced hospital costs, although the effects varied across states. During the 1970s cost growth per day and admission was 2 to 3% lower in states with rate-setting programs. The empirical results also suggest that rate setting reduced hospital expenditures over the long run by 10 to 20% (Sloan). There is less compelling evidence, however, that rate-setting programs reduced the growth in per capita health care spending. If true, this suggests that any reductions in inpatient hospital costs were offset by similar increases in unregulated sources of revenue. These findings are similar to the experience with PSROs discussed above.

Although implementation of rate-setting programs reduces cost growth on average, their performance varies widely across states. These effects have ranged from none to reductions exceeding 6% per year (Coelen & Sullivan). Much of the variations across programs stem from important design issues that define payment levels. Key design issues identified from previous studies as associated with their effectiveness include frequency in which the base year is moved, scope of revenue covered, number of payers included, and the construction of the trend factor (Thorpe & Phelps).

The Process of Cost Reductions

Effective rate-setting programs provide incentives for hospitals to adjust their "behavior" across many dimensions. Most notably, rate-setting programs provide incentives for hospitals to reduce the service intensity of medical care. In an earlier section, increased service intensity was identified as a major factor accounting for real increases in yearly health care costs. Reductions in service intensity are possible through lower staffing levels, a less expensive mix of personnel (e.g., the substitution of licensed practical nurses for registered nurses), slower adoption of new technology, or all of the above. The early literature on rate setting found evidence of adjustment across all dimensions (Cromwell & Kanak).

More effective rate-setting programs reduced costs by limiting the inputs (most notably technology) used to produce medical care. Hospitals in rate-setting states adopted new technologies at slower rates. Among the diffusion patterns examined were such major expense items as intensive care units, open-heart surgery, coronary artery surgery, obesity surgery, and burn care units (Romeo, Wagner, & Lee). Moreover, other technologies, most notably imaging devices such as CT, were adopted by hospitals at a slower pace in rate-setting states.

Rate setting also resulted in reduced hospital payroll expenses per patient day (Kidder & Sullivan). These "productivity" increases were achieved through both reductions in staff per adjusted day and changes in the mix of personnel. In some instances, particularly in teaching hospitals, administrators reduced their ancillary staff component, including intravenous and phlebotomy teams, messenger/transporters, and clerks, among others. Their tasks were generally absorbed by resident physicians, nurses, or both.

Although rate-setting programs during the 1970s achieved some of their goals, some dysfunctional side effects were evident. Rate setting programs that focused solely on the day of care often led to increases in the average length of a hospital stay (Sloan). In some cases, average hospital occupancy rates also increased. As a result, per capita days of care remained relatively stable after the implementation of rate-setting programs, blunting the full cost-containment potential. As noted earlier, the first rate-setting programs appeared less effective in reducing per capita health care spending. This led many observers to speculate that hospitals merely shifted their fixed costs to other, unregulated payers (often termed cost shifting) or unregulated sources of revenue (e.g., outpatient care) (Eby & Cohodes). The ability of hospital administrators to escape the full regulatory potential of the rate-setting laws created increased demand for alternative cost-containment strategies. Sharp increases in charges to unregulated payers—who were largely commercial health insurers—created growing allegations that they bore the burden of any cost savings enjoyed by regulated (generally, government) payers (Sloan & Becker). The growing differential between "costs" reimbursed by regulated payers and "charges" to unregulated payers raised concerns about the overall effectiveness and equity of rate-setting programs. These concerns were largely responsible for the subsequent generation of rate-setting programs, competitive bidding schemes, and alternative delivery systems described below.

Efforts to Control Health Care Costs (1983–present)

Informed by the early experience with hospital rate-setting, attempts to control rising health care costs changed in four important aspects during the mid-1980s. First, private payers and employers increased their efforts to develop cost-containment programs. Second, state governments and Medicare experimented with new approaches to hospital rate setting. Third, both the public and private sector created incentives for hospitals to compete on the basis of price, rather than other dimensions. Finally, the cost-containment debate was extended to physician payment in addition to institutional payment reforms.

Role of Private Payers

Facing sharply rising health insurance premiums during the early 1980s, private payers extended their efforts to control health care costs (particularly, hospital costs) in three important directions. First, private payers and employers increased efforts to "manage" the utilization of health care. Second, dissatisfied with the ability of private health insurance carriers to control costs, a growing number of employers decided to "self-insure." Third, using their purchasing power for leverage, private payers increasingly negotiated rates of payment with health care providers.

Growth in Managed Care

During the early 1980s the HMO concept assumed a prominent role in the health care delivery system. The key features of the HMO concept include (1) serving a defined population voluntarily enrolled in the plan, (2) the assumption of contractual responsibility and financial risk by the plan to provide a stated range of services, and (3) the payment of a fixed annual or monthly payment by the enrollee independent of the actual use of services (Luft). The intent of the HMO concept was to shift some financial risk to providers (rather than to patients under various cost-sharing schemes). Risk shifting would, in theory, create incentives for the plan to provide appropriate levels of medical care in general and preventive care in particular. Payment of a fixed annual fee also limited the ability of providers to thwart the intent of the cost controls through shifting costs to unregulated payers or costs.

Enrollment in HMOs grew rapidly during the 1980s, increasing to 29.3 million by 1987, a 300% rise in just 8 years (Interstudy). Moreover, private payers adopted selected elements of HMOs, developed to control utilization, for use in more traditional fee-for-service plans. Most important was the growing reliance on controlling the use of "inappropriate" medical care. Growth in the number of employers and private payers developing "managed" care plans during the 1980s has been impressive. Of those receiving health insurance through the workplace, over 70% are enrolled in some type of managed-care plan (Gabel et al.). Over 43% of insured employees and their dependents are enrolled in some type of managed-care, fee-for-service plan; another 18% are enrolled in HMOs, and 11% are in plans with negotiated payment rates (i.e., preferred provider arrangements [PPAs]).

The interest of corporate America in managed-care plans is not without merit. Several studies have documented the wide variation in medical practice patterns, many of which result in costly and inappropriate patterns of medical care (Wennberg, 1984). Estimates of the magnitude of this inappropriate use vary widely. Some estimate that up to 30% of all health care costs result from unnecessary medical and surgical tests, treatments, and procedures (Chassin).

Among the most popular of the managed-care options is the HMO. The spectacular growth in HMO enrollment noted above was enhanced by their well-documented ability to reduce total health expenditures. Early, nonexperimental experience placed the magnitude of these cost savings between 20 and 40% compared to those enrolled in more traditional health care plans (Luft). At issue was whether the observed reductions in expenditures stemmed from a different style of medicine practiced by physicians in HMOs, a favorable selection of enrollees, or both. Indeed, there was mounting evidence that healthier, younger individuals were more likely to join HMOs. Thus, the observed savings may simply represent self-selection rather than real savings.

Evidence from the Rand Health Insurance Experiment (HIE) provided insight into the selection issue. Using an experimentally controlled population, the HIE found that, compared to a free, fee-for-service plan, HMOs reduced total expenditures by 29% (Manning et al., 1985). The magnitude of these reductions was impressive, similar to those observed under a 95% co-insurance rate. Thus, the experimental results indicated that HMOs did not require favorable selection to achieve their large apparent cost savings. Remaining at issue, however, is whether these savings represent one-time or continued reductions in health care spending. One early comparison of premium growth among traditional plans with that of HMOs found little difference in rates of increase (Newhouse, Schwartz, Williams, & Witsberger). If these results are valid, they suggest that HMO savings, although substantial, may be transitory.

Spurred by the studies documenting their effectiveness, selected aspects of HMOs, such as second surgical opinion, preauthorization of selected hospital admissions, concurrent review, and outpatient surgery and testing requirements, assumed standard roles in many health plans (Jensen, Morrisey, & Marcus). In some cases, immediate reductions in health care spending resulted. Although evaluations of the cost savings traced to private sector utilization programs are rare, one study provided some early insight. For the large private health insurer examined, hospital utilization review (which included preadmission certification and on-site and concurrent review) reduced admissions 12.3%, inpatient spending 11.9% and total per capita expenditures 8.3% (Feldstein, Wickizer, & Wheeler, 1988). Other, company-specific evaluations have found similar expenditure reductions accompanying the introduction of utilization review programs. Whether these limited programs generate spillover savings (or additional costs) to other payers is not clear.

Growth in the Number of Self-Insured Companies

Frustration over the inability of more traditional third-party payers to control the rise in health insurance premiums led many companies to self-insure. Between 1981 and 1985 the number of full-time employees working in companies that self-insure nearly doubled, rising from 22 to 41.9% (Jensen & Gabel, 1988). A number of factors account for the rapid growth in self-insured firms. Self-insured plans are exempt from state mandated-benefit laws that require group health insurance plans to include specific benefits. Many of the mandated benefits receive little criticism. Others, such as chiropractic services, catastrophic coverage, and more esoteric benefits (e.g., wigs, acupuncture), are often criticized and are thought responsible for a portion of the continued rise in health care premiums. The growth in the number of mandated health benefits has been spectacular, rising from approximately 40 in 1970 to nearly 700 by 1988 ("Health Insurance Premiums"). Thus, some of the continued rise in group health insurance premiums stems from the proliferation of mandated benefits.

In addition to avoiding state benefit mandates, there are additional incentives to self-insure. For instance, self-insured funds are not subject to state premium taxes or to laws governing capital and financial reserve requirements. Moreover, self-insured funds do not contribute to state "risk pools," designed to finance insurance for high-risk, low-income individuals through state taxes.

Growth in the number of self-insured plans is also symptomatic of the longer-term trend away from "community"-rated plans and toward "experience" rating. Built into traditional group health insurance premiums are costs stemming from uncompensated care, insurance company profits, and cross-subsidies of high-cost policyholders. The rising number of uninsured individuals and uncompensated care has accounted for a portion of the yearly increases in health insurance premiums. Firms that self-insure avoid these additional costs, which are built into a typical group health insurance premium. In this sense, self-insuring eliminates any cross-subsidies included in health insurance premiums. However, the move to self-insuring also transfers all (or in some cases most) of the financial risk of catastrophic cases from private insurers to firms.

Despite the benefits accruing to firms that self-insure, the comparative ability of such plans to contain costs remains unproved. One recent study compared the level and rate of increase in costs among self-insured commercial and Blue Cross plans. The results found no significant differences in expenditures across plans between 1981 and 1985 (Jensen & Gabel, 1988). Moreover, firms self-insuring during this period actually experienced sharper increases in health care spending compared to commercial and Blue Cross plans. Although our experience with self-insured plans is relatively new, their ability to significantly reduce cost growth relative to more traditional payers appears questionable.

Growth in PPAs

Finally, private payers and self-insured firms have increasingly used their purchasing power to negotiate payment rates with providers. Under a PPA arrangement, private payers negotiate a discounted rate, often guaranteeing the provider a specified volume of business. For hospitals suffering from low occupancy rates (generally in California, Colorado, and Florida), the arrangements are quite attractive. The number of PPAs increased from 42 in 1982 to over 700 in 1988. More than 34 million individuals are enrolled in plans with some type of PPA.

Although the sponsorships, form, and incentives found in PPAs differ widely, today's PPAs share four common characteristics:

1. PPAs represent an organized network of providers (e.g., hospitals, physicians) available to provide care.
2. Patients enter the PPA network through financial incentives in their benefits, a physician gatekeeper, or both.
3. PPAs negotiate discounts from providers from prevailing market payment rates.
4. PPAs include a variety of managed-care elements, usually including physician gatekeepers, utilization review, and second-opinion programs.

The early PPAs focused on negotiating reduced rates of payment to both hospitals and physicians. Little attention was directed toward including checks on utilization. As a result, early experience with PPAs provided mixed results. Although unit costs fell, the volume of services often increased, reducing the success of the ventures. More recently, insurers have developed hybrid programs incorporating utilization-control features along with negotiated payments. The utilization-control features in these hybrid plans are similar to those found in most HMOs. A central feature of these plans in the use of a "gatekeeper" primary care physician. The primary care physician in essence manages the patient referral process. Most hybrid plans include financial incentives for the gatekeeper to monitor utilization by setting specific targets for hospital admissions, total hospital days, and outpatient surgery. Since these hybrid plans are so new, few empirical analyses have assessed their impact on health care expenditures. One recent study, however, examined the impact of a PPA for a large western company. The study found no discernible difference in spending among these enrolled in the PPA compared to other employees. Whether these results will generalize to other settings remains unknown.

Innovations in Hospital Rate Setting—the Growth in Diagnosis-Related Group Payment Systems

Perhaps the most important change in hospital rate setting during the 1980s was Medicare's shift from a retrospective cost-based program to a prospectively determined payment based on diagnosis-related groups (DRGs). Under this system, hospitals are paid a preestablished amount per case treated, with payment rates varying by type of case. The DRGs measure hospital output by originally classifying patients into 23 major diagnostic categories (MDCs), based on major body systems. The MDCs are divided further into more than 470 diagnostic groups based on the patient's diagnosis or surgical procedure used, and on age, sex, and other clinical information.

Three aspects of this approach differ from Medicare's previous payment methodology. First, the payments are determined in advance and are fixed. Second, the unit of payment changed from per day to per admission. Finally, payment rates were eventually divorced from each hospital's own cost experience.

The new payment scheme implemented by Medicare applies only to inpatient, operating costs. Excluded are payments for capital (which Medicare continues to reimburse at levels slightly below interest and depreciation expenses), direct medical education (e.g., salaries for attending physicians and residents), and outpatient and emergency departments. Also left intact is Medicare's fee-for-service payment system for physician payment (discussed below). Not all hospitals were included in Medicare's case payment system. Some specialty hospitals, such as children's, long-term-care, rehabilitation, and psychiatric hospitals, were exempt. Also exempt were four states (New York, Massachusetts, Maryland, and New Jersey) receiving waivers from the HCFA to develop their own experimental payment programs. However, by 1986, only Maryland and New Jersey retained their waivers.

Payment that an individual hospital receives for treating Medicare patients in a given DRG depends on the DRG's "cost" weight (i.e., its cost relative to an average Medicare admission) multiplied by a "standardized" average cost for all Medicare patients. The standardization process includes adjustments for interhospital differences in wages, teaching status, and amount of care provided to low-income patients. Different rates are also set for urban and rural hospitals. In addition, payment amounts to hospitals are adjusted each year by a trend factor, consisting of a measure of the price of goods and services purchased by hospitals and a discretionary adjustment factor to account for changes in new technology and productivity.

The original plans called for a gradual phase-in of the case payment system over 3 years. In the first year (1984), 75% of a hospital's per-case payments were to be based on its own cost experience. This level gradually declined over time, and by 1988 payment rates (known as prices) to hospitals were based on national "standardized" average costs per admission. Movement to a pricing system divorced payment rates from each hospital's costs.

Medicare's experience with the DRG system has produced mixed results. Initially, hospitals responded quite dramatically to the altered incentives created by the DRG payment system. The payment of a fixed price per admission provided hospitals clear incentives to reduce costs. Any savings stemming from these reductions could be retained by the hospital. The new opportunity to earn short-term profits resulted in impressive changes during the early years of the program. During the first year of the program (federal fiscal year 1984), inpatient expenditures declined as the number of full-time equivalent (FTE) employees fell 2.3%, reversing the trend of earlier years (see Table 11.1). Although lengths of stay among the elderly had been falling for years, the DRG program accelerated the decline. Finally, total admissions fell 2.6% during the first year of the DRG program, again reversing a long trend toward increased admissions.

Table 11.1 Percent Change in Medicare Inpatient Expenses, Hospital Staffing, and Hospital Volume, 1980–1987

Year	Medicare inpatient expenses	Total inpatient expenses	Total hospital FTEs[a]	Length of stay	Admissions
1980	—	16.8%	4.7%	–0.1%	6.7%
1981	—	18.4	5.4	–0.1	3.0
1982	—	15.6	3.7	–2.3	4.1
1983	—	9.6	1.4	–4.5	4.7
1984	–4.4%	3.5	–2.3	–7.6	–2.6
1985	3.0	4.1	–2.3	–2.0	–5.2
1986	6.5	7.1	0.3	0.3	–1.2
1987	—	6.1	0.7	1.1	0.4

[a]FTEs, full-time equivalent employees.
Source: American Hospital Association, National Panel Survey. Prospective Payment Assessment Commission, Annual Report to Congress.

Falling lengths of stay, admissions, and employment levels resulted in slower hospital expenditure growth. Total Medicare inpatient operating costs decreased 6 percentage points during the first year of the program. Inpatient cost per admission increased slightly, approximately 1.3%, significantly below the 4.7% update factor allowed during the first year. With cost growth slower than increases in revenue, hospital operating margins rose sharply. By 1984 the median hospital's margin was 11.3%, the highest in nearly two decades (AHA).

Unfortunately, the expenditure reductions were short-lived. Many of the trends observed in the initial year of the program were reversed in subsequent years. Total Medicare operating costs increased 3% during fiscal year 1985 and 6.5% during 1986 (see Table 11.1). The latter increase was cause for concern, as it exceeded the allowed increase in revenues (e.g., the trend factor) by 6 percentage points. Although the factors accounting for the more recent rise in Medicare spending are unknown, hospitals may simply have reinvested large portions of their "profits" back into hospital operations. If true, this would account for the cost growth bubble observed in fiscal year 1986.

Lengths of stay also increased during 1986 and 1987, although admissions continued to fall. However, since the average acuity of patients admitted to hospitals increased, adjusted (for case mix) lengths of stay did not rise. In contrast to the initial decline, total hospital employment increased during 1986 and 1987. The bulk of the increase occurred in hospital outpatient departments, with employment levels on the inpatient side continuing to fall.

The new DRG payment system also provided strong incentives for hospital administrators to "unbundle" services. This included encouraging physicians to complete tests and procedures outside the hospital (which are not subject to the payment controls). Moreover, recent changes in medical technology, most notably surgical procedures, have accelerated the trend toward outpatient care. These incentives and changes in technology resulted in substantial increases in Medicare's spending for outpatient services. For instance, by 1987 Medicare expenditures for outpatient services increased 21%, more than five times the rate of increase observed for inpatient expenditures (Physician Payment Review Commission). The large increase in outpatient department expenditures blunted the full cost-containment potential of the DRG program.

In addition to the most recent rise in Medicare spending, the DRG program had uneven impacts on hospital expenditure growth. As discussed above, a central element of the new system was the use of predetermined "prices" for hospital payment. These prices were based on national average Medicare costs per discharge standardized for teaching status, share of low-income patients treated, wage rates, and urban/rural location. Because payments were no longer based on historic hospital costs, payments to some hospitals were lower and others higher than their average costs. Hospitals with payment rates set lower than average costs were thought less efficient and were the initial targets of the regulatory program. However, large numbers of hospitals initially benefited from the program because payment rates exceeded their average costs.

Use of the pricing methodology led to an uneven response by hospitals to the DRG payment system. On average, total inpatient costs growth was initially attenuated under the DRG system. To a more modest extent, the DRG system reduced the rate of increase in total (both inpatient and outpatient expenditures) through 1986. The reduced growth in costs, however, was generally limited to those hospitals with payment rates set below costs. Among these hospitals, inpatient cost growth was over 4.4 percentage points lower than the overall average (Feder, Hadley, & Zuckerman). In contrast, compared to the most tightly constrained hospitals, expenditures for hospitals least constrained were some 7 percentage points higher. Thus, the redistributive effect of the pricing system limited the full cost-containment potential of the DRG program.

Most recently, reforms of the DRG system have focused on a variety of "technical" adjustments to the payment rates as well as adjusting the methodology used to reimburse for capital expenses. Medicare currently reimburses hospitals a percentage (less than 100) for all depreciation and interest spending. Failure to include capital payments in the prospective payment system has likely reduced the potential effectiveness of the DRG program. A capital pass-through ensures that hospital spending decisions are insensitive to interest rates or less costly methods of expansion. Moreover, the pass-through also provides incentives for hospitals to inefficiently substitute capital for labor. The debate over an appropriate payment policy for capital will attract broader discussion over the next 5 years.

Growth and Subsequent Decline in All-Payer Rate-Setting Programs

State experiments with innovative hospital rate-setting programs expanded during the 1980s. Until then, most state rate-setting programs set prospective per diem rates for Medicaid and Blue Cross plans. In some cases, commercial payers were also included. However, Medicare payments to hospitals were outside the prospectively determined rates. Beginning in 1977, Maryland obtained a waiver from the HCFA allowing the state to develop its own payment rules for Medicare. This allowed the state to include all sources of third-party inpatient revenue under the state's rate-setting rules. Three other states—New Jersey, Massachusetts, and New York—subsequently obtained Medicare waivers during the early 1980s. Like Maryland, each state included Medicare payments within its historic rate-setting programs.

The genesis of these four all-payer systems was complicated. They included concern over both continued escalation in hospital costs within these states as well as issues regarding the equity of payment rates facing private payers. As discussed below, use of the rate-setting process to achieve both cost reductions and distributional objectives distinguished the all-payer approach from previous efforts (Thorpe). Each state adopting the all-payer approach had previous rate-setting programs covering some portion of inpatient revenues. Although these programs were often successful in reducing cost growth among some payers (and in the case of New York, all payers), costs among unregulated payers continued to climb. Price controls on Medicaid and Blue Cross plans created incentives for hospitals to increase charges—often referred to as cost or charge shifting—to unregulated commercial payers. As a result, the difference between charges and costs for commercial payers escalated rapidly during the late 1970s and early 1980s. Thus, protecting commercial payers against cost shifting assumed an important role for all-payer systems.

Growth in the number of uninsured individuals over this period created another set of pressures. Between 1979 and 1984 the number of individuals without health insurance increased 20% to more than 34 million individuals (Congressional Research Service, Table 4.7). Growth in the number of individuals without health insurance increased the volume of bad debt and charity care provided by hospitals. For those hospitals unable to recover such costs through commercial payers (through increased charges) or state and local governments (in the case of public hospitals), a serious deterioration of operating margins resulted. Deteriorating hospital financial conditions, combined with the growing number of uninsured patients, created pressures on state governments to provide some financial relief.

The growing demands of the commercial insurance industry to limit legislatively the difference between charges and costs (e.g., the differential), combined with the mounting requirements of hospitals to finance uncompensated care, presented a dilemma. Limiting the size of the differential would eliminate one traditionally passive method of financing a portion of uncompensated care. Thus, some alternative and more explicit financing method would be required. Moreover, the growth in the differential created a common perception that commercial payers were assuming an unfair burden in financing care for the uninsured (Meyer, Johnson, & Sullivan). Thus, to distribute the costs of uncompensated care more evenly, each state developed some type of uncompensated-care pool. Although methods of collecting revenue and distributing it to hospitals differed across states, the burden of financing uncompensated care was more widely distributed.

Finally, experience with the "partial" payer approaches used by most state rate-setting programs during the 1970s provided mixed results. As noted above, cost growth among regulated payers was often attenuated, although per capita cost growth was generally stable. Thus, the all-payer approach was also designed to provide a uniform inpatient revenue cap, reducing the ability of hospitals to escape the intent of the regulatory controls. Although the programs provided a comprehensive inpatient rate cap, payment methods for outpatient services in each state were largely left intact.

The four state all-payer programs described above generally achieved their intended results. Relative to the "unwaivered" states, the all-payer states were able to reduce total cost growth. Inpatient costs per admission were 2 to 3 percentage points lower between 1982 and 1985 in waivered states relative to unwaivered states (Schramm, Renn, & Biles). More impressive perhaps was the 2-percentage-point reduction in total costs per admission (adjusted for outpatient visits).

Lower cost growth among the all-payer states was achieved through reductions in labor, rather than reduced admissions or length of stay. The number of FTE personnel in the waivered states grew at significantly slower rates than observed elsewhere (Schramm et al.). Thus, the comprehensive regulatory controls appeared to increase the productivity of hospital care. Fewer labor inputs per patient day were also accompanied by slower rates of technological diffusion. As noted in an earlier section, slower adoption rates were especially pronounced in New York. Although growth in hospital personnel in all-payer states proceeded at a significantly slower pace, changes in average length of stay between the waivered and unwaivered states revealed few discernible differences.

The all-payer states were also successful in limiting the differential between private charges and costs. Each state enacted a statutory limit on the magnitude of each hospital's allowed difference between costs and charges. In New York this reduced the differential from a statewide average of 30% to less than 15% by 1985 (Thorpe). Similarly, the all-payer program in Massachusetts reduced the magnitude of the differential by 1.4% in its first year and steadily lowered it to approximately 7.5% by 1985. The magnitude of the differential in these states was significantly lower than the national average of 25% (AHA).

Finally, the regulatory approach adopted by the all-payer states raised a significant volume of revenue to finance hospital uncompensated care. More than $300 million was raised each year in New York and Massachusetts, with similar amounts (relative to total state hospital costs) in the other states. The pool revenues allowed financially strained hospitals to maintain, and often increase, the volume of care they provided the medically indigent. Moreover, the significant influx of revenues raised by the pools improved the operating margins of many hospitals. In New York, for example, the magnitude of the statewide hospital operating deficit was over $600 million less during the experiment relative to deficits projected without the pools (Thorpe). Thus, the redistributive goals of the all-payer programs were largely fulfilled.

The success of the all-payer programs in simultaneously reducing cost growth and internally redistributing revenues to fiscally distressed facilities ironically led to their near elimination. Hospitals in each state were quick to compare the expected revenue under their waivered systems with revenues expected under the national DRG program (Hospital Association of New York State). For instance, the hospital association in New York State projected a $400 million influx of Medicare revenues in 1986 should the state switch from its waivered system to the DRG program. Similar projections of higher revenues flowing to the waivered states also were developed in other states. In partial response to industry interests in switching to the DRG program, New York and Massachusetts did not extend their waivers, thus joining Medicare's DRG payment programs.

Growth in Competitive Bidding

A final payment innovation during the 1980s was the growth in competitive bidding schemes designed to create incentives for providers to compete on a price basis. As discussed in an earlier section, competition among providers in the health care industry has traditionally occurred along nonprice dimensions (e.g., service intensity, technology, and amenities). Those interested in promoting price competition were quick to highlight the shortcomings of the regulatory approach (Enthoven). According to this school of thought, vigorous price competition among health care plans and providers would provide the only "practical" solution to the health care cost crisis.

While other states moved to increase the scope of hospital revenue regulated, others moved to competitive bidding. The California Medi-Cal program implemented the most notable bidding scheme, known as selective contracting, in 1983. Under this program hospitals would submit price bids to the state contracting "czar" to provide services to Medi-Cal beneficiaries. Except in emergencies, hospitals not receiving contracts could not receive payment from the state. Two other state Medicaid programs followed California's lead: Illinois in 1985 and, most recently, Washington State.

The early experience with selective contracting in California has produced favorable results (Melnick & Zwanziger). In contrast to earlier research results that found higher cost growth in the most competitive markets, the opposite held for California hospitals after the implementation of selective contracting. Between 1983 and 1985, real (adjusted for general inflation) inpatient costs increased an average of 1% for hospitals in less competitive markets, compared to an 11.3% decrease among hospitals in more competitive markets (Melnick & Zwanziger). In keeping with the empirical results noted above, the state estimated savings exceeding $1 billion during the selective contracting program.

Both the selective contracting program implemented in California and the all-payer rate-setting systems discussed above were able to reduce cost growth. Still at issue is their relative ability to contain costs. Is competitive bidding the salvation or the imposition of more comprehensive and binding rate-setting programs? Recent studies provide at least an initial insight. Based on a national study, all-payer rate regulation reduced cost growth by 16.3% in Massachusetts, 15.4% in Maryland, and 6.3% in New York between 1982 and 1986 relative to a set of control states (Robinson & Luft, 1988) Cost growth in New Jersey was similar to that observed among the control states. In comparison, cost growth among California hospitals using the selective contracting strategy was 10.1% lower compared to states without rate-setting or competitive bidding. Thus, based on these results, it appears that, on average, the more comprehensive rate-setting programs and selective contracting have similar impacts on cost growth. Whether the longer-term performance of these decidedly different approaches is similar requires continued monitoring.

Reform of Physician Reimbursement

As this chapter illustrates, efforts to reduce health care costs have often focused on limiting institutional payment (especially to hospitals). Often excluded from these regulatory efforts were payment for hospital capital and outpatient and physician services. Much of the recent policy debate has focused on extending payment reform to these three expenditure items.

At the forefront of the discussion is physician payment reform. Although expenditures on physician services account for less than one quarter of all spending, physicians potentially influence over 70% of all health care spending (Fuchs). Thus, the focus on physician incentives and payment issues is not myopic. Traditionally, most third-party payers have reimbursed physicians using a modified fee-for-service method. Medicare's customary, prevailing, and reasonable (CPR) payment methodology is typical of these fee-for-service methods. Under the CPR method, payments for each service performed are based on the lower of the physician's historic charge, the billed charge, or an average charge of similar physicians in the area. Payment rates are also limited to yearly increases in the Medicare economic index. The current fee structure has been roundly criticized as inflationary and complex (Physician Payment Review

Commission). Moreover, the CPR method may distort the service mix provided by physicians, as well as specialty and location choices.

The criticisms aimed at the CPR payment system are not without some merit. For instance, total Medicare expenditures increased an average of 15.5% between 1975 and 1987 (Physician Payment Review Commission). Payments for physicians' services represented one of the fastest-growing components of this increase, rising an average of 18% during the same period. In addition, higher payment rates (relative to costs) for specialists and those performing complex procedures (relative to those completing more cognitive tasks) have frequently been cited as influencing physician specialty choices. The apparent "surplus" of surgeons and subspecialties projected over the next 20 years has often been traced to this payment system.

Two policy options have frequently been advanced to address both the cost growth and specialty choice issues. The first payment option is to expand the number of providers paid on a capitated basis. Capitation refers to the receipt of a fixed payment over a defined period regardless of the number of services or procedures completed by the physician. This is essentially the style of payment successfully used by many HMOs to control cost growth. The role of capitation in addressing cost growth was discussed earlier.

A second option often discussed is a new fee schedule for physicians. One recently developed fee schedule is based on the resources used by physicians to produce services and procedures. This particular relative value scale, a resource-based relative value (RBRV), has three components: a measure of total "work" by the physician, an allowance for practice costs, and an allowance for time in specialty training (Hsiao et al.). A major objective of the RBRV is to develop a more equitable method of reimbursing physicians. In contrast to the CPR method, payments and costs for services and procedures under an RBRV would be equated. This could eliminate the distortive effect the current system has on specialty choice and service mix.

Full implementation of an RBRV system could substantially redistribute income among physicians. Under current payment rules the price-cost margin for surgeons (e.g., profit) is the highest. As a result, they would be the largest losers under such a system, perhaps losing over 40% (in the case of ophthalmologists) of their revenue (Hsiao et al.). In contrast, those with the lowest price–cost margins, generally family practitioners and internists, would enjoy the largest increases in revenues, over 60% in some cases. The magnitude of these redistributions is substantial and obviously has drawn intense scrutiny by the relevant specialty societies as well as policymakers.

Although an RBRV would redistribute large volumes of physician revenue and is often viewed as a more equitable method of reimbursing physicians, its ability to reduce costs is not known. By itself the RBRV does little to control the volume of procedures completed by physicians. At issue is the likely response of physicians receiving either large increases or decreases in their fees. Previous experience with physician fee schedules produced mixed results. In most cases, reductions in *all* fees resulted in significant increases in the volume of procedures (Physician Payment Review Commission). Whether changes in *relative* fee levels produce similar results is not known.

Area-wide limits on total physician expenditures have recently been suggested in conjunction with the RBRV to augment the ability to control physician expenditure growth. In addition to the skepticism over its ability to control costs, others wonder whether implementation of an RBRV would alter the service mix to yield a net increase in patient health. In its best form, such an index would be linked to some measure of the efficacy or appropriateness of the procedure or service. Despite these uncertainties, it seems apparent that some type of payment reform is high on the policy agenda.

Summary and Conclusions

Despite 20 years of regulatory controls, health care spending continues to grow relative to the GNP. The inability to reduce the national rate of expenditure growth continues to frustrate both public and private payers. Indeed, in spite of growing efforts to reduce costs, health care spending now accounts for 11.1% of the GNP, up from 9.1% in 1980. Even though the United States spends more on health care as a percentage of GNP than does any other industrialized country, more than 37 million Americans remain uninsured. Frustration over the sustained rise in health care costs and a 25% increase in the number of uninsured since 1980 has increased interest in more fundamental changes in our financing system. For the first time in decades, polls report that most Americans want a fundamental shift in the direction of U.S. health policy. Indeed, one recent poll indicates that 61% of Americans indicated they would favor a comprehensive national health insurance system like Canada's (Blendon). This mounting sentiment for change will likely continue, creating pressure for more innovative methods of addressing health care cost issues.

The continued rise in health care costs indicates that our attempts to address the problem have failed. This failure may be traced to a mismatch between the underlying problem and previous interventions. Our earlier discussion indicated that the fundamental force driving up health care costs was the diffusion of new technologies. Of the estimated sevenfold real increase in health care spending since 1950, new technologies and practice patterns account for up to 90% of the growth (Manning et al., 1987). Innovations in medicine have been nothing short of remarkable. Our capacity to increase average life expectancy and its quality reflect these developments. The growth in transplant capacity, diagnostic imaging, and drugs represents a few of these medical innovations. If this increase in spending had generated commensurate increases in benefits, then the "problem" of health care cost growth would be illusory. In short, that we spend 11.1% of our GNP in the health care sector may simply reflect societal preferences to direct limited resources to health rather than to other areas.

At the center of the debate over the growth of health care costs is whether the same level of health could be purchased for less. A growing body of research indicates that substantial savings could be achieved without significant changes in the health of our population. Critical examination of the "appropriateness" of various medical procedures indicates that health care spending could be reduced by $50 billion without a deleterious impact on health. At issue is the appropriate intervention to address the underlying problem of health care cost growth. The push of new technology suggests that more centralized, rather than fragmented, approaches underlie any solution. This would require the multiple public and private payers to reach some consensus concerning a comprehensive strategy to address the technology issue. One promising proposal is the development of a national technology assessment commission empowered to conduct clinical trials of new technologies before they are widely diffused. Another would move us closer to the Canadian budget-cap system. Although the precise path is not evident, what is clear is that failure to match the next generation of interventions with the technology and costly variation in practice patterns will continue to thwart our efforts to contain costs.

References

Aaron, H., & Schwartz, W. *The Painful Prescription: Rationing Hospital Care*. Washington, D.C.: Brookings Institution, 1984.

American Hospital Association. *National Hospital Panel Survey*. Chicago: AHA, 1988.

Blendon, J. "Three Systems: A Comparative Survey." *Health Management Quarterly*, *11*(1) 2, 1989.

Chassin, M. "Does Inappropriate Use Explain Geographic Variation in the Use of Health Care Services? A Study of Three Procedures." Santa Monica, CA: Rand Corporation, 1987. (N-2748).

Coelen, C., & Sullivan, D. "An Analysis of the Effects of Prospective Reimbursement Programs on Hospital Expenditures." *Health Care Financing Review*, Winter, 1, 1981.

Congressional Budget Office. *The Impact of PSROs on Health Care Costs: An Update of CBO's 1979 Evaluation*. Washington, D.C.: U.S. Government Printing Office, 1981.

Congressional Research Service. *Health Insurance and the Uninsured: Background Data and Analysis*. Washington, D.C.: U.S Government Printing Office, 1988.

Cromwell, J., & Kanak, J. "The Effects of Hospital Rate-Setting Programs on Volume of Hospital Services." *Health Care Financing Review*, 4(2) 47, 1982.

Eby, C., & Cohodes, D. "What Do We Know About Rate-Setting?" *Journal of Health Politics, Policy and Law*, Summer, 299, 1985.

Enthoven, A. C. *Health Plan*. Reading, MA: Addison-Wesley, 1981.

Feder, J., Hadley, J., & Zuckerman, J. "How Did Medicare's Prospective Payment System Affect Hospitals?" *New England Journal of Medicine, 317,* 867, 1987.

Feldstein, P., Wickizer, T., Wheeler, J. "The Effects of Utilization Review Programs In Health Care Use and Expenditures." *New England Journal of Medicine,* May 19, 1988, pp. 1310–1314.

Freeland, M., & Schendler, C. E. "National Health Expenditure Growth in the 1980s: An Aging Population, New Technologies and Increasing Competition." *Health Care Financing Review,* March, 1, 1983.

Fuchs, V. *Who Shall Live?* New York: Basic Books, 1974.

Gabel, J., et al. *Trends in Managed Health Care.* Washington, D.C.: Health Insurance Association of America, 1989.

Health Care Financing Administration. *HHS News,* November 18. Washington, D.C.: Health Insurance Association of America, 1988.

"Health Insurance Premiums to Soar in '89." *Wall Street Journal,* p. B1, October 25, 1988.

Hospital Association of New York State. *Modelling Alternative Reimbursement Systems.* Albany, N.Y.: HANYS, 1985.

Hsiao, W., et al. "Resource-Based Relative Values: An Overview." *Journal of the American Medical Association, 260,* 2347, 1988.

Interstudy. *National HMO Census, 1987.* Excelsior, MN:, 1988.

Jensen, G., Gabel, J. "The Erosion of Purchased Health Insurance." *Inquiry, 25*(3), pp. 328–343, 1988.

Jensen, G., Morrisey, M., & Marcus, J. "Cost Sharing and the Changing Pattern of Employer-Sponsored Health Benefits." *Milbank Memorial Fund Quarterly, 65*(4) 521, 1987.

Joskow, P. *Controlling Hospital Costs: The Role of Government Regulation.* Boston: MIT Press, 1981.

Kidder, D., & Sullivan, D. "Hospital Payroll Costs, Productivity and Employment Under Prospective Payment." *Health Care Financing Review, 4*(2) 89, 1982.

Luft, H. *Health Maintenance Organizations: Dimensions of Performance.* New York: John Wiley, 1981.

Manning, W., et al. *A Controlled Trial of the Effect of a Prepaid Group Practice on the Utilization of Medical Services.* Santa Monica, CA: Rand Corporation, 1985.

Manning, W. G., et al. "Health Insurance and the Demand for Medical Care." *American Economic Review, 77*(3), 251, 1987.

Melnick, G., & Zwanziger, J. "Hospital Behavior under Competition and Cost-Containment Policies." *Journal of the American Medical Association, 260*(18), 2669, 1988.

Meyer, J., Johnson, W., & Sullivan, S. *Passing the Health Care Buck: Who Pays the Hidden Cost?* Washington, D.C.: American Enterprise Institute, 1983.

Mullen, P. "Big Increases in Health Premiums." *Health Week,* December 27, 1988, p. 1.

Newhouse, J. P., Schwartz, W., Williams, A., & Witsberger, C. "Are Fee-For-Service Costs Increasing Faster than HMO Costs?" *Medical Care, 23*(8), 960, 1985.

Office of Technology Assessment. *Medicare's Prospective Payment System: Strategies for Evaluating Costs, Quality and Medical Technology* (OTA-H-262CDC). Washington, D.C.: U.S. Government Printing Office.

Pauly, M. "Taxation, Health Insurance and Market Failure in the Medical Economy" *Journal of Economic Literature,* 629, 1986.

Pauly, M., & Satterthwaite, M. "The Pricing of Primary Care Physicians' Services: A Test of the Role of Consumer Information" *Bell Journal of Economics,* 488, 1981.

Physician Payment Review Commission. *Annual Report to Congress, 1988.* Washington, D.C.: U.S. Government Printing Office, 1988.

Robinson, J., & Luft, H. "The Impact of Hospital Market Structure on Patient Volume, Average Length of Stay, and the Cost of Care." *Journal of Health Economics,* 4(4), 333, 1985.

Robinson, J., & Luft, H. "Competition, Regulation and Hospital Costs, 1982–1986." *Journal of the American Medical Association,* 2676, 1988.

Romeo, A., Wagner, J., & Lee, R. "Prospective Reimbursement and the Diffusion of New Technologies in Hospitals." *Journal of Health Economics,* 3(1), 1, 1984.

Salkever, D., & Bice, T. "The Impact of CON Controls on Hospital Investment." *Milbank Memorial Fund Quarterly, 54,* 185, 1976.

Schramm, C., Renn, S., & Biles, B. "New Perspectives on State Rate-Setting." *Health Affairs,* 5(3), 22, 1986.

Sloan, F. "Rate Regulation as a Strategy for Hospital Cost Control: Evidence from the Last Decade." *Milbank Memorial Fund Quarterly, 61* (Spring), 195, 1983.

Sloan, F., & Becker, E. "Cross-Subsidies and Payment for Hospital Care." *Journal of Health Politics, Policy and Law,* Winter, 670, 1984.

Sloan, F., Valvona, J., & Perrin, J. "Diffusion of Surgical Technology: An Exploratory Study." *Journal of Health Economics,* 5(1), 31, 1986.

Thorpe, K. E. "Does All-Payer Rate Setting Work? The Case of the New York Prospective Hospital Reimbursement Methodology." *Journal of Health Politics, Policy and Law, 12*(3), 391, 1987.

Thorpe, K. E., & Phelps, C. E. *Regulatory Intensity and Cost Growth. Journal of Health Economics,* forthcoming 1990. Boston: Harvard School of Public Health, 1989.

Wennberg, J. E. "Dealing with Medical Practice Variations: A Proposal for Action." *Health Affairs,* Summer, pp. 6–32, 1984.

12

The Government's Role in Health Care

Charles Brecher

The government is a "major player" in the health care industry. It spends over $207 billion, or more than $4 of every $10 spent on care; it employs over 1.6 million people to deliver health care directly; and it regulates private providers by determining who shall be entitled to practice medicine and what the standards for that care shall be. Without an understanding of what government does, and why, students would be ignorant of an important part of what happens in health care.

This chapter provides an introductory perspective on the nature of the government's role. The first section identifies the key questions to be addressed and presents some concepts essential for answering them. The second section describes the functions governments perform, and the third analyzes why government health care policies change. The final section considers alternative ways of specifying what the government's role ought to be in the future.

Key Questions and Concepts

In light of the vast and diverse nature of government activities, some particular perspective should be chosen for considering the role of the public sector. Three distinct, but not mutually exclusive, approaches to the subject can be taken.

The first is descriptive. It asks simply, what is the government's role? Much of this chapter will be devoted to answering this question.

A second approach seeks to go beyond knowing what government currently does to understanding what causes government to act in certain ways. It asks, why does government do certain things? It is based on a recognition that government activities vary among units of government (the United States's public sector role differs markedly from that of Great Britain) and over time (the public sector role in the United States today is markedly different from what it was 25 years ago).

A third approach considers not what is but what might be. It asks whether the government's role conforms to some normative standard of what is a desirable set of public activities. Because reasonable individuals differ over the best role for government, the answers to this question vary widely. Yet it is possible to reach some judgments after making explicit the value assumptions that underlie them.

The next three sections of this chapter examine these three types of questions in successive order. But to answer them in a sophisticated fashion it is necessary to use a few key concepts. One set relates to the fragmented nature of American government; a second set relates to the multiple possible roles government can play.

Multiple Governments

In the United States there is no single government; rather there are multiple governments with distinct roles in a federal system. The nation has one national government entity, but 50 states and 82,290 units of local government within the states (see Table 12.1). Not all of these units are involved in health care, but many are. The federal government and virtually all of the states play some role in health care financing and delivery. Of the local governments, many of the 3,041 counties and some of the larger cities are involved in health care activity, and most of the 14,851 school districts also have some health education and health delivery functions.

The federal nature of American government has important implications for how the key questions identified above can be answered. Descriptive questions need to be answered separately for each level of government; the answers to causal questions may vary among units of government; and normative arguments

Table 12.1 Governmental Units in the United States, 1982

Type of government	No. of units
U.S. government	1
State governments	50
Local governments	82,290
County	3,041
Municipal	19,076
Township	16,734
School district	14,851
Special district	28,588

Source: U.S. Department of Commerce, Bureau of the Census, *1982 Census of Governments,* Vol. 1, Washington, D.C.: U.S. Government Printing Office, 1983, Table A, p. 61.

about the proper role for government need to specify not just what *government* should do but which *level of government* should do it.

Potential Roles

In any industry, including health care, government activity can be considered along three dimensions: financing, delivery, and regulation. The extent of government activity can vary along each dimension, and units of government most active on one dimension need not be active on another. Moreover, the same roles are played in varying degrees by the private sector.

Government financing of an activity typically takes the form of levying a tax to raise funds and then appropriating the funds to purchase or provide the service. However, financing may be separated from delivery. Tax funds can be used to purchase care from the private sector or to pay the salaries of civil servants employed to provide care. As will be seen, American governments follow both courses. It is also worth noting that governments could provide care without financing it. Governmental units established to provide care can and do operate without appropriations of tax dollars; they can "earn" revenues from private purchases or from insurance programs sponsored by other organizations. Examples of such arrangements in health care include some local public hospitals that operate without direct governmental subsidies.

Regulation is the setting of standards for those engaged in the delivery of care. Regulations include licensing of occupations as well as facilities, setting standards for the process of care, and imposing restrictions on capital investments. The extent to which governmental entities engage in each form of regulation, and the particular standards they set, may vary.

It is worth noting that these roles are not unique to the public sector. Obviously, private individuals and firms engage in the financing and delivery of care; they also engage in regulation. Private insurers set standards for receipt of payment and engage in utilization review; private health maintenance organizations (HMOs) set standards for practice by their physicians and monitor utilization. Thus, there is tremendous potential variation in the way in which roles are divided, both between the public and private sectors and among units of government within the public sector.

What Are the Governments' Roles?

The key concepts of federalism and multiple potential roles can be combined to create a framework for describing governments' roles. As summarized in Table 12.2, the federal government plays a major role in financing health services, serves as a direct deliverer only for selected specialized populations, and engages in relatively little regulation. The states show tremendous variation in their roles,

Table 12.2 Summary of Governments' Major Health Care Roles

Financing	Delivery	Regulation
Federal		
Large role through Medicare and Medicaid; other categorical programs	Operates facilities for veterans and indians	Sets standards for Medicare providers; determining what drugs and devices may be sold; prohibits discrimination by providers
State		
Funds Medicaid, mental health, medical education and public health programs	Operates mental hospitals, health deparments, and medical schools	Regulates insurance industry; Licenses facilities and personnel; establishes health codes
Local		
Subsidizes public hospitals; funds local health departments	Operates count and municipal hospitals; operates local health departments	Establishes local health codes

but an aggregate summary is that they play a substantial role in financing; they are important direct providers of mental health and professional education services; they vary widely in regulatory activity but typically license providers, set standards for insurers, and are otherwise the dominant source of restrictions on the private sector. Similarly, local governments vary in their health activities, but they typically provide relatively little funding, especially for general medical care, and establish few local regulations. However, many cities and counties operate hospitals and clinics to ensure access to care for poor residents. This summary description provides an introduction to a more detailed analysis of the ways in which government units perform each role.

Governments as Financers

More complete information about the public sector's financial role is presented in Table 12.3. In 1987 (the latest year for which data are available), government was the source of 41% of all expenditures for health care. Within the public sector the federal government played the largest role, accounting for 70% of government spending.

The trend in governments' financing role is a sharp increase from the early 1960s to the mid-1970s and relative stability since. In 1965 government accounted for just 26% of health care spending, but by 1975 the figure was 42%. It remained at that level through the early 1980s and has been about 41% since 1983. Of course, the recent stability in *share* of funding has occurred in the context of rapid increases in total spending, causing the absolute amount of

Table 12.3 National Health Expenditures, Selected Years, 1965–1987

Sources	1987	1986	1985	1984	1983	1980	1975	1970	1965
					Amount (in billions)				
Total	$500.3	$455.7	$419.0	$388.5	$357.2	$248.1	$132.7	$75.0	$41.9
Private	293.0	266.8	244.0	228.8	209.7	142.9	76.4	47.2	30.9
Public	207.3	188.9	175.0	159.6	147.5	105.2	56.3	27.8	11.0
Federal	144.7	132.8	123.1	112.0	102.7	71.0	37.0	17.7	5.5
State & local	62.7	56.1	52.0	47.7	44.8	34.2	19.3	10.1	5.5
					Percent distribution				
Total	100.0	100.0	100.0	100.0	100.0	100.0	100.0	100.0	100.0
Private	58.6	58.5	58.2	58.9	58.7	57.6	57.5	63.0	73.8
Public	41.4	41.5	41.8	41.1	41.2	42.4	42.5	37.0	26.2
Federal	28.9	29.1	29.4	28.8	28.8	28.6	27.9	23.6	13.2
State & local	12.5	12.3	12.4	12.3	12.5	13.8	14.5	13.5	13.0

Source: Health Care Financing Administration, U.S. Department of Health and Human Services, press release, November 18, 1988.

public spending to rise dramatically. Between 1975 and 1987, public spending jumped from $56.3 billion to $207.3 billion, or 268%.

Much of the public spending is accounted for by two programs—Medicare and Medicaid. The passage of these two programs in 1965 and their subsequent implementation explains much of the trend in government spending. Nonexistent in the early 1960s, these two programs accounted for $130.6 billion in spending in 1987, or 63% of the government total.

Medicare is a two-part program designed to help pay the medical care costs of the elderly. (Certain disabled individuals also have been made eligible.) Part A covers most hospital and some nursing home care; part B covers physician services. Legislation passed in 1988 extended Part A benefits by eliminating most caps on hospital coverage and limiting co-payments for hospital care, and it extended Part B coverage to prescription drugs on a phased-in basis over the period 1990–1993. Part A benefits are financed primarily through a payroll tax, although elderly persons not qualifying for federal retirement benefits are obliged to pay a premium, and the extended benefits established in the 1988 legislation are paid for through a surcharge on the income tax liability of the elderly. Part B is financed through a combination of federal general fund appropriations and premiums paid by elderly enrollees. Both parts are administered by the federal Health Care Financing Administration (HCFA), a division of the Department of Health and Human Services.

Medicaid is a joint federal–state program to pay for medical care of the indigent. The federal legislation authorized the federal government to reimburse states for the cost of providing such care. In the years following enactment in 1965 most states established such a program, with Arizona being the last to do so in 1982. The states must cover persons receiving public assistance and may cover other persons with low income. States must provide certain basic services, including hospital care, family planning, skilled nursing care, and physician services; they have the option of receiving federal reimbursement for additional services. Benefit structures vary widely because of the extent to which states include the optional benefits and because states' provision of the mandatory services vary in the number of days of hospital or nursing home care covered and the rate at which the benefits are paid for. Thus, in effect, Medicaid is 50 different programs having different eligibility criteria and different benefit structures. The share of the poor covered by the program varied from 104% in Hawaii to just 17% in South Dakota, and the average cost per beneficiary varied from $2,897 in New York to $793 in West Virginia (Ruther et al., p. 97).

Both Medicare and Medicaid are modeled on private insurance programs. Few of the benefits are provided directly by government agencies; most are purchased from private vendors. Medicare Part A pays hospitals directly at rates established by the federal government (the basis for setting the rate was shifted from per diem to per admission in 1983). Part B pays physicians directly if they agree to accept government-established fees, or it reimburses patients for the established amounts if they choose to pay the provider directly. Medicaid only pays providers directly, but the basis for setting rates varies widely among the states. Some states have adapted the Medicare payment standards; others have established less generous rates; still others have been imaginative in designing innovative payment schemes to encourage more efficient delivery. Arizona, for example, relies almost exclusively on capitation to apply for acute care and is extending the concept to long-term-care benefits. New York has designed a Resource Utilization group (RUG) patient classification system to pay for nursing home care that builds on the experience of the diagnosis related group (DRG) classification system for acute care.

Because the states have so much discretion in designing their Medicaid programs, it is important to note that the aggregate spending figures cited earlier understate the role of state governments. Although they raise only 46% of the $49.4 billion of Medicaid expenditures, state governments substantially control the entire sum, including the federal portion. In this sense the states control expenditures amounting to fully 28% of all public expenditure for health care.

The benefit structures of the Medicare and Medicaid programs strongly influence the distribution of government spending among different types of health care services. Although it is 41% of the total, government spending is just 31% of spending for physician services and fully 53% of hospital expenditures. The full payment of hospital cost by Medicare and the heavy use of hospitals by the elderly make government the predominant source of hospital revenues. In contrast, the more uniform use of physician services among age groups and the less generous role of Medicare in paying for the elderly's doctor bills leaves the bulk of physician services to be paid for from private sources. Nursing home care is almost evenly divided between the public and private sectors, but within the government's share Medicaid dominates. It accounts for 45% of nursing home expenditures, compared to Medicare's 1%. The restrictions on eligible nursing home care under Medicare have kept its share of nursing home payments strongly in check. However, amendments passed in 1988 may expand Medicare's role in financing nursing home care because some restrictions were removed.

Governments as Deliverers

In assuming a strong role in financing health care, governments have typically followed an insurance model and avoided operating medical care facilities and employing physicians and other providers. However, there are important exceptions to this pattern. Each level of government has assumed responsibility for delivering either certain types of care or more comprehensive care to a specific subset of the population.

The federal government selected three population groups for which it funds and delivers services: veterans, Indians, and merchant seamen. The medical care program operated by the federal Veterans Administration (VA) is one of the largest health delivery systems in the world. Its 1989 budget for health care programs, including the operation of 172 medical centers, was over $11 billion (Kosterlitz, 1988).

The VA program has evolved through a special Congressional concern for veterans. In addition to providing pension and cash disability benefits, Congress sought to provide veterans' health care. Like hospitals generally, the VA's hospital system initially grew as an extension of homes for the aged and disabled. Homes were authorized for indigent and disabled Civil War veterans, and after World War I this system was expanded to include a separate hospital system. After World War II the system was dramatically expanded and integrated with more advanced medical technology through a program of affiliations with medical schools. About 40% of the current stock of VA hospitals was built between 1946 and 1966, many near medical schools. In 1965 nursing home benefits were broadened, and the system was expanded accordingly, although much VA nursing home care is purchased from private homes rather than provided in VA-operated facilities (Congressional Budget Office, 1984.)

Initially, VA medical care benefits were limited to those who developed conditions during their wartime service. A 1924 law broadened eligibility to include those who suffer from a condition likely to have been linked to military service even if it did not require treatment or become evident until later. Subsequently, any veteran who testified he or she was unable to pay for care became eligible, and in 1970 benefits were extended to any veteran past age 65 regardless of income or nature of condition. It is estimated that in 1990 the number of veterans over age 65 will total about 7.2 million, more than twice the number in 1980. The aging of World War II and Korean war veterans and the extension of benefits to all veterans over age 65 has and will continue to markedly increase the number of people eligible for VA care.

However, the VA system is not based on an insurance model with benefits funded as an "entitlement." Instead, each year Congress appropriates a fixed sum to the VA for provision of care at its facilities. The VA does establish priorities among veterans in deciding whom to serve. First priority is given to individuals with a service-related condition and to treatment for that condition. Second priority is for individuals with a service-related condition requiring care for an illness or injury that is not service-related. Lowest priority is for veterans without a service-related condition who require some medical care. Currently, about 70% of VA hospital patients have no service-related conditions, and the agency reports it is able to care for all those requesting services. However, the rapid growth of the eligible population has required large budget increases for the VA, and the continuation of its programs is considered to be jeopardized by insufficient funds.

The wisdom of continuing to operate a separate public health care system for veterans has been questioned. A prestigious 1977 report from the National Academy of Sciences recommended the gradual integration of VA facilities with the nation's general medical care system. However, this policy is opposed by VA employees, veterans relying on the system, and medical schools benefiting from their affiliations with the VA hospitals. Together these constituencies have been politically strong enough to thwart any efforts to dismantle the system despite recommendations from outside bodies.

A second group to whom the federal government provides care directly are Indians living on reservations. Federal appropriations to the Indian Health Service (IHS), a division of the Department of Health and Human Services (DHHS), totaled over $41.0 billion in 1988. The agency operated 50 hospitals and 340 clinics to serve nearly 1.1 million Indians. (Wagner).

Federal responsibility for health care to Indians was first established in 1911, when the Bureau of Indian Affairs in the Department of the Interior was given an appropriation for this purpose. The Bureau gradually expanded its commitment, and in 1955 a separate unit to provide care to Indians was established within the Public Health Services (PHS). On January 1, 1988, this unit, the IHS, was elevated from its status as a subunit of the PHS to that of an independent unit within the DHHS.

Since there is no "mainstream" system serving Indians, the need for a separate federal system seems self-evident. However, there are efforts to integrate the IHS facilities into the larger medical system through referrals. Since many of the IHS facilities are necessarily in rural areas and have low volume, they often refer cases to other providers for specialized care. Almost one-fifth the IHS budget is spent for care at private facilities that is not available at the IHS facilities. In addition, legislation passed in 1976 gave tribal governments the right to assume responsibility for operating IHS facilities. Tribes wanting to do so can contract with the IHS for operation of hospitals and clinics. Currently, 6 of the 50 hospitals and 294 of the 340 clinics are managed by tribes under these contracts, and the contracts represent over $200 million, or about 20% of the IHS budget. The IHS seems committed to promoting tribal self-determination, and the policy of tribal management of health facilities is likely to be expanded.

A third federal delivery system, that for merchant seamen, has been largely dismantled. The federal responsibility in this area dates from the 1798 act creating the Marine Hospital Service. Subsequently, the responsibility for care of foreigners in quarantine was added, and in 1889 a separate quasi-military personnel system, known as the commissioned corps, was established within the federal PHS. To provide this care separate PHS hospitals were constructed. However, the PHS expanded its responsibilities in other areas after World War II, including research and control of communicable diseases. The PHS hospitals became vestigial organs as the need for care of seaman and foreigners declined. Eventually, budgetary pressures led to the PHS hospitals being either closed or transferred to private control. The commissioned corps of the PHS remain a group of federal employees who engage in health care activities, but few provide direct personal care; they primarily work in communicable disease control.

Despite its disengagement from delivery of personal health care, the PHS remains an important federal agency within the DHHS. It operates the National Institutes of Health, a major source of funding for research and of intramural research. Its Centers for Disease Control are the nation's major source of intervention in control of communicable diseases; its Food and Drug Administration (FDA) regulates these substances; its Health Resources and Services Administration and its Alcohol, Drug Abuse, and Mental Health Administration have as their major activities the distribution of federal grant funds to states and private organizations to expand the capacity of the health care system.

In general, the federal government has restricted its role as direct provider at the same time that it has expanded its commitments as a financer. The PHS hospitals have been eliminated; the IHS is relying more on private contracting and management by tribal organizations; the VA also is increasing its reliance on private purchase of care, although it remains strongly committed to maintaining a separate delivery system, including VA hospitals affiliated with medical schools.

State governments are involved in the direct provision of medical care in three important ways: the operation of state mental hospitals, the conduct of medical education, and the maintenance of state (or often combined state and local) health departments. States' roles in the provision of mental health services date from the late-19th-century movement to identify insanity as a medical or mental condition requiring treatment rather than confinement in either poorhouses or prisons. The reformers successfully encouraged state governments to create mental institutions, usually in remote areas, where the ill could be removed from sources of stress and receive available treatment. However, the facilities were underfunded and became notorious "snake pits," providing only minimal treatment and low-quality food and shelter. The poor conditions, together with the availability of drug treatment in the 1950s, led to a movement toward "deinstitutionalization." The population of state mental hospitals peaked in 1955 and has been declining since (Mechanic).

The initial impetus for deinstitutionalization was accelerated in the 1960s through expanded federal financial resources for alternative modes of care or, at least, residence. The federal Community Mental Health Centers Act in 1963 funded outpatient care in facilities located closer to patients' previous homes; the Medicaid and Medicare programs funded psychiatric care and nursing home care for many previously supported in state facilities by state appropriations; the federal Supplemental Security Income program passed in 1972 provides direct cash benefits for the aged and disabled that permitted many to reside in private homes rather than be placed by their relatives in state institutions (Clarke). As a result of these medical and policy changes, the population in state mental hospitals dropped from 558,000 in 1955 to under 110,000 in 1987 (AHA).

Despite the shrinkage, state mental hospitals remain major institutions in the American health care system. In 1987 these 224 hospitals accounted for 119,319 beds. Their budgets totaled more that $4.9 billion, and they employed approximately 184,000 workers (AHA). Such hospitals are often a major source of employment within state government, and their historic location in small communities often makes them a dominant source of employment for communities with little other major economic activity. As a result of these political pressures, as well as a serious need to upgrade the facilities, employment at state mental hospitals has not shrunk at a pace anywhere near that of their bed capacity.

A major problem associated with the deinstitutionalization of the mentally ill has been a lack of corresponding investment in outpatient care for those sent home or not admitted. States have tended to rely on local governments to provide the outpatient care and have not typically shifted resources to the localities to assist them in meeting the expanded need. There is poorly planned, coordinated, or supervised outpatient care for many of the mentally ill. As a consequence, they too often end up on the streets, homeless and unmedicated. States vary widely in the extent to which they have undertaken, by themselves or in cooperation with localities, a system of outpatient mental health serivces; and in some states the design and implementation of such a system remains a major policy failure (Blum & Blank).

States are also important supporters of medical education, and because medical education has a significant clinical component, this requires states to become involved in direct delivery of care. State appropriations comprise nearly 17% of total revenues for all medical schools; and state governments, through their public university systems, sponsor 73 of the nation's 127 medical schools (Jolly, Taksel, & Beran). Often the state medical schools have a general medical care hospital attached to them that also is operated by the state.

These state general-care hospitals typically combine two roles. They provide medical students access to patients, and they provide the medical school faculty a place to admit private patients. The two roles are sometimes quite divergent: The patients with whom medical students obtain clinical training are typically poor and dependent on the state subsidy to the hospital for their access to care; the faculty's private patients are often commercially insured, and their fees provide the faculty with a significant source of private income. In some instance the two roles are performed satisfactorily at the same facility, but often the state's general hospitals serve only one of these functions. Where it is primarily a source of clinical experience for students, the medical school typically lacks an affiliation with a large voluntary hospital; where it is primarily a source of income for faculty, the medical school typically has an affiliation with another hospital (often public) that has a large patient volume, but the faculty do not use that facility as the preferred site for their private patients.

State health departments are another area of direct government provision. In this area it is often difficult to distinguish state from local efforts. The relations between states and localities in structuring a public health department are often complex; some states establish subunits that are identified as local entities, whereas others primarily fund local governments to conduct activities. However, it is clear that the combined network of state and local health departments provides a significant volume of medical care along with engaging in regulatory and other public health activities (Miller & Moos). The personal care delivery is typically oriented to maternal and child health, vaccinations and other communicable disease control activity, and treatment for chronic conditions. Although sometimes available to all citizens, the state health department services are more typically targeted to low-income residents (Davis & Millman).

Health departments provide these services directly because they believe the services would not otherwise be available. Even when other agencies or programs fund services, there may not be delivery capacity available in a community in the private sector. Reluctance or an inability of private practitioners to treat indigent (even Medicaid-enrolled) patients with multiple disabilities or psychiatric or substance abuse problems, plus the need to have outreach services for many poorly educated potential patients, often justify continued health department provision of personal services.

The major remaining form of government involvement in direct delivery of care is local governments' operation of general care hospitals. The last comprehensive examination of these hospitals in the late 1970s found that they comprised more than one-third of all community hospitals, nearly one-quarter of all community hospital beds, and 28% of community hospital outpatient department visits. Moreover, they account for a major share of health professions education, including a disproportionate share of graduate medical education (Commission on Public General Hospitals).

The most troubled and widely publicized of these public institutions are those located in the nation's largest cities. A recent survey found that 48 of the 100 largest cities had a local public hospital, and another 23 had a state government hospital (Altman et al.). Such urban public hospitals are often characterized by political controversy because of their staffing and financing arrangements, but they play a major role in providing care to the urban indigent. Cities with public hospitals were found to provide more care to the uninsured poor than was available in cities without such hospitals, although private hospitals did somewhat increase their uncompensated care in areas that lacked public hospitals (Thorpe & Brecher).

Governments as Regulators

The ability to regulate private behavior is inherent in government authority and is not derived from the public sector's role as financer. Government legally can call the tune, even when it does not pay the piper. In its role as regulator of otherwise private behavior, the government is generally seeking to protect the consumer.

Because private individuals have little basis on which to determine if a seller of medical goods or services is competent and honest, the government sets standards for such providers. Many government regulatory activities derive from this distinct legal authority (Levin).

Government's major role as financer is a second source of regulatory activity. As a purchaser of care, the government has set standards that providers must meet before public funds will be paid to them. The setting of such conditions for participation in public programs is another type of regulatory activity. Because Medicare and Medicaid are the leading sources of public financing, they have also been the major source of this type of regulation.

The leading example of federal regulation intended to protect consumers in otherwise private transactions is the role of the FDA. This agency's authority dates from the 1906 Pure Food Act, which responded to scandals arising from the unsanitary methods used to produce some food products (Grabowski & Vernon). Regulatory authority was extended to drugs and cosmetics by 1938 legislation, this time in response to the death of more than 100 children due to a drug company's use of a toxic chemical in creating a liquid form of sulfanilamide. The FDA was given authority to set standards that pharmaceuticals must meet before being marketed.

Important amendments to the law were passed in 1962, again following large-scale tragedy. Limited testing of thalidomide in the United States and its more widespread use in Europe revealed that its use among pregnant women led to the birth of deformed babies. The well-publicized tragedy led Congress to establish extensive requirements for premarket testing of drugs.

The standards for drug testing that the FDA now administers are a source of controversy. It is believed that they provide little or no additional protection over the prior 1962 standards, but they add substantially to the cost of developing new drugs and the time required before they can be widely used (Statman). As a result, the United States often lags behind other countries in the use of new drugs, and American pharmaceutical firms are at a disadvantage in developing new products. The spread of AIDS and a consequent sense of urgency in developing treatments for AIDS have produced additional pressures to alter the extensive premarket requirements (Panem).

Another form of consumer protection regulation is the licensing of health care practitioners and facilities. This licensure activity is conducted by state governments. The scope of state licensure authority varies, but virtually all states require that physicians, nurses, optometrists, chiropractors, and podiatrists meet state standards to obtain a license before practicing in that state. Some states recognize the licenses granted by other states in order to facilitate mobility among professionals, but this is not always the case.

Although the principle of licensure as a form of consumer protection is well established, its practice by state governments has been criticized on two grounds (Begun). First, the standards are not well enforced. The record of state agencies in locating and disciplining practitioners who violate professional standards is poor. Relatively few licenses are revoked each year despite evidence of more widespread professional misconduct. Second, licensing sometimes seems to protect the "turf" of selected professionals and thereby thwarts more effective delivery of care. Physicians have been accused of using state laws to prevent nurses, physician assistants, and optometrists from assuming broader responsibilities in delivery of care. Reforms designed to make state licensing efforts more effective include the appointment of more consumers and nonphysicians to the state boards setting and enforcing licensing standards.

State government regulation of the insurance industry is another example of consumer protection efforts. Initial public regulation of the insurance industry was intended to protect consumers from firms, particularly life insurance firms, that might sell policies and then disappear with the premium income before paying benefits. To protect consumers, firms were required to establish reserves for future benefit payments and meet other standards.

These regulatory requirements have been applied to private sales of health insurance as well. In addition, some states have extended their scope of regulation to include minimum benefit standards. These requirements were initially designed to protect consumers from believing they were well protected when benefits were actually very poor. Thus, minimum numbers of days of hospital inpatient coverage and other standards were set for health insurance products. This concept has been extended by some states to require certain types of benefits or prohibit certain types of exclusions, such as maternity benefits or alcoholism treatment.

Federal government regulations established for participation in the Medicare and Medicaid programs in some ways complement state regulations and in other ways expand the scope of government regulations. The complementary nature of the two types of activity is evident in the standards set by the federal government for providers; they generally defer to state licensing requirements and recognize physicians, hospitals, and other providers licensed by a state as eligible.

The federal government also has relied on state governments to implement its regulatory program for hospital capital investments. Between 1974 and 1986 the federal government required that a hospital or nursing home receive approval from a state planning agency before making a major hospital investment in order for that capital expense to be reimbursed by Medicare and Medicaid. The federal government abandoned this form of regulation in 1986, but some states continue to regulate the capital investments of providers within their borders despite the absence of federal requirements to do so and of federal funds to underwrite the effort. Both the aborted federal programs and the continuing state programs are justified, not on grounds of consumer protection but on grounds that excessive capital investment, especially in hospital bed capacity, leads to unnecessary costs that will be financed by government funds and by private consumers through higher insurance premiums.

Federal Medicare and Medicaid regulations also work independently of state governments. A particularly dramatic example was the requirement that hospitals and nursing homes desegregate in order to be eligible for funds under the programs. When the legislation was passed in 1965, many facilities in the south remained racially segregated, and there were no state laws prohibiting this. The federal requirements for racial integration of hospitals (for patients and medical staff) were widely perceived as helping to speed integration in the south.

A final form of Medicare and Medicaid regulation worth noting is the programs' utilization review requirements. Beginning in 1972 the federal government authorized and financed independent organizations to review hospital services for which federal funds were sought to determine if they were medically necessary. The organizations, originally called professional standards review organizations (PSROs), regulated the quality of care by reviewing hospital records to see if more care than necessary (i.e., a longer stay) was provided or if the entire admission itself was unnecessary. At the peak of the program there were 182 regional PSROs operating, and the program received $150 million in federal appropriations (Lohr & Brook).

The program was substantially revised in conjunction with changes in the Medicare program that shifted hospital payments from a per diem to a per admission basis. The new payment approach was expected to provide hospitals with economic incentives to decrease lengths of stay, so regulation of this aspect of hospital utilization was deemphasized. Instead, greater attention was given to assuring the accuracy of diagnostic information (because the payment per admission varied with the type of condition treated) and verifying the medical necessity of the entire admission. Accordingly, PSROs were reorganized into a smaller number of professional review organizations (PROs), and these entities were expected to review hospital services, with emphasis on minimizing inaccurate diagnostic data and unnecessary admissions.

The requirements for review of hospital stays by PSROs and PROs have subjected physicians to far more scrutiny of their practice than was previously the case. These requirements, together with trends in malpractice litigation, have obliged physicians and hospital personnel to be more diligent and detailed in making entries in medical records and to document the reasons for medical decisions more extensively than before. These requirements are associated, often unfavorably, with government regulations.

Causes of Change and Variation

The previous section illustrates that governments' roles change over time and vary among places. In the past quarter-century major new federal programs have been enacted and significantly modified several times; the practices of states and localities in financing and delivering services and in regulating providers vary widely. For example, as noted, Medicaid is in many ways 50 different state programs rather than a single, uniform national program.

Explaining change and variation in government activity is a major focus of political science, and political scientists have applied their conceptual tools to the analysis of health policy. Two broad (and hence not entirely accurate) types of theoretical explanations are the Marxist approach and the interest group (or pluralist) approach (Marmor, 1983). Both theories see change arising from conflict within society, but they differ over the sources of those conflicts. Marxists see the conflicts as essentially economic and as between two inherently hostile economic groups (or classes): those who own the means of production (capitalists) and those who work for them (labor). The public sector is seen as serving the interests of capitalists in the United States and other non-Communist nations. Fundamental change can occur only after violent revolution places control of the government in the hands of the labor class. Pending such revolutionary change, reforms are made by the ruling capitalist class only as necessary to appease workers and to ensure peaceful compliance with government rules that serve capitalist interest.

Interest group theory sees conflict arising from a more diverse set of interests than only economic positions. Individuals perform multiple social roles and may belong to numerous social groups. Those groups have diverse interests, and their efforts to promote their particular goals through government action draws opposition from other groups. The groups and their competing interests have many different sources besides economic class, including place of residence, ethnic identity, religious beliefs, and occupational roles. Decisions of government are seen as shaped by the relative influence different groups bring to bear on elected officials (Truman).

In American society variations of interest group theory have proved more useful than Marxist theory for explaining change and variation. The emergence of a large middle class with substantial influence and income derived from service as opposed to capital-intensive manufacturing industries, the effectiveness of elections in promoting the interests and legislative agenda of labor organizations as well as middle-class citizens, and the concentration of social and economic problems among an "underclass" that is largely outside the world of regularized work have reduced the relevance of classic Marxist theory and led its revisionists to adopt modifications that closely approximate variations of interest group theory. Thus, the concept of changing or different balances of influence among competing groups is a more useful conceptual framework for analyzing American health care policy.

Changes in Federal Policy

From a broad perspective, federal health care policy can be seen as divided into three periods. Prior to 1960 the federal government avoided large-scale participation in the financing of personal health care services; from 1960 to the mid-1970s the federal role expanded rapidly; since approximately 1975 the federal role has been relatively stable, with some efforts at contraction. It is possible that the federal role will again expand in the future.

These shifts in policy can be related to broad shifts in patterns of interest groups' influence. In the first two periods the same types of groups were active, but their relative influence shifted; the third period is associated with the partial withdrawal of one type of interest and the emergence of a new, influential group. The prediction of a possible new phase is related to the emergence of additional new influential groups as well as greater strength of others.

For much of this century national health care politics was a battle between proponents of national health insurance and its opponents (Marmor, 1973). Proponents included most working Americans, who promoted their cause through union political activity. Their cause was championed by the Democratic party. Opponents were many physicians and other providers, including hospitals, who feared the consequences of government involvement in their income flow; private insurance companies that feared a loss in their market for health insurance; and business organizations that feared the tax burden associated with a government funding program.

Until 1960 the opponents were highly successful. Efforts to include a health insurance program in the original 1935 Social Security Act were dropped by President Roosevelt because he feared strong physician opposition would jeopardize the entire program. Post–World War II efforts by President Truman to add national health insurance to the nation's social security system led to a large-scale, well-funded campaign against it by the American Medical Association and organizations representing business. The victory of a Republican in the 1952 presidential election led to an 8-year period of little action or prospect for change in federal health care policy.

The presidential election of 1960 saw a revival of interest in federal efforts. This time the Democrats, supported by labor organizations, advocated hospital insurance for the elderly only, rather than immediate enactment of a universal system. The Democratic presidential candidate won, but the legislation that emerged from Congress reflected major compromises with more conservative legislative leaders. The Kerr-Mills Act of 1961 established a program to pay for the medical expenses of the poor elderly that was closely linked to joint state–federal welfare programs, rather than a broader program linked to federal Social Security.

The landslide victory of the Democrats in the 1964 national elections made possible the passage of broader legislation. The 1965 amendments to the Social Security Act added Titles XVIII and XIX, Medicare and Medicaid. As described earlier, these programs provide relatively comprehensive health insurance for the elderly and opportunities for states to create relatively extensive programs for the indigent.

In response to the initial success of Medicare, the opponents—including physicians and many business leaders—changed their position on national health insurance. By 1974 Democrats and Republicans in Congress appeared to have reached agreement on programs that would cover all Americans through a combination of Medicare for the elderly, a more uniform national version of Medicaid for the poor, and mandatory employment-based insurance for others (Rivlin). However, the impending impeachment of President Nixon diverted Congressional attention, and improved prospects for the Democratic party in the 1976 elections undermined the compromise and ended prospects for national health insurance.

Since the mid-1970s federal efforts have focused on controlling the rising cost of Medicare and Medicaid rather than on expanding their scope. As noted earlier, this shift was first evident in 1972 with the creation of utilization review organizations for the programs. The health planning legislation of 1974 established a system of regulation for capital investments also intended to promote efficiency. The federal Health Maintenance Organization Act of 1973 also sought to promote these organizations because they were viewed as cost-saving delivery mechanisms.

The election of a Democrat to the White House in the 1976 elections did not lead to renewed pressure for national health insurance. Instead, President Jimmy Carter sought to create an effective mechanism for controlling hospital costs before expanding government financing of the industry. His 1977 proposal for a national system of price controls for hospitals was defeated in Congress as a result of strong lobbying efforts by the hospital industry (Hughes et al.). Initiatives to redefine the administration's position after this defeat never came to fruition but led to exploration of greater emphasis on competition among providers as a means for cost control.

The triumph of conservative Republicans in the 1980 national elections and the reelection of President Ronald Reagan in 1984 gave greater energy to efforts to curb spending under Medicare and Medicaid as well as virtually all other forms of domestic federal policy. Health policy, like most domestic policy, became a subtheme of budget policy. Expenditure reductions for Medicaid were sought by measures that limited growth in federal reimbursement to states and that gave states greater freedom in structuring their programs. States have pursued some of these options and innovated in designing new ways to pay providers to encourage efficiency, but the states have relied on other policies as well. Specifically, states have reduced enrollment in the program by failing to adjust Medicaid income eligibility limits for inflation. As a result, the share of the poor covered by Medicaid nationwide fell from 74% in 1979 to just 59% in 1984 (Holahan & Cohen, p. 45).

Reagan administration efforts to curb Medicare spending led to the new prospective payment system in 1983. This changed the basis on which Medicare pays hospitals: from cost reimbursement based on average per diem costs to a national price system that establishes standardized rates for different categories of hospital admissions. Under the new system the federal government has been able to curb Medicare benefit payment growth and better control expenditures under Part A.

The apparent success of the prospective payment system for hospitals has led to new efforts to revise the payment system for physicians (Holahan & Etheredge). Rapid increases in Medicare Part B expenditures led to a freeze on physician fees in 1984 and 1985. With the recognition that a freeze was not a viable long-term policy, Congress created a Physician Payment Review Commission in 1985. The commission made recommendations for a new system for paying physicians in 1989.

The shift in emphasis of federal policy from a period of expansion in federal financing to one of cost control has been linked to changes in patterns of interest group influence. In the initial two periods, the battles were largely between groups seeking expansion of federal policy and those opposed; the dormant period of 1935–1960 resulted from stronger influence by the opponents, and the expansion from 1960 to 1974 represented greater influence by the proponents. However, the post-1974 shift to cost control has seen a new actor become prominent and develop new relations with the old opponents.

The new actors in federal health politics are bureaucrats administering the federal programs. Lodged in the HCFA and the Office of Management and Budget, these professionals administer programs on behalf of taxpayers. They bargain with providers in a pattern political scientist Lawrence Brown (1985) calls "technocratic corporatism." Professionals hired by the government interact with representatives of provider organizations to shape health policy. This pattern was evident in the creation of the prospective payment system in 1982 and is emerging as the pattern for shaping revisions of physician payments under Medicare. Health care politics in the period of cost containment have been battles between professionals representing taxpayers and the providers of services.

The prospects for a new period of expansion in health care politics is linked to the emergence of another type of interest group (Tierney). Consumer groups (other than labor unions) have been organized and have gained in strength. These groups include organizations such as Ralph Nader's Health Research Group. But by far the most influential new consumer group is the elderly—Medicare beneficiaries—represented by the powerful American Association of Retired People (AARP). Although founded in the 1950s, AARP recently has grown to have a membership of over 27 million and an annual budget of $185 million (Kosterlitz, 1987). Because many of its members have direct economic dependence on the federal government through cash Social Security benefits as well as Medicare, they vote in national elections at high rates and give great attention to domestic policy positions, including health care issues.

The influence of the AARP is linked to the most recent significant expansion of Medicare, the Medicare Catastrophic Coverage Act of 1988. At a time when budget deficits were leading to expenditure reductions for most federal programs and when tax increases were politically unacceptable, Congress nonetheless passed a program with added annual costs projected at $10.6 billion to be funded with higher premiums and a new surcharge on personal income tax liabilities for the elderly. The new benefits can be attributed largely to the effective efforts of the AARP.

The political pressures to expand benefits to the elderly may lead to further expension of federal financing of health care. The major benefit now excluded under Medicare is long-term care of chronic conditions. States provide some of these benefits under Medicaid, but the means testing required under Medicaid is resented by many needy elderly and their working-age children. Consequently, pressure is rising for a national long-term-care program. Expansion of such services would be very expensive, but the growing political clout of the elderly could lead to such a program. At the same time that basic hospital benefits are unavailable to many poor children and unemployed workers, the elderly seem capable of achieving greater federal commitments for their care.

Variations in State Policy

The substantial variation in health care activity among the states is related to three sets of factors: levels of economic development, general political culture, and patterns of interest group activity. The first two are general state characteristics; the third is distinct for the health care arena.

Studies of a wide range of state policies have demonstrated that states with higher levels of income and urbanization tend to be more active (Gray et al.). In general, per capita spending by states for most functions rises with average per capita income. Wealthier states provide their citizens with relatively more public services than do poorer states. This generalization applies to health care.

However, the relationship between economics and state government activity is influenced by political forces. The degree of party competition in states, the division of responsibility between states and their localities, and the balance of political values among citizens between moralistic and traditionalistic values have been found to be important influences on state expenditure levels for a variety of services, including health.

Finally, the nature of interest group activity also shapes state health policy. The principal competing interests within state capitols typically are provider groups, business groups concerned with tax levels, local government officials involved in financing or delivering care, and, more recently, state employees analogous to the federal "technocrats." However, the relative influence of these groups and the resulting policies vary widely among states.

The different patterns of state health politics can be illustrated by analyzing important decisions for state Medicaid programs recently enacted in Arizona, California, and New York. Arizona was the last state to establish a Medicaid program, a decision not reached until 1982 (Brecher, 1984). The absence of a program was largely the result of sentiment among conservative business interests. They felt that state taxes should not be increased to finance health care for the poor; rather, this should be either a private concern or one of local governments. The pressure to change this policy came from local government officials who faced great difficulty in financing local programs when statutory limits were placed on revenues from the property tax. To obtain federal aid for care for the indigent, the local officials successfully pressured the state legislature for a Medicaid program. Health care provider groups played little role in shaping the program, which mandated enrollment in capitation programs.

In California the same interests interacted differently. California established a relatively generous Medicaid program early, and its expenditures increased rapidly. The program was supported by local officials and health care providers with little opposition. However, a state budget crisis in the early 1980s led to major reforms in which the business community played a strong role. The reforms changed the way the state pays hospitals for its Medicaid enrollees, with the intention of lowering payments to hospitals, and they altered the distribution of financial responsibility between the state and localities for care to the indigent in a way that obliged localities to do more. These changes resulted from business interest intervention in a policy area previously let largely to the localities and the providers. As one observer put it:

> With the passage of this remarkable legislation, the relationship among interest groups, units of state and local government, and private medical care systems were changed, perhaps permanently. The California Medical Association and the California Hospital Association, previously undisputed winners of the legislative game, had been crowded off the board by pressures from the budget, by the newly activated business coalitions, and by the insurance companies. [Bergthold, p. 213]

In contrast, Medicaid reforms in New York in the 1980s have been more responsive to providers', particularly hospitals', concerns (Brecher, 1986). In 1975, in response to state and local budgetary pressures, New York began to regulate tightly payments to hospitals on a prospective basis. The hospitals did not respond with necessary expenditure reductions and soon faced severe operating deficits. Ater several years of such deficits many hospitals were facing contraction or bankruptcy. In response, the state established a new payment system that included extra revenues for hospitals providing care to the uninsured poor. This substantially improved the financial position of the providers (although it did little to improve coverage for the uninsured poor). Providers obtained additional concessions after the federal government switched Medicare to a prospective payment basis. The state abandoned its waiver under Medicaid in order to permit hospitals in the state to participate in the new federal program because the state hospital association had calculated members' revenues would be greater under the new federal system than under a continued state-controlled system (Thorpe.)

As these examples suggest, a state's health policy is shaped by more than the state's levels of economic development. Competition between local officials, providers, business groups, and others leads to a wide range of compromises. Within the federal system, states respond to these competing pressures in different ways, with widely differing benefits for the interests represented as well as for the low-income consumers who are often unrepresented at the bargaining tables.

Values and Policy Preferences

The political competition among interest groups produces divergent policies in different states and localities and leads to a steadily changing federal policy. How does one judge whether one policy is better than another or whether proposals for change should be judged as steps forward or backward?

The answer inevitably obliges a citizen to consider his or her personal values. Often choices about the governments' roles are choices between competing values. In a broad sense, the conflicting values are typically efficiency and equity. Efficiency often requires that rewards or benefits be linked to economic output, whereas equity seeks to ensure that all citizens receive some minimum standard of goods and service regardless of their economic output. When a proposal for government action enhances (or reduces) both efficiency and equity, it clearly is preferable (or undesirable). But when proposals promote one value while reducing another, citizens must make more difficult choices.

In the next few years a number of public policy issues are likely to arise regarding the governments' roles in health care. They involve the more difficult types of choices between competing values, so only individual values can determine what is right. But considering such issues with respect to each of governments' roles can help individuals make informed decisions.

Government as Financer

Three issues relating to government's role as financer are now or recently have been subjects of public debates. The first relates to proposals to provide insurance for the approximately 18% of Americans who lack health insurance (General Accounting Office). This group consists of unemployed people ineligible for Medicaid under current state rules and employed people who are not offered group health insurance by their employer and cannot afford to buy private insurance individually.

The existence of a large group of uninsured citizens poses multiple problems. In some cases they are able to get needed care through the charitable efforts of voluntary organizations or through local public hospitals subsidized by city or county taxes. But these forms of assistance vary widely across the country and leave many people without access to services. The absence of health insurance coverage reduces the utilization of services among this group.

Numerous different proposals have been made to alleviate this problem. Proposals include mandating employer-based benefits, expansion of Medicaid coverage, and special funding for hospitals providing care to the uninsured. The advantages of the proposals are the improved equity they would yield by helping an underserved group and assuring them a minimum standard of care. The perceived disadvantages are economic difficulties for business firms, which would have higher costs and be less competitive because of the mandated coverage or higher tax burdens for the currently employed and insured in order to pay for the new public programs. Resolving these conflicting goals is likely to remain a major national health care issue.

A second emerging issue is the financing of long-term-care services. (Rivlin & Wiener). As previously mentioned, Medicare does not provide these benefits, and private insurance is not widely available for such services either. As a result, most people suffering from chronic disability must deplete their assets, rely on friends or family for health assistance, and/or suffer discomfort and in-convenience because of a lack of assistance. The unfortunate circumstances of many frail elderly (and the prospect for many others of eventually being in this position) have led to proposals that government play a greater role in financing long-term care.

The advantages of such public financing include protection from catastrophic expenses for those who have saved during their working life and assurance of some minimum level of services for those without savings or relatives able to assist. The disadvantages are that citizens other than the disabled (i.e., the working-age population) would face increased taxes to pay for the benefits. Moreover, it is likely that much of the added public financing would finance services by paid home care providers who would replace or reduce the care now being given to the frail elderly by their friends and relatives. The challenge for policy analysts in the coming years will be to design a long-term-care financing program that reconciles the needs of the elderly with the concerns of working-age taxpayers that much of the new funding would go for care that otherwise would be provided voluntarily or might not be necessary.

A third financing issue concerns so-called tax expenditures for health care (Congressional Budget Office, 1982). The federal income tax provides deductions for certain types of expenses. Businesses are allowed to deduct payments made for employee health insurance. These and similar deductions are referred to as tax expenditures because they represent revenue forgone by the government. If the deduction did not exist, the government would collect taxes on these sums. Recent estimates are that the tax expenditures (i.e., forgone tax revenue) related to deductions for health insurance expenses total $88 billion annually.

The wisdom of these expenditures has recently been questioned, and the questioning is particularly relevant because of the large federal deficits. The criticisms of these government subsidies in the form of tax expenditures are that they promote more generous health insurance packages than individuals would choose if they were spending their own taxable income and that the benefits are distributed inequitably, with higher-income individuals receiving proportionately more of the benefits than lower-income citizens, more in need of assistance, do. Defenders of the tax expenditures generally acknowledge that these points are true but present a case based on historical circumstances and the need to abide by previous agreements between government and workers. That is, the growth of employer-based health insurance followed restrictions on wages during World War II, and after the war the government encouraged employer-based insurance and created a national system of collective bargaining that facilitated the growth of these benefits. A sudden reversal of this policy and the taxing of benefits previously negotiated with employers would impose new and unexpected burdens on workers.

Government as Deliverer

A general direction of American health care policy has been expansion of government financing without expansion of government delivery. Political leaders debate the merits of various national health insurance proposals but rarely consider creation of a national health service such as exists in Great Britain.

The aversion to public sector delivery is rooted in ideological beliefs that private organizations can do the job more efficiently. Yet despite this bias, many American governments are deeply involved in delivering health care. As noted earlier, for example, there is a large federal system for veterans, and many local governments operate hospitals serving the urban poor.

A recurring issue in health policy is whether some or all of these public sector delivery roles should be shifted to the private sector. In the case of the VA system, the issue seems to have been resolved after considerable controversy in the late 1970s. Despite recommendations for elimination of the separate, government-run system, those preferring its continuation were successful in Congress.

The history and prospects for local government hospitals are different. A prestigious commission reporting on this subject in the late 1970s recommended the continuation of these institutions because of the important roles they play in providing trauma care, services to the indigent, and sites for graduate medical education (Commission on Public General Hospitals). Without such public institutions it was believed these roles would not be performed as well by the private sector.

Despite the commission's recommendations, there have been strong pressures to close or contract out the management of local public hospitals in some communities. Local political leaders sometimes believe they can save local tax funds through these measures. As noted earlier, however, in the case of closure these savings are likely to be associated with reduced access to care for the uninsured poor. The evidence on the results of contracting the management of public hospitals to private firms is more mixed (Shonick & Roemer). Private management is not associated with greater efficiency in the sense of lower unit costs, but it often yields local taxpayers savings through greater cost shifting to consumers or third parties.

Government as Regulator

Government regulation is a frequent target of criticism as an enemy of efficiency. Often competition and regulation are presented as alternatives, but reality is quite different. Effective competition generally requires some regulation; standards of behavior must be set and enforced for market competition to work. Efforts to promote competition in the health care industry are likely to go hand and hand with new forms of regulation.

One federal initiative is greater monitoring of the quality of care in order to provide consumers with more information with which to select providers. Perhaps the most controversial example is the publication by the HCFA of hospital-specific mortality rates for Medicare patients with selected conditions (Blumberg). The intent was to identify hospitals that did especially well or especially poorly and to let the public know these findings. The effort was widely criticized for being misleading, but the concept that the government should monitor quality of care is gaining broader acceptance. As more emphasis is placed on consumer choice and concern grows over the quality of care, governments' roles are likely to be expanded.

Another important regulatory issue relates to technological innovation. A case has been made that the FDA's requirements for bringing new drugs and devices to market slows innovation, and reform of their approach seems warranted. However, a related issue is whether new devices and procedures, once approved, should be paid for by public payers without any restrictions or whether expensive new technologies should be regulated or, perhaps more accurately, rationed (Hillman). For example, widespread availability of heart transplants and similar medical advances would be very expensive. But the concept of government officials setting a quota on the number of procedures or treatments to be paid for is anathema to many. If the development of medical technology continues to lead to expensive treatments for relatively widespread conditions, this issue will become especially prominent. Some balance between the amount taxpayers collectively are willing to devote to medical care and the need of individuals for treatment will have to be reached. Such societal decisions about rationing health care seem to be an inevitable consequence of the trends of greater public financing and increased costs resulting from technological innovation.

References

Altman, S. H., Brecher, C., Henderson, M. G., & Thorpe, K. E. *Competition and Compassion*. Ann Arbor, Mich.: Health Administration Press, 1989.

American Hospital Association. *Hospital Statistics*. Chicago: AHA, 1988.

Begun, J. W. *Professionalism and the Public Interest*. Cambridge, MA: The MIT Press, 1981.

Bergthold, L. "Crabs in a Bucket: The Politics of Health Care Reform in California." *Journal of Health Politics, Policy and Law, 9*(2), 1984.

Blum, B., & Blank S. "Mental Health and Mental Retardation Services." In G. Benjamin & C. Brecher (ed.), *The Two New Yorks*. New York: Russell Sage Foundation, 1989.

Blumberg, M. S. "Comments on HCFA Hospital Death Rate Statistical Outliers," *Health Services Research, 21*(6), 715, 1987.

Brecher, C. "Medicaid Comes to Arizona." *Journal of Health Politics, Policy and Law, 9*(3), 411, 1984.

Brecher, C. "Progress in New York State Hospital Payment Policy." *Bulletin of the New York Academy of Medicine, 62*(1), 115, 1986.

Brown, L. D. "Technocratic Corporatism and Administrative Reform in Medicare." *Journal of Health Politics, Policy and Law, 10*(3), 579, 1985.

Clarke, G. J. "In Defense of Deinstitutionalization." *Milbank Memorial Fund Quarterly, 57*(4), 461, 1979.

Commission on Public General Hospitals. *Readings on Public General Hospitals*. Chicago: Hospital Research and Educational Trust, 1978.

Congressional Budget Office. *Containing Medical Care Costs through Market Forces*. Washington, D.C.: Author, 1982.

Congressional Budget Office. *Veterans Administration Health Care: Planning for Future Years*. Washington, D.C.: Author, 1984.

Davis, E. M., & Millman, M. L. *Health Care for the Urban Poor*. Totowa, N.J.: Rowman and Allanheld, 1983.

General Accounting Office. *Health Insurance: A Profile of the Uninsured in Ohio and the Nation* (HRD-88-83). Washington, D.C.: Author, 1988.

Grabowski, H. G., & Vernon, J. M. *The Regulation of Pharmaceuticals*. Washington, D. C.: American Enterprise Institute, 1983.

Gray, V., Jacob, H., & Vines, K. N. (Ed). *Politics in the American States: A Comparative Analysis*. Boston: Little, Brown, 1983.

Hillman, B. J. "Government Health Policy and the Diffusion of New Medical Devices." *Health Services Research, 21*(5), 681, 1986.

Holahan, J. F., & Cohen, J. W. *Medicaid: The Trade-Off between Cost Containment and Access to Care*. Washington, D.C.: Urban Institute Press, 1986.

Holahan, J. F., & Etheredge, L. M. *Medicare Physician Payment Reform: Issues and Options*. Washington, D.C.: Urban Institute Press, 1986.

Hughes, E. F. X., et al. *Hospital Cost Containment Programs: A Policy Analysis*. Cambridge, Mass.: Ballinger Publishing Company, 1978.

Jolly, P., Taksel, L., & Beran, R. "U.S. Medical School Finances." *Journal of the American Medical Association, 260*(8), 1077, 1988.

Kosterlitz, J. "Test of Strength." *National Journal, 19*(42), 2652, 1987.

Kosterlitz, J. "Graying Armies." *National Journal, 20*(11), 664, 1988.

Levin, A. (Ed.). *Regulating Health Care*. New York: Academy of Political Science, 1980.

Lohr, K. N., & Brook, R. H. *Quality Assurance in Medicine: Experience in the Public Sector*. Santa Monica, CA: Rand Corporation, 1984.

Marmor, T. R. *The Politics of Medicare*. Chicago: Aldine, 1973.

Marmor, T. R. *Political Analysis and American Medical Care*. New York: Cambridge University Press, 1983.

Mechanic, D. "Correcting Misconceptions in Mental Health Policy." *Milbank Quarterly, 65*(2), 203, 1987.

Miller, C. A., & Moos, M. *Local Health Departments: Fifteen Case Studies*. Chapel Hill, N.C.: American Public Health Association, 1981.

National Academy of Sciences. *Study of Health Care for American Veterans*. Washington, D.C.: U.S. Government Printing Office, 1977.

Panem, S. *The AIDS Bureaucracy*. Cambridge, MA: Harvard University Press, 1988.

Rivlin, A. M. "Agreed: Here Comes National Health Insurance." *New York Times Magazine*, July 21, 1974, pp. 8, ff.

Rivlin, A. M., & Wiener, J. M. *Caring for the Disabled Elderly: Who Will Pay?* Washington, D.C.: Brookings Institution, 1988.

Ruther, M. et al, *Medicare and Medicaid Data Book, 1984* Baltimore: U.S. Health Care Financing Administration, HCPA Publication No. 03210, June 1986.

Shonick, W., & Roemer, R. *Public Hospitals under Private Management*. Berkeley, CA: Institute of Governmental Studies, 1983.

Statman, M. *Competition in the Pharmaceutical Industry*. Washington, D.C.: American Enterprise Institute, 1983.

Thorpe, K. E. "Health Care." In G. Benjamin & C. Brecher (ed.), *The Two New Yorks*. New York: Russell Sage Foundation, 1989.

Thorpe, K. E. & Brecher, C. "Access to Care for the Uninsured Poor in Large Cities: Do Public Hospitals Make a Difference?" *Journal of Health Politics, Policy and Law, 12*(2), 313, 1987.

Tierney, J. T. "Organized Interests in Health Politics and Policy Making." *Medical Care Review, 44*(1), 89, 1987.

Truman, D. *The Governmental Process*. New York: Alfred A. Knopf, 1960.

Wagner, L. "Blending Old Traditions with Modern Medicine." *Modern Health Care*, August 26, 1988, p. 22.

13

Planning for Health Services

Roger Kropf

Planning involves selecting and carrying out a series of actions designed to achieve stated goals. It could be argued that such planning should take place for health services at every level—national, state, and local.

In fact, the history of planning for health services in the United States shows great disagreement about whether national or even state planning for health services is necessary and what the role of government should be. Some of the issues are the following:

1. Who should define the goals? The federal government? State or local government? Consumers? Hospitals? Physicians?
2. What actions can government prevent or force anyone to take in order to achieve a goal? For example, can it prevent a hospital from being built?
3. Do the actions of individual hospitals and physicians, unregulated by government, lead to the achievement of goals for the community such as improved health?

Government at both the national and state levels has given different answers to these questions since the end of World War II.

The process of planning health services in the United States as we arrive at the end of the 1980s is largely in the control of private hospitals (both not-for-profit and for-profit), physicians, and health maintenance organizations (HMOs). Private companies that manufacture medical equipment and drugs must also plan for the development, production, and distribution of their products. Insurance companies, both for-profit and not-for-profit, that have invested in the HMOs and other providers also are involved in planning health services.

The role of government in planning is very limited. The Reagan administration and many states viewed government as another purchaser of health care in what was expected to be a marketplace controlled by supply and demand. Only in the areas of medical research and the fight against major diseases such as AIDS was there a consensus in Congress and in the Reagan administration that the federal government must act forcefully and commit substantial resources, although there were disagreements about how much money to spend in a time of large budget deficits.

The major objective of this chapter is to convey the current state of planning for health services in the United States and to describe the events that have led to a major role for private organizations and a limited role for government. We shall first trace the history of planning for health services since World War II and describe some of the major debates that have led to the current state of planning.

The process of planning hospital services will then be described, hospitals being the most numerous and most active planners of health services in any community. Within the hospital community a debate continues about the importance of "strategic" planning and marketing. Both will be defined, and the differences between them will be examined. This will be followed by discussion of a range of techniques for planning health services, to convey what planners and managers actually do, regardless of whether they work in a hospital, for a private physician's group, or in an HMO.

Planning: Politics and Analysis

Planning is not a science in which conclusions emerge solely from mathematics, computers, and data. It also should not be only a political process in which the conclusions depend entirely on which groups or individuals have the most money or influence. Regardless of whether planning is carried out in a for-profit hospital or a state government, it must involve both politics and analysis. The analysis is necessary to educate those making decisions, whereas politics determines what actions are feasible.

Those who take the position that planning has nothing to do with politics or nothing to do with analysis often become disillusioned with planning. For those who hold that politics should not be involved in planning, the failure to achieve a plan for political reasons leads to disillusionment with the planning process. And for those who see no real role for analysis, the failure of programs when facts are ignored makes planning seem irrelevant. The best chance for success comes when informed decision makers take actions that are feasible within the political environments in which most managers operate. For this reason, both planning techniques and the politics of planning will be stressed in this chapter. The two are not contradictory but equally important for those who plan health services.

History of Health Planning in the United States

The history of health planning since 1946 can be described as a debate over (1) whether government should be directly involved in planning a health care system that is largely in private hands, (2) which levels of government should have the authority, (3) what means of control should be allowed, and (4) what role citizens in local communities should have. A rapid rise in national health care expenditures has greatly influenced the debate because the federal government plays a major role in financing the care of millions of poor and elderly Americans.

To understand the current situation, the history of planning since America emerged from the Depression and World War II must be understood. In 1945 America emerged as a more prosperous country than it had been during the 1930s and one in which spending for domestic programs had largely been postponed. A tremendous need for hospitals was evident, and the question was what action the federal government would now take after having been actively involved in planning and providing a wide range of services during the war and depression years.

The Hill–Burton Act and Its Successors

The Hospital Survey and Construction Act of 1946 (P.L. 79-725), known as the Hill–Burton Act, authorized the appropriation of funds for new hospital construction. Each state was to receive a minimum allocation of funds, the amount varying according to population. Rather than establishing a central planning authority in Washington, it set requirements for health facilities planning across the nation and mandated a combined federal and state planning process. Each state had to designate a single state agency to undertake hospital planning and had to submit a plan that prioritized the needs.

The Hill–Burton Act and its later revisions therefore embodied the principle that the federal government should not directly plan for hospital services. Its authors believed that since a national government could not know all the health care needs of people in thousands of cities and towns, planning needed to be carried out in each state. Once it was told what the needs were, the national government could then allocate funds to meet those that were most critical. Amendments in 1954 broadened the program to include nursing homes, rehabilitation facilities, chronic disease facilities, and diagnostic and treatment facilities.

By 1961, facilities housing 238,946 hospital beds had been constructed. Criticism of the lack of coordination among hospitals in providing services increased. In response, the Community Health Services and Facilities Act of 1961 (P.L. 87-395) made federal demonstration grants available for "areawide" or local planning, a recognition of the fact that state governments could not be aware of local health needs and that some coordination of hospitals at the local level was needed.

The Hill–Harris Act of 1964 (Hospital and Medical Facilities Amendments, P.L. 88-443) allocated funds for a grant program to assist not only in the new construction but in the modernization or replacement of facilities. Project grants also were authorized for development of comprehensive regional, metropolitan, and other local plans for health and related facilities.

Comprehensive Health Planning Act

The Comprehensive Health Planning (CHP) and Public Health Service Amendments Act of 1966 (P.L. 89-749), also known as the Partnership for Health Act, authorized grants to agencies at the state (Section 314a, or "A" agencies) and regional (Section 314b, or "B" agencies) levels. Funds also were provided to establish a State Health Planning Council, which would include representatives of state and local agencies and consumers concerned with health.

In addition to developing plans, "B" agencies also had the right to "review and comment" on local proposals, including federal grant applications and applications under state laws that required a "Certificate of Need" for the construction of health facilities or the establishment of certain health programs.

"B" agencies had no legal authority to implement their plans; they could only advise the state government in carrying out its regulatory programs. Results were supposed to be achieved by increasing the participation of both consumers and providers, by assistance to groups that could establish needed health services, and by assisting in negotiations among competing interests in local communities.

The National Health Planning and Resources Development Act

The National Health Planning and Resources Development Act of 1974 (P.L. 93-641) authorized funds for the establishment of regional Health Systems Agencies (HSAs) to replace "B" agencies. Funds also were provided for State Health Planning and Development Agencies (SHPDAs) and State Health Coordinating Councils (SHCCs).

The new HSAs were given an ambitious number of objectives, including the following:

1. Improving the health of residents of a health service area.
2. Increasing the accessibility, acceptability, continuity, and quality of health services provided to residents of the area.
3. Restraining increases in the cost of providing residents with health services.
4. Preventing unnecessary duplication of health resources.
5. Preserving and improving competition in the health service area.

Concern over the rising cost of medical care soon dramatically altered federal priorities in regard to health planning. The new regional HSAs were asked to focus on controlling unnecessary expenditures for health services and health facilities. However, they were not given more authority to do so. They still could only advise state and federal agencies on the need for health services.

The major impact of P.L. 93-641 was to create more uniformity in health planning across the United States. The entire country was divided into health systems areas, with CHP "B" agencies covering only selected areas. Plans were required of both HSAs and the new SHPDAs.

In some ways, however, the appearance of uniformity masked deep differences across the country in the willingness of communities and states to accept the new mandate to control health care costs. The difference was not only between politically conservative and liberal areas. Local communities in relatively liberal states like Massachusetts, New York, and New Jersey found it difficult to accept a federal mandate that the rise in health care costs needed to be slowed down through reduced expenditures for health facilities and programs when citizens perceived a need for the modernization of hospitals and for additional services (e.g., long-term-care and mental health services).

Many HSAs continued to concern themselves with issues such as access to health services for poor and rural residents, environmental pollution, mental health services, and other causes of deep interest to their local communities. Increasingly, however, the test being applied by critics of the health planning program was whether HSAs were helping to slow the increase in health care costs.

The Health Planning Act continued to be funded, however, during the Nixon, Ford, and Carter administrations. Proponents during the Nixon and Ford years argued that it was too early to tell whether such a complex program was working, and in any case support for local and state, as opposed to national, planning was consistent with Republican principles. When President Carter failed to win passage of a hospital cost-containment act that would have established a national system for setting payments to hospitals, the Health Planning Act became one of the few remaining devices for potentially lowering the rise in hospital costs.

The Reagan administration felt differently from all three previous administrations. Direct support to local communities for planning violated conservative principles concerning the primacy of the states in directing certain activities within their borders. The health planning program had been passed during the Carter years primarily because of strong Democratic support within the Congress. When the Democrats lost the Senate, a program now desired only by the majority Democrats in the House was unlikely to win favor in the Reagan administration, which was in the midst of searching for social programs to cut.

Also, a number of studies had concluded that Certificate of Need laws, the main tool available to state planning agencies, for slowing the increase in hospital costs, were not effective. Although a report by the Congressional

Budget Office (1982) noted the methodological and other problems with these studies, they were used by critics to undermine support for renewal of the Health Planning Act.

P.L. 93-641 had authorized appropriations for health planning until fiscal year 1977. P.L. 96-79 then reauthorized support for health planning until September 30, 1982. Although Congress failed to pass legislation in that year, funds continued to be appropriated under continuing resolutions until 1986, when all federal support for the health planning system ceased. Legislation was passed in 1986 terminating support for HSAs, SHPDAs, and SHCCs. HSAs in most states closed. Many states ended Certificate of Need legislation as well, allowing hospitals and other health care providers to build facilities and start services whenever and wherever they wanted. A few states, such as New York and Massachusetts, have continued active Certificate of Need programs; New York State has even provided HSAs with funds to continue operations and provide the state with advice and data on local conditions, which the state feels is vital for both its Certificate of Need program and for planning health services in the state.

In the Congress and the Reagan administration, however, the idea of a national health planning program based on local definition of needs but following national priorities failed to find a constituency. Why? Perhaps it was because of lack of effectiveness. Contradictory research studies appeared and continue to appear about the efficacy of Certificate of Need—the main tool available to state regulators in lowering capital expenditures. A program designed to meet a list of goals was ultimately judged by its effectiveness in attaining a goal for which no adequate tools were offered. Although lacking the authority to stop health care expenditures, HSAs were evaluated on their ability to reduce them. Achievement in other areas (e.g., better coordination of planning among hospitals) was both harder to measure and less of a priority in Washington in the face of large increases in Medicare and Medicaid expenditures and massive budget deficits (Institute of Medicine, 1981).

Perhaps it was because the program was caught between two contradictory forces. On the one hand, Americans want quick, effective action. On the other hand, we don't want government telling us what to do. To cut the rise in health care expenditures by reducing the money spent for hospitals and new health care programs would mean saying no to important people and organizations in hundreds of communities across America. In the abstract, the money saved would return to citizens in the form of higher wages, higher stock dividends, and lower taxes. No one could, however, keep an accounting of where the money went, whereas the loss of a new hosptial wing or piece of medical equipment was an immediate, painful loss. State health departments, armed with the legal authority to deny applications for Certificates of Need, were often unable to resist the pressures from governors and legislatures who were besieged by angry voters, hospital associations, and physicians demanding approval of a project. Voters increasingly demanded no tax increases and even tax reductions, but this did not create a constituency for reductions in unused hospital beds and less duplication of medical equipment.

Health planning as a tool for controlling health care costs also was challenged by a new system for setting the payments made to hospitals that was believed to be not only effective but flexible enough to allow the marketplace to decide which services would be offered. Competition in a "free market" would bring supply and demand into balance at the lowest cost. The government itself would participate as a buyer in this free market, using its considerable buying power to change both the services available and their price.

The Free Market Model

The assumption that individuals acting alone in a market free of government control will, in the long run, produce the maximum benefits at the lowest cost is part of what economists call the 'free market model'. In this view, planning is best done by private individuals and organizations. The free market model justified the government's not having a set of goals for health care, a plan, or even a planning process at the national level during the Reagan administration. Government's role would be to act to prevent certain failures in the market-place—for example, fraud—that prevented the free market from working.

Economists have noted that a condition for a free market to exist is that there be many buyers and sellers in the marketplace, with no buyer or seller dominating the market enough to fix supply or prices. The federal government, however, is the major purchaser of hospital services in the United States. Proposals were made to increase the number of buyers in the marketplace. One proposal was to give each Medicare or Medicaid recipient a voucher that would allow him or her to purchase health insurance from competing firms. The needed legislation was never passed by Congress. A program to encourage the development of "competitive medical plans" that would compete to insure Medicare recipients and then negotiate for their health care in the open market has grown very slowly and represents a tiny fraction of total Medicare expenditures.

The situation in the United States in the 1980s therefore suggested that the free market model would not work without considerable intervention by government. While continuing to support the concept of competition rather than regulation, the Reagan Administration worked to put into effect a broader range of regulatory controls than the Carter administration had suggested. These included (1) a system of fixed prices for hospital care provided to Medicare recipients, (2) temporary controls on the fees that physicians could charge for services to Medicare recipients, (3) a revamped federally supported program to monitor the quality of medical care by Professional Review Organizations (PROs), and (3) continued use of the federal government's authority to deny payment under Medicare for new procedures and technologies whose effectiveness was viewed as inadequate when compared to the additional cost. Control over what physicians and hospitals were paid became in effect the major tool for influencing what services were provided by whom and in what quantities.

Hospital Rate Setting

P.L. 98-21, the Social Security Amendments of 1983, authorized a system for setting in advance the prices the federal government would pay for hospital services provided to those eligible for Medicare. It set a fixed price for each Diagnosis Related Group or (DRG). Hospitals would be allowed to keep the difference between the DRG price and its actual cost, or would sustain a loss.

The federal government would then not need to get involved in decisions concerning how many hospital beds existed and what services would be provided. Hospitals would open or close facilities and begin or cease to provide services depending on the profits they made.

The goals that were set by the federal government concerned annual increases in Medicare spending rather than improvements in health. It was assumed that hospitals and physicians would use the money they were given to provide what people needed to restore or improve their health. The federal government would look for fraud and would not pay for any new drug, surgical procedure, or test until its usefulness was proved. It would not, however, interfere in the matter of where hospitals and physicians were located or in determining which services were most needed in a community.

The dilemma would then be solved. The federal government would not tell states and local communities what services to offer. On the other hand, the rise in the cost of hospital care to Medicare recipients would decrease because the federal government would not rapidly raise prices.

It is now widely believed that the new prospective payment system based on DRGs resulted, perhaps in conjunction with other factors, in a rapid decrease in hospital admissions and shorter stays in the hospital for Medicare recipients. No evaluations have been made of whether Medicare recipients are healthier as a result. The federal government has devoted resources to determining and publishing the rates at which Medicare recipients die in individual hospitals in order to begin studying the effects of paying hospitals for each case they treat and letting them keep any profits that result. The new system provides an incentive to provide fewer rather than more services, which is desirable as long as the outcome (e.g., recovery from an illness, prevention of death or disability) is the same.

At first glance the new system seems to solve a number of problems, but a number of questions remain:

1. Will the new system result in the highest-quality, as opposed to the most profitable, providers staying in business? Does a review of the quality of

care require a local organization to assist the federal government? Who should control that organization?

2. Should the federal government be pursuing other goals, such as increased disease prevention, and who will carry out the necessary actions to achieve them?

National Health Planning Today

What we have ended up with in the late 1980s is a federal government that provides massive sums of money to be used by state governments, private for-profit and not-for-profit hospitals, physicians, and other professionals. The U.S. Department of Health and Human Services, the federal government's major health agency, does not, however, have a plan for what services should be provided with the money, how many hospitals should exist and where, or how many physicians should practice in various cities and states.

It could be argued that no one could write such a plan in such a complex system. On the other hand, the spending of billions of dollars has the impact of moving the health care system in some direction, whether planned or not. The idea that thousands of hospitals and physicians acting independently in response to the current system of financing will produce a better result than conscious planning would is a matter of faith rather than fact.

For some, the concept of central government control is so repugnant and frightening that the cost in inefficiency of a free market system is a small price to pay for freedom. For others, the loss in efficiency is too high. So far, those in the latter group are a minority in Congress and the state legislatures, and the free market system of planning (or not planning) receives at least tacit support.

Americans want health services that produce better health; they also want low taxes and a government that does not often tell people what they can and cannot do. They want government to be a prudent buyer with taxpayers' money. All of this requires planning in a general sense. The major questions are who shall do the planning and how shall we decide when the desires of individuals and private organizations need to take second place to what government believes is needed to reach widely shared goals. The answers may change as we understand the positive and negative impact of the hospital rate-setting system now being used to purchase hospital care in behalf of millions of older Americans.

Hospital Planning in the United States

An examination of hospital planning since World War II will show how private organizations responded to a changing environment and federal legislation. Although other organizations plan health services, hospitals have a longer history of formal planning, so changes in their behavior over the last 40 years can be assessed by looking at the plans they have produced and how they have carried out the planning process (Kropf & Goldsmith). Hospital planning affects every community in the United States. Other organizations that have a long history of formal planning (e.g., some HMOs such as Kaiser-Permanente in California) have been concentrated in specific regions of the United States and serve a much smaller percentage of Americans.

Hospital Planning Responds to a Changing Environment

Hospital planning in the 1950s and 1960s reflected the emphasis on construction and modernization that was made possible by the availability of federal funds under the Hill–Burton Act and its successors. Hospital planning was facilities planning, and building design and construction were the focus of that planning.

With the passage of Certificate of Need legislation in the late 1960s and 1970s, emphasis began to shift to the documentation of the need for hospital services in the community and in a particular hospital. Hospital planning had to combine both community and facilities planning.

The shift in emphasis by the federal government to control of hospitals through reimbursement, the repeal of many state Certificate of Need laws, and the failure of Congress to pass a national health planning act again altered hospital planning in the 1980s. At the same time, hospital admissions began to decrease, and lengths of stay continued to decline—a trend that started in the 1970s (Moss & Moien). The result was a decline in occupancy rates, with community hospitals in the United States averaging 65% occupancy in 1987 (American Hospital Association).

Hospital managers now searched for a way to fill the empty beds. Facilities planning had taken for granted that whatever services were available would be used. Community planning assumed that the government would grant a franchise to the "best" hospitals, limiting supply, and that services would then be used. In the new environment, neither approach seemed relevant.

Hospital managers searching for something new and relevant could draw on two management approaches that had been developed in the general business community: "strategic" planning and marketing. Both assumed that firms competed for customers in a market where supply often exceeded demand and where rapid technological change continually produced new products They both therefore fit the new environment faced by hospitals.

Strategies in the 1980s

Strategic planning requires that managers use resources to put their organization in a favorable position in the marketplace. Such a position might be (1) having the largest share of the demand in a market; (2) being the most technologically advanced company, whose products command a higher price; or (3) being a high-volume, low-price company, which is very profitable. The major strategies used by hospitals during the 1980s to achieve a favorable market position are *vertical integration, horizontal integration,* and *diversification.*

An "integrated" firm includes a number of businesses that are related either because they produce the same product or service ("horizontal" integration) or because they carry out a number of stages in the manufacturing process ("vertical" integration). Marriott is a horizontally integrated corporation because it owns a number of hotel chains. General Motors is vertically integrated because it owns companies that produce components for automobiles as well as those that assemble, market, and finance the purchase of automobiles.

There are many advantages and disadvantages to vertical and horizontal integration (Porter; Harrigan; Smith, & Reid). In the hospital industry, horizontal integration was viewed as potentially advantageous because a chain of hospitals might be able to purchase supplies and services at a volume discount, hire specialized staff at the corporate level to increase expertise, raise capital less expensively on the securities markets, and market hospital services under a single brand name in a number of communities.

A vertically integrated health care "system" can include outpatient or office services for routine and preventive care, diagnostic services to detect disease, and treatment services to cure patients. Nursing home care and rehabilitation and mental health care also may be included. The potential advantages of a vertically integrated system are that the consumer—both patients and referring physicians—never has to leave the system to get the health services needed. Revenues are kept in the system while the patient's care is managed to assure that the needed services are provided.

Diversification simply means adding services not usually found in a hospital. These may include home care, physical fitness centers, prevention and detection services provided at the workplace, and residential drug and alcohol treatment services. The potential advantage of diversification is that revenues are not lost to other organizations. The hospital's reputation in the community provides it with an advantage over companies that may move in and offer the same services.

Horizontal integration proved the easiest strategy to carry out. Chains of for-profit hospitals (such as Hospital Corporation of America) grew, their growth financed by investors who thought they saw a profitable trend in the hospital industry. Chains of not-for-profit hospitals also emerged and actually remain the most numerous. Some of the chains, however, simply involved agreements to cooperate (e.g., in purchasing supplies) rather than actual ownership of all of the hospitals by a single company. The largest "multihospital system" of not-for-profit hospitals, Voluntary Hospitals of America (VHA), was formed when hospitals agreed to invest in a new corporation that would start new businesses (and return profits to investors), negotiate favorable purchase agreements with suppliers, and take other actions that would benefit hospital investors. VHA doesn't own any hospitals, however.

Vertical integration was far less common in the 1980s. The examples that are most widely known—the Kaiser-Permanente Medical Plans, the Cleveland Clinic Foundation, the Mayo Clinic—were all formed much earlier. Even in these organizations the full continuum of services is not provided. Long-term nursing home care, for example, is rarely provided by these organizations.

Diversification was more common than vertical integration. Hospitals diversified and provided those services that market analysis showed might be profitable.

As hospitals approach the 1990s, considerable disillusionment with all three of these strategies has developed. Although volume purchasing has resulted in real savings to chains of hospitals, the other advantages of horizontal integration are less apparent. Several hospital chains have sold off hospitals to raise capital and improve their profitability. Doubts are being expressed about whether the additional expertise is worth the extra costs of a central corporate office. As profits have fallen, both for-profit and not-for-profit chains are paying more to raise capital. Managers of profitable community hospitals that have a healthy share of a local market are not sure that remaining independent will hurt them in the long run, a common assumption in the early 1980s. Whereas joining a group of hospitals to obtain discounts on supplies and services still makes sense, selling the hospital to a chain is now more difficult to justify to boards of trustees.

Hospitals have lost considerable money trying to start health maintenance organizations (HMOs), the most common attempt at vertical integration. Diversification into other businesses has frequently resulted in long periods during which the new businesses had to be subsidized, with smaller profits than had been expected (Freudenheim).

Professional journals and lecturers at conventions have begun to discuss whether a new strategy is needed—a "back-to-basics" strategy. Hospitals, it is argued, should seek to provide the traditional range of inpatient and outpatient services but with a new emphasis on quality, measured in both improved health and higher levels of patient and physician satisfaction (Kropf & Szafran; Perry; Peterson).

Although this may seem attractive to many groups within a hospital, it will not be an easy strategy to pursue. Most hospitals have always believed they provide high-quality services. Unless they can document and communicate to patients and physicians that they do in fact provide higher-quality services, they may be left investing in improvements that fail to produce significant changes in volume. Some dimensions of quality are very difficult to measure, and others are subjective. Proving that a hospital offers higher-quality services may be very difficult, although the goal is admirable. Whether it produces the bottom-line results that hospital managers are seeking is not clear.

Focus on Marketing Tactics. In military jargon a strategy is an idea that results in winning a war, whereas tactics are actions that win battles. A military strategist is not alarmed about losing a battle if an effective strategy continues to be implemented.

A number of hospitals, alarmed at actual or projected drops in patient volume and revenues, have pursued advertising, sales, and other tactics of marketing in an attempt to reduce anxiety and produce better end-of-the-year results. The results have been disappointing for many hospitals. Marketing experts have countered that hospitals have neglected market research and overlooked the development of market strategies in the pursuit of tactics to produce quick results. They also have criticized the tactics as inappropriate for the kinds of problems that hospitals were actually facing (Powills).

For many hospitals, marketing meant advertising. For a smaller number, it meant sales through sales forces paid on a commission basis.

For the first time many hospitals began advertising their "products." Marketing professionals already knew, based on years of experience in a variety of businesses, that advertising alone does not produce large increases in demand. In order to achieve a change in the behavior of customers, repeated exposure to the message is necessary (Robertson & Wortzel). Advertising campaigns that reach a large number of people with a message many times are very expensive. Some hospital managers appear to have thought that a few ads in the newspapers would produce a significant increase in demand. When the increase did not occur and bills for thousands of dollars of advertising arrived, the result was disillusionment with marketing. Hospital experience with sales forces and commissions is too recent to assess, but it also reflects a focus on market tactics rather than strategy.

Notable missing is an emphasis on market research prior to deciding on strategy and tactics. American industry spends huge resources on market surveys in an attempt to understand consumer behavior. Hospitals have spent much more on advertising than on market research. Consultants and marketing professionals report very little concern in hospitals about the concepts that underlie much of marketing strategy, particularly market position (how consumers perceive a product in relation to its competitors).

What explains this approach to marketing? Part of the reason may be that some senior managers of hospitals have no experience in other industries, and were trained in academic programs that placed little emphasis on marketing because of the very different environment hospitals faced in the 1960s and 1970s. Also, hospitals are relatively small organizations that cannot compete with major industries in salary and career advancement for trained marketing professionals. Hospital staff placed in charge of marketing either have no formal training in that area or have come from sales and public relations positions in other industries.

The research and strategy-development skills and knowledge are available in marketing firms but at a cost that far exceeds what hospitals have wanted to pay.

For example, a "focus group" involving a 1- to 2-hour discussion among 6 to 8 consumers, a full transcript, and an analysis of significant comments would cost a hospital $5,000 to $10,000 if done by a professional marketing firm.

The development of a marketing strategy—including careful and professional market research, a consensus among hospital decision makers on the position the hospital should seek to obtain in the market, product and personnel changes to implement the strategy, and a multiyear advertising and public relations campaign to communicate to the desired market—is time-consuming, expensive, and likely to result in conflict in the complex, highly political environment of a hospital. It is perhaps not surprising then that some hospital managers without previous experience and training in marketing would opt for tactics such as advertising rather than market strategy development and implementation.

What Should Hospital Planning Include? The hospital industry has arrived at the end of the 1980s without a widely accepted model for how hospital planning should be carried out. It would have been possible at the end of the 1970s to have described what a hospital plan looked like and what a hospital planner did. At the end of the 1980s there is far greater diversity but also a great deal of frustration among hospital managers. Just what should hospitals be doing—more marketing? more strategic planning?

In an industry composed of so many organizations, different answers will be given to this question. We are likely to see considerable anxiety among hospital managers about whether their hospital is doing the right thing. To understand the choices facing an individual hospital, it is important to understand what strategic planning and marketing are, as well as the differences between them.

Strategic Planning

Strategic planning involves the allocation of resources to achieve an organization's long-range goals. It involves selecting among alternative uses, of resources and among alternative goals. It also involves forecasting future conditions under alternative scenarios (Kropf & Greenberg).

The major debates about strategic planning, in both the hospital and other industries, concern (1) who should carry out the strategic planning process, (2) whether a plan is necessary or desirable, and (3) whether the term "strategic management" would be a more appropriate description of what managers need to do in turbulent environments.

Numerous case studies have shown that planning that does not involve the real decision makers does not result in changes in the organization's behavior. Although no one will argue that planning is not a responsibility of boards of directors and the president or CEO of a company, the reality is that planning as an organizational function in large organizations often becomes the name of a department headed by a middle-level staff person. When this occurs, considerable time and money can be spent on activity about which the board and the senior executive are only vaguely aware. The result is often wasted effort. The middle-level staff member does not understand what the board/president wants and will accept, and the board/president is not interested in what the planning department produces.

Reinforcing this message is research showing that many plans are not implemented because they are incorrect and irrelevant by the time they are produced. In industries in which the environment changes weekly, a plan that took 2 years to prepare is rarely useful. The central role of forecasting in the development of plans is being questioned because forecasts of many variables are highly suspect.

It is now frequently argued that strategic planning should be one of the day-to-day activities of top managers. Mintzberg (1987) has coined the term "crafting strategy," using an analogy to the way a potter creates a vase or bowl. Based on day-to-day contact with the reality in which the organization operates, the senior manager crafts the strategy of the organization, rejecting one idea for another as events unfold.

The term that has emerged for this dynamic, flexible style of strategic planning carried out directly by the senior manager is "strategic management." It responds to the major criticisms of strategic planning but at the same time leaves open some questions. How does the senior manager locate and draw conclusions from the vast amount of data about the organization and its environment and still get all of his/her other jobs done? Is there a role for staff? How does the manager communicate the content and rationale for the organization's strategy to key decision-makers such as the board of trustees? Is a written plan necessary or desirable?

In seeking the answer to the question of what hospital planning should become, the concept of strategic management needs to be carefully considered. It suggests that hospital managers are going to have to incorporate more long-range thinking into their daily activities, that they are going to have to develop information systems that are responsive to ther needs of senior managers, and that communication about what the hospital's strategy is as it develops will have to become a formal activity.

Marketing

It is easy to exaggerate the differences between strategic planning and marketing by emphasizing the tactics of marketing, especially advertising, public relations, and sales. On the other hand, popular textbooks used at graduate business schools have titles like "strategic marketing" and "strategic market management." The point is that marketing, like strategic planning, requires a vision of where the organization wants to go in the future and also a plan for getting there.

The rationale for both marketing and strategic planning is that an organization will not automatically achieve its goals and objectives—and will not meet customer needs and desires as effectively—unless a formal process of selecting among alternative uses of resources is carried out.

A major difference is the points from which strategic planning and marketing often begin. Strategic planning begins by asking what the organization's mission and goals are. Marketing begins by asking what the needs and desires of consumers are. Both must consider these two issues at some point. Both proceed in very similar ways until the question of tactics arises. Marketing may turn more frequently to its well-developed tactics, including advertising, whereas strategic planning more frequently considers alternatives suggested by economics (e.g., diversification, and horizontal and vertical integration).

This suggests another difference between strategic planning and marketing: their theoretical roots. Marketing professionals are far more likely to use the terms and concepts of human psychology, whereas strategic planners draw on those of economics. For example, Kotler and Clarke (1987) use Maslow's hierarchy of needs to understand which of the individual's basic needs might be served by a product. They note that it would be futile to offer activities such as jogging and exercise classes to the very poor who lack food and shelter. Activities such as these will more likely appeal to those seeking to fulfill the higher social, esteem, and self-actualizing needs.

Michael Porter (1980), a prominent writer on strategic planning, focuses on what he calls the "value chain" to explain why organizations and individuals purchase goods and services. The value chain is the series of activities that the purchaser must go through—for example, travel to where a service is provided. By increasing the value of the good or service at any point along the chain, the chances that the purchase will be made are increased. For example, providing a physician with the report of an x-ray procedure faster adds value to the service because the physician wishes to inform a patient, especially about any negative results. The value chain concept can be applied to a range of health services (Kropf & Szafran). It should be noted, however, that Porter has simply borrowed the concept of "value-added" from economics (i.e., that manufacturing involves the addition of value at each step of the process) and made the assumption that people are primarily motivated by their calculation of the monetary value of the services they purchase.

The theoretical roots of strategic planning and marketing are therefore different. Both processes, however, draw on a wide range of concepts and techniques from many disciplines.

Techniques for Planning Health Services

Techniques are needed to produce the information to be used by decision makers and to manage the process of decision making by the individuals who must agree before action is taken. Information is needed about the needs and desires of the people to be served, other organizations that provide health services, and the general environment in which the health care organization must operate—especially what actions government and other third-party payers are likely to take.

In this section a number of techniques for investigating the needs and desires of consumers are presented:

1. Describing the *health* of the population.
2. Describing what people *desire*, regardless of need.
3. Describing *past utilization* of health services.

Techniques for managing part of the process of decision making in a group are then presented. These include the following:

1. A technique for determining perceptions of the *strengths, weaknesses, opportunities*, and *threats* facing an organization. Agreement on these subjects is necessary before a group can decide on how to allocate resources.
2. The Nominal Group Process, a technique for assuring that all viewpoints are heard by the group prior to making a decision. This is likely to increase the chances that a plan of action will be successfully implemented.

Measuring Health Status

The extent to which people are healthy or ill is valuable information for planning. Much has been written, however, about the difficulties of defining health and illness, as well as the methodological and cost problems of measuring the extent of health or illness in a population (Berg; Goldsmith).

For example, if we define health as the absence of organic illness (e.g., the absence of infection, cancer, malfunction of an organ or body system), this would leave out the feeling of well-being that many individuals associate with feeling "healthy." An overweight individual who got little exercise and felt lethargic could still be "healthy"—that is, free of organic illness. Even if we expand our definition to include body weight and muscle tone charactertistics considered ideal, it would leave out the perception of well-being commonly associated with good health.

On the other hand, if we expand the definition of health to include other dimensions—for example, "emotional well-being," how do we define and measure what is good health? Such a definition would lead us to define health as what is perceived by the individual to be positive, which is highly subjective and vastly different from person to person.

Regardless of whether good health is defined in terms of absence of disease or a feeling of physical and emotional well-being, the problems of measurement remain. How do we know in the absence of extensive medical testing if an individual is free or organic disease? Individuals free of symptoms may in fact be at high risk of a heart attack, for example, because of blocked arteries. Determining physical and emotional well-being would require extensive interviews that are costly to carry out.

While the debate continues on how to measure health status, individuals involved in planning health services continue to rely on measures that are believed to be closely related or correlated to the level of health, such as infant mortality, total mortality, and mortality from specific causes that are preventable or treatable (Dever). Measures that use the death rate require data that are available from public records for almost all deaths in a community.

The reliance on death rates, however, is particularly troublesome for health care organizations seeking to become more responsive to consumer demand. Such organizations are more likely to rely on data concerning the use of health services, rather than on death data, as an indication of both need and demand for health services (Rice & Creel; Tseng). When the investment (and the risk) is large enough, surveys and other forms of consumer research are more likely to be undertaken to determine with more certainty how consumers feel about their health and what services they want.

Consumer Analysis: Understanding What Physicians and Consumers Want

Until the 1980s, individuals responsible for planning health services at all levels paid surprisingly little attention to the subject of what consumers' and physicians' wants and desires were in regard to health services. Planning for health services focused on the question of need. Most health care professionals accepted the idea that what the consumer wanted was at best a secondary consideration to providing for consumers the services that physicians and other professionals thought they should have.

The competitive environment described earlier produced a great change in this attitude among some health services managers whose organizations faced significant underutilization. The issue now became how to determine what consumers desired so that their organization could provide it. A significant number of pregnant women, for example, wanted alternatives to the hospital labor and delivery rooms that they did not, in the minds of many obstetricians, "need." A number of hospitals therefore established birthing centers and other new arrangements for labor and delivery to boost sagging utilization in maternity services, or to win a greater share of patients in the community.

Because a physician's advice has a major impact on the decisions made by consumers, what referring physicians wanted also became a major concern. Hospitals developed a range of programs in response, including courier services to get test reports to physicians faster, more formal arrangements for providing specialty consultations, and even links to the hospital's computer to allow information sharing.

To understand what its consumers (including physicians) wanted, hospitals and other health care organizations looked at the techniques being used by other industries that had made analysis of consumer desires and behavior a major part of their planning processes (Berwick & Weinstein; Ross et al.).

Market Segmentation. A fundamental concept in marketing is the *market segment* (Kotler & Clarke), a group of individuals who are distinguished by one or more characteristics believed to affect their purchasing behavior. Consumers might, for example, be segmented by age, and the over-70 market segment identified as behaving differently from other age groups. Within this over-70 segment, those with high income could be segmented and offered different services, such as luxury accommodations while in a hospital.

Two important points need to be made. First, market segmentation should be based on research rather than logic. Second, segments need to be determined for specific products or services because it is purchase behavior we are trying to predict.

Consumer Research. In order to identify market segments, research must be conducted to determine how consumers behave and the attitudes, knowledge, and beliefs that may affect that behavior. Telephone, mail, and personal interview surveys are frequently used to gather data. Formal discussion groups called focus groups are a popular way of gathering preliminary data to be used in preparation for more formal research.

Tools for Analysis. Computer technology has had a major impact on the ability of an analyst to follow a line of questioning. General purpose programs for analyzing survey data, such as the Statistical Package for the Social Sciences (SPSS) (Nie et al.) are available to assist the analysis. Several firms (such as HBO & Company in Atlanta, the Sachs Group in Evanston, Illinois, and SysteMetrics in Santa Barbara, California) have developed computer systems that allow the analysis of market-related data and produce tables, maps, and graphs that combine census data, data on utilization from bills and discharge abstracts, and survey research data.

Impact. Analysis of consumer behavior, attitudes, knowledge, and beliefs is changing the way some health care organizations plan for new services. For some organizations, the major question has become "What do our consumers want?" rather than "What do consumers need that we want to offer?" How many organizations have changed their way of thinking is hard to tell, but the number of new programs being offered that emphasize life-style change, disease detection, and alternatives to traditional hospital care suggest that some organizations have changed their behavior.

Analysis of Health Services Utilization

Data Sources. The number and type of health services used by consumers is critically important information for planning. The necessary data are usually obtained from national surveys, bills and related forms that are completed in order to receive payment, and special surveys undertaken at the local level (Kropf & Greenberg). The most important national surveys are undertaken by the National Center for Health Statistics (NCHS) of the U.S. Department of Health and Human Services. The National Health Interview Survey, for example, provides self-reported data on the physician and hospital services used by individuals in approximately 40,000 households. Data is available for more than 20 years, allowing the planner to look at trends over time, which is extremely important for forecasting.

Since NCHS surveys are samples of the entire U.S. population, in most cases they cannot provide local data (i.e., for an individual city, town, county, or state). Data from bills and related forms can be aggregated to provide such data. In states such as New York and Massachusetts, the state government requires that hospitals submit a copy of the hospital bill and a discharge abstract for each patient in a form that can be read by a computer. The number of times that people in an individual area were hospitalized and the reason can be determined. Because only a minority of states require that such data be submitted, the only truly national data source on hospitalization comes from the Medicare program, and that covers only people over the age of 65. However, the U.S. Department of Health and Human Services has been reluctant to release these data to anyone but researchers because of concerns about violation of the confidentiality of patients.

In order to collect data on a range of topics other than hospital stays, private organizations and local governments sometimes pay for surveys that are conducted over the telephone, through the mail, and, more rarely, in individual households. Such surveys are, however, expensive.

In summary, local data on how many and what type of hospital inpatient services consumers use are available in a minority of states, although the federal government possesses such data for all states for Medicare recipients. Local data on what occurs outside the hospital are scarce for all age groups; no state has yet mandated that physicians and/or insurance companies submit copies of bills for services outside the hospital. The federal government has not made local data on the services used by Medicare recipients outside the hospital available to hospitals and other organizations that plan health services.

Tools for Analysis. Computer technology has vastly changed how the data just described can be analyzed (Dever; Kropf & Greenberg). The major impact has been to allow the analyst to follow a line of questioning as information is received rather than being forced to accept a fixed series of tables. As each question is raised, the computer allows the analyst to ask for tables and graphs. In response to this new information, a new question(s) can be asked and new tables and graphs requested.

Mobile Mammography for the Corporate Customer: A Case Study in Planning

To illustrate how the techniques that have just been described might be used, the situation faced by an organization—a hospital or a physician group practice—wishing to establish a mobile mammography screening program aimed at employees of corporations will be discussed (Kettlehake & Malott).

Mobile mammography screening is an attractive option for some organizations seeking to increase their volume of patients because

1. It brings the organization into contact with women who may not have personal physicians and will use the organization for other services.
2. It can locate women who have cancer and therefore need specialized services that the organization can offer.
3. It increases the visibility of the organization to all those who come into contact with the promotional materials for the program.
4. It can enhance the public image of the organization.
5. It can serve as the entry point into a corporation, resulting in later sales of other services.

Mobile mammography screening involves the use of specialized x-ray equipment, placed in vans and driven to an office or factory location, or portable equipment set up inside a building. Employees are offered the opportunity to register and receive a mammogram, which is read by radiologists. The report is then returned to the woman's personal physician, or an appointment is made with a physician affiliated with the sponsoring health care organization. The employer's role is to offer the opportunity to employees by allowing them access—for example, use of company internal mail and facilities. The employer may or may not subsidize the cost of the mammogram.

Health Status. Current American Cancer Society (ACS) statistics indicate that 1 in ten women will develop breast cancer at some time during their lives. It was estimated that there would be 135,000 new cases of breast cancer detected in 1988, and 42,000 women would die of the disease.

Analysis of data on breast cancer mortality suggests that annual screening of women over 50 could reduce mortality by 30% or more when followed by appropriate treatment (Kolata). Evidence on the impact of routine screening on women 40 to 49 is mixed; some experts suggest that the cost is not justified for women who have no symptoms and whose mother or sister(s) have not had the disease (Kolata). Current ACS guidelines suggest that a baseline mammogram be taken between ages 35 and 39 to facilitate the detection of later changes and that a mammogram be taken every 1 to 2 years for women aged 40 to 49 and every year for symptomless women age 50 and over.

An organization considering offering such a service could use data from death certificates collected by all states to determine the number and ages of women who die from breast cancer in particular towns, cities, and counties.

Consumer Analysis. The ACS guidelines suggest that market segmentation by age is essential. Women under 35 need to be advised that mammography is not advisable. The message communicated to women 35–39, 40–49, and over 50 will be different because of their differing professionally defined needs. The next question is what other segmentation of the market should be undertaken.

The organization could hold one or more focus groups to suggest what differences in attitudes, beliefs, and desires exist among women in each age group. Because a large amount of research suggests that the use of preventive services is strongly related to education and income, the organization also may wish to investigate (through focus groups or surveys of samples of women) the differences among women in various employment categories within the organization (e.g., managerial, clerical, manufacturing).

The purpose of focus group research is to suggest topics that should be explored in more formal personal interviews or in mail or telephone surveys. How much research is carried out will depend on the size of the investment to be made, the willingness of the corporation to allow customization of the program to fit the desires of groups of workers, and prior experience in offering screening programs.

Following are some research results that might be seen:

1. Younger women express a greater desire for the procedure.
2. Higher-paid, better-educated workers have greater knowledge of the procedure.
3. Most women have a friend or relative who has had a mammogram and told them what to expect (Seago).

If survey research is undertaken and yields a large number of responses, the organization or a consultant will probably analyze the data, using a computer program to examine the relationship between responses. For example, does age or employment category better explain differences in the expressed desire for the service?

This kind of consumer analysis could be reflected in the content of promotional material. Simplified descriptions of the need for the procedure and how it will be carried out could be distributed to lower-paid, less-educated women who need basic information. Higher-paid, better-educated women could be given materials that focus on the qualifications of the organization, the amount of radiation they will be exposed to, and other subjects that are shown to be of interest to this group. Consumer analysis also could have an impact on how the service is provided. Only female staff may be used because of concerns expressed about being seen by men (Seago) and because it is assumed that women nurses and technicians will be viewed as more sympathetic to the anxieties and concerns of women.

Analysis of Utilization. One of the problems faced by an organization that considers offering this service is the absence of data on the number of women in local communiities who have had mammograms. Data from the National Hospital Discharge Survey for 1986, the latest year available, show that 214,000 women were discharged with a diagnosis of "malignant neoplasm" or cancer of the breast (National Center for Health Statistics). Local data on hospital utilization would be available in those states in which hospitals are required to submit discharge abstracts to state government. This would allow the organization to determine not only the number of discharges but the patients' ages and places of residence and what percentage were treated in each hospital in the community and outside the area.

Data from the National Health Interview Survey for January–June 1985 (the latest data available) indicate that 34% of women aged 30 to 44 practice breast self-examination once a month or more. Thirty-seven percent of women 45–64 do so (Thornberry et al.). This suggests that a substantial majority of women do not follow current ACS guidelines. The ACS estimates that only 28% of women over 40 have annual mammograms and that an additional 14% have mammograms every 2 to 4 years. The ACS does not have data on how many of these women are over 50 (Kolata).

Other Planning Tasks. This discussion of the information that might be collected as part of the planning process is not meant to suggest that data collection and analysis are the only tasks to be undertaken. The current activities of competitors must be examined. The willingness of the board or owners of the organization to devote resources must be determined. The willingness of employers to promote the use of this service must be assessed. Equipment, personnel, and supplies must be obtained.

Asking questions about what the needs and desires of consumers are has been stressed because it is a task that many health care organizations are less familiar with. Before any action can be taken, however, the decision makers in an organization must agree on many issues, including the best way to allocate resources.

Group Process Techniques

Decisions are made by people, not computers. The highest-quality information is useless if it has no impact on the thinking of the individuals who must approve the allocation of resources.

Planning health services involves the selection of a process for arriving at a decision on how resources are to be spent and for what. Since it is rare in health care organizations that a single individual has the sole authority to allocate major resources, the most relevant techniques for arriving at a decision are those used with groups.

The final method for decision making is, of course, most likely to be the vote of a board of directors or trustees. The question is how this group of individuals arrives at decisions about what the major facts are, what the options are, and which options are most attractive given the mission, goals, and capabilities of an organization.

SWOT Analysis. A simple technique for moving closer to a consensus on the current environment is a Strengths–Weaknesses–Opportunities–Threats (SWOT) analysis (Peters). The board would be asked to meet for an extended period (e.g., a weekend) to discuss these four topics with an experienced discussion leader brought from outside the organization to facilitate the discussion.

Members of the board would be asked during a series of meetings to answer the following questions:

1. What are the major *strengths* of the organization?
2. What are its major *weaknesses?*
3. What *opportunities* in the environment should the organization take advantage of?
4. What *threats* exist to the achievement of the organization's mission and goals.

Consensus on the answers to these questions within a short time is highly unlikely. Each individual probably will have a different level of knowledge of the "facts." If all agree on the facts, they may not agree on the implications of those facts. For example, members of the board may arrive with different ideas about the extent to which their competitors' hospital beds are full or empty. When given the best estimate, they may still disagree on what the numbers imply that their own organization should do.

The job of the discussion leader is to help the members of the group define the information they need, apply it to their situation, expose the differences in values and beliefs that explain differences in opinion, and lead the group over time to a consensus on what needs to be done. There are certainly no fixed rules for carrying this process to a successful conclusion, and some organizations may never reach the required consensus. Over the years, however, consultants and professional planners have developed some techniques that appear to facilitate at least part of the decision-making process.

The Nominal Group Process. The Nominal Group Process is one such technique (Spiegel & Hyman). Research by sociologists and psychologists has shown that some individuals will not speak in a group discussion. Other people will use the situation to express their views and attempt to dominate the group. The end result is that the group does not reach a consensus because (1) the opinions of some members have never been revealed and opened to scrutiny and/or (2) opinions are rejected simply because they are voiced by members whose attempt to dominate the group is resented by others.

The Nominal Group Process seeks to solve the problem by asking each member of the group to write a response to one or more specific questions on index cards. The question might be one of the four listed above for a SWOT analysis. The discussion leader then goes in clockwise order around the room and asks each participant for a response, for example, a strength of the organization. The group is asked not to comment until the end of the process. Each response is written on a large piece of paper and posted for everyone to see. A number of rounds is completed until all responses are out in the open. The discussion leader then leads the group in a discussion—of which responses are similar, for example, and which are true or not true. The virtues of this process are that each person contributes, the contribution is not evaluated until all responses are known, and no one can dominate the discussion until everyone's opinion is known.

Although the technique is not perfect, it offers advantages over an un-structured discussion that have made it popular with planners. Other techniques are available to fit different objectives and environments (Spiegel & Hyman).

Should We Merge with Metro? A Case Study in Board Decision Making

To understand how these decision-making techniques might be used, let us consider the situation faced by the board of directors of a small rural HMO that was faced with a major decision.[1] It had received an inquiry from Metro Health Plan, one of the nation's largest HMOs, concerning a merger. The HMO was not-for-profit and consumer-controlled (i.e., a majority of the board members were not physicians, nurses, or other providers of health services). The HMO had experienced slow growth in the 10 years it had been in operation, and it operated in only three sites, all located within a 10-mile radius of each other.

---

[1]This case was prepared for teaching purposes, although the situation was one actually faced by a rural HMO.

Table 13.1 SWOT Analysis

Strengths
    Loyalty of current members
    High level of employee satisfaction
    Stable financial condition
    High quality of service as perceived by both providers and consumers
Weaknesses
    Stagnation in membership growth
    Limited ability to borrow funds for expansion
    Limited range of expertise in current administration (e.g., no attorney on staff)
Opportunities
    Become the largest high-quality, rural HMO in the state by remaining independent and
        Using its current reputation for quality and consumer satisfaction to market the plan
        in adjacent communities
        Being the first HMO to start operations in a number of rural areas in the state
        Using the knowledge of its board and members to design facilities and programs
        that would appeal to rural communities
    Join a much larger organization whose resources would allow the HMO to dominate
    an expanded market area
    Merge with another HMO and develop a statewide HMO that would be locally
    controlled but have sufficient resources to grow and dominate an expanded market
    area
Threats
    Metro or another HMO would enter rural communities first and sign up members, who
    would be reluctant to change plans later
    The HMO could not expand fast enough and compete with other HMOs because of
    the lack of capital and management expertise.

The board decided to hire an experienced consultant to lead them in a weekend retreat to consider the offer. The consultant recommended that they meet and for the first 4 hours carry out a SWOT analysis. Table 13.1 shows the list produced by the end of the session.

A consensus was reached that the strengths, weaknesses, opportunities, and threats listed in Table 13.1 summarized the situation faced by the HMO. The board then went through another Nominal Group Process to reach consensus on its options, which included a merger with Metro, a merger with a smaller HMO in a rural part of the state, and conversion to a for-profit corporation in order to sell stock to raise capital. Eventually, the board voted for a merger with Metro Health Plan.

Issues and Comments

The role of the federal government in planning services is likely to remain indirect and focused on problems that are perceived to be high-priority, such as

AIDS. The cost of health care is likely to remain the major focus of the federal government, although efforts may be made to correct the problems that federal cost-control efforts do not affect or that they make more serious. This includes the lack of health services in rural and inner-city areas and the concentration of poor patients in public hospitals.

The extent to which state government is involved in planning health services has varied dramatically and is likely to continue to do so. Prosperous states with long traditions of actively pursuing solutions to health problems (e.g., New York, Massachusetts) are likely to continue to plan and to implement those plans through regulation and state spending. Other states are likely to view health services as local and federal issues and be active only in the traditional public health functions (e.g., disease control and the maintenance of birth and death records).

Is a change in this scenario needed? Will pressure build for a national health insurance program that requires explicit government planning to assure the availability of services. The answer at this time appears to be no, but it will depend on the new administration in Washington, the economy, and public opinion.

The prediction made in the early 1980s that most hospitals would eventually be owned by a few large hospital chains has yet to come true. The critical assumption was that central management would make hospitals more efficient, more attractive to patients and physicians, and therefore more profitable. However, much of the capital to make acquisitions has come, and probably will continue to come, from investment by buyers of stocks and bonds. These funds are likely to remain in short supply because of the perception that the federal government and large employers are serious about reducing the increase in expenditures for hospital care and that they will act to pay hospitals less. Unless managers can prove that large gains in efficiency and lower costs (and therefore profits) are still possible, investors are likely to conclude that the days of high profitability and gains in stock prices are over. As of today, rapid growth in multihospital systems that own their hospitals appears unlikely.

Growth may be greater in chains of not-for-profit hospitals that offer their members group purchasing arrangements and other services. As hospitals are further pressed to lower their costs and find new services to offer, they may turn to organizations that offer solutions. Whether multihospital systems turn into multiproduct firms, offering their members solutions to management problems, will depend on the quality of leadership in both member hospitals and the systems themselves.

The local hospital is likely to retain its role as the major planner of health services in most communities. If demand for inpatient hospital services continues to decline, hospital planning probably will remain focused on creating services outside the hospital and making the remaining inpatient services attractive to patients and physicians. If public interest in health promotion and prevention continues to increase, the hospital may find itself planning, marketing, and providing a much wider range of services. However, because of the limited funding for health services for the poor, much of this planning will be for the middle-class population who can afford to pay.

Under a competitive, free market system, many middle-class Americans are likely to be served by a much more consumer-oriented hospital industry than has existed in the past. What happens to consumers who cannot pay out-of-pocket or with private insurance will depend on the actions of government in response to pressures from citizens and employers. The poor need an array of health services, which can be delivered in a way that is sensitive to their personal desires. The question is who will pay for it.

References

American Hospital Association. *Hospital Statistics* (1988 Edition) Chicago: American Hospital Association, 1988, p. xxvi.

Austin, C. J. *Information Systems for Health Services Administration.* Ann Arbor, MI: Health Administration Press, 1988.

Berg, R. L. (Ed.). *Health Status Indexes.* Chicago: Hospital Research and Educational Trust, 1973.

Berwick, D. M., & Weinstein, M. C. "What Do Patients Value? The Willingness to Pay for Ultrasound in Normal Pregnancy." *Medical Care, 23,* 7, 1985.

Congressional Budget Office. *Health Planning: Issues for Reauthorization.* Washington, D.C.: Congressional Budget Office, 1982.

Dever, G. E. A. *Community Health Analysis: A Holistic Approach.* Rockville, MD: Aspen, 1980.

Freudenheim, M. "Hospital Ventures: Some Successes." *The New York Times,* August 23, 1988, p. D2.

Goldsmith, S. B. "The Status of Health Status Indicators." *Health Services Reports, 87,* 212, 1972.

Harrigan, K. R. *Strategic Flexibility.* Lexington, MA: Lexington Books, 1985.

Institute of Medicine, Committee on Health Planning Goals and Standards. *Health Planning in the United States: Selected Policy Issues.* 2 vols. Washington, D.C.: National Academy Press, 1981.

Kettlehake, J., & Malott, J. C. "Mobile Screening Mammography for the Corporate Customer." *Radiology Management, 10,* 2, Spring 1988.

Kolata, G. "Breast Cancer: Anguish, Mystery and Hope." *The New York Times Magazine,* April 24, 1988, p. 43.

Kolata, G. "Doubts Increase on Need for Early Mammogram." *The New York Times,* March 11, 1988, p. A10.

Kotler, P., & Clarke, R. *Marketing for Health Care Organizations.* Englewood Cliffs, N.J.: Prentice-Hall, 1987.

Kropf, R., & Goldsmith, S. B. "Innovation in Hospital Plans." *Health Care Management Review, 8,* 2, 1983.

Kropf, R., & Greenberg, J. A. *Strategic Analysis for Hospital Management*. Rockville, MD: Aspen Systems, 1984.

Kropf, R., & Szafran, A. "Developing a Competitive Advantage in the Market for Radiology Services." *Hospital and Health Services Administration*, Summer 1988, p. 213.

Mintzberg, H. "Crafting Strategy." *Harvard Business Review*, July–August 1987, p. 66.

Moss, A. J., & Moien, M. A. "Recent Declines in Hospitalization, United States, 1982–6. *Advance Data from Vital and Health Statistics*, No. 140. (DHHS Pub. No. PHS 87-1250). Hyattsville, MD: Public Health Service, September 24, 1987.

National Center for Health Statistics. "1986 Summary: National Hospital Discharge Survey." *Advance Data From Vital and Health Statistics*, No. 145. (DHHS Pub. No. PHS 87-1250). Hyattsville, MD: Public Health Service. 1987.

Nie, N. H. et al. Statistical Package for the Social Sciences. New York: McGraw-Hill, 1975.

Perry, L. "The Quality Process: Hospitals Begin to Emphasize Quality in Devising Strategic Plans." *Modern Healthcare*, April 1, 1988, p. 30.

Peters, J. *A Strategic Planning Process for Hospitals*. Chicago: American Hospital Association, 1985.

Peterson, K. *The Strategic Approach to Quality Service in Health Care*. Rockville, MD: Aspen, 1988.

Porter, M. *Competitive Strategy*. New York: Free Press, 1980.

Powills, S. "Hospitals Call a Marketing Time-Out." *Hospitals*, June 5, 1986, p. 50.

Rice, J., & Creel, G. *Market-Based Demand Forecasting for Hospital Inpatient Services*. Chicago: American Hospital Association, 1985.

Robertson, T. S., & Wortzel, L. H. "Consumer Behavior and Health Care Change: The Role of Mass Media." *Advances in Consumer Research*, 5, 1984, p. 50.

Ross, C. K., et al. "The Role of Expectations in Patient Satisfaction with Medical Care." *Journal of Health Care Marketing*, 7, 4, 1987.

Seago, K. "Breast Imaging Centers and Patient Emotions: Niceness Counts." *Applied Radiology*, November/December 1986, p. 59.

Smith, H. L., & Reid, R. A. *Competitive Hospitals: Management Strategies*. Rockville, MD: Aspen, 1986.

Spiegel, A. D., & Hyman, H. H. *Basic Health Planning Methods*. Rockville, MD: Aspen Systems, 1978.

Thornberry, O. T., et al. "Health Promotion and Disease Prevention, Provisional Data from the National Health Interview Survey: United States, January–June 1985." *Advance Data From Vital and Health Statistics*, No. 119. (DHHS Pub. No. PHS 86-1250). Hyattsville, MD: Public Health Service, May 14, 1986.

Tseng, S. "Community Demand Analysis for Hospital Ambulatory Care Services." In Meshenberg, K. & Burns, L. (eds.), *Hospital Ambulatory Care: Making It Work*. Chicago: American Hospital Association, 1983.

14

The Quality of Care: Assessment and Assurance*

Beth C. Weitzman

"There are differences in the quality of care given by physicians and hospitals. We can measure those differences and that information should be conveyed to the public" ("US Plans"). Rarely does a statement provoke as much heated debate as the one above, issued by Dr. William L. Roper, administrator of the Health Care Financing Administration, in 1988. But then few health care issues have engendered as much controversy as have recent discussions of quality assessment and quality assurance. Although it is agreed that quality health care is desirable, there continues to be substantial disagreement about its definition, its measurement, and methods for ensuring its occurrence. Both quality assessment—that is, the measurement of the extent to which the care provided is of high quality—and quality assurance, guaranteeing the provision of quality care, are central to current discussions on the future of health care delivery in this nation.

Quality-of-care problems are diverse; they include excessive or inappropriate surgery, variable outcomes of surgical procedures, inappropriate diagnosis or treatment of common acute conditions, and excessive or inappropriate use of prescription drugs (Lohr et al.). Whether one is discussing the relative merits of health maintenance organizations (HMOs), the seriousness of the shortage of nurses, or the introduction of new technologies, questions of quality must be addressed.

Historically, there has been surprisingly little concern about the quality of care provided. "Do no harm," taken from the Hippocratic Oath, served as the guiding principle. However, increased health care costs and government financing of health care, coupled with increased consumer dissatisfaction and malpractice litigation, have contributed to a growing concern about quality. This chapter will

*Much of the section on quality assurance is adapted from earlier editions of this chapter authored by Steven Jonas and Stephen N. Rosenberg.

begin with a brief review of the history of quality assessment and assurance. Definitions and methods of measuring quality health care will then be explored. This will be followed by a discussion of the strategies for quality assurance.

History of Quality Assessment and Assurance

Although concern with quality has only recently become a focal issue for the health care community, the stage for this discussion was, in fact, set well over 100 years ago. In the early 1860s, Florence Nightingale helped lay the groundwork for medical care evaluation by suggesting a uniform format for collecting and presenting hospital statistics (Christoffel). At the turn of the century a Boston surgeon, Dr. Ernest Codman, encouraged the collection and evaluation of systematic information on the end results of patient care activities (Christoffel). Entitled "end result analysis," it was introduced at Massachusetts General Hospital in 1900 and featured a careful analysis of cases for which treatment was unsuccessful. Like many current systems of quality assurance, end result analysis featured data collection on large numbers of patient outcomes and a recognition that a poor outcome might result from a range of factors. Codman's ideas failed to gain widespread acceptance in the earliest years of the 20th century, a period characterized by rapid gains in medical science, growth in medical professionalism, and limited consumer knowledge.

Despite the initial lack of enthusiasm for end result analysis, one of the foremost agencies for quality assurance, the Joint Commission on Accreditation of Health Care Organizations (JCAHO), traces its inception back to Codman's original proposal (Roberts). Dr. Edward Martin believed that the American College of Surgeons should be established to implement and introduce Codman's end-result idea. In 1917 the college formally established and published the *Minimum Standard for Hospitals,* which contained the first formal requirements for the review and evaluation of the quality of patient care. The Minimum Standard required clinical review and addressed such issues as the quality of the medical record, the quality of clinical performance, and the requirements for medical staff membership. Quality of care in hospitals that participated in the Hospital Standardization Program improved noticeably (Shanahan). In 1951 the American College of Surgeons joined with the American College of Physicians, the American Hospital Association, the American Medical Association (AMA), and the Canadian Medical Association to establish the Joint Commission on Accreditation of Hospitals (JCAH). JCAH's function was to oversee the minimum standards; by this time more than half of all hospitals in the United States were approved (Roberts). In recognition of the growing diversity of health care provider settings, the JCAH broadened its scope in the 1980s to become the JCAHO.

With the funding of hospital facilities through the Hill–Burton Act and, more dramatically, with the enactment of Medicare and Medicaid in the 1960s, the role of the federal government in health care grew dramatically. As it became a major source of health care dollars, the federal government took on a more active role in quality assessment and assurance. Quality standards for participation in federal programs were established. By the 1970s, because of the large federal deficit and increasing federal expenditures, cost containment and its relationship to quality emerged as key issues in health care (Thurow). Emphasis was placed on the elimination of unnecessary procedures and overutilization of health care services; such excessive care is both high in cost and low in quality. Further-more, in order to attain the often-stated goal of providing the best possible care at the lowest possible cost, it became essential to identify what was meant by the best possible care. The quest for quality became tied to the drive to contain costs. Much of the federal health care legislation of this era had cost containment as its main goal but also provided new impetus to improve quality.

Traditionally, the focus of quality assurance programs has been on hospital care both because it is so expensive and because hospitals are more amenable to organizational constraint (Donabedian, 1985). Only recently have such programs been applied widely to ambulatory care.

Definition of Quality

According to *Webster's New Collegiate Dictionary,* quality may be defined as "degree of excellence" or "superiority in kind." This concept of quality is certainly not unique to health care. As consumers we must assess the quality or degree of excellence of a broad range of products and services. Whether we are selecting a restaurant, purchasing an article of clothing, or making a reservation with an airline, consumers, like providers, use available information to try to identify the best-quality product relative to its cost. Yet in few cases is this assessment of quality more difficult than in regard to health care. The concept of health embraces physiological, psychological, and social components. Care may refer to an individual practitioner, a given institution, or an entire health care system. And quality may be defined relative to the technical aspects of care, the interpersonal relations between patient and practitioner, or the amenities of care and the setting in which it is offered. Quality may be defined against absolute standards or against individual or social needs. The broad range of services and activities that comprise health care delivery and the complexity intrinsic to quality have led many to conclude that there is not one quintessential definition of quality but rather several legitimate definitions. Yet planners, managers, and policymakers must work from some definition that is consensually accepted before quality of care can be assessed and assured.

The Components of Quality

Such widely agreed upon components of quality do indeed exist. Quality care aims to promote, preserve, and restore health. Quality care is delivered in a manner that is satisfying to patients and in an appropriate setting. Quality refers to the extent to which possible improvements in health status are realized. It is not an assessment of the state of medical science but rather an assessment of the application of existing knowledge (Donabedian, 1980). The quality of health care embraces (1) the patient's health status and attitudes on entry to care; (2) the suitability of the stable characteristics, or structure, of care; (3) the processes of care; and (4) the outcomes of the processes of care (Blum).

According to the AMA's Council on Medical Services (1986), high-quality care is that "which consistently contributes to improvement or maintenance of the quality and/or duration of life." The definition goes on to stress that quality care produces optimal improvement in physiological state, physical function, and emotional and intellectual performance. It should emphasize health promotion and disease prevention and be delivered in a timely manner. The AMA's definition also notes that quality care must include the patient as an informed participant, and it should be delivered with sensitivity. Finally, quality care should make efficient use of resources and allow for continuity of care. This comprehensive definition of quality health care underscores the complexity of the concept; application of this definition is likely to result in an emphasis on some aspects over others.

In trying to define and measure precisely what can be called quality care, there is a dilemma or tension between focusing on that which is unacceptable or poor-quality care and that which is optimal or highest-quality care. For many purposes, good-quality care is seen as that which is free of incidences or evidence of poor quality; this is a standard that focuses on the minimal requirements for quality. Such definitions are often employed because they are relatively easy to use and measure. In other cases, the definition aims to characterize an optimal or ideal standard of high quality. Often this sort of definition, of which the AMA's definition of quality is an example, can be difficult to use in a meaningful way.

Competing Definitions

As already noted, quality can be defined in relationship to technical care, management of the interpersonal relationship between practitioner and patient, and the amenities of care. Research has indicated that one's role in the health care delivery process is likely to influence how one defines quality. Traditionally, quality of care has been defined by clinicians, primarily in terms of the technical delivery of care: "the application of the science and technology of medicine, and of the other health sciences, to the management of a personal health problem" (Donabedian, 1980, p. 4). From early in the development of medical practice in the United States, and especially since the beginning of the 20th century, society has delegated the establishment of quality standards to the medical profession (Caper). Even though most quality assurance efforts have been aimed at institutions (especially hospitals), the standards for those institutions have been developed by physicians. Peer review—the assessment of the work of colleagues by those within the same profession—has been placed at the center of quality assessment and assurance efforts. The medical profession's peer review efforts have emphasized the scientific aspects of quality; appropriate drug prescription, postoperative infection rates, and accuracy of diagnosis are among the measures of quality that have been used.

In contrast to the physician's emphasis on the technical aspects of care, most patients tend to focus on interpersonal aspects of care in assessing quality. Lacking technical expertise, clients most typically judge the quality of technical care indirectly, by evidence of the practitioner's interest in and concern for the patient's health and welfare (Donabedian, 1985, p. 5). Also, patients may assume technical competence, especially in university-affiliated settings, and thus assess quality in terms of interpersonal relationships and the amenities of care (Donabedian, 1985, p. 12). Research has suggested that "consumers' ratings of care do reflect, at least in part, how many services they received" (Davies and Ware, 1988). Hospital quality is often assessed in regard to the care and concern demonstrated by the nursing staff.

Until very recently, patients' assessments of the quality of care have typically been overlooked or dismissed as too subjective and unreliable. However, the importance of client satisfaction and the interpersonal relationship to the quality of technical care must be considered. First, there is a significant body of research indicating that the quality of the patient–practitioner interaction may be a major contributor to treatment success (Danziger; Svarstad). Second, comparisons of the viewpoints of clients and practitioners suggest that there is, in fact, a great deal of similarity between the two (Donabedian, 1980, p. 73). Finally, the viewpoint of patients must be understood because client satisfaction is in itself an important component of the quality of care and is also important as an assessment of the quality of care. Clients' assessments of quality guide them through the competitive market of health care providers.

Administrators, nurses, and other health care personnel emphasize different aspects of quality from that stressed by physicians and patients. Administrators, for example, tend to focus on the amenities of care, perhaps because this is the area over which they have greatest control. Nurses present something of a middle ground—looking both to indicators of technical competence and interpersonal relations. Recognizing and integrating the legitimacy of these various definitions is essential to the success of current quality-assurance efforts. As health care becomes more of a team effort and as more nonphysician professionals begin to practice independently, the entire focus of quality of care must broaden (Lohr et al.). Definitions of quality in health care can no longer be left solely to physicians and cannot emphasize the technical management of care to the exclusion of its other dimensions. Furthermore, whereas there has been a tendency to define quality in terms of the attributes of facilities and clinicians and of their behavior (Donabedian, 1980, p. 72), there is growing recognition of the need to define quality in terms of the consequences of care.

Quality of Care versus Quantity of Care

Despite certain perceptions to the contrary, more care does not necessarily equal better care. Quality of care may be confused with quantity of care, as exemplified by the finding that consumer ratings of quality do reflect, at least in part, how many services are received (Davies & Ware). Yet closer examination reveals that although there are times when more care does equal better care, there are also times when more is not better but is in fact worse.

The precise relationship between inputs and benefits is not clear in health care. When care received is insufficient to bring about the realizable benefits in patient health and welfare, the care is clearly poor in quality because of quantitative inadequacy (Donabedian, 1980). Such inadequacy is exemplified by an incomplete vaccination series; more care is needed before benefits can be realized. In underdeveloped areas of third world nations, for example, more is almost always definitely better (Maxwell). In such cases, where the existing quality of care is low because of the inadequate quantity of care, improving quality necessarily costs money. Increments in the quality of care require additional services and skills. Eventually, however, a point is reached at which increments in services are unlikely to improve the quality of care. Care can become excessive and even harmful; such care is costlier but of equal or poorer quality. Many would place heroic measures for the terminally ill elderly in this category.

There are many good examples of care that may be simply excessive or unnecessary. Annual Pap smears (Benedet et al.) and routine use of fetal sonograms in low-risk pregnancies (Luthy et al.; McCusker) have been criticized on these grounds. A study of routine annual laboratory screening in an institutionalized elderly population found few additional diagnoses or resulting changes in medical service (Domoto et al.). Such care is excessive but with little attendant risk. It is wasteful in that it is costlier but without corresponding increases in quality (Donabedian, 1980, p. 7). Costs for unnecessary care are hard to justify; resources could be better spent elsewhere.

There are other situations in which additional care is not only excessive or wasteful but also harmful. Routine chest and annual dental x-rays provide good examples of care that is more intensive and expensive yet of poorer quality. Such "ritualistic" care may appear to be of good quality because additional services are being provided, but it offers no real benefit to the patient and introduces potential danger to the patient's physical well-being. Eliminating the use of unnecessary and potentially dangerous medical procedures has been the focus of many cost-containment programs such as "second surgical opinions."

In addition to unnecessary and excessive care, sometimes care is produced inefficiently. In such cases, reducing the costs of care can be achieved not by reducing the quantity of intensity of care per se but rather by producing it more efficiently. Quality need not be sacrificed. Substitution of a nurse-practitioner for a physician visit and use of ambulatory rather than inpatient surgery are two examples of strategies aimed at maintaining quality while reducing costs.

The risks, as well as the financial costs, associated with treatment have often been ignored or glossed over by the medical community. When risks are not considered, it is easy to mistake quantity for quality care. Alternatively, Thurow (1985) suggests that we need to convert the medical community from its traditional reliance on the principle of "do no harm" to one of "employ a treatment only when you are sure that it will make a noticeable improvement."

In contrasting the quality of care with the quantity of care, it is necessary to distinguish between individual and societal needs. There may be times when the extra "unit" of health care cannot be justified in terms of the social good, even if the individual believes it can be justified in terms of personal good. In the debate over annual Pap smears, the discussion focuses on whether the yield from additional screening (identification of women with positive test results) is sufficient to justify the cost. The overall costs are weighed against the overall risks; but for the individual woman whose cancer has gone undetected, one would presume this cost-benefit ratio to be different. As another example of this split between individualistic and communal definitions of quality, some might believe cosmetic surgery to be a form of unnecessary care, even if of high quality in the technical sense.

Donabedian's (1980) "unifying" model represents an effort to bring together the issues of costs, benefits, and risks in assessing the quality of care. At first, benefits of care increase rapidly while the risks of such care remain small. As more services are added, however, the increased or marginal benefits become smaller while the increased or marginal risks become greater. Theoretically, the optimal point—perfect quality—is reached when the benefits minus the risks is greatest (see Figure 14.1). Increased monetary costs may eventually be accompanied by poorer quality, as risks begin to outweigh benefits.

Because it is difficult to objectively identify the "optimal" point in Donabedian's model—where benefits are maximized and risks are minimized—individual consumers, providers, and policymakers must routinely make their own assessments of the trade-off between quality and quantity of care. Such decisions are essential to addressing questions like the following: At what age should women begin routine screening for breast cancer? And at what point do the risks of x-ray exposure from the mammography and the costs of the screening become justified by the ability to identify and treat cancer in its early stages? In trying to assess benefits relative to risk, one must consider the likelihood and magnitude of the potential benefits and risks. Unfortunately, our knowledge of risks and benefits tends to be very limited. We may have some sense of the risks and benefits to large groups, but we possess extremely limited ability to project the risks and benefits in individual cases (and therefore medicine must often be practiced as an "art," not as a "science"). Our ability to make such assessments for groups or individuals is dependent on the availability of accurate information about the risks and benefits associated with procedures and treatments. Such information is the desired product of quality assessments; only by linking care with its consequences can informed decisions be made.

Measuring Quality

Structure, Process, and Outcome

Defining what is meant by the term *quality* in only the first step toward assessing the delivery of health care. Appropriate variables must be identified for assessing the degree to which quality is present. Structure, process, and outcome are the three most commonly defined approaches to gathering information on the presence or absence of the attributes that constitute or define quality. Structure has been defined as "the relatively stable characteristics of the providers of care, of the tools and resources they have at their disposal, and of the physical and organizational settings in which they work" (Donabedian, 1980, p. 81). We may view structure as those things that exist prior to and separate from interaction with patients. Structural indicators that are commonly used include board certification for physicians, nurse/bed ratios for hospitals, and availability of laboratory facilities for HMOs. Structure is an indirect measure of quality; it is useful to the degree that structure can be expected to influence the direct provision of care.

Process concerns the set of activities that go on between practitioners and patients; it may be seen as the object of assessment. Process measures may be used to assess the quality of the technical management of care (e.g., was the appropriate laboratory test ordered?), as well as the interpersonal aspects of care (e.g., was the medical history taken in a sensitive and caring manner?). Process may be viewed as what is done to patients, whereas outcomes are what happens to them (Hogness). Outcome refers to a change in a patient's current and future health status that can be attributed to antecedent health care (Donabedian, 1980, p. 83). Outcome measures include mortality rates, postoperative infection rates, and rates of rehospitalizations.

The Causal Model. Before we can use structure, process, or outcome measures to assess quality, it is important that we understand something about the relationship among all three. The underlying *causal model* in most quality assessments is that structure influences the process of care, which has an impact on the outcome of care. In other words, the basis for the judgment of quality is what is known about the relationship between the characteristics of the structure and processes of the care that is delivered and their subsequent impact on the health and welfare of individuals and of society. Most definitions of quality assume that the application of the appropriate process of care will maximize patient outcomes (Lohr et al.). However, the validity, or justifiability, of this inference must be established; there is considerable disagreement about cause and effect in health care.

Scientific research methods, especially those of program evaluation, are used to establish the links between particular structures and processes and the desired outcomes. Scientific methods are used to test whether changes in health status (outcome) are really the result of the care given. Are board-certified physicians (structure) more likely to make appropriate use of laboratory tests (process)? And does the appropriate utilization of laboratory tests have an impact on patient recovery (outcome)? Do second surgical opinion programs (structure) influence the use of surgery (process)? And does this have an impact on patient health (outcome)? Once the relationships between structure, process, and outcome are established, we can choose to focus on one area of measurement and have greater confidence that it is, in fact, providing a good indicator of quality.

"Structure 7 . . . is relevant to quality in that it increases or decreases the probability of good performance" (Donabedian, 1980, p. 82). Despite the fact that structure has been a commonly used indicator of quality, there is insufficient information about the relationship between structure and performance. We know relatively little about when and how structural indicators (e.g., board certification for physicians, bachelor's degrees for nurses, university affiliation for hospitals) influence the processes and outcomes of care. Structure is, at best, a crude measure of quality because it can address only general tendencies. However, information on structural indicators is generally easy and inexpensive to access and measure, whereas information on the process and outcomes of care is often unavailable, incomplete, or expensive. Therefore, in those cases in which there is sufficient information to link structural characteristics with the quality of care that is provided, structure can provide an important measure of protecting and promoting high-quality health care.

As already noted, process is the most direct measure of quality. A great virtue of process evaluation lies in the broad clinician involvement and education that is a consequence and may subsequently result in improved practices (Blum). Process measures tend to be more timely than outcome measures. But their validity as a measure is limited to the extent that their relationship to outcomes has been well established. When the link between process and outcome has been validated, process indicators become an important tool for assessing and assuring quality in a direct and timely fashion. Because we know that immunizations are critical to the promotion of children's health, we know that completed immunization series (or lack of completion) provide a valid process indicator for assessing the quality of pediatric practice. Too often what is described as high-quality care has not been demonstrated to have much of an impact on the health status of the patients. The Congressional Office of Technology Assessment has estimated that only 10 to 20% of clinician practices are supported by randomized controlled trials (Eddy & Billings, 1988). In other words, for most health care practices there is a lack of proof of the efficacy of the treatment. Use of process indicators, in the absence of a scientifically tested causal model, can result in the perpetuation of expensive and ineffective practice.

Whereas the validity of elements of process depends on the contribution of process to outcome, outcomes tend to be inherently valid because change in health status and patient well-being is the ultimate goal of health care. When high-quality care is delivered, we expect improvement in such outcomes as mortality, morbidity, or social functioning. But before outcomes are used to make inferences about the quality of care, it is necessary to establish that the outcomes can be attributed to that care. Intervening factors must be ruled out; were the changes in health really the result of the care that was provided? Health care is but one factor influencing an individual's or community's health status. We must have some confidence that the change in outcome that is identified can be seen as resulting from the care that has been given. Would the improvement in the patient's health have occurred without the treatment? Conversely, poor resulting outcomes must not be simplistically attributed solely to current failures of the health care organization or process (Blum). Release of hospital-based mortality rates by the federal government's Health Care Financing Administration (HCFA) has been criticized on these grounds; there is insufficient evidence to attribute the mortality to poor hospital performance. Rather, differences in the patient mix (one aspect of structure) may be the cause for many of the differences in mortality rates. The HCFA has acknowledged that "preventable deaths" would be a more valid indicator of quality of care (Roper & Hackbarth). Yet current plans are "to measure the performance of individual physicians by seeing how well their patients do" ("US Plans"). Health outcomes are presented as a valid indicator of the quality of care that has been provided, but without scientific evidence testing this assumption the linkage may be tenuous at best.

Examples of Research Studies. Numerous research studies have tried to link structure with process, and process with outcome. One recent study compared the complication rates (outcome) for first-trimester abortions performed by physician assistants (PAs) and physicians (structure) (Freedman et al.). The researchers found no difference between the PAs and physicians with respect to overall, immediate, or delayed complications. However, one of the two abortion procedures (process) that was studied was associated with an increased number of delayed complications regardless of provider type. In this case the structural factor did not seem to have an impact on the process or outcome of care. The process did, however, make a difference in terms of health outcome. Dissemination of these findings can enhance the quality of care that is provided.

In another study, process and outcome criteria were separately applied for evaluating the quality of hypertension care. No statistically significant association was detected between process and outcome. "[C]omparisons between the proportion of all process criteria items completed and the outcome by level of diastolic blood pressure at follow-up examination" did not indicate that improved outcomes could be attributed to high-quality process (Nobrega et al., p. 147). Despite low physician compliance with established criteria, the outcome of care among the group of hypertensive patients was rather good. This demonstrates the potential danger of using either process or outcome measures without validating the relationship between them.

As indicated earlier, quality also may be influenced by patient characteristics. Many studies of quality have linked process and outcome with patient characteristics. For example, one study found that older patients receive inadequate treatment for breast cancer, even when controlling for stage of disease, co-morbidity, and functional status (Greenfield et al.). The patient's characteristics influenced the process to be used.

Formulation of Criteria and Standards

Whether one decides to approach the assessment of quality via indices concerning structure, process, or outcome, specific criteria or standards must be formulated. Before we can assess or monitor the quality of care, the abstract construct of quality must be translated into concrete variables, and those variables must be made measurable, or "operationalized." Differences in structure, process, and outcomes across practitioners, institutions, or regions do not, in and of themselves, indicate the appropriate level or highest quality of care. Rather, these standards must be established through scientific study or consensus.

Measurement is important to the assessment and assurance of quality, for it is through measurement that we can make precise comparisons of benefits and risks. In selecting appropriate quality measures, note that no single indicator can capture the entire concept of quality or even any major component of it. Indeed, there may be certain aspects of quality that are all but impossible to measure. Therefore, it is important to use multiple operational definitions or measures that can account for the broadest understanding of quality. For example, in a study comparing costs and benefits of hospice and conventional care for terminally ill cancer patients, a broad range of criteria and measures had to be developed, including measures of pain, symptoms, and activities of daily living, as well as patient and family satisfaction (Kane et al., p. 159). Any single measure would have provided an incomplete and misleading assessment of the quality of care provided.

The criteria or measures that are selected in conducting a quality assessment or program of quality assurance can themselves be assessed in regard to a number of desirable attributes. Measures should be both valid and reliable. Reliability concerns the accuracy of observed score; how well does the measure reflect the true score? Reliable measures do not fluctuate randomly from one moment to the next; this is called test–retest reliability. Reliable measures yield the same results regardless of who is making the rating; this is called interrater reliability. Mortality data tend to be highly reliable; psychiatric and social assessments do not.

The validity of a measure concerns how well it really reflects the concept being assessed. A reliable measure is not necessarily a valid one. Although a yardstick is a highly reliable measure (two people using the same yardstick are likely to come up with the same measure), it would not be a valid measure of weight. Analogously, although mortality data are considered highly reliable, they may be invalid indicators of quality of care. The validity of a measure may be considered in terms of its correlation or convergence with other measures of the same concept; if several different measures of the same concept all lead to the same conclusions, we can have greater confidence that the individual measures are valid. If we were trying to rate physician performance, we might include a review of lab tests ordered, an assessment of the medical histories taken, and a judgment of the quality of the medical record; if all three measures led to the same conclusion about the physician's performance, we would have greater confidence about the validity of any one measure. Validity of measures also may be considered in terms of their ability to distinguish between cases that are known to differ and in terms of their predictive power.

The scientific validity of a measure is based on a demonstrated causal relationship, as described above. However, in the absence of a scientifically demonstrated relationship, "normative validity" is often substituted. Normative validity rests on the presence of professional consensus (e.g., agreement among physicians), so it also might be called consensual validity (Donabedian, 1980). In conducting an assessment of the quality of care, process elements may be used if there is general agreement that certain procedures are appropriate for certain situations, even though there is no "scientific proof" of appropriateness (Donabedian, 1980). The problem with relying on measures that have normative validity, as compared to scientific validity, is that it can lead to the perpetuation of ineffective process. Process measures, which typically possess normative or consensual validity, evaluate conformity to a given standard of performance but do not evaluate the adequacy of the standards themselves (Flood & Scott).

As a result of the lack of information linking process to outcomes, there is also a tendency to apply the criterion of potential benefit. In this framework a practice is considered appropriate if it *might* have benefit (Eddy & Billings, 1988, p. 27). The appeal of the criterion of potential benefit is that it is easy to apply and it deals smoothly with the uncertainty that surrounds many practices. As an example, in some hospitals fetal monitors are used in all pregnancies, not just high-risk deliveries, because it can be difficult to assess risk, and there might be some rare cases where otherwise unidentified problems would be found. Unfortunately, the criterion of potential benefit translates easily into "when in doubt, do it." The criterion is sorely lacking in those cases in which the benefits do not clearly outweigh the potential risks.

Explicit or implicit criteria may be used in operationalizing a variable. Implicit criteria include unguided, individual judgments of quality or unstructured observations. Quality assessments—particularly peer reviews—often rely on the implicit judgment of physicians, who may review a medical record or observe a patient encounter and, without any stated guidelines, make an assessment of quality. This can be contrasted with explicit criteria, which are preformulated and provide the rater with clear guidance in making an assessment. "Preformulated explicit criteria and standards are meant to ensure that the best professional opinion is used uniformly and consistently in judging the quality of care" (Donabedian, 1985, p. 184). In some cases the criteria may fall between the two extremes; record review with guidance provides an example of guided or structured implicit criteria (Donabedian, 1985).

Sources of Information

To determine the kinds of measures that should be used to assess and ensure quality of care, it is necessary to consider the possible sources of data. Data may be gathered through interviews, observations, or record review. Each method of data collection has its strengths and limitations. Data collection methods may be compared in terms of costs, acceptability, reliability, and validity (Gerbert). Generally, the method becomes more expensive and less feasible if it requires information that is not routinely collected. However, routinely gathered data may not have quality assessment and assurance as its primary focus; the available information may be only an indirect and incomplete measure of quality. Furthermore, in comparing data collection strategies we need to distinguish techniques of rating performance from those of reporting performance; the former involves a value judgment (e.g., a patient may be asked to assess the quality of a physician visit), whereas reporting concerns the presentation of the objective details of an interaction (e.g., a physician is asked to report on all lab tests performed during a visit).

Structural Measures. Structural measures tend to be the easiest for which to obtain data. Many structural measures involve simple counts of things—number of beds, number of RNs, number of board-certified surgeons—and such data collection has become a routine part of accreditation and certification procedures (discussed in greater detail below). Structural information on health care institutions is regularly compiled by a range of public and not-for-profit agencies and is often available in computerized form. However, obtaining information about the process and outcomes of care is more difficult. To assess the process of care one must know how the practitioner conducts himself or herself. Gaining insight into the process of care must typically be gathered in an indirect manner.

The Medical Record. Medical records are the most commonly used source of information on the quality of the process of care. Record review or chart audit is an integral part of many quality-assurance and cost-containment programs, such as utilization review. Ideally, the medical record provides information on patient symptoms, the tests and procedures that were undertaken, and patient progress. It should provide an accurate and detailed report of the medical process. Unfortunately, in reality, medical records rarely reach the ideal standard because they tend to be incomplete. Medical record keeping is local and uses practice-specific terminology; this fragmentation means that information on diagnosis, treatment, and outcomes cannot be linked across settings (Lohr et al.). Problems with the medical record are especially acute in ambulatory care settings, which are less likely to be subject to institutional constraints. Rating the process of care based on the medical record can be questionable given the incomplete nature of reporting practice.

Access is the most attractive characteristic of the medical record. The information is routinely gathered; using it for quality assessment involves limited additional expense or time. In addition to the medical record, insurance claims, drug prescriptions, and malpractice suits also may provide readily accessible information on the process of care. One advantage of such information over the medical record is its greater uniformity. The chief disadvantage is limited focus; quality can be measured only in relatively narrow terms. However, use of information such as insurance claims, if properly organized, can permit relatively inexpensive, large-scale quality assessment and assurance activities. Recognizing the potential benefit of such a system of information, a General Accounting Office (GAO) report suggested that "a centralized medical malpractice information system would help identify recurring problems, including problems with individual medical care providers, and focus attention on needed corrective and preventive actions" (Baines).

Observations of Process. Another method of obtaining data on the process of care is via direct observation. Several studies have been undertaken to observe, and in some cases videotape, the physician–patient interaction. Because the observation allows actual viewing of the process of care and the videotape provides a record of that process, it has often been assumed that this method would provide a perfect report of the care provided. However, videotaped observations have been found to be time-consuming, costly, and difficult to standardize (Gerbert et al.). Of even greater importance, even if such time and cost concerns were eliminated, recent studies have indicated that "videotaped observation does not adequately capture the content of visits to the physician in areas of medication regimen, patient signs and symptoms, tests and treatments recommended, and patient education" (Gerbert et al., p. 530). Finally, there has been limited discussion about the degree to which observation biases the process of care. That is, does a provider (and a patient) change his or her practice style (behavior) when under observation?

Patient and Practitioner Interviews. In addition to chart or record audit and direct observation, information may be obtained by directly interviewing providers and patients. It has been suggested that the provider is the most accurate source of reported information regarding the process of care (Gerbert et al). But physician interviews are a very expensive source of information and may not be a good source of information on the nontechnical aspects of care. In contrast, getting information from consumers of care may be no more expensive, and under many circumstances it is less expensive than traditional sources such as the medical record (Davies & Ware). There is also good evidence that the information reported by patients is valid and reliable. The consumer seems to be able to distinguish poor-quality from high-quality care, especially for common problems. Most crucially, the consumer is probably in the best position to rate the interpersonal aspects of care.

Methods of Assessment

Researchers in the area of quality assessment have developed a broad range of techniques and methods for conducting quality assessments. Overall, methods may be characterized in terms of those that assess the quality of care relative to a positive standard (i.e., what should have been done or what should have occurred) and those that assess it relative to a negative standard (i.e., what should not have been done or what should not have occurred). In regard to the former, we are trying to define and measure good-quality care; in the latter we are looking for evidence of poor-quality care. Generally, it is agreed that it is easier to define and identify cases of poor quality than of high quality. For example, we can look for interventions that are either obsolete or so rarely indicated that their mere use is reason enough to question the quality of care (Donabedian, 1985). Prescription patterns can be especially useful after drugs that are ineffective or hazardous have been identified.

Assessments that focus on unnecessary or inappropriate care can be conducted prospectively (that is, before care is provided) or retrospectively (after care is provided). For example, if we are interested in using unnecessary surgical procedures as an indicator of poor quality of care, second surgical opinions would provide a prospective means of approach (how often does the second opinion contradict the first physician's recommendation?). Tissue analysis provides a retrospective method of using the same indicator, unnecessary surgery (how often does the tissue analysis indicate that a healthy organ was removed?).

Assessments focusing on the use of inappropriate techniques and interventions have found poor quality of care to be concentrated; that is, a very small percentage of physicians tend to account for a large proportion of poor-quality care (Donabedian, 1985).

Utilization review is another example of quality assessment and assurance that identifies cases of poor-quality or inappropriate care. Inappropriate hospital utilization may arise from inappropriate admissions, delayed discharges, or extra days during which services are not fully provided (Donabedian, 1985, p. 78). Utilization review tends to emphasize the "overstay," not the "understay," as an indicator of poor quality.

Williamson's (1978) health accounting method focuses on "achievable benefits" rather than process indicators of quality care. It looks at patient groups to see if the quality of care is adequate. Acceptable outcome standards are set for the group, and if there are substantial failures, corrective action is to be taken. Stress is placed on those areas of care most likely to be deficient and most amenable to change.

Prospective outcome analysis is another method, or system, that has been suggested for using outcomes to assess quality (Blum). It also sets positive standards for overall outcomes. Aimed at institutional self-assessment as a means of quality assurance, a medically expert committee selects the most important conditions to be studied—based on such criteria as prevalence, cost, and danger—and establishes standards or best expectations of specified outcomes for selected conditions. If the outcomes on a sample of cases are significantly worse than expected, the committee then does a critical analysis of each case with a poor outcome. Quality assurance grows from this assessment process as the institution changes to avoid failures and continues checking outcomes against its standards until the desired outcome is reached.

Quality Assurance

Measuring or assessing the quality of care does not, unfortunately, result in immediate improvements in that care. Simply defining what is meant by "high quality" care does not guarantee its implementation. Quality-assurance activities are intended to translate the concepts and findings of research assessments into programs that will ensure that the care that is delivered is of the highest quality possible. The emphasis shifts from measurement to control.

Efforts at quality assurance take place at the local and the national level. They are geared toward both individuals and institutions. Currently, professional associations, health care institutions and organizations, government, private external quality-review organizations, and group purchasers of care all play a role in quality assurance. Professional associations use such means as specialty board certification and continuing medical education requirements for recertification. Hospitals and HMOs have their own internal quality-assurance programs (e.g., JCAHO). State governments operate through licensure of individuals and institutions. The federal government imposes its quality-assurance standards though Medicaid and Medicare reimbursement. But regardless of the organization or its focus, quality-assurance activities are in flux. The dynamic nature of quality-assurance activities results, at least in part, from our insufficient knowledge about the effectiveness of various methods for assuring quality care.

Organizational Considerations in Assuring Quality

To assure good-quality care, we need to know something about changing or modifying the behaviors of providers and the organizations in which they practice. And organizational change creates strains and tensions; it raises conflict between the norms of professional freedom and bureaucratic autonomy (Hetherington).

Professional autonomy may represent one of the most important impediments to health institutions' becoming more fully accountable for the care they provide. Doctors have traditionally operated as free agents within the hospital structure. In contrast, nurses have traditionally been accountable to physicians. As quality-assurance activities have grown, hospitals (as well as other health care organizations) have imposed new restrictions and requirements on physicans. Resistance is an expected by-product of these changes. In recent years, as the accountability obligations of health institutions has been formalized, the potential for conflict between institutional goals of self-regulation and the autonomy requirements of clinicians has grown.

Despite resistance and the obstacles posed by the tradition of autonomy, it is possible to improve the quality of care and to hold clinicians and organizations accountable for the care given. Even within the context of a change-resistant environment, we know a great deal about the ways in which health care delivery can be shaped or modified. For example, we know that quality-assurance activities are more likely to succeed when professionals have played an active role in developing and administering the regulations. There is also evidence to suggest that to change physician behavior, information must come from a credible source (e.g., a professional organization) and should be backed with financial incentives (Ball). In accordance with these ideas, the American College of Physicians has taken an unusually active role in setting and disseminating standards for care and guidelines for reimbursement (Ball). It is easier to change behavior when there is considerable consensus about what constitutes quality care. In one study, researchers attributed the success of an on-side educational program to reduce inappropriate use of x-ray pelvimetry to the considerable consensus surrounding the use of this procedure (Chassin & McCue). Institutional commitment to change also may play a role in modifying providers' behaviors. Slenker et al. (1985) looked at the impact of establishing procedural guidelines for physicians, nurses, and allied health professionals in the diagnosis and treatment of cancer. Factors contributing to program success were hospital commitment to the program, ready availability of guidelines, and mandatory participation in the educational program.

It also may be important to target quality-assurance activities at those areas that most need improvement. One institutional quality-assurance program in hypertension, which employed concurrent and peer comparison feedback, found that the program had no impact. However, the program failed because the providers were already committed to controlling blood pressure and aware of modern approaches to improving compliance (Winickoff et al.). Before we attempt to improve the quality of care given, we need to be certain that such change is really necessary.

General Approaches to Quality Assurance

Licensing, accreditation, and certification are three general approaches to quality assurance. They are similar in that they assess an individual's or institution's ability to provide quality care on the basis of meeting established criteria at a particular time. The underlying assumption of these approaches is that education and current knowledge, as measured by a written examination, are good predictors of future performance—or in the case of health care organizations, that the presence of certain equipment, personnel, and organizational arrangements promises the delivery of high-quality care over an extended period of time.

General approaches tend to use structural criteria for assessing quality, and as a result, structure is perhaps the most important single factor in what is typically called quality assurance. Licensing, accreditation, and certification represent most of the earliest quality-assurance activities. They aimed to ensure quality by guaranteeing the presence of certain fundamental structural characteristics of the institution or individual.

Licensing. Licensing may be distinguished from all other quality assurance activities because it is backed by the force of law. The states have been empowered under the U.S. Constitution to license both individuals and institutions; that is, the state is permitted to restrict certain activities (e.g., the performance of surgery or a dental exam) to those individuals and institutions it has determined to possess acceptable standards. Thirty-five different health professions and occupations are currently licensed by one or more states, as are a broad array of health care facilities (Wilson & Neuhauser).

Individual and Medical Licensure. In licensing individuals, the state enters into a compact with a professional group. The professional group assumes responsibility for controlling the quality of work provided, and the state grants the professional group the right to control entry into the professional group and, in many cases, to define the content of that work. Licensing grants the professional group a legal monopoly over that area of work, a monopoly backed by the state's law enforcement power. Licenses are granted to a wide range of occupations. Among the occupations that are licensed by all states are medicine, dentistry, pharmacy, nursing, nursing home administration, and podiatry. In some states occupations such as laboratory technicians, midwives, and psychologists also are licensed. Generally, the professional organization (e.g., nursing) establishes standards based on educational attainment, experience, and performance on a written exam. Once a license is granted, it is typically valid for life; in the absence of egregious conduct, licenses are rarely suspended or revoked.

The use of licensure as a method of ensuring quality is a source of great controversy. There is ample evidence that licensure serves, first and foremost, to foster guildism; that is, rather than protecting the public, there is evidence that licensure protects the professional group and its members from competition and public scrutiny. Licensing makes it difficult to change occupations within the health care sector. As a result of licensing restrictions, the most qualified labor-room nurse may not be able to take responsibility for a baby's delivery. Licensing also makes it difficult for a professional to move from one state to another. A highly qualified physician from New York may not be able to practice in Florida. Most significantly, there is little evidence to indicate that the criteria used in licensing actually predict the quality of care to be delivered.

Even if the criteria used for licensing were valid, it is unreasonable to expect that they would be valid throughout a person's life. In a dynamic field, knowledge at the time of graduation from medical school is unlikely to be a good indicator of knowledge 20 years after graduation. Licensing for life is beginning to give way to periodic reevaluation. For example, the New York State Board of Regents is reviewing a plan whereby doctors, who now receive a single lifelong license from the state education department, would be required to submit to peer review or a written exam every 9 years. Those who fail to pass either the review of the examination could have their licenses revoked. Under this plan, those not in active practice, such as administrators or retired doctors, could put their licenses in "escrow" and reactivate them by taking an exam if they returned to practice. As one might guess, the medical profession has strongly opposed this plan ("State Readies").

The issues posed by licensing are especially complicated in the case of physicians. Physicians are in an unusual professional position; they do not merely control their own work but are also the dominant professional group throughout the health care arena (Freidson). This position of professional dominance has effectively shielded doctors from public scrutiny and accountability. There is a growing belief that the public has not been well served by this isolation.

One area of "self-policing" that has received considerable attention is the disciplinary actions of the state medical boards, which are responsible for licensure. Although increasing in number, such disciplinary actions continue to be the exception. One recent study indicated that the number of reprimands and censures has grown. However, revocations and suspensions of licenses remain relatively constant, despite an increase in the number of practicing physicians (Kusserow et al.). That is, the rate of suspending licenses has actually decreased. In this study it was also found that most reports to state medical boards are provided by consumers and law enforcement agencies, not by health care professionals, hospitals, or peer review organizations. Three-quarters of all disciplinary actions are for inappropriate prescription writing. The state licensing procedures were criticized because they permitted doctors to voluntarily give up licenses in one state and resume practice in another. In order to make licensing an effective tool in the pursuit of quality care, it is critical to encourage the sharing of information among states, to close loopholes that permit interstate movement and continued participation in the Medicaid and Medicare programs, and to increase the funds available to state disciplinary boards (Kusserow et al).

Institutional Licensure. All states license hospitals (short- and long-stay, general, and/or psychiatric), nursing homes, and pharmacies (Wilson & Neuhauser). States also typically license such facilities as homes for the mentally retarded. Certain services such as ambulances and home health care also are licensed in some states.

Licensing of facilities is usually accomplished directly by a state agency—for example, the state health department. Institutional licenses may be granted for a period of 1 or more years. The criteria for licensing typically emphasize structural elements like bed/nurse ratios and the presence of appropriate equipment. Licensing boards for institutions tend to be less completely dominated by providers from the regulated institution than are those for licensing individuals.

Accreditation and Certification. Although licensing is critical to understanding the role of government in the assurance of quality, voluntarism has long characterized the prime approach to quality assurance in health care (Luke & Modrow, 1983). Voluntary self-regulation is reflected in both accrediting boies (like the JCAHO) and professional certification boards. Accreditation is limited to institutions, whereas certification applies to individuals.

The basic principles of accreditation are similar to those of licensure; it is assumed that if the institution meets certain standards of physical and organizational structure, then good-quality care will be delivered at that time and the future. In the case of accreditation, groups of like institutions or organizations with mutual interests come together to set up an organization, establish standards, and proceed to inspect and "accredit" themselves on a periodic basis. Although accreditation is not a legal procedure, there are strong legal and financial incentives for undergoing accreditation. For example, the Medicare laws restricts payments that may be made to unaccredited hospitals, and state education departments will not recognize diplomas from medical schools that are not accredited.

The recently renamed JCAHO is perhaps the oldest and best known of the accrediting bodies in health care. Changes in accrediting standards issued by the Joint Commission over the past two decades are reflective of the changing nature of quality assurance. Traditionally reliant on minimal structural standards, in 1966 JCAH's board of commissioners voted to rewrite the standards to raise them from "minimal essential" to "optimal achievable" standards. In 1975 numerical requirements for audit were established to ensure optimal care (Shanahan). In 1979 new standards were issued that eliminated the numerical audit requirement and directed hospitals to develop a hospital-wide program that integrates all quality-assurance activities (Roberts). The new requirements for accreditation deemphasize specific approaches and emphasize flexible ongoing quality-assurance activities and coordinated systems. In the most recent version each hospital must provide a written plan for a coordinated, comprehensive system for quality assurance that includes problem identification and resolution.

Medical school education is another area in which accreditation plays a critical role. Medical schools are accredited by the Liaison Committee on Medical Education. The AMA and the Association of American Medical Colleges are equally represented on the committee. Separate accrediting bodies review postgraduate medical education and accredit residency programs. Training for other health care occupations also takes place in accredited programs or schools; accreditation is carried out by a range of boards and agencies representing such fields as dentistry, medical technology, and health services administration.

Certification, like accreditation, represents a form of voluntary self-regulation. And although certification is not backed by law, there are incentives that encourage individual practitioners to seek certification. For example, some third-party payers will reimburse visits only to certified social workers. Of great consequence, most hospitals limit privileges to board-certified specialties. Certification uses standards of education, experience, and achievement on examinations to determine qualification.

A great diversity of health care occupations have certifying bodies. In nursing alone there are 23 different organizations that offer certification in nursing or one of its subspecialties (Scofield). These include the American Nurses Association, the Oncology Nursing Certification Corporation, and the Association of Operating Room Nurses.

Within the field of medicine, certification plays a critical role in the designation of specialists. Certification is granted by specialty boards approved by the AMA through its Council on Medical Education. These medical specialty boards rely entirely on structural criteria of assessment, and certification of medical specialists is, typically, for life.

Specific Approaches to Quality Assurance

Specific approaches to quality assurance look at discrete instances of provider–patient interaction. Whereas general approaches typically focus on structure, specific approaches emphasize process and outcome. Specific approaches include medical staff review committees, peer review organizations, and malpractice litigation. They also include reimbursement review, such as second opinion programs and preadmission review, by third-party payers.

Review Committees. Hospital medical staff review committees are the most common of the specific approaches used for quality assurance in the United States. The JCAHO requires that the hospital medical staff be organized to provide for the review of the quality of care, utilization of hospital services, products of surgery, use of therapeutic agents, medical records, blood and blood products, infection control, disaster plans, and hospital safety (Fifer, 1983). Despite their prevalence as a mechanism for quality assurance, little is known about the activities of review committees or their impact on the quality of services provided. However, a lack of communication across committees has been noted; this hinders quality improvement and recognition of problem areas. There is also indication that hospitals have been reticent to engage actively in problem identification, perhaps for fear that litigation will result.

PSROs and PROs. Professional Standards Review Organizations (PSROs) were established by the 1972 amendments to the Social Security Act. They represented a major step toward institutionalizing peer review of individual instances of physician care and the quality of care provided outside the hospital setting. The purpose of the law was to involve local practicing physicians in the ongoing review and evaluation of health services covered by Medicare, Medicaid, or the Maternal and Child Health programs of the Department of Health and Human Services. PSROs were charged with the dual role of quality assurance and utilization review (which had previously been the function of the medical staff review committees). Most PSRO activity focused on utilization review, rather than overall quality assurance, and cost containment became the hallmark of the PSRO's own measure of success. Established in 195 geographic areas, the PSROs were limited in their efficacy as a tool for quality assurance by physician protectionism, lack of concern for the nontechnical aspects of care, and overemphasis on cost containment.

Despite campaign promises to abolish PSROs, the Reagan administration encouraged the passage of legislation that created the successor to the PSRO system. Peer Review Organizations (PROs), which went into operation in 1984, can be distinguished from PSROs in a number of ways. PROs review only Medicare; Medicaid review was to be left to the states. The law called for one PRO per state, greatly reducing the number of organizations involved. Physician-based organizations were given a prominent role in the control of the PROs. Under the PRO system, disciplinary procedures were simplified, and a ban was placed on delegating review functions to hospitals.

Perhaps of greatest importance to the achievement of quality standards, PROs are awarded fixed-price contracts that specify, in numerical terms, the results to be achieved. For example, some of the PROs' objectives focus on reducing inappropriate admissions; others focus on reducing admissions overall. Because of the specific nature of the objectives, PROs were given an increased incentive to actually try to change physician behavior.

Malpractice Litigation. Malpractice litigation also can be seen as a specific approach to quality assurance. Malpractice is one measure of patient satisfaction (or, more accurately, dissatisfaction) with the care received. Malpractice focuses on extreme cases of poor-quality care, rather than trying to assure ongoing high standards of care. Using malpractice as a tool for quality assurance shifts the focus away from frequent but low-cost errors to infrequent and high-cost ones. Malpractice is not an effective tool for trying to control the overprescription of antibiotic drugs, for example, because the damages accruing to any one individual are generally not of the magnitude to instigate a legal suit.

Although not a new problem per se, malpractice litigation is seen as a growing problem in the United States, threatening the solvency of some institutions and the practice of some physicians. It is not clear, however, the degree to which the malpractice "crisis" is a function of a more litigious society, dishonest practices by insurance companies, declining patient–provider relations, or the unwillingness of the medical profession to engage in effective quality control, especially in regard to disciplining those physicians responsible for a significant share of practice error. Consumer advocate Ralph Nader wrote that "the root cause of the malpractice insurance crisis is malpractice compounded by very weak disciplining of incompetent or negligent physicians who should not be practicing medicine at all" (Fuchsberg).

A number of solutions to the malpractice crisis have been suggested, including tort reforms, which have been implemented in several states. For example, in Georgia, immunity has been granted to providers who give care without compensation and to medical students. Virginia gives immunity to providers who render emergency care without pay (Burda, 1987). New York State has passed legislation limiting malpractice premiums and has considered establishing a "medical indemnity fund" for future medical expenses over $100,000 (Fuchsberg). Other suggestions have included upper limits on the dollar amount that can be awarded for pain and suffering and shorter statutes of limitations. Both consumer and attorney groups have fought such restrictions on malpractice litigation, arguing that tort reform begs the question of reducing the incidence of malpractice.

By contrast, the use of "early warning systems" to identify potentially compensable hospital events has proved to be a successful method of averting liability claims. Such systems have helped hospitals to identify recurring problems and to diffuse some situations (Burda, 1986).

Representing new federal action in this area, Congress enacted the Health Care Quality Improvement Act of 1986 (1) to moderate the incidence of malpractice, (2) to allow the medical community to demonstrate new willingness to weed out incompetents, and (3) to improve the base of timely and accurate information on medical malpractice (Waxman). The law, which was supported by a number of medical and hospital organizations, provides broader legal protection to hospitals and physicians engaging in peer review activities. Doctors who are disciplined as a result of peer review may not sue their reviewers. In exchange, the law requires professional societies, health care organizations, and insurance companies to report to a national data base all disciplinary action taken against physicians and all settlements and verdicts in medical malpractice cases (Iglehart). Further, hospitals must regularly request information on their physician staff from this clearinghouse. The act represents Congress's belief that "peer review has been used as a shield for activities that had an anticompetitive effect and purpose" and has served the self-interest of physicians and hospitals rather than the public interest (Waxman).

Economic Approaches. Third-party payers also have initiated a number of activities that can be viewed as specific approaches to quality assurance. Although such activities are often primarily concerned with cost containment, they serve a quality-assurance function to the degree that they reduce unnecessary or excessive use of care. Second surgical opinion programs, preadmission review, and diagnosis related groups (DRGs) all aim to reduce costs by eliminating unnecessary or excessive care. In addition to third-party payers, employers and unions who must foot the bill for insurance premiums also have begun to play a role in this dual area of cost containment and quality assurance. For example, the Ford Motor Company has been working with Southeast Michigan Hospital Council to reduce costs through reductions in unnecessary medical treatment and by examining quality review programs (Powills).

Unfortunately, there is limited reason to be optimistic about the potential of cost-containment efforts to enhance quality. Economic solutions seem to impact as much on appropriate care as they do on inappropriate care (Brook, 1988). Evidence from the Rand Health Insurance Experiment suggests that cost sharing for inpatient and outpatient care reduces the use of effective and presumably needed services about as much as it lowers the use of ineffective or unnecessary services (Lohr et al.). Before cost-containment efforts can be expected to have a positive impact on quality, economic solutions must be coupled with medical solutions. Some argue that medicine must begin to be codified (in what Brook [1988] has termed a "gourmet cookbook") and that physicians must be rewarded for appropriate medical practice. Recent history suggests, however, that those who pay for care, whether governmental or private, may be more interested in cost containment than in quality assurance (Lohr et al.). Concerns about the overuse of care have shifted to concerns about underuse (e.g., the "quicker and sicker" phenomenon). There is growing debate about whether financial incentives to shift or control expenditures will lead to the underprovision or underuse of needed and appropriate services and, in turn, to adverse effects on health outcomes and patient well-being (Lohr et al.).

Some Further Issues

Quality Assurance or Cost Containment?

As has already been suggested, health care policymakers, program managers, and practitioners are experiencing a growing tension between the goals of cost containment and quality assurance. Whereas the earliest attempts to contain cost could readily be coupled with efforts to enhance quality (i.e., by eliminating excessive and unnecessary care), we may have reached a point in the evolution of the U.S. health care system at which efforts to contain costs will have a negative impact on quality. The public and their representatives will be faced with hard choices in trying to assess the pros and cons of these trade-offs.

Early in this chapter it was noted that before one can try to assure quality, one must be able to identify it. This continues to be the critical dilemma. If costs are to be reduced without hindering quality care, we must be able to weed out the good from the bad. Our abilities in this area remain weak. The HCFA's use of mortality data as an indicator of hospital quality has been criticized as inappropriate and misleading because it does not adequately control for variations in the patient mix. Yet the called-for measures of unjustifiable deaths (as compared with all patient deaths) remain elusive.

Quality Assurance and Staff Shortages

Limitations in our ability to identify the necessary components for providing quality care also will impinge on our ability to respond effectively to the changing nature of the health care delivery system and the environment in which it operates. In particular, how can we maintain quality care during a period when staff shortages are endemic. If falling medical school enrollments continue, the shortage of nurses may soon be accompanied by an unexpected physician shortage, especially in primary care areas. How can we effectively respond when we continue to be uncertain about the elements of structure (e.g., nurse-to-bed ratios) necessary to ensure good outcomes?

The Costs of Quality Assessment and Assurance Activities

Finally, there is rising concern about the costs incurred when engaging in quality-assurance activities. In a time of increasingly limited health care resources, are the costs associated with quality assessment and quality assurance justified by cost savings or improvements in quality (Thompson, et al.)? We must be diligent to see that quality assessment and assurance activities continue to play key roles in solving the problems of the health care system and do not themselves become part of the problem.

References

American Medical Association Council on Medical Service. "Quality of Care." *Journal of the American Medical Association, 256,* 8, 1986.

Baines, D. P. "DOD Health Care." Statement given by the General Accounting Office before the U.S. House of Representatives Subcommittee on Military Personnel and Compensation, July 21 1987.

Ball, J. R. *Physician Payment: Why Money Doesn't Buy Quality.* Presentation made at the Association for Health Services Research, San Francisco, June 1988.

Benedet, J. L., et al. "Cervical Cancer Screening: Who Needs a Pap Test? How Often?" *Postgraduate Medicine, 78,* 8, 1985.

Blum, H. L. "Evaluating Health Care." *Medical Care, 12,* 12, 1974.

Brook, R. H. *Physician Payment: Why Money Doesn't Buy Quality.* Presentation made at the Association for Health Services Research, San Francisco, June 1988.

Burda, D. "Law." *Hospitals, 60,* p. 33, May 20, 1986.

Burda, D. "New Tests Reform." *Hospitals, 61,* 8, 1987.

Caper, P. "Defining Quality in Medical Care." *Health Affairs, 7,* 1, 1988.

Chassin, M. R., & McCue, S. M. "A Randomized Trial of Medical Quality Assurance." *Journal of the American Medical Association, 256,* 8, 1986.

Christoffel, T. "Medical Care Evaluation: An Old Idea." *Journal of Medical Education, 51,* 2, 1976.

Danziger, S. K. "The Use of Expertise in Doctor-Patient Encounters During Pregnancy." In P. Conrad & R. Kern (eds.), *The Sociology of Health and Illness,* New York: St. Martin's Press, 1986.

Davies, A. R., & Ware, J. E., Jr. "Involving Consumers in Quality of Care Assessment." *Health Affairs, 7,* 1, 1988.

Domoto, K., et al. "Yields of Routin Annual Laboratory Screening in the Institutionalized Elderly." *American Journal of Public Health, 75,* 3, 1985.

Donabedian, A. *Explorations in Quality Assessment and Monitoring: Vol. 1. The Definition of Quality and Approaches to Its Assessment.* Ann Arbor, MI: Health Administration Press, 1980.

Donabedian, A. *Explorations in Quality Assessment and Monitoring: Vol. 3. The Methods and Findings of Quality Assessment and Monitoring.* Ann Arbor, MI: Health Administration Press, 1985.

Flood, A. B., & Scott, W. R. "Professional Power and Professional Effectiveness: The Power of the Surgical Staff and the Quality of Surgical Care in Hospitals." *Journal of Health and Social Behavior, 19,* 3, 1978.

Freedman, M. A., et al. "Comparison of Complication Rates in First Trimester Abortions Performed by Physician Assistants and Physicians." *American Journal of Public Health, 76,* 5, 1986.

Freidson, E. *Profession of Medicine.* New York: Harper and Row, 1970.

Fuchsberg, A. "Editorial: Ralph Nader Calls on Governor Cuomo to Stand Tall." *Trial Lawyers Quarterly, 19,* 20, 1988.

Gerbert, B. *Validity of Patient Report: A Comparison with Other Methods of Physician Quality Assessment."* Presentation made at the Association for Health Services Research conference, San Francisco, June 1988.

Greenfield, S., et al. "Patterns of Care Related to Age of Breast Cancer Patients." *Journal of the American Medical Association, 257,* 20, 1987.

Hetherington, R. W. "Quality Assurance and Organizational Effectiveness in Hospitals." *Health Services Research, 17,* 2, 1982.

Hogness, J. R. "What About the Patient." *New England Journal of Medicine, 313,* 11, 1985.

Iglehart, J. "Heatlh Policy Report." *New England Journal of Medicine, 316,* 5, 1987.

Kane, R. L., et al. "A Randomised Controlled Trial of Hospice Care." In L. Aiken & B. Kehrer (eds.), *Evaluation Studies Review Annual, Vol. 10.* Beverly Hills, CA: Sage Publications, 1985.

Kusserow, R. P., et al. "An Overview of State Medical Discipline." *Journal of the American Medical Association, 257,* 6, 1987.

Lohr, K. N., et al. "Current Issues in Quality of Care." *Health Affairs, 7,* 1, 1988.

Luke, R. D., & Modrow, R. E. "Professionalism, Accountability, and Peer Review." In R. D. Luke, J. C. Krueger, & R. E. Modrow (eds.), *Organization and Change in Health Care Quality Assurance,* Rockland, MD: Aspen Publications, 1983.

Luthy, D. A., et al. "A Randomized Trial of Electronic Fetal Monitoring in Pre-Term Labor." *Obstetrics and Gynecology, 69,* 5, 1987.

Maxwell, R. J. "Resource Constraints and the Quality of Care." *Lancet, 2,* 8461, 1985.

McCusker, J., et al. "Association of Electronic Fetal Monitoring during Labor with Cesarean Section Rate and with Neonatal Morbidity and Mortality." *American Journal of Public Health, 78,* 9, 1988.

Nobrega, F. T., et al. "Quality Assessment in Hypertension: Analysis of Process and Outcome Methods." *New England Journal of Medicine, 296,* 3, 1977.

Powills, S. "Ford Seeks to Define Quality." *Hospitals, 61,* 8, 1987.

Roberts, J. S. "A History of the Joint Commission on Accreditation of Hospitals." *Journal of the American Medical Association, 258,* 7, 1987.

Roper, W. L., & Hackbarth, G. M. "HCFA's Agenda for Promoting High-Quality Care." *Health Affairs, 7,* 1, 1988.

Scofield, R. "Certification: What Does It Mean?" *Current Concepts in Nursing, 2,* 1, 1988.

Shanahan, M. "The Quality Assurance Standard of the JCAH: A Rational Approach to Patient Care Evaluation." In R. D. Luke et al (eds.), *Organization and Change in Health Care Quality Assurance,* Rockville, MD: Aspen Publications, 1983.

Slenker, S. E., et al. "Increasing Physicians' and Nurses' Compliance with Treatment Guidelines in Cancer Care Program." *Journal of Medical Education, 60,* 11, 1985.

"State Readies Legal Defenses in Plan for Licensing Doctors." *New York Law Journal,* March 2, 1988, p. 3.

Svarstad, B. L. "Patient-Practitioner Relationships and Compliance with Prescribed Medical Regimens." In L. H. Aiken & D. Mechanic (eds.), *Applications of Social Science to Clinical Medicine and Health Policy.* New Brunswick, N.J.: Rutgers University Press, 1986.

Thompson, M. S., et al. "Resource Requirements for Evaluating Ambulatory Health Care." *American Journal of Public Health, 74,* 11, 1984.

Thurow, L. C. "Medicine Versus Economics." *New England Journal of Medicine, 313,* 10, 1985.

"US Plans to Rate Doctors Treating Medicare Patients." *New York Times,* June 12, 1988, p. 1.

Waxman, H. A. "Medical Malpractice and Quality of Care." *New England Journal of Medicine, 316,* 5, 1987.

Wilson, F. A., & Neuhauser, D. *Health Services in the United States* (2nd ed.). Cambridge, MA: L. Ballinger, 1987.

Winickoff, R., et al. "Limitations of Provider Interventions in Hypertension Quality Assurance." *American Journal of Public Health, 75,* 1, 1985.

15

Technology Assessment in Health Care

H. David Banta

Technology assessment, defined simply, refers to evaluating technology for its effects. Within the health field, the effects of primary concern are health benefits (efficacy) and financial costs. At the same time, broad social implications of both specific technologies and medical technology in general become more and more apparent (Banta, Behney, & Willems, pp. 137–156). The rather definitive Institute of Medicine report (1985) defined it as follows: "any process of examining and reporting properties of a medical technology used in health care, such as safety, efficacy, feasibility, and indications for use, cost, and cost-effectiveness, as well as social, economic, and ethical consequences, whether intended or unintended" (p. 2).

Technology assessment is also sometimes considered as a type of policy research (Banta & Behney; Office of Technology Assessment, 1976). In this formulation, the goal of technology assessment is to provide policymakers with information on policy alternatives, such as allocation of research and development funds, formulation of regulations, or development of new legislation. Whether this more specific definition or the more general one is used is not particularly important. It *is* important to realize that medical technology can be evaluated very much from a clinical perspective, or from the standpoint of the broader society as part of a decision-making process. This chapter will emphasize the second sense, that is, as a form of policy analysis.

Technology is broadly defined in this chapter. Galbraith (1977) states that technology "means the systematic application of scientific or other organized knowledge to practical tasks" (p. 31). In other words, technology is not merely machines. All commentators on technology agree on this point. For example, Mesthene (1977) supports this broad definition, saying, "It is in this broader meaning that we can best see the extent and variety of the effects of technology on our institutions and values. Its pervasive influence on our very culture would be unintelligible if technology were understood as no more than hardware" (p. 158). Because of these considerations, medical technology has been defined as "the drugs, devices, and medical and surgical procedures used in medical care, and the organizational and supportive systems within which such care is provided" (Office of Technology Assessment, 1978a). However, systems of care are the subject of this entire book. For that reason, the discussion in this chapter will be dealing primarily with clinical technology, that is, the drugs, devices, and procedures of medical care.

The Value of Medical Technology

Medical technology has transformed the face of modern medicine within the recent past (Bennett; Mushlin). A wide variety of infectious diseases now can be prevented and/or treated. Many chronic diseases also have become controllable, and rates of conditions such as heart disease are falling in this country. Modern medicine has a panoply of diagnostic technologies. Thus there is no real question that medical technology has contributed greatly to the health of the population of the United States and the rest of the world.

At the same time, it is important not to overestimate the benefits of medical technology. McKeown's analysis, discussed in Chapter 2, shows that medical care historically has had a limited impact on death rates. At the same time, many technologies of benefit have other effects besides preventing death. For example, the growing use of hip joint implants leads to restored function and diminished pain (National Institutes of Health, 1982).

It is important to remember the broad spectrum of disease and the possible applications of technology. Much of health care is taken up with psychological problems and physical complaints that have no immediate visible cause. Simple technology may be effective in these conditions. Whether or not caring is a technology is a matter of definition, but counseling patients and achieving their cooperation with therapy surely is a technology, under the definition just given.

Many other factors influence health besides technology, as discussed in Chapter 2. Health must include how one feels about life. What are the effects of racism in a society on one's feeling healthy, or how does one react to a high unemployment rate? At the personal level, studies have demonstrated direct associations between employment rates and mortality rates (Brenner). Such factors fall outside the direct responsibility of the health care system but must be considered in promoting health. An important factor is people's own behavior, which can be influenced by health and medical care (Russell). There is no necessary conflict between technological interventions and attempts to control one's own life and health, but in a society that overvalues technological procedures and pays little attention to the general social and cultural context, such conflicts seem to occur frequently. Providers need to keep in mind that the health of the client is at stake; it is up to the client to make the important decisions.

Concerns about Medical Technology

The greatest concern about technology, at least within the policy arena, is the costs that its use engenders. During the 1970s and early 1980s, health care costs rose at an average rate of about 15% a year (see Chapter 10), almost double the rate of general inflation. The percentage of the gross national product going to health care rose from 6.0% in 1965 to above 11% in 1987. Expenditures in the Medicare program rose even faster (Office of Technology Assessment, 1984c).

A number of analyses have examined the contribution of medical technology to rising costs. Estimates of the effect of technology on per diem hospital cost increases range from about 33% to 75%, depending on the definition of technology, the period of time, and method of calculation (Banta & Gelijns, 1987b). An analysis by the Office of Technology Assessment (1984c, p. 48) found that increases in service intensity (a partial measure of new technology) contributed 24% to the rise in hospital costs during the period between 1977 and 1982.

Scitovsky and McCall (1979) traced the change in costs of treating 11 conditions at a large medical clinic, over time. Between 1951 and 1964 the real costs of treating fell for only two conditions: otitis media and pregnancy/delivery. From 1964 to 1971, the real cost of treating 5 of 11 conditions fell, but aggregate costs rose. The general increases in diagnostic tests and therapeutic procedures per diagnosis were especially striking. Laboratory tests per case of perforated appendicitis, for example, rose from 5.3 in 1951 to 31.0 in 1971. Scitovsky (1982) subsequently updated her work to 1981. She found that the net effects from 1971 to 1981 were cost-saving in eight conditions, cost-raising in seven, and neutral in one. The largest differences were in breast cancer and myocardial infarction, where new "big-ticket" technologies increased costs considerably. The other large difference was in the increasing use of cesarean section with its high costs. Showstack et al. (1982, 1985) had similar results in their research, emphasizing the important role of intensive treatments for the critically ill in rising costs.

These rising costs have raised questions about the benefits being derived from the increased use of technology. Early studies assumed that more services were synonymous with better-quality care; however, recognition has grown that many technologies are used extensively in situations where they may not be appropriate. The focus of the debate has shifted away from analysis of technology and medical expenditures in overall categories to the benefits and costs of specific technologies applied in particular circumstances.

How much benefit is gained under what circumstances remains relatively unknown. Concerns have been raised about the benefits of a great many modern technologies that are used routinely in the United States. For example, questions have been raised about electronic fetal monitoring (Banta & Thacker), other obstetric practices (Chalmers & Richards), and oral drugs for diabetes (Knatterud et al.). The most-quoted case of lack of benefit is gastric freezing, which came into widespread use in the 1960s as a treatment for peptic ulcer, promoted by a renowned surgeon and a commercial enterprise, and then just as quickly fell out of use when it turned out to be dangerous and of no benefit (Fineberg). A number of surgical treatments for coronary artery disease were developed and used widely before the advent of bypass surgery (Preston). The rising rate of cesarean sections mentioned above is probably without significant benefit, as is much of intensive care, which is reviewed in more detail below. Particularly expensive and useless procedures are focused at the extremes of life, in very small babies and in very old adults near death.

At the same time, all technologies are associated with risks. In many cases, these risks are small and perhaps can be ignored if benefits are significant. The risks of many medical technologies are also significant, however, and one is often left with the impression that they are not sufficiently taken into account. Drug risks have been most publicized, as in the cases of thalidomide and estrogen use during pregnancy (Dowling; Lambert). Although the risks of these drugs were dramatic, the more typical risk is probably similar to that which often accompanies drug treatment for hypertension: dizziness, impotence, and general tiredness. Surgery is obviously associated with risks, including mortality and morbidity from such causes as thrombophlebitis (clots in the leg veins). However, many risks are not so obvious, as in the case of carcinogenic effects of x-rays and certain drugs.

Finally, while costs and benefits are the most obvious and direct effects of medical technology, many technologies are also associated with important social consequences. Perhaps the most important social question today is how to provide decent medical care to everyone, given the limitation of resources for the health care area. At the same time, the ethical questions surrounding the lack of access that many people have today to such care are important to consider. Another important social question concerns the overall role of medical technology in the health care system, given its tendency to depersonalize care. Finally, specific technologies raise serious ethical questions. How does one turn off a respirator when a patient's brain appears to be dead? What is the impact on quality of life of renal dialysis three times a week for as long as the patient lives? The rapid pace of change in the area of genetics, with genetic screening and the possibility of genetic engineering, raises a variety of social and ethical issues (Holtzman). These concerns all need to be more effectively addressed by the society. Technology assessment is one tool for improving society's ability to deal with such issues. The sections that follow briefly describe the process and methods of technology assessment. The interested reader may consult a series of

Office of Technology Assessment publications for more details (OTA, 1976, 1978a, 1980, 1982, 1984a).

Evaluating Efficacy and Safety

Efficacy and safety are the basic starting points in evaluating the overall utility of a medical technology. If a technology is not efficacious, it should not be used, and if its efficacy is unknown, statements about its value cannot be made. In addition, speaking of financial costs has relatively little meaning without knowledge of efficacy. The question of interest is how much benefit is derived from the cost incurred.

Efficacy may be defined simply as health benefit, but its evaluation requires attention to four factors: (1) the benefits to be achieved, (2) the medical problem giving rise to use of the technology, (3) the population affected, and (4) the conditions of use under which the technology is applied (OTA, 1978a).

The question of benefits is not as simple as it seems at first. Outcomes have usually been measured in terms of mortality and morbidity; however, psychosocial and functional factors have become recognized as important outcome. As mentioned in Chapter 3, the measurement of health status has progressed greatly in the last few years.

Each technology is associated with a range of outcomes. This may be illustrated by the case of diagnostic technologies, such as CAT scanners, which can be examined at five levels (Fineberg et al.):

1. *Technical capability:* Does the device perform reliably and deliver accurate information?
2. *Diagnostic accuracy:* Does use of the device permit accurate diagnoses?
3. *Diagnostic impact:* Does use of the device replace other diagnostic procedures, including surgical exploration and biopsy?
4. *Therapeutic impact:* Do results obtained from the device affect planning and delivery of therapy?
5. *Patient outcome:* Does use of the device contribute to improved health of the patient?

Often those using diagnostic technology seem to be most interested in the diagnostic outcome, while the outcome for the patient is surely the most important factor. At the same time, evaluating the impact of various diagnostic technologies on patient outcomes is very difficult. Definition and measurement of benefit are often difficult for other classes of technologies as well. For example, coronary bypass surgery may extend life in some patients but is used to relieve chest pain in others. Likewise, technologies are addressed to different medical problems and populations. And, as indicated previously, the outcome of application of a technology is partially determined by the skills, knowledge, and abilities of physicians, nurses, and other health personnel and by the quality of the drugs, equipment, and institutional settings. Similar surgical procedures, for example, can have quite different outcomes, depending on the skill and experience of the surgeon.

Efficacy is differentiated from *effectiveness*. *Effectiveness* is the benefit achieved by the use of a technology under average or community conditions, while efficacy is a measure of benefit under ideal or experimental conditions of use. Thus, a technology with demonstrated efficacy in a university hospital may turn out to be ineffective in the community setting, for a number of reasons. There have, however, been few studies of effectiveness.

Safety, like efficacy, is a relative concept, since no technology is ever completely safe or efficacious. A safe technology does not cause undue harm. It requires value judgments, however, to determine what is undue or acceptable. As with efficacy, the medical problem to which the technology is applied must be defined, the population affected must be specified, and the conditions of use must be stated.

The measurements of efficacy and safety often require quite different study methods. In assessing efficacy, a study is usually oriented to a limited number of specific benefits. The measurement of safety, however, usually involves a study design that is able to identify a broad range of risks, some of which are unknown or unexpected. Side effects of technology often occur in a small percentage of individuals and may occur far in the future.

There are methodological principles that guide the design, conduct, and interpretation of any particular study. Randomized clinical trials (RCTs) are considered the most definitive experimental method for evaluating the efficacy of a technology. An essential element of an RCT is randomization. Patients in an RCT are assigned randomly to one of at least two groups: (1) a study group, of which there may be several, in which subjects are exposed to the experimental treatments, and (2) a comparison group, in which subjects are exposed to a control condition. The control condition can be either no treatment, the then-current standard treatment, or a variation of the experimental treatment. If effects are observed in the experimental group and not in the comparison group, the effects can be attributed to the treatment technology.

In many cases, RCTs are difficult to organize and expensive to carry out. This situation has led to alternative methods of evaluating efficacy. Control groups can be formed retrospectively, for example. However, one always has to be cautious in interpreting such studies.

As mentioned already, examination of safety requires alternative methods, especially observational studies and applications of epidemiology. Case control studies, in which individuals with particular conditions are compared to others without the particular condition, are particularly useful for investigating the relationship between a commonly used drug and a rare adverse event.

It should be stressed that study design depends on multiple factors, including the developmental stage of the technology, the purpose of the study, ethical considerations, the population available, and budget constraints. Seldom is assessment a one-time event. A single study seldom establishes a clear relationship between a suspected cause and a particular effect. Ideally, a strategy of assessment should be laid out so that each new study builds on the previous ones, toward a total assessment of the technology.

Evaluating Costs and Cost-Effectiveness

While costs alone can be evaluated, such studies have little meaning without knowing the benefits derived from the investment. This section, therefore, will concentrate on evaluating cost-effectiveness. *Cost-benefit analysis* is probably a more familiar term than *cost-effectiveness;* however, cost-benefit analysis requires putting all costs and benefits into the same units, usually money, so that the answer is a ratio. Since health outcomes such as life or death are hard to express in such terms, cost-benefit analysis has lost favor in the health area during the past few years. Cost-effectiveness analysis allows one to express effectiveness in different units from costs. For example, the result of a study might be stated in terms of years of life saved per $1,000 investment.

Cost-effectiveness analysis is gaining more and more visibility as a potential help to policymaking (Klarman; Warner & Luce). Policymakers have long referred to the need to understand more about the cost-effectiveness of interventions in the health care areas. In response the cost-effectiveness literature has rapidly increased in size (Warner & Hutton). Nonetheless, there are still relatively few high-quality cost-effectiveness analyses and little evidence that they have made much impact on health policy.

There are a number of reasons why this is so. As mentioned, few good cost-effectiveness analyses have been performed. The Office of Technology Assessment (1983) found that studies by recognized experts were inadequate with respect to the relevancy/usefulness of the results, the validity of the methods, the tenuousness (or error) in the key assumptions, and the validity of the data used. At the same time, like a good RCT, a high-quality cost-effectiveness analysis is expensive and takes time. Policy decisions do not necessarily wait on formal analysis. Thus, OTA concluded that, formally applied, this analytical method could often be too complex, expensive, and time-consuming if used routinely in public-policy decision making.

Nevertheless, the logic behind using cost-effectiveness analysis is important in decision making. Simpler, "back-of-the-envelope" analyses are common within the policy setting and clearly have influenced decision making. OTA (1980) has developed a set of principles of cost-effectiveness analysis that should be used in all situations, whether the analysis is long and expensive or short and cheap:

1. Define problem.
2. State objectives.
3. Identify alternatives.
4. Analyze benefits/ effects.
5. Analyze costs.
6. Differentiate perspective of analysis.
7. Perform discounting.
8. Analyze uncertainties.
9. Address ethical issues.
10. Interpret results.

If these 10 principles are followed consistently, one can have more confidence that one's conclusions are valid.

Evaluating Social Concerns

The social aspects of medical technologies are some of the most difficult to evaluate. There are several reasons for this. It is difficult to tell in advance which of the thousands of medical technologies will have serious social implications and for whom. At the same time, there has been little interest overall in this form of evaluation, so methods have not been developed and defined (Banta & Gelijns, 1987a; Institute of Medicine, 1985; OTA, 1976).

Clearly, the relationship between medical technology and social values is reciprocal. Technologies affect values, as when technology allowed the definition of "brain death" to supersede the earlier standard life endpoint: heart stoppage. Society still has not been able to grapple effectively with the issue of what to do for a person whose heart and lungs are artificially supported but whose brain is "alive." At the same time, values affect medical technology and its development, use, and evaluation. Social values and technology interact in a very broad sense. For example, what value does society place on health, on innovation, on financial security, on technology itself? It often seems that the present society overvalues technology and undervalues human supports and caring.

Specific technologies also have social effects, as well as being subject to broad social forces. The most visible social impact is on costs. How will society cope with the ever-increasing cost of health care? Will we decide to use some formal criterion such as "social worth" to decide who shall have access to expensive life-saving technologies? Every technology is fed into a delivery system that historically discriminates, in terms of access and distribution, against poor people, minorities, the aged, and other groups. Thus, technological advances can be in part the cause of, in part the catalyst for, and in part the mechanism for continued inequities.

U.S. society has not dealt with such issues effectively and indeed often seems overtly to avoid dealing with them. There are few, if any, examples of a broad technology assessment done of a medical technology, for purposes of policymaking. Perhaps the best example is a study done of the artificial heart by the National Institutes of Health in 1972 (National Heart and Lung Institute). That report analyzed the broad social consequences of having a workable heart. According to NIH staff close to the decisions, the report helped lead to an emphasis on left-ventricular assist devices and a deemphasis of the totally implantable heart. In 1976, OTA used this report and other sources to develop a list of questions that could be applied to any technology used in health care. In 1979, the Health Care Financing Administration delayed the decision on whether or not to pay for heart transplants through the Medicare program until a broad study of the consequences of the technology could be completed by Batelle (Evens, et al.). With the growing concern about such social consequences, this field of inquiry seems certain to grow and develop.

The Process of Technology Assessment

Until now this chapter has dealt with original research aimed at evaluating medical technology. Research results often do not affect policy or clinical decisions very directly, however, as policymakers and clinicians do not tend to read research reports and often lack the skills to interpret them, in any case. To assure that assessment results affect decisions on technology requires a more systematic approach.

The components of a medical technology assessment process can be seen as including four stages of assessment (OTA, 1982):

1. *Identification:* Monitoring technologies, determining which need to be studied, and deciding which to study.
2. *Testing:* Conducting the appropriate analyses or trials.
3. *Synthesis:* Collecting and interpreting existing information and the results of the testing stage, and usually, making recomendations or judgments about appropriate use.
4. *Dissemination:* Providing a synthesis of the information to the appropriate parties who use medical technologies or make decisions about their use.

A decision to conduct a technology assessment clearly must be preceded by the identification of technologies that should be assessed and the setting of priorities among candidates for assessment. Identifying technologies for assessment is done by a number of federal and private organizations; however, there is no one program or agency with this responsibility.

Testing includes stimulating, requiring, funding, or conducting studies. Shortcomings in this area center around four issues: (1) the quality of methods used in assessment; (2) the level of financial support, particularly for controlled clinical trials; (3) the relative appropriateness of the questions and technologies being studied; and (4) the number of personnel qualified to conduct such research. Again, existing activities are rather limited in scope, but two most important are found in the Food and Drug Administration (FDA) and the National Institutes of Health (NIH).

Synthesis of information is a necessary step to providing a convincing and responsible basis for decisions made during all phases of a technology's life cycle. This activity falls into two broad areas: (1) synthesis of the results of individual research studies and (2) synthesis of a body of research findings with various concerns such as risk or social, ethical, or cost factors. The first type of synthesis addressed questions of safety, efficacy, or effectiveness and is oriented toward clinicians. The American College of Physicians' Clinical Efficacy Program is an excellent example of a private program that does such synthesis. The second type is more policy-oriented and often seeks to set guidelines or standards for medical practice or health policy. The oldest program doing synthesis related to policy concerns in this country is the Office of Technology Assessment (OTA), a part of the U.S. Congress. By 1985 OTA had published about 60 health-related case studies covering the entire spectrum of medical and health policy (OTA, 1984d). Another program worth noting is the Consensus Development Program of the NIH (Perry & Kalberer). The NIH program uses synthesis of the literature but also includes a multidisciplinary group as part of the process that attempts to arrive at a consensus and give recommendations on the specific technology. It has examined more than 50 technologies.

Finally, dissemination deals with questions of who should have the highest priority in receiving information. At a minimum, information must reach decision makers involved with the technology in various aspects of its use. This means industry officials, clinicians, policymakers, and/or the general public. Unfortunately, communication activities are highly flawed and have actually been cut back in recent years. Little is known about how technology is adopted or how information is acquired and used.

The Institute of Medicine (1985) estimated that the entire U.S. expenditure for medical technology assessment in 1984 was $1.3 billion, or about 0.3% of the national health expenditure. The federal government invested about $450 million, including $250 million for clinical trials (primarily from the NIH) and $100 million to 150 million for health services research (IOM, 1985, p. 3). The greatest expenditure was by the drug industry, which must fund clinical trials to obtain approval of its products and which also funds postmarketing surveillance activities; the estimated expenditure from this source is about $700 million. Less than $50 million is spent on activities devoted to synthesis and interpretation of primary evaluative data (IOM, 1985, p. 5). Its analysis of this issue led the Institute of Medicine (1985) to conclude that funding for medical technology assessment should be increased by $300 million "by instituting new contributions from payers and providers for health care" (p. 6).

Some Examples of Technology Assessment

The Computerized Axial Tomography (CAT) Scanner

The CAT scanner is a diagnostic device that combines x-ray equipment with a computer and a cathode-ray tube to produce images of cross-sections of the human body. Following its development in the late 1960s, the CAT scanner was hailed as the greatest advance in radiology since the discovery of x-rays, and it was rapidly accepted. The scanner was of concern to policymakers from the beginning, however, because of its rapid spread and use and the expenditures associated with that use.

The first technology assessment done in the health area by OTA was of the CAT scanner (OTA, 1978b). The first draft of OTA's evaluation was widely circulated in late 1976, but diffusion of scanners during 1977 and 1978 was nevertheless very rapid. The main conclusion of OTA's draft was that little research had been done on evaluating possible improvement in health outcomes resulting from the introduction of CAT scanning. As noted earlier in the chapter, this is a critical issue in evaluating diagnostic technologies. OTA's final report was published in 1978. It included a comprehensive analysis of federal government policies that could be used to control the spread of scanners. In 1981, OTA updated the CAT scanner report, focusing on changes in numbers of scanners and in federal policies since the 1978 report. Reports on CAT scanners also have been done by the Institute of Medicine (1977), the Consensus Development Program (National Institutes of Health, 1981), and institutions in a number of other countries.

These reports seem to have had a limited impact in the United States. One reason for this is that the profits associated with using a CAT scanner were extremely high in the early years. OTA estimated average profits per machine in 1976 to vary from $51,000 to $283,000, with an investment for the scanner itself that averaged around $500,000 (OTA, 1978b). In addition, the CAT scanner did give the medical care system a diagnostic tool that was unique. However, in other countries that have more effective methods for controlling the spread of technology, its introduction and use expanded much more slowly. For example, in 1979 the United States had 5.7 scanners per million population. Whereas the Netherlands had only 1.4 per million (Banta; by 1986, the United States had approximately 12.8 scanners per million, and the Netherlands had 3.2 per million (Groot).

Thus, an early lesson for assessors was that the assessment itself might make no difference to the subsequent adoption and use of a technology. A more important factor might be the effectiveness of government programs, such as those planning for the purchase and siting of medical machines.

The Electronic Fetal Monitor

Electronic fetal monitoring (EFM) of the fetal heart rate during labor and delivery was developed as an alternative to auscultation by stethoscope (fetoscope). It was introduced into obstetric practice during the 1960s and spread rather quickly. By 1980 it was used in 48% of deliveries in the United States (Placek et al.).

By 1977, EFM had become controversial because it tended to replace a human being (usually a nurse or midwife) with a machine. Many women did not like this change, and the women's movement made such depersonalization an issue. Because of this controversy, an RCT was initiated at the University of Colorado, Denver (Haverkamp et al., 1976). The trial, while small, found no benefit to the fetus from EFM, compared with auscultation. At the same time, other trials were under way. In 1977, OTA (1978a) did an assessment of EFM that was published as part of a larger report. The full assessment was also published by the National Center for Health Services Research and in an obstetrics journal (Banta & Thacker). By that time, three other RCTs had been published, none showing clear-cut benefit. By 1986, nine controlled clinical trials had been completed in six countries, including one involving 35,000 women from Dallas (Leveno et al), with no benefit except a decrease in the occurrence of neonatal seizures of unknown significance in the EFM group (Thacker). In addition, the OTA analysis showed that the use of EFM added considerably to costs. Much of this increase was due to increased rates of surgical deliveries, especially cesarean sections, confirmed by pooled data from the nine trials (Thacker).

Nonetheless, EFM has continued to be used. Why? There are a number of reasons. One is that younger obstetricians have all been trained to use the machine, and many have limited auscultation skill. Another is that malpractice suits have been brought against obstetricians who did not use EFM with their patients. From the standpoint of the policymaker, there are few ways to affect the use of EFM. The machine itself is relatively inexpensive and too small an item to be subject to direct health planning, and FDA's mandate is too limited to allow it to remove EFM from the market. All the same, the negative or equivocal assessments have been quoted in many news articles and magazines, and one has the impression that its use is falling slowly. If this is true, perhaps the lesson is that consumers can use assessment to promote change in health care, when they are committed to such change.

Intensive Care Units

The intensive care unit has been called the hallmark of the modern hospital. It developed during the past 25 years, first as an expansion of the surgical recovery room and subsequently as an outgrowth of respiratory care units made possible by the development of the mechanical ventilator. Today, almost 80% of short-term general hospitals have at least one intensive care unit. Overall, 5.9% of total hospital beds in nonfederal, short-term community hospitals in 1982 were beds in intensive and coronary care units. Other types of special care units, including pediatric, neonatal, and burn units, add another 1% to this total (OTA, 1984b).

Intensive care is expensive. The average national per diem charge in 1982 for an ICU bed was $408, compared to a regular-bed per diem of $167. Based on such figures, it has been estimated that intensive care represents about 14% to 17% of total hospital costs (OTA, 1984b).

An NIH-sponsored consensus panel found it impossible to generalize about whether ICU care improves outcome for the varied ICU patient population (NIH, 1983). At one end of the patient spectrum are those who are very sick and who often do not survive but who pay a large share of the ICU charges. At the other end of the spectrum are patients in the ICU primarily for monitoring in case of the development of a life-threatening complication. Many of these patients could be cared for safely in regular hospital wards. One of the most critical issues with intensive care is when to stop it. The NIH group concluded that it is not appropriate to devote limited ICU resources to those patients who do not have a reasonable prospect of significant recovery or where the effect simply is to prolong the natural process of death. Many ICU patients do fall into those two categories.

Intensive care has been evaluated from many different perspectives. In 1984, OTA completed an assessment summarizing available data on distribution, costs, utilization, and efficacy of ICU care (OTA, 1984b). A major conclusion is that ICU care is often used with patients who have nominal hope of surviving and with people who need early monitoring for potential problems. Nonetheless, ICU use continues to grow. Why? One important reason is that the reimbursement system pays well for intensive care. Another is the natural desire on the part of physicians to provide the best care for their patients, even if it is at a standard not strictly required medically. It should be noted, moreover, that few good evaluations of ICU care have been done because most clinicians feel that RCTs of intensive care would be unethical, since it is the accepted standard of care.

Pneumococcal Vaccine

In 1978, a new vaccine against the pneumococcus, aimed at the prevention of pneumococcal pneumonia, was marketed. The vaccine had been approved by FDA on the basis of proven efficacy in experimental studies, but many groups and individuals were cautious about widespread use of the vaccine because it had not been tested in high-risk groups such as the elderly. In 1979, OTA published a cost-effectiveness analysis of the vaccine, in which it was concluded that the Medicare program would incur a net cost per elderly beneficiary vaccinated of about $5 if the program covered 100% of the vaccination cost and that each vaccination would produce a gain of .004 healthy days of life. If 21.5% of the population were vaccinated, Medicare would spend about $26 million over the lifetimes of those vaccinated, and 22,000 years of healthy life would result. Since Medicare does not pay for all medical expenses of the elderly, however, the actual results would be even more favorable. This analysis led to a congressional act in 1981 providing for coverage of the vaccine under the program. The findings of a reanalysis by OTA in 1984, using the actual experience of the Medicare program, were similar to those of the earlier study (OTA, 1984d). Nonetheless, only about 25% of the high-risk target group has received the vaccine. This indicates that, while financial coverage for technology is important, it is not the only factor in use.

Another important lesson from this case is that technology assessments are more likely to be directly influential when a specific policy decision is involved. Cost-effectiveness analysis has been widely applied in the case of vaccines, probably because immunization programs are developed by the government and are funded with public monies. Other than the pneumococcal vaccine, Medicare, by law, has never covered preventive measures from the time of its passage in 1965 to the mid-1980's. Congress has recently incrementally added coverage of hepatitis B immunization for high-risk beneficiaries and of biannual screening mammographies.

Impact of Technology Assessment

Evaluation is not a new area of medicine, but the RCT is a product of this century. Other forms of assessment are even newer. For example, a random sample of articles from general medical journals found no RCTs in 1946, while 5% of the articles were reports of RCTs in 1976 (Fletcher & Fletcher). The literature on the impact of technology assessment is small and focuses on the impact of RCTs. By the mid-1970s, the literature had begun to grow, and in 1983 OTA reviewed the literature on the impact of RCTs on policy and practice (OTA, 1983).

Most authors conclude that the impact of RCTs on medical practice has been less than optimal or that their impact is exceedingly slow to develop. The literature as a whole demonstrates great variation in the use of RCTs and in their influence in different medical areas. Recent articles have identified some of the reasons for lack of influence of RCTs, including (1) poor quality of many RCTs, (2) poor dissemination of the results of RCTs, (3) lack of an overall system for assessing medical technologies, (4) less-than-optimal use of RCTs in policy decisions, and (5) different traditions and practices in different areas of medicine (internists are more accustomed to such evidence than surgeons, for example).

Assessments have also had a limited impact on policy. In part, this is related to the small efforts aimed at producing information for policymaking (that is, synthesis activities). In part it is related to the lack of primary data. For example, the Office of Health Technology Assessment (OHTA) assessed 26 technologies for the Medicare program in 1982 and found that randomized clinical trials were available for only 2 (IOM, 1985, p. 5).

What, then, is the value of technology assessment in health care? Although it is difficult to document, one important use is what might be called "strategic," in which the analysis includes consideration of what the individual, the group, or the organization is attempting to achieve (Smits et al). An example might be the repeated conclusions of the Office of Technology Assessment during the 1970s that the nature of the payment system for technology was one of the most important policies leading to inappropriate use of medical technology. Such reports surely helped prepare the way for policy changes in the payment system in the Medicare program, including the development of the Diagnostic-Related Groups (DRG) program, a change from retrospective cost reimbursement to prospective payment.

Technology assessment also can be used as part of operational decisions. It has a long-established role in the area of drug regulation as part of the premarketing approval process. A newer role is as a part of payment decisions. In 1978 Congress established a National Center for Health Care Technology, one of whose purposes was to establish a more systematic approach to technology assessment; although the Center ceased to exist in 1982, the OHTA carries on this function. A number of other organizations, including Blue Cross/Blue Shield, also carry out assessments as a guide to payment decisions. When decisions have been based on technology assessment information, they seem to have saved the organizations much more than the cost of the assessments (Perry).

It would be premature to say that health care technology assessment has demonstrated its own cost-effectiveness. It may be too early to ask for such evidence because investments have been small and activities have begun to be rationally organized only during the past decade. Nonetheless, experience thus far is promising enough to lead a number of groups and individuals to support an expansion of such activities, along with the development of national systems (Banta & Gelijns, 1987a; Feeny, Guyatt, & Tugwell; IOM, 1985).

Experiences of Other Countries

Other countries have had experiences with medical technology similar to those of the United States. Almost all industrialized countries have experienced rapidly rising health care costs, which has led to rapid changes in policies toward medical technology (Banta & Kemp; Groot).

Until fairly recently, the major involvement of governments in medical technology was to promote a new technology's development and adoption actively, through such means as funding biomedical research and technology development or assuring payment for the technology under a national health plan. In recent years, however, governments have become more and more concerned with whether or not new technologies were being used efficiently. Without making a judgment about the efficacy of the technology, governments have intervened to encourage greater efficiency in the production and use of a technology. This has been a major orientation of health planning, for example. With increasing concerns about the cost-effectiveness of technology, governments also have begun to question and test the benefits of medical technologies. A number of governments, especially those in Western Europe, now have new programs to assess medical technology, and funds available are increasing rapidly. Finally, some governments have gone further, by limiting the diffusion of technologies to a level that strikes a balance between the benefits to be gained and the costs of achieving them. England is an example of a country that seems to have moved to this stage.

Summary and Conclusions

The major problem with technology assessment in medicine in the United States is the lack of a system for doing so that would assure timely, high-quality assessment. In 1978 Congress passed legislation establishing the National Center for Health Care Technology, which was a step in that direction. The center was a victim of Reagan administration budget cuts, however, and ceased to exist in 1981. During the period between 1981 and 1984, the National Center for Health Services Research funded a small amount of research in the area, and the Office of Health Technology Assessment carried on the task of giving advice to the Medicare program regarding which technologies to pay for.

Many people were concerned about this situation, including Congress. In 1982–1983, OTA analyzed the problem in depth and pointed out the need for a systematic approach (OTA, 1982). In 1983 the Institute of Medicine of the National Academy of Science also identified this problem as a critical one and proposed the establishment of a public/private consortium to serve as a clearinghouse for technology assessments in medicine (IOM, 1983). In late 1984, Congress responded to these reports and their own concerns and passed legislation changing the name of the National Center for Health Services Research to the National Center for Health Services Research and Health Technology Assessment, earmarking about $3 million for health technology assessment. The same statute authorized funding of a new Council on Health Care Technology at the Institute of Medicine. The council was appointed in 1986 and has begun to develop its information systems and to support conferences and other activites.

These fragments, however, do not make up a system that can carry out identification, testing, synthesis, and dissemination on all technologies. Resources available for assessment are small. The 1985 report from the Institute of

Medicine recommended a greatly expanded federal role in addressing these problems. Whatever the immediate results of these actions, it seems clear that technology assessment in medicine is becoming more and more an integral part of decision making at both the policymaking and the clinical levels.

References

Banta, D. "The Diffusion of the Computed Tomography (CT) Scanner in the United States." *International Journal of Health Services, 10,* 2, 1980.

Banta, D., & Behney, C. "Policy Formulation and Technology Assessment." *Milbank Memorial Fund Quarterly, 59,* 3, 1981.

Banta, D., Behney, C., & Willems, J. *Toward Rational Technology in Medicine: Considerations for Health Policy.* New York: Springer Publishing Co., 1981.

Banta, H. D., & Gelijns, A. G. *Anticipating and Assessing Health Care Technology: Vol. 1. General Considerations and Policy Conclusions.* Boston: Martinus Nijhoff Publishers. 1987a.

Banta, H. D., & Gelijns, A. G. "Health Care Costs: Technology and Policy. In C. J. Schramm (Ed.), *Health Care and Its Costs: Can the U.S. Afford Adequate Health Care?* (pp. 252–274). New York: W. W. Norton, 1987b.

Banta, D., & Kemp, K. (Eds.). *The Management of Health Care Technology in Nine Countries.* New York: Springer Publishing Co., 1982.

Banta, D., & Thacker, S. "Assessing the Costs and Benefits of Electronic Fetal Monitoring." *Obstetrical and Gynecological Survey, 34,* 627, 1979.

Bennett, I. "Technology as a Shaping Force," *Daedalus, 106,* 125, 1977.

Brenner, M. H. "Health Costs and Benefits of Economic Policy. *International Journal of Health Services, 7,* 581, 1977.

Chalmers, I., & Richards, M. "Intervention and Causal Inference in Obstetric Practice." In T. Chard & M. Richards (Eds.). *Benefits and Hazards of the New Obstetrics.* London: Heinemann Medical Books, 1977.

Dowling, H. *Medicines for Man.* New York: Alfred A. Knopf, 1970.

Evens, E. W., et al. *The National Heart Transplantation Study: Final Report.* Seattle, WA: Battelle Human Affairs Research Centers, 1984.

Feeny, D., Guyatt, G., & Tugwell, P. *Health Care Technology: Effectiveness, Efficiency and Public Policy.* Montreal: Institute for Research on Public Policy, 1986.

Fineberg, H. "Gastric Freezing—A Study of Diffusion of a Medical Innovation." In Committee on Technology and Health Care, *Medical Technology and the Health Care System.* Washington, DC: National Academy of Sciences, 1979.

Fineberg, H. et al. "Computerized Cranial Tomography: Effect on Diagnostic and Therapeutic Plans." *Journal of the American Medical Association, 238,* 224, 1977

Fletcher, R., & Fletcher, S. "Clinical Research in General Medical Journals." *New England Journal of Medicine, 301,* 180, 1979.

Galbraith, J. *The New Industrial State.* New York: New American Library, 1977.

Groot, L. M. J. *Study on Regulatory Mechanisms of the Diffusion of Expensive Health Technology in the Member States of the EC.* Report to the European Commission, Brussels, Belgium, 1986.

Haverkamp, A., et al. "The Evaluation of Continuous Fetal Heart Rate Monitoring in High-Risk Pregnancy." *American Journal of Obstetrics and Gynecology, 125,* 310, 1976.

Holtzman, N. A. *The Application of Recombinant DNA Technology to Genetic Testing: Promise and Peril.* Manuscript submitted for publication.

Institute of Medicine. *Computed Tomographic Scanning.* Washington, DC: National Academy of Sciences, 1977.

Institute of Medicine. *A Consortium for Assessing Medical Technology.* Washington, DC: National Academy Press, 1983.

Institute of Medicine. *Assessing Medical Technology.* Washington, DC: National Academy Press, 1985.

Klarman, H. "Application of Cost-Benefit Analysis to the Health Services and the Special Case of Technology." *International Journal of Health Services, 4,* 325, 1974.

Knatterud, G., et al. "Effects of Hypoglycemic Agents on Vascular Complications in Patients with Adult-Onset Diabetes." *Journal of the American Medical Association, 217,* 777, 1971.

Lambert, E. C. *Modern Medical Mistakes.* Bloomington, IN: Indiana University Press, 1978.

Leveno, K. J., Cunningham, F. G., Nelson, S., Roark, M., Williams, M. L., Guzick, D., Dowling, S., Rosenfeld, C. R., & Buckley, A. "A Prospective Comparison of Selective and Universal Electronic Fetal Monitoring in 34,995 Pregnancies." *New England Journal of Medicine, 315,* 615, 1986.

Mesthene, E. "The Role of Technology in Society." In A. Teich (Ed.), *Technology and Man's Future.* New York: St. Martin's Press, 1977.

Mushlin, S. *Biomedical Research: Costs and Benefits.* Cambridge, MA: Ballinger, 1979.

National Heart and Lung Institute. *The Totally Implantable Artificial Heart.* A Report of the Artificial Heart Assessment Panel. Bethesda, MD: National Institutes of Health, 1973.

National Institutes of Health. Consensus Development Conference Statement. *Computed Tomographic Scanning of the Brain.* Bethesda, MD: National Institutes of Health, 1981.

National Institutes of Health. Consensus Development Conference Statement. *Total Hip Joint Replacement.* Bethesda. MD: National Institutes of Health, 1982.

National Institutes of Health. Consensus Development Conference Statement. *Critical Care Medicine.* Bethesda, MD: National Institutes of Health, 1983.

Office of Technology Assessment, *Development of Medical Technology: Opportunities for Assessment.* Pub. No. OTA-H-34. Washington, DC: U.S. Government Printing Office. 1976.

Office of Technology Assessment. *Assessing the Efficacy and Safety of Medical Technologies.* Pub. No. OTA-H-75. Washington, DC: U.S. Government Printing Office, 1978. (a)

Office of Technology Assessment. *Policy Implications of the Computed Tomography (CT) Scanner.* Pub. No. OTA-H-56. Washington, DC: U.S. Government Printing Office, 1978. (b)

Office of Technology Assessment. *A Review of Selected Federal Vaccine and Immunization Policies.* Pub. No. OTA-H-96. Washington, DC: U.S. Government Printing Office, 1979.

Office of Technology Assessment. *The Implications of Cost-Effectiveness Analysis of Medical Technology.* Pub. No. OTA-H-126. Washington, DC: U.S. Government Printing Office, 1980.

Office of Technology Assessment. *Policy Implications of the Computed Tomography (CT) Scanner: An Update.* Pub. No. OTA-BP-H-8. Washington, DC: U.S. Government Printing Office, 1981.

Office of Technology Assessment. *Strategies for Medical Technology Assessment.* Pub. No. OTA-H-181. Washington, DC: U.S. Government Printing Office, 1982.

Office of Technology Assessment. *The Impact of Randomized Clinical Trials on Health Policy and Medical Practice.* Pub. No. BP-H-22. Washington, DC: U.S. Government Printing Office, 1983.

Office of Technology Assessment. *Abstracts of Case Studies in the Health Technology Case Studies Series.* Pub. No. OTA-P-225. Washington, DC: U.S. Government Printing Office, 1984. (a)

Office of Technology Assessment. *Intensive Care Units (ICUs)—Clinical Outcomes. Costs, and Decisionmaking.* Pub. No. BP-HCS-28. Washington, DC: U.S. Government Printing Office, 1984. (b)

Office of Technology Assessment. *Medical Technology and the Costs of the Medicare Program.* Pub. No. OTA-H-227. Washington, DC: U.S. Government Printing Office, 1984. (c)

Office of Technology Assessment. *Update of Federal Activities Regarding the Use of Pneumococcal Vaccine.* Pub. No. OTA-TM-H-23. Washington, DC: U.S. Government Printing Office, 1984. (d)

Perry, S. "The Brief Life of the National Center for Health Care Technology." *New England Journal of Medicine, 307,* 1095, 1982.

Perry, S., & Kalberer, J. T. "The NIH Consensus-Development Program and the Assessment of Health Technologies: The First Two Years." *New England Journal of Medicine, 303,* 169, 1980.

Placek, P., et al. "Electronic Fetal Monitoring in Relation to Cesarean Section Delivery, for Live Births and Stillbirths in the U.S., 1980." *Public Health Reports, 99,* 173, 1984.

Preston, T. *Coronary Artery Surgery: A Critical Review.* New York: Raven Press, 1977.

Relman, A. S. "Assessment of Medical Practices." *New England Journal of Medicine, 303,* 153, 1980.

Russell, L. B. *Is Prevention Better Than Cure?* Washington, D.C.: The Brookings Institution. 1986.

Scitovsky, A. A. "Estimating the Direct Costs of Illness. *Milbank Memorial Fund Quarterly/Health and Society, 60,* 4623, 1982.

Scitovsky, A., & McCall, N. "Changes in the Cost of Treatment of Selected Illnesses. 1951–1964–1971." USDHEW Pub. No. (PHS) 79-3216. Hyattsville, MD: National Center for Health Services Research and Bureau of Health Planning, 1979.

Showstack, J. A., Hughes Stone, M., & Schroeder S. A. "The Role of Changing Clinical Practices on the Rising Costs of Hospital Care. *New England Journal of Medicine, 313,* 1201, 1985.

Showstack, J. A., Schroeder, S. A., & Matsumoto, M. F. "Changes in the Use of Medical Technologies, 1972–1977: A Study of 20 Inpatient Diagnoses. *New England Journal of Medicine, 306,* 706, 1982.

Smits, R. E. H. M., Leyten, A. J. M., & Guerts, J. L. A. The Possibilities and Limitations of Technology Assessment—in Search of a Useful Approach. The Hague, The Netherlands: Staatsuitgeverij, 1984. (Summary in English.)

Thacker, S. B. *The Effectiveness and Safety of Intrapartum Electronic Fetal Monitoring.* Unpublished manuscript, 1987

Warner, K., & Hutton, R. "Cost-Benefit and Cost-Effectiveness Analysis in Health Care." *Medical Care, 18,* 1069, 1980.

Warner, K., & Luce, B. R. *Cost-benefit and Cost-effectiveness Analysis in Health Care: Principles, Practice, and Potential.* Ann Arbor, MI: Health Administration Press, 1982.

16

Governance and Management

Anthony R. Kovner

Put simply, governance in health care organizations (HCOs) is the system for making important decisions, and managers are the group responsible for implementing those decisions. Governance and management are important, as health care is being provided increasingly in large organizations, where these functions are partitioned among trustees, managers, and clinician leaders. In small HCOs, such as some doctor's offices and nursing homes, owners and operators often govern, manage and provide care.

This chapter is divided into two parts. The first, on governance, covers how power is distributed; it describes the role, structure, and function of governing boards, and it examines current issues and approaches toward more effective governance. The second part of this chapter is on management; it describes what managers do and how they are trained; it examines the managerial contribution to HCO performance, and it explores important current issues in management.

Governance

Governance is direction, control, and exercise of authority. Authority is the power or admitted right to command or act. The difference between the concepts is this: governance describes those who have power and how it is exercised; authority explains the bases of such power. Governance may be dominated by a few individuals or by many; it may be exercised in an authoritarian or in a democratic way. Those who govern have the final say and are accountable for what an HCO does.

How the governance of HCOs is viewed depends on how one views their mission. HCOs may be seen as existing primarily to satisfy those who use or consume their services, those who own or work in the organization, or some combination of both. Those who govern make decisions that affect organizational policy or, by not making decisions, they allow others to influence what the HCO chooses to do and how. HCOs are dependent on the resources they require to achieve their purposes and survive. Such resources include patients, clinicians, facilities, and legitimacy. Governance influences the supply of resources as well as their allocation and use. Health care is increasingly provided by organizations rather than by solo practitioners. How HCOs are governed influences the futures of those who work in and are served by them.

Level of Analysis

There are several levels at which health care policy can be determined. Decisions can be made at the national level that affect local activities. For example, as a result of the Medicare legislation of 1965, general hospitals provided older Americans with more inpatient services per capita than previously and with more health care financing relative to other age groups. This decision was, in essence, determined not by each general hospital but by the elected representatives of the American people, who would now have government collect and reimburse more adequately for inpatient services provided to the elderly. Decisions affecting HCOs are also made at the level of the clinician or the consumer.

Here governance will be examined at the level of the HCO rather than that of the industry or the individual provider. HCOs are defined as organizations engaging in the direct provision of health care. By this definition, a hospital, a nursing home, and a group practice are included, but an insurance company, a drug company, and a government regulatory agency are not. Within the HCO the focus is at the level at which policy is determined rather than that at which policy is implemented.

Policy and Administration

The content of policy decisions varies widely among HCOs. What are policy decisions for one HCO are administrative or routine decisions for another. For example, the duties of family health workers in a community health center may be a policy decision, whereas the operation of a laundry facility with other centers is not. The reverse may be true for an urban general hospital, because the objectives of the two HCOs are different. Policy decisions are those that affect objectives. If an objective of a community health center is to provide primary care to a local population, the way in which family health workers are trained is likely to affect the objective, whereas lowering the cost per pound of laundry done does not. If a hospital objective is to reduce operating losses for certain diagnostic related groups (DRGs), however; then, sharing laundry services with other hospitals may involve policy, whereas reconfiguration of the duties of health care workers in the ambulatory care department does not.

Certain types of organizational decisions usually involve policy. Such decisions include long-range planning, the allocation of resources, and the selection and evaluation of top management. Decisions in these areas all have an important effect on organizational objectives. Long-range plans determine which programs will be provided at what level by the HCO and therefore how resources will be allocated. For example, the need for inpatient beds in a large mental hospital may decrease because of improved methods of treatment. This results in a long-range planning decision to emphasize rehabilitative rather than custodial care. Changing organizational objectives, however, often causes conflict within an organization. A new priority of rehabilitative care may be resisted by mental hospital staff because behavior that had been acceptable and perhaps even desirable when custodial care was a primary objective of the mental hospital is unacceptable and undesirable when rehabilitative care becomes a primary objective.

Organizational objectives are also often affected by the allocation of resources. For example, a group practice may weigh its salary structure heavily in favor of senior partners, thereby influencing the kinds of physicians attracted to the group and hence the ability of the group to attract new patients. The group is therefore able to increase revenues primarily by providing additional services to those already using its services. If a hospital increases its budgetary allocation for management or social services, this may indicate that the hospital no longer places the same emphasis on meeting the needs of physicians in their private practice and that it will place a higher priority on coordination of services or meeting the service needs of the disadvantaged.

Another type of policy decision concerns the selection and evaluation of top management, including supervising clinicians in their managerial role. The interests and enthusiasms of a hospital chief of surgery may conflict with those of the governing board. The chief may wish to raise money to invest in facilities and staff to perform open-heart surgery, whereas the board's long-range plan is to establish a prepaid group practice to provide primary and secondary care. Alternatively, the board may place heavy emphasis on the provision of tertiary care, but the chief of surgery may prefer that department to perform a high volume of simple surgical operations.

Governance and Management

Although those who govern are supposed to make policy and those who manage are supposed to administer policy, there is no clear-cut boundary between governance and management. In practice, those who manage are often key participants in governance, as they have the necessary time and information to define a problem or to limit the policy alternatives. This is, in large part, what those who manage are paid to do. On the other hand, those who govern the organization often carry out policy or manage as well, as they have the power and the will to do so. A more useful distinction between governance and management may therefore involve the importance and nature of the decisions for the HCO. Decisions involving who governs and those involving organizational mission are governance, not management, decisions. Decisions regarding day-to-day operations, such as who should do what and when in the operating room or the personnel office are management decisions.

Governing Boards

This section focuses on HCO governance through a detailed look at the structure and function of HCO governing boards. We shall look at HCOs in which there is a specialized structure such as a board, a group, or a committee that determines policy and in which a substantial number of policy decisions are made by the HCO. These *two conditions* are generally found in general hospitals, health maintenance organizations (HMOs), and large group practices and nursing homes.

The Legal Basis of the Governing Board

In HCOs there is generally a governing body of designated persons who have legal responsibility for the conduct of the organization. Corporations are required to make such designations as a condition of incorporation by the state in which their home office is located.

Hospital or nursing home bylaws usually outline the purposes of the organization, the composition and duties of the governing board, the requirements for meetings of the board and notice of meetings, the duties and nature of corporate officers and the method of their selection, the nature and purpose of board committees, and how the bylaws can be amended. A physicians' partnership agreement may typically include the responsibilities of partners, how net income is shared and losses borne, disability provisions, termination of a partner's agreement, and the composition of the executive committee or board and its functions.

The legal powers of the governing board, suggested in a model constitution and bylaws for voluntary hospitals published by the American Hospital Association (1981) are the following:

> The general powers of the corporation shall be vested in the governing board, which shall have charge, control and management of the property, affairs, and funds of the corporation; shall fill vacancies among the officers for the unexpired terms; and shall have the power and authority to do and perform all acts and functions not inconsistent with these bylaws or with any action taken by the corporation. [p. 11]

These bylaws could be those of any corporation, health care or otherwise, for-profit or not-for-profit.

In theory, the governing board has the responsibility for making policy for the organization. In practice, the power and function of governing bodies in HCOs varies widely, depending on the HCO's history, key resources required for the HCO's survival and growth, the nature of the local power structure, and so forth. Policy in various areas may be formulated and decided on by different groups in different organizations. For example, questions of capital funding may be decided by the board of the multiunit organization of which a hospital is only a part; the scope of services may be decided by the hospital governing board; clinician educational programs may be decided on by the professional staff, and issues of local marketing and community relations decided by management.

The role of the governing board in the HCO is more ambiguous when there are no shares to be sold as in business, it is more complex in HCOs where the medical staff are not employees.

Selection of Board Members

The functions and powers of a governing board are influenced by its composition and its method of selecting members. When a hospital or a group practice is first established, the governing board usually consists of the founders, those who are contributing key resources to begin the enterprise. Officers are selected by the members of the governing board. In the case of investor-owned institutions, this is done formally by voting of shares. In nonprofit organizations and large partnerships, all full members generally have an equal vote. The board members themselves select additional members or replacements, or they are chosen from larger corporate bodies whose membership may be self-selected by those making a contribution of a certain sum to the corporation. In consumer-dominated HMOs or neighborhood health centers, some or all members of the governing board may be elected by health plan subscribers or residents of areas served by the organization,

In 1985 approximately 46% of the average hospital board's membership had backgrounds in business or finance. About 30% of board membership was made up of health care professionals, particularly of physicians (HRET). There was a wide difference in board composition by the type of control. Unsurprisingly, government and religious hospitals had a greater proportion of governmental officials and religious officers on their boards. Osteopathic hospitals had a greater proportion of doctors on their boards.

Board members may be "insiders"—HCO managers or clinicians—or "outsiders" chosen for some special expertise, status, or access to resources. The type chosen will depend, in large part, on the functions and role of the board. If the primary function of the board is to raise money or give advice and counsel to the chief executive officer (CEO), then outsiders are more likely to be selected. If the primary function is to decide policy, then the directors should have detailed knowledge of HCO operations and environment, and insiders may be preferred.

Table 16.1 Sample Position Description for the Hospital Board of Directors

General functions

Establish and maintain the organization's mission

Act as trustee for the assets and investments of the shareholders or owners in the nonprofit corporation

Select, advise, and audit the CEO.

Grant physicians staff privileges and ensure that quality medical care is provided.

Provide broad direction for the affairs of the hospital and ensure the development and growth of the institution's services.

Specific duties

Prepare for board and committee meetings by whatever study and preparatory work are necessary to deliberate intelligently with co-directors

Attend meetings of the board and committee appointments

Execute board assignments on time.

Maintain confidentiality and security regarding hospital information

Contribute positively to board discussions, assisting the board in reaching conclusions

Serve as a consultant to the CEO and, with his or her approval, to others in the organization

Acquire a working knowledge of those functional activities for which he or she has committee assignments

Develop a broad knowledge of today's hospitals and future trends in health care

Be alert to new program opportunities and assist the organization on specific programs when requested

Avoid interference in hospital operations

Avoid conflict of interest whenever an issue arises, and abstain from board discussions when matters in which he or she has a personal interest are being considered

Adapted from J. Witt, *Building a Better Hospital Board.* Ann Arbor, MI: American College of Healthcare Executives, 1987, pp. 64–65.

Governance of hospitals has been dominated by outsider trustees, governance of nursing homes by manager outsiders, and governance of group practices by insider physicians.

A sample job description for hospital boards and board members is given in Table 16.1.

Except in large investor-owned HCOs, most board members are not paid for their time, although Witt (1987) and Kovner (1985) believe they should be. Board members serve for a variety of reasons: community service or fiduciary responsibility, status, access to medical care, or because they believe their skills and experience are vital to HCO mission attainment.

Board Structure and Function

Governing boards vary in internal structure and function. Information is not generally available concerning the number of boards with restrictions on terms of office and mandatory retirement age, nor concerning the length and frequency of meetings or the nature of participation by few of many members. In regard to size, governing boards range from fewer than 10 to more than 200 members. A 1985 American Hospital Association (AHA) survey revealed that the average hospital board consisted of 14 members, almost all of whom had voting privileges. Not-for-profit hospitals averaged 19 members, and boards of investor-owned and public hospitals were half of that size (HRET). Witt (1987) suggests that no board, no matter how large the hospital, should have more than 15 members and that hospitals with revenues of $20 million or less should have no more than 5 to 7 members.

Board committees are generally of two types: standing, or permanent, committees, and special committees, which are discharged on completion of a task. Typical standing committees for a hospital board are executive, finance, medical staff, nominating, and long-range planning. Executive committees usually have power to act between regular meetings of the governing board. A large group practice may have a separate committee on personnel, which is concerned with defining responsibilities and benefits of partners, a committee on hospital relations, and one concerned with recruiting physicians. Focusing on large business corporations, Mintzberg (1983) has suggested the following seven functions for governing boards.

1. Select the chief executive officer.
2. Exercise control during a crisis.
3. Review managerial decisions and performance.
4. Co-opt external influences.
5. Establish contracts and raise funds.
6. Enhance the organization's reputation.
7. Give advice and technical assistance.

A significant omission from this list is "make strategic decisions." Mintzberg argues, and I agree, that part-time board members know less than full-time managers and that deferring too many decisions to the board raises questions about the ability of top managers to run the organization.

The Changing Role of the Board

Views of the role of governing boards differ and are changing. More than 30 years ago, Burling, Lentz, and Wilson (1956) stated that the governing board in a hospital has a responsibility to provide and maintain the hospital to serve a community need according to the wishes of the donors. Underwood (1969) has viewed the governing board as a referee between the interests of the hospital administrator and the medical staff. Pelligrino (1972) has seen the governing board as designated by the community to oversee the process of medical care within the hospital. Perloff (1970) has viewed the responsibility of the board as creating an environment in which health care workers can provide services to patients. To Umbdenstock (1987), the board must be the "organization's conscience, constantly assessing proposed directions . . . in light of what these steps mean for the implementation of a mission to serve and care for all (p. 12)." He divides work between the board and the CEO as follows: "whereas the board is concerned primarily with whether or not the hospital will do something, the administrator is responsible for how it will be done once the board gives the go-ahead" (Umbdenstock, 1983, p. 12). Some HCOs such as veterans hospitals or state mental hospitals do not have any governing boards; they are managed by administrators reporting to state officials and legislatures.

There is probably no one best way to allocate functions between board and management. Rather, what is important in any particular HCO is clarification and agreement as to who in the organization decides what on the recommendations of whom. Otherwise, the political cost of making timely strategic decisions is too high, and the probability of implementing such decisions is too low.

Relation to Medical Staff. In general hospitals, the governing body delegates to the medical staff the authority to evaluate the professional competence of staff members and applicants for staff privileges. Medical staff bylaws, rules, and regulations are subject to governing board approval, which, according to the Joint Commission on the Accreditation of Hospitals, shall not be unreasonably withheld. The Joint Commission also mandates that the governing board "shall require that the medical staff . . . to implement and report on the activities and mechanisms for monitoring and evaluating the quality of patient care for identifying and resolving problems, and for identifying opportunities to improve patient care" (JCAH, p. 50).

The bylaws of hospital governing boards deal with medical staff principally in three areas: (1) organization, appointments, and hearings for medical staff, (2) medical care and its evaluation, and (3) medical staff bylaws. The board's bylaws may include paragraphs dealing with organization and bylaws *of a medical and dental staff.* The AHA's suggested bylaws approach the problem of hospital appointment by recommending the following:

> The governing board shall consider recommendations of the medical staff and appointment to the medical staff, in numbers not exceeding the hospital's needs, physicians and others who meet the qualifications for membership as set forth in the bylaws of the medical staff. Each member of the medical staff shall have appropriate authority and responsibility for the care of his patients, subject to limitations as are contained in these bylaws and in the bylaws, roles and regulations for the medical staff and subject, further, to any limitations attached to his appointment. (AHA)

The bylaws then deal with the appointment procedure and the renewal of appointments without formal reapplication (hospital appointments are generally made for a period of 1 year). Then a paragraph may be devoted to opportunity for a hearing if any change is proposed in the appointment to assure due process and afford full opportunity for the presentation of all pertinent information. A key paragraph in the second section dealing with medical care and its evaluation suggests that "the medical staff shall conduct an ongoing review and appraisal of the quality of professional care rendered in the hospital, and shall report such activities and their results to the governing board" (AHA, p. 18). With regard to medical staff bylaws, the AHA suggests that only those bylaws adopted by the governing board shall become effective.

In hospitals, physicians commonly expect governing boards to keep the organization financially solvent, to avoid "interfering" with the practice of medicine or curbing physicians' freedom, and to respect the contribution physicians make as practitioners. Some of the expectations commonly held by hospital governing boards for physicians include showing loyalty to the hospital by admitting their patients, practicing good medicine, understanding that the hospital is not merely a doctor's workshop, and acknowledging that they as physicians may lack the information to make certain important decisions such as scope of services or compliance with government regulations.

Some of the reasons that physicians' expectations are not met include the following: Boards increasingly believe that the practice of medicine can have an important impact on hospital solvency; other clinicians, such as nurses, have claims that conflict with those of physicians; and board members may feel that some physicians' benefits from hospital practice far outweigh their contribution to the hospital's objectives.

Some of the reasons that boards' expectations are not met include the following: Some physicians compete against the hospital with which they have a primary affiliation; some physicians do not always meet the standards of adequate medical practice; and some physicians may feel that the medical staff should be a separate organization contracting at arm's length with the hospital to provide medical services.

Lack of Consensus on Board Role. As HCOs become larger and more complex and as the environment in which they function becomes more competitive, consensus on the role of the governing board tends to break down. And many HCOs may have difficulty in adapting to changed requirements for survival and growth. In response to public discontent with the cost and responsiveness of hospitals, some may urge governing boards to assume a legislative role, making policy in a way analogous to governmental legislatures and representing the consumers of services, or to assume merely an advisory role, ceding decision-making power to top executives who can presumably "get things done."

In the face of increasing competition, the governance function may become more critical to accomplishment of HCO performance objectives. The leadership of medical group practice, for example, may become increasingly specialized, with some clinicians devoting increasing time to, and developing expertise in nonclinical functions such as adapting to competition from HMO, interfacing with government agencies, keeping practicing physicians aware of the pressures facing the group, and the appropriate alternative organizational responses necessary for group survival and growth.

Current Issues

Some current key governance issues include the following: (1) Who should own HCOs? (2) To what extent does board performance need to be improved? (3) What kind of autonomy should HCOs have? (4) How and to what extent should HCOs be accountable to those whom they serve and whom they potentially serve?

Preferable Ownership Patterns

With the increasing role of government in the health care sector of the economy, ownership of HCOs has become an issue. Should HCOs be owned by government or by for-profit or by nonprofit corporations? A separate question, also a current issue, is whether or not there are sufficient significant differences between not-for-profit and for-profit ownership of HCOs to justify tax exemption for the former (Gray; *Utah County v. Intermountain Health Care, Inc.*).

There is insufficient evidence to make categorical statements regarding the effect of ownership per se on the cost or quality of medical care. Those who argue against for-profit ownership maintain that the motivation of proprietary owners is profit rather than community service: For-profits concentrate on providing only those services that are profitable, leaving the not-for-profits and public HCOs to provide care for those who lack adequate insurance. A corollary argument is that for-profit HCOs build facilities only in expanding high-income communities, leaving not-for-profit and governmental HCOs to provide services to the urban and rural poor; the monies allocated to shareholders of for-profit HCOs could be better reinvested in the delivery of services; and health care is of lower quality in for-profit HCOs than in nonprofit or governmental HCOs.

Counterarguments have been made in favor of for-profit ownership: Even allowing for profit, these HCOs are more efficient because of the profit incentive, and they pay taxes; consumers should be charged the costs of the services they use rather than overcharging certain consumers because others cannot pay, as is the case in nonprofit HCOs; for-profits can respond more quickly and more flexibly in meeting community demand; and the quality of care provided in most for-profits is adequate and in some for-profits is higher than that provided in certain HCOs under nonprofit or governmental auspices.

Regarding governmental ownership, the following arguments are made in its favor: Total costs and unit costs are lower, signifying greater efficiency; everyone gets treated similarly, based on health needs and regardless of income or disease status; and the quality of care is not lower than that provided in HCOs under other auspices. The following arguments are opposed to government ownership: Primary emphasis is in keeping total costs low rather than upon providing adequate health care; governmental management is bureaucratic and inflexible; and, the quality of care is lower in governmental HCOs.

Arguments in favor of nonprofit ownership are the mirror image of those made in favor and against for-profit and governmental HCOs. Those in favor of not-for-profit HCOs praise their high quality of care and the high level of community service; those opposed cite the high cost. For specific nonprofit HCOs, opponents add that the quality of care is low and the community services nonexistent. This has led to the suggestion that there ought to be clearly articulated standards for what it means to deserve the special "voluntary" description whether these standards are sponsored and regulated by the Joint Commission on the Accreditation of Hospitals, the Internal Revenue Service, or the hospital or health care industry (Seay & Vladeck).

In order to evaluate these arguments, research must be conducted relating ownership to performance. To do such research it is required that conditions other than ownership, such as size of the HCO, be held constant. Also required is a greater consensus about adequate and effective performance in various HCOs.

Performance of Governing Boards

Peters and Tseng (1983) note some characteristics of boards of well-managed hospitals: the boards are active and working, they have a clear understanding of their own and management responsibilities, and they are viewed by management as an ally in managing change. There is, however, disagreement about what the board's contribution to hospital performance should be and even about hospital performance itself, other than avoidance of bankruptcy and retention of accreditation.

Kovner (1985) has specified four key problems in hospital governance: board inability or unwillingness to specify objectives, inefficient and ineffective decision-making, lack of strategy development, and inability to deal with conflict over functions of board, medical staff, and management. One of the chief advantages that investor-owned HCOs have is the clarity of their organizational objectives. In 1984 Hospital Corporation of America (HCA), a large investor-owned corporation, expected an after-tax return of at least 17% on average equity and growth on annual earnings per share, after general inflation, of at least 13% (HCA). Most HCOs do not specify measurable objectives in advance because board, management, and medical staff cannot or will not agree on either the objectives themselves or on a desirable level of attainment. In hospitals, conflict probably stems from the only partial integration of the medical staff into the organizational structure, with a resultant lack of clarity over whose hospital it is.

There are several possible reasons for inadequate decision making by boards: The board may be too large; too many groups and individuals may be involved in strategic decision making; too many levels of groups may be involved; those who make strategic decisions may not be adequately informed; and it may be unclear which group at what level is supposed to make which decisions. The following description of decision making in a teaching hospital is a good example of such ineffectiveness.

> First, there are two boards that govern the hospital, each with different orientations and separate reporting lines and with few guidelines to determine how decisions are allocated between them . . . Second . . . the hospital's director continues to be subject to the university. Third, the hospital director and the dean of the medical school share line authority over the same chiefs of the hospital's clinical services, who are also chairpersons of academic departments within the medical school. Finally, each line executive's bureaucratic authority is countered by a collegial body of subordinates who advise the executive in matters affecting their vital interests. [Allison & Dalston, 1982, pp. 11–12]

According to Ritvo (1980), hospital boards cope with actual problems rather than anticipating future issues. In identifying concerns, they rely heavily on internal data rather than on data regarding competitors. In the past, boards and managers have tended to allocate resources to the acquisition of new technology rather than to the development of planning and marketing capabilities. When developed, plans and programs are often lacking in political reality; they are delayed, rejected, or watered down by medical staff and therefore are not effectively implemented.

It must be clear what group in an organization is supposed to make which decisions. According to Dayton (1984), "every time you find a business in trouble, you find a board of directors either unwilling or unable to fulfill its responsibilities." And according to Pfeffer (1972), "corporations who fail to use their boards as links to their environments pay penalties in reduced profits." If the board is to review and approve management's decisions, management must be informed and willing, and the board must be able to evaluate the competence of management.

Toward improved hospital board performance, the following recommendations have been made by Kovner (1985): Integrate medical leadership into hospital governance, largely through the employment of accountable clinician managers; streamline the process of making strategic decisions, largely through a unified organizational structure that focuses responsibility on front-line manager and clinician leaders; foster board support for management in making changes;

and encourage the board to focus and energize itself around key issues of mission, such as scope of services, competitive strategies, and financial support required to successfully implement management plans.

The Extent of Organizational Autonomy

To what extent should an HCO be allowed to determine what services to provide to whom at what price? This issue relates to the role of the governing board, regardless of the type of ownership, and to the scope and depth of its powers. The powers, or autonomy, of HCO governing boards have been shrinking since 1960. Federal and state governments have passed legislation forbidding discrimination against patients who seek admission or persons seeking employment and invalidating a requirement that staff physicians of a voluntary hospital be graduates of a medical school approved by the AMA and members of the county medical society. They have removed the exemption of hospitals from state labor laws, specified standards to be met by HCOs in order to be licensed by a state or reimbursed by Medicare, and forbidden construction of hospitals, nursing homes, and related facilities in some states without prior approval by state planning authorities. More recent limitations on the autonomy of HCOs that have been enacted by government include limiting payment for new technology under Medicare and Medicaid; imposing requirements for community services for hospitals to retain not-for-profit status; requiring, in West Virginia, community representation on governing boards; and capping revenues in some states or limiting reimbursement under Medicare (by DRGs) to average payments for length of stay regardless of cost.

There is no simple answer to the question of HCO determination of services, prices, and population served. Too little autonomy for the HCO board will result in withdrawal of high-quality individuals from leadership positions and of voluntary energies that have been a strength of not-for-profit HCOs. Excessive standardization and centralization of decision making in governmental bureaucracies will result in decreased HCO innovation and eventually in decreased productivity. On the other hand, too much autonomy for HCOs may have been responsible, at least in part, for the present situation of uneven age-adjusted mortality and morbidity rates by race and income, overutilization of hospitals and underutilization of long-term care, uneven productivity and service, and high cost. One suggestion for appropriate centralization and decentralization is the regionalization of HCOs. However, that is also subject to similar criticisms of involving too much or too little centralization.

Accountability to Those Served

Whatever the scope of HCO activities and their regulation by government, what should be the extent and nature of governing board accountability to users and potential users of services? Some of those who advocate more formal accountability argue that this can be assured only by a governing board controlled by consumer representatives. Opponents argue that such control will lead to ineffective decision making at the board level and eventual withdrawal of community resources from health care. The opponents ask, furthermore, what evidence there is that the newly chosen representatives will be any more accountable. In what ways would they be more accountable and to whom? Consumers desire health care that is reasonably priced, accessible, provided in a humane, personal way, and technically of high quality. The great majority do not wish to make policy for HCOs, either directly or indirectly through their representatives, as long as they can obtain satisfactory health care. Advocates respond that consumers will not obtain satisfactory health care until governing boards are dominated by consumer representatives.

Regardless of the debate at the governing-board level, appeal mechanisms should be available for consumers at the level at which services are received, especially in large HCOs. In many HCOs consumers lack voice when they are dissatisfied with the manner of the provider, the wait for services, and the explanations they receive about what is wrong and about the alternative courses of treatment and their pertinent costs and benefits. They may be told to seek service elsewhere, or they can sue for malpractice. Consumers who are poor or institutionalized lack even these often-unsatisfactory alternatives. Proposals have been made and implemented regarding a variety of appeal mechanisms—the special board committee, the externally appointed ombudsman, the patient advocate—all specialized mechanisms for helping the patient who is unfairly treated by the HCO. Other, more general mechanisms include consumer advisory councils, focus groups and market surveys, and holding the chief executive personally accountable for responding to consumer complaints. As with all solutions, there are difficulties in implementing appeal mechanisms and limitations to their usefulness. To whom does the consumer appeal if he or she is dissatisfied with the response of the appeal mechanism, which may be, after all, a creation of the HCO? Appeal mechanisms may be costly in relation to the benefits obtained by the consumer. And there are many aspects of care that consumers (and providers) find objectionable but about which little can be done at the level of the HCO, such as obtaining high-quality accessible outpatient services for the uninsured. Finally, appeal mechanisms may serve only as buffers that satisfy the occasional vocal complainant but do little to change the system of care that may be the cause of much more unspoken dissatisfaction among many.

Management

This part will focus on what managers do in HCOs, how they are trained, their contributions to effective HCO performance, and current issues in health care management.

The Organization of Managerial Work in HCOs

In simple organizations such as the physician's office, clinicians themselves perform managerial functions such as billing patients or contracting with an outside vendor to bill patients (see Figure 16.1A). In a group practice the hiring, paying, and firing of physicians is done by clinicians who manage and who also practice medicine. Other work such as billing is supervised by non-clinician managers. In the large hospital or HMO, specialized staff managers support clinician and nonclinician managers. Specialized departments include human resource, finance, security, and marketing, among others. In multiunit organizations of several hospitals, nursing homes, and/or group practices, the manager of the individual HCO reports to the division manager of a geographical area such as the northeastern United States. Division managers, in turn, are accountable to corporate headquarters management. In these large organizations certain management functions are divided among headquarters, divisions, and HCOs. Headquarters functions may include legal services, construction, capital financing, and corporate public relations. Other functions, such as quality assurance and production standards, are partitioned among the three organizational levels.

A relatively new development in the organization of managerial work in HCOs is the concept of product-line management. The large hospital or group practice can be reorganized into several product lines, such as women's health services, emergency care, cancer care, and rehabilitation services, each with its own manager and budget. The logic behind such reorganization is that these services can be more effectively managed as separate "businesses" than as parts of a large HCO. Whether or not this is really so is unproven. (For a comparison with traditional organization, see Figure 16.2.)

What Managers Do

Positions and Functions

A job or position description is one way of looking at the work that managers do. The position description of an outpatient manager in a hospital is shown in Table 16.2.

Implicit in this job description are managerial functions, each of which comprises a group of activities. Longest (1980) views the basic managerial functions as

- Planning, which involves the determination of objectives.
- Organizing, which is the structuring of people and things to accomplish the work required to meet the objectives.
- Directing, which is the stimulation of members of the organization to meet the objectives.

Figure 16.1 Organization of Managerial Work in HCOs

A. Doctor's office

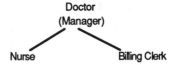

B. Group Practice

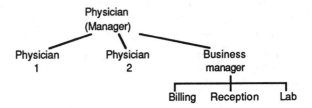

C. Hospital

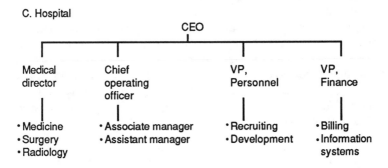

D. Multiunit hospital corporation

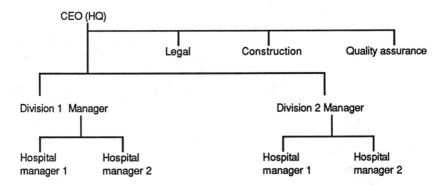

Table 16.2 Position Description of Outpatient Manager

Title of Direct Supervisor: *Assistant V.P. for Ambulatory Care*
Purpose

To manage the administrative staff and functions and to coordinate the professional, clerical, and support services of all nonpsychiatric units in the Outpatient Department for the purpose of optimizing delivery of ambulatory patient care.

Description of duties
- Manages day-to-day operations of all ambulatory, medical/surgical, Ob/Gyn, adult and pediatric clinics, subspeciality clinics, private ambulatory service for related services.
- Supervises a staff of approximately 30 clerical and supervisory employees; hires, fires, takes disciplinary action.
- Plans and oversees training and orientation of employees; evaluates performance on a periodic basis; establishes standards, goals, and performance criteria; initiates personnel action as appropriate.
- Determines staffing needs and establishes schedules to ensure appropriate administrative coverage.
- Prepares, maintains, and controls the administrative operating capital budget for the Outpatient Department; designs and installs appropriate expense and manpower controls to measure budget adherence; makes adjustments as necessary and coordinates allocation of resources with other related cost centers.
- Plans and requisitions supplies and services for Outpatient Department.
- Collaborates with nursing, medical and administrative staff to formulate and implement policies for the Outpatient Department.
- Establishes and coordinates systems and procedures that support efficient delivery of medical and support services to the patient and that maintain quality patient care.
- Updates Outpatient Department procedural manuals; distributes information to staff.
- Evaluates all systems and procedures periodically for appropriateness and efficiency in meeting goals.
- Coordinates functions of and serves as a liaison with the hospital departments providing services to the Outpatient Department, such as pathology, radiology, and medical staff administration, to ensure effective and smooth interdepartmental operations.
- Investigates, reviews, and responds to patient complaints.
- Develops periodic statistical analyses and prepares departmental reports.
- Oversees environmental matters; coordinates with support departments to insure proper maintenance of Outpatient Department facilities.
- Assists Assistant Vice President for Ambulatory Care in preparing grant proposals; prepares all budgetary aspects of proposals.
- Participates in outside activities, including conferences and workshops.
- Represents hospital center in dealings with community groups and outside agencies, such as the Association for Ambulatory Care and the Hospital Association Ambulatory Care Project.
- Ensures that the Outpatient Department complies with standards of agencies such as JCAH and the city Department of Health.
- Manages Outpatient Department's quality-assurance program.
- Assists the Assistant Vice President in performing other related duties and projects as needed.

Education required

B.A./B.S. degree with courses in management; master's degree preferable.
Experiences and/or skills required

A minimum of 3 years experience in an ambulatory care administrative position, preferably in a hospital setting; experience in third-party reimbursement systems and budgeting.

Figure 16.2 Traditional versus Product-Line Organization

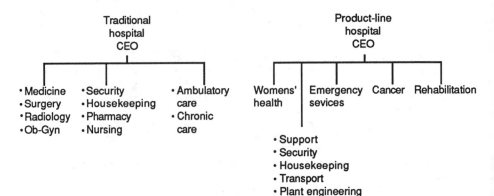

- Coordinating, which is the conscious effort of assembling and synchronizing diverse activities and participants so that they work toward the attainment of objectives.
- Controlling, in which the manager compares actual results with objectives to provide a measure of success or failure.

Managerial Roles

Another way of conceptualizing what managers do is in terms of roles, which are aspects of behavior that can be isolated for analytical purposes, such as leading, or handling disturbances. Managers settle conflicts, inspire other workers, and represent the organization to outside groups. An individual manager's roles can thus be abstracted. This helps in understanding how managers contribute to organizational effectiveness and the constraints and opportunities they face in their work.

Because of the fragmented authority structure of many HCOs, managers often must lead by persuasion rather than by directive. Leadership is a relational rather than a personal characteristic, and therefore effectiveness as a leader is measured by what followers do rather than by how managers behave. The health care manager, especially in public and voluntary organizations, is constantly involved in testing the positions of other inside and outside the HCO and in confronting claimants for organizational resources. The manager must constantly persuade physicians, nurses, and others that the organization has good reasons for not doing what they want or for doing what they object to. External regulatory agencies may compel or allow certain actions desired by claimants. What claimants want may not be equitable. Some claimants may demand unequal treatment because the organization is unequally dependent on them.

An example of this is the demand by a hospital department head of inhalation therapy, supported by the chief of pulmonary medicine, for an increase in salary beyond the general guidelines for department heads. Either the hospital administrator must deny the request and convince these two individuals that the denial is fair, or the administrator must approve the request and convince other department heads that the increase *is* fair, or at least that the decision was arrived at fairly.

Disturbances in HCOs sometimes involve life-and-death issues, such as providing emergency services to victims of a natural disaster, responding to a bomb threat, or confronting deranged employees or aggrieved relatives. In such cases, managers must act quickly and appropriately, as if they know what to do. Managers should plan in detail their responses to possible emergency situations and should test their responses before emergencies occur.

Even when a life-and-death issue is not involved, patients and their families often have intense feelings about what is happening—for example, about death and dying or about diagnosis of infectious disease. It is the manager's job to deal with conflicts and problems that arise in treating such patients and in disturbances among workers of different backgrounds and skills in a labor-intensive organization. Kovner (1984) has reconceptualized managerial roles into four sets: motivating others, scanning the environment, negotiating the political terrain, and generating and allocating resources.

Motivating Others. Managers spend a great deal of their time recruiting and retaining managerial and supervisory staff and in making decisions about rewards and promotions, work procedures, and development and training. To carry out these activities they use communications and analytical skills. Managers assist subordinates in doing what is required and in doing what subordinates want to do, within organizational limits. This can be difficult if managers have not recruited subordinates (and recruitment is more of an art than a science). An excellent batting percentage in recruitment may be more like .600 than .850.

An example of motivating others is managerial development and training. Managers in new organizations or in new positions in existing organizations must be developed and trained by their supervisors. Such development and training can assist in the subordinate's learning process. Managers can aid those who work with them by identifying the skills that must be learned and the experience that must be acquired for effective job performance. Seniors can also help juniors become more aware of their own values, how they are perceived by others, and how the values of others affect their job performance in this position in this HCO.

Scanning the Environment. Effective managers scan or search the environment for potential problems and targets of opportunity. Scanning activities include market and product research, long-range planning, and quality assessment. The development of management information systems may be essential for effective scanning. In large HCOs scanning activities are usually performed by special units of marketing, quality assessment, development, and planning. In smaller organizations managers may scan the environment themselves or with the assistance of subordinates or colleagues. Information about what similar organizations and managers do is available from journals, books, newsletters, and advertisements. Managers attend continuing education and trade association meetings where colleagues and experts discuss organizational and managerial opportunities and problems. Managers visit similar organizations to learn at firsthand about possible ways to improve effectiveness and efficiency. Openness to such visits is characteristic of public and voluntary HCOs.

Negotiating the Political Terrain. Effective managers maintain trust and build alliances with groups and individuals. A positive political climate contributes to effective decision making and implementation. New managers must find out "who is doing what to whom" in their organization; or, put another way, "What is the ball park in which I am playing, who are the players, and what are the rules?" Managers learn the informal organizational power structure by reading and listening. The operative rules are not always easy to ascertain. They vary by organizational setting, and they depend on the issue being discussed. Decision makers involved in establishing a management information system are different from those who decide to establish a renal dialysis unit.

Activities the manager undertakes in this set of roles include public relations, lobbying, labor negotiations, influencing decisions made by governing boards and medical staffs, arbitrating between internal units and departments, and negotiating with other organizations.

Generating and Allocating Resources. Effective managers spend a great deal of time analyzing organizational efficiency and finding ways to increase revenues and decrease expenses. In doing this, managers must consider past performance in this organization, present performance in like organizations, and industry standards.

Effective managers attempt to improve financial performance, for example, by making decisions about buying procedures, efficient securing of long-term and working capital, effective maintenance of buildings and equipment, appropriate price changes, and new construction. Effective managers attempt to understand whatever special circumstances may influence preferences among alternative objectives and strategies, and they listen closely to explanations and analysis by subordinates and clinicians.

Effective managers continually make decisions about generating and using resources. This occurs as part of the budgetary process and in response to emergency or extraordinary requests. Less tangible resources, such as staff time, must also be allocated, as must resources that may be less amenable to negotiation, such as space.

Tasks

Another way of looking at what managers do is in terms of the tasks or activities they perform, such as recruiting professionals and determining buying procedures. Managerial tasks can be grouped and analyzed as episodes of work, which can be examined in relation to organizational objectives, outcomes achieved, and resource costs involved. An example of what a hospital CEO does on a particular day is shown in Table 16.3 (Kovner, 1988).

Table 16.3 Episodes and Activities for Chief Executive Officer (CEO) T. Grover on Monday (12.25 hours)

Episodes and Activities	Time Spent
1. CEO is informed by Chief Operating Officer (COO) of phone threat to V.P. for Human Resources.	Brief (less than 10 min)
2. CEO is informed by COO that applicant has accepted offer as new Chief of Genetics.	Brief
3. CEO is informed by COO of office space mix-up involving physician whom the hospital is attempting to terminate.	Brief
4. CEO is informed by clinical chief about perceived ineffective behavior of another clinical chief.	Brief
5. CEO responds that he will meet state surveyors after being informed by COO of preparation underway for the state Health Department Inspection Survey.	Brief
6. CEO requests information from COO concerning drop in census.	Brief
7. CEO informs COO about the progress in planning hospital budget reductions.	Brief
8. CEO informs COO regarding implementation of changes in the hospital's fringe benefit plan.	Brief
9. CEO informs COO about MRI (magnetic resonance imaging) lease.	Brief
10. CEO informs COO about progress on a second site construction budget.	Brief
11. CEO is informed by COO about cost/productivity information that may be available for each hospital cost center.	Brief
12. CEO informs COO re continuation of captive malpractice insurance company involving other hospitals as well.	Brief
13. CEO informs COO re arrangements for delayed payments to pension fund.	Brief

Table 16.3 (*continued*)

Episodes and Activities	Time Spent
14. CEO informs COO that he will review Executive Committee meeting later with Chief Financial Officer (CFO).	Brief
15. CEO informs other hospital CEO and consultant of merger and is informed by them: he requests and is asked for further information.	Very long (more than 1 hr)
16. CEO requests CFO obtain information regarding obtaining increased state reimbursement after CEO informs re progress in rate adjustment by the state.	Brief
17. CEO requests from COO of second site the channeling of a donation through the hospital development program in response to being informed of such a donation.	Brief
18. CEO is informed by the COO about awards ceremony at second site.	Brief
19. CEO responds to trade association secretary that he can't attend a meeting after being informed about proposed state malpractice insurance rates and legislation.	Brief
20. CEO responds to secretary of medical disease organization affirmatively to requested use of his name to sponsor charitable luncheon for another organization.	Brief
21. CEO tells secretary that he cannot attend a medical school consortium meeting.	Brief
22. CEO responds to CEO of other hospital with his preferences after being informed of options in reorganizing state payment for uncompensated care.	Brief
23. CEO is informed by VP of Medical Affairs regarding planned dismissal of a physician.	Brief
24. CEO is informed by Assistant Administrator re implementation of hospital's quality assurance program.	Brief

As shown in Table 16.3, managers perform a great quantity of work and must continue beyond customary working hours. Their jobs are characterized by brevity of interactions with others, variety, and fragmentation. They favor verbal over written contact. Scheduled meetings consume more of managers' time than any other activity (Hales, 1986).

Skills and Experience

What are the skills and experience needed to obtain and perform managerial jobs in HCOs? Managers use communications and analytical skills in their work. Communications skills include reading, writing, speaking, and listening. Analytical skills include judging and deciding.

Communication Skills. Managers spend more time communicating than they spend deciding. In understanding what managers do, communication skills are probably underemphasized relative to analytic skills. As Urmy indicates,

> Hospital administration is not about sitting in your office with a calculator. . . . About ten percent of the job is pushing paper, bureaucratic work. . . . Although I may have gone to six meetings and put in a ten-hour day, sometimes I feel I didn't get anything done. . . . The primary function of a hospital administrator is to provide integration and coordination within the hospital. . . . This means meeting and talking with people. [Kovner, 1984, pp. 193–195]

Although communicating and deciding can take place simultaneously, lengthy communication often takes place before decisions are made and while they are being implemented.

Managers receive and send out a great deal of written material. Some managers compensate for limited reading and writing capability by doing most of their work in person or by phone. Reading, of course, includes analyzing numbers as well as concepts or service plans. Being able to interpret numbers critically is an important skill for health services managers.

Reading and writing skills can be learned. Managers should have learned them as part of an elementary and high school education, but unfortunately some have not. Many colleges and graduate schools have instituted special remedial writing courses and workshops. Speed reading courses are widely available as well.

Listening and speaking effectively are even more important for managers than skill in reading and writing. Many managers are not even aware that listening and speaking skills (other than public speaking) can be learned. However, managers can learn to make focused yet personal phone calls. They can learn to conduct meetings that accomplish goals yet make attendees feel that their points of view have been listened to and their feelings have been adequately taken into account.

Analytical Skills. Perhaps more clearly identifiable than communications skills are the analytical skills of judging and deciding. Brown (1966) has defined judgement as "knowledge ripened by experience." Many managers feel that skill in judging and deciding can come only from experience, that it cannot be taught in school. Others argue that by analyzing and responding to managerial situations such as structured cases or simultations, with students taking parts or playing roles of different participants, judgmental and decisional skills can be assessed and improved.

Before managers can judge or decide, they must, of course, be able to define a problem, gather data, structure alternatives, and calculate benefits and costs for each alternative. Each step of this problem-solving approach involves judging and deciding. For example, how valid is the manager's definition of the problem relative to that of key clinical chiefs? How much time should the manager spend gathering what data?

Computational skills are also required—for example, in making decisions regarding appropriate scheduling of patients for appointments, discounting the value of money over time to assess the true cost of capital financing, or pricing services to different payers so that revenues can be maximized.

Experience. Like other professions, skill as a manager involves learning through practice and being coached by others on how to avoid mistakes and achieve better outcomes. Participating in meetings and writing memos can be learned by self-analysis and feedback from peers, superiors, and subordinates. Experience also can be gained as a student in reading, listening, writing, computing, and interpreting data or in working as a member of a team doing a project for a local HCO.

Persona

The effectiveness of managers is determined as much by who they are and how they manage as by what they do. Managers are trusted, at least in part, based on how they are perceived by others. Managers are likely to think that how they manage—rather than race, sex, age, or beliefs—affects how others view their contribution. However, workers tend to feel more comfortable with, and more trusting of, persons whom they see as similar to themselves.

Superiors, subordinates, and peers sometimes react to managers primarily in terms of the question "Is the manager one of us or is he part of some outside group whom we dislike or fear?" The group practice administrator in a rural community in west Texas may have great difficulty gaining the trust of her board of directors if she is well educated and from New York City. Or a west Texas graduate of a small religious school will have a similarly hard time gaining the confidence of the medical and administrative staff in a public hospital in New York City serving Hispanics and blacks.

People trust one another partly because of what they think others believe. "If she believes in the same things that I do, perhaps it doesn't matter so much whether I like her. I can trust her because she is likely to do what I would do in a similar situation for her own reasons."

Registered nurses distrust managers when they see managers as being interested only in money, with little or no perceived commitment to providing high-quality patient care. Such distrust may or may not be justified, but it is usually dissipated only over time, as managers' actions indicate what their beliefs really are relevant to a particular work situation.

Educating Health Care Managers

How do people learn to be health care managers? Can health care management be taught? Is it a science, an art, or a craft? What can best be learned at school and on the job?

Graduate Programs. Graduate education is increasingly being required of persons seeking employment as health care managers. There are over 100 graduate programs in health care management in the United States today. Such programs may be called health care or medical care administration, health planning and policy, hospital administration, nursing home administration, medical group practice management, and public health administration. Many graduate programs are members of the Association of University Programs in Health Administration (AUPHA), headquartered in Washington, D.C. Of the 61 AUPHA American and Canadian members in 1986, 19 graduate programs are housed in graduate schools of business management or public administration, 18 in schools of public health, and 24 in one or more of the following schools: business, allied health, community health, and medicine.

In the academic year 1986–1987, a total of 4,188 students enrolled in 59 AUPHA graduate programs; slightly more than half were full-time. Of these students, 62% were women, and 10.5% were members of minority groups. In the same year 4,665 persons applied to the programs, and 56.5% were accepted. Master's degrees were awarded to 1,386 students.

As of 1986–1987, 52 programs had been accredited by the Accrediting Commission on Education for Health Services Administration (ACEHSA). ACEHSA is sponsored by AUPHA, together with the American College of Healthcare Administrators, the AHA, and the American Public Health Association. For accreditation, ACEHSA requires that the curriculum of a graduate program cover the following areas:

- Social-behavioral disciplines: economics, sociology, psychology, and political science.
- Determinants of health, disease, and disability: the study of what health is, how it is measured, patterns and characteristics of illness, and interventions possible with a health care system.
- Elements of personal health systems and their interrelationships: evaluation, governance, financial structure, organization, function and structure, quality assessment, and social accountability.
- Management and administrative skills and their applications: organizational behavior, quantitative methods, financial management, information systems, law, strategic planning, and health regulation.

In addition to curricular requirements for accreditation, ACEHSA sets criteria in the following areas: program eligibility, resources, objectives, faculty, students and alumni, research, community service, continuing education, and program evaluation.

Most graduate programs include an academic and a practice component, which may involve employment with or without pay in an HCO for a period of 3 to 12 months. Some programs do not require a practice component at all. As the supply of graduates increases in relation to demand, programs may extend the formal training period to 3 years, 1 year of which would be a residency.

Undergraduate Programs. Undergraduate programs in health care administration are a more recent development. As of 1985, 31 undergraduate programs in the United States were members of AUPHA, with 639 graduates in that year. The movement in undergraduate education began between 1965 and 1970, when some programs were established to train students for entry-level positions in the health care field.

Most of the undergraduate programs attempt to produce managers for intermediate-level positions in hospitals and for top-level positions in those health services organizations that have been found less attractive to graduates of the master's degree programs. The curriculum offered by the undergraduate programs is generally similar to that offered by graduate programs. Courses that are generally required include introduction to the health care field, economics, health law, administrative theory, personnel administration, financial management, health planning, medical sociology, quantitative methods, system analysis, and management of specific types of health care facilities.

Continuing Education. In addition to graduate and undergraduate programs, there is a great variety of continuing education programs in health services management. They are of various lengths and cover various subjects. Some continuing education programs are offered by the university programs themselves. Others are offered by centers of continuing education that are freestanding or that have been sponsored by professional associations or corporations that sell equipment and services to health services organizations. Still others are offered by the large HCOs themselves.

On the Job. Much of what managers learn about what works in an organization and about how they can best work with physicians and nurses is done on the job. This includes what managers say, how they write, how they look, and how they influence others. Superiors, subordinates, and peers can assist managers in teaching about an HCO.

Managerial Contribution to Effective Performance in HCOs

HCOs are seldom formally evaluated in terms of their own preset specified goals. Part of the reason is the difficulty of securing agreement among the various parties of interest as to what these goals are, what acceptable standards of performance are, and who should evaluate performance and by what methods. Yet the basic problem in public organizations, according to Drucker (1973), is not high cost but lack of effectiveness: "Only if targets are defined can resources be allocated to this attainment, priorities and deadlines be set, and somebody be held accountable for results."

Measuring Organizational Performance

One reason for attempting to specify effective or acceptable organizational performance is to focus attention on whose organization it is. If performance is acceptable to managers, physicians, and trustees, does it matter what anyone else thinks? If it does matter, what are others going to do if they find performance unacceptable?

Another reason for developing measures of organizational performance has to do with the distribution of organizational resources. In order to adjudicate claims on resources among claimants, questions may need to be raised about the organization's purposes. For example, "How is the HMO doing? How does what we do compare to what our competitors do? How does what we do compare with what our doctors, nurses, trustees, customers, and potential customers think we ought to be doing?"

Prior agreement about standards of performance facilitates agreement on performance evaluation. Otherwise, performance is not measurable in terms such as excellent, acceptable, and unacceptable. Statements such as "The hospital operated at a $100,000 surplus this year, one percent of the patients made formal complaints, and our turnover rate in nursing was 15 percent per year" are uncertain indicators of performance unless they can be related to agreed-upon standards and purposes. The standards of performance for which the organization and its managers are to be held accountable must be made clear in measurable terms and in advance. Of course, targets can be adjusted for fully explained reasons as circumstances change.

Putting Performance Requirements into Operation

Standards can be developed regarding performance requirements. Certain standards, such as financial ratios, are easier to quantify than others, such as commitment of physicians and nurses to organizational performance requirements. Yet commitment can be quantified in terms of turnover and absenteeism rates; unit costs per clinical service relative to industry standards; nurses' attitudes, as measured by surveys; and physician commitment measured by attendance at key committee meetings and contributions to fund-raising campaigns. Whether the effort and cost of putting such requirements into operation and then measuring performance is "worth it" is, of course, a separate and not a trivial question.

Griffith (1978) has argued that guidelines need to be developed for hospital performance in the face of national concern about rapidly increasing health care costs. Accordingly, there should be a few, well-understood measures of hospital care—uniformly available and designed to permit each community to compare itself to other, similar communities, its state, its region, and the nation as a whole.

Reasons for Not Specifying Objectives. One of the difficulties in measuring organizational performance is that, according to Perrow (1982), the concept of organizational goals as a major influence on organizational behavior is "only a convenient fiction," and much of what happens in organizations results from

> "happenstance, accidents, misunderstanding, and even random, unmotivated behavior. . . . Programs are started for a variety of vague and conflicting reasons, with the help of a lot of trivial or even accidental events. . . . Decision makers do not look for optimal solutions, have trouble discovering what they want, and settle for the first acceptable solution that come along, which is usually what the organization has been doing. That is, they settle so long as some important person or group doesn't want to change what the organization is doing and how the organization has been doing it."

Goal specification may not be necessary to achieving acceptable performance results, at least not in the eyes of major contributors of resources. Specification costs may be high in relation to projected benefits. It may be easier to accommodate diverse interests if goals are not specified. Competing members of a coalition may rarely see conflict among organizational objectives until goals are specified, at which time they may be forced to recognize and deal with the conflict. It may be easier to shift organizational direction if the proposed change does not have to meet criteria that have been previously defined and agreed to. Finally, trustees, managers, and clinicians may choose not to specify goals in order to avoid accountability and to maximize discretion or authority.

Results of Not Specifying Goals. Not specifying or targeting organizational performance requirements may result in lower levels of performance than would otherwise occur. By not focusing on particular goals and levels of attainment, the organization may fail to perform satisfactorily. Strong members of a coalition may gain more power or resources at the expense of the weak than they would have if the goals of the weak had been considered formally by all participants.

When performance requirements are not specified and opportunistic interests prevail, long-term survival of HCOs may be threatened, or short-term organizational crises may become more frequent and more severe. Without goal specification, it may become more difficult to make and implement policy decisions—that is, to the extent that there is disagreement regarding effective performance requirements among the controlling coalition.

Not specifying performance requirements favors retention of the present power structure. And as long as the organization can continue to obtain necessary and appropriate inputs and sell or dispose of adequate quantities of outputs, the status quo will tend to be perceived as a satisfactory level of goal attainment.

The environment that many HCOs will be facing in the 1990s is expected to be increasingly competitive and problematic. Hospitals are competing for patients with physicians on their own medical staffs. Attending physicians are in conflict with staff nurses about nurse functions. Nurses are in conflict with managers and trustees regarding pay and working conditions. In these circumstances goal specification may be increasingly perceived by effective HCOs as less costly than direct conflict over limited resources. Evidence of a trend toward goal specification may be found in the startling growth of investor-owned corporations, some of which have well-developed internal systems specifying performance requirements by unit or department.

Measuring Managerial Contribution

Managers disagree regarding how and whether they should be evaluated by whom, and it is indeed difficult to isolate managerial contribution to organizational performance, about which there is also disagreement. For example, despite substantial managerial contributions, an organization may be floundering because of a hostile environment or poor decisions by previous managers. Or the reverse situation may be occurring: despite little or ineffective managerial contribution, an organization may be growing rapidly or raising quality standards and performance because of lack of competitors or excellent management in the past and excellent physicians and nurses now.

Reasons for Evaluating Managers. Generally, health services managers are evaluated to avoid setting them apart from all other employees who are evaluated, to determine continued employment and terms of employment, to set prospectively agreed-upon managerial performance requirements and to assess how these requirements may be accomplished, and to force self-examination in regard to managerial performance and improvements that would enhance managerial performance. A manager may be evaluated relative to what he or she has accomplished previously or relative to what managers in like organizations contribute, assuming a correlation between managerial and organizational performance.

Evaluation is a way of communicating to managers how superiors feel about them and of learning from managers how they feel about superiors' assessments. This can serve as a basis for desired changes in behavior by managers, or it may stimulate superiors to make certain changes that would enable managers to perform as desired. The evaluation process can make both superiors and managers focus on the most important organizational objectives for the time period ahead and can stimulate efforts to generate additional resources necessary to attain goals. Evaluation of managers also serves as a standard for managerial evaluation of others in the organization.

Formal evaluation may not be necessary for a high level of managerial performance or for a high level of satisfaction with managerial contribution by superiors. Nor is formal evaluation of the manager a panacea for effectively adjudicating political conflict between board members and physicians. Formal evaluation can avoid misunderstandings about what constitutes satisfactory managerial performance. The process can facilitate specification of managerial performance requirements that are realistic yet responsive to organizational constraints and opportunities.

Current Issues

Some key issues in HCO management for the 1990s include the following: (1) What should managers do in HCOs? (2) Is too much money spent on managing HCOs? (3) How should managers be trained? (4) To what extent does management performance need to be improved?

Functions of HCO Managers

Should HCO managers basically support the work of more or less independent clinicians, or are managers responsible for integrating the HCO with its environment and coordinating work in the organization? What should be the relationship of line and staff managers in large HCOs? For example, to what extent should a local HMO manager be responsible for marketing relative to the marketing specialists in the HMO central headquarters? How should front-line managers best spend their time—attending internal meetings and writing memos or listening to customers and influencing legislation?

Assuming again that the health care sector is becoming increasingly competitive, with too much capacity relative to demand, there will be an increasing need for managers to be skilled in the production of care and the sale of services in order to gain market share in a competitive situation. This means being the low-cost producer or else providing a differentiated service for which customers are willing to pay higher prices.

If this is so, there will be an increasing requirement in HCOs to specify objectives with regard to cost, quality, and market share and for managers to spend more of their time in activities that contribute to attainment of these objectives. This means more time spent in listening to customers, determining their perceptions and preferences, and in developing production standards to assist clinicians and others in meeting standards.

Resources Spent on Management Functions

Is too much money spent in HCOs on management relative to provision of care? Do managers make too much money relative to their contribution as compared with clinicians, technicians, and nonprofessional workers? How should managers be paid, and to what extent should pay be related to performance?

Himmelstein and Woolhandler (1986) estimated the total cost for health care administration in 1983 at $77.7 million, 22% of all spending for health care. They divided expenditures into $15.6 million for program administration and insurance, $31 million for hospital and nursing home administration, and $31.1 million for physicians' overhead. They argue that institution of a national health service as in Great Britain would generate substantial savings of $38.4 million by eliminating the entire private health insurance industry, much of the hospital and nursing home bureaucracy, and some of the expenses of doctors' offices (Himmelstein & Woolhandler). Their critics can argue that, yes, the British system is cheaper; but no, that is not the kind of health care system that Americans want.

Proponents of paying managers more can argue that health care is increasingly a competitive sector of the economy as patients are increasingly being steered away from high-cost and low-quality HCOs and toward those of low cost and high quality. The management function may be generally responsible for keeping costs down and quality high in large complex organizations, and managers must be attracted to work in health care as opposed to other organizations.

In the United States payment to workers is largely determined by market forces. Markets, of course, are influenced by reimbursement policies of payers, subsidies to suppliers, and governmental licensing of providers. So what managers earn relative to orthopedic surgeons, pediatricians, nurses, x-ray technicians, nurse's aides, and accountants is determined by what HCOs must pay to hire the type of staff they require to perform in variably competitive local markets. Hospital and other HCO managers are not licensed; nursing home administrators are licensed in certain states. Whether earnings of health care managers are too high, too low, or just right relative to other workers may depend on their relative contribution to organizational performance as determined by the board of directors. Obviously, different health care workers will answer this question differently, depending on different interests and perceptions.

Training of HCO Managers

Should managers be trained in business schools, schools of public health, medical schools, schools of public administration, or schools of allied health professions? Should managers of hospitals or group practices be physicians, lay managers, or nurses with management training? What kind of management training should managers receive?

There are no simple answers to any of these questions because of the variability of HCOs and the jobs of managers within them. Trends in the industry are toward a greater supply of physicians to population (hence, more physicians interested in management) and increasing surveillance of physicians, increased competition among HCOs, fewer and larger HCOs, and better-trained HCO managers. Given the tremendous changes taking place in the industry, this means a greater need for management training for those already working in HCOs compared to those entering the HCO managerial labor market.

What the industry trends imply for management training is that more physicians will want and require management training. Such training need not be the same as that required for lay managers, particularly if the managerial jobs of physicians so trained consist largely in supervising and recruiting other physicians while continuing to practice.

Increased competition among HCOs has implications for management curriculum that include more emphasis on economics, marketing and planning, information systems, and accounting and reimbursement, as well as on production of care that meets quality standards and is responsive to consumer preferences.

Increased size of HCOs implies increased standardization and specialization of work, including managerial work. Large HCOs will spend more on managerial training and have more in-house training programs for new managers to teach them about the values, policies, and skills required in these HCOs.

Managerial Performance

To what extent does managerial performance in HCOs need to be improved? Does the health care sector require more MBAs, and would business managers do a better job of running HCOs than do those who currently manage them? Should expectations be any different for managers of particular types of HCOs, such as public hospitals and health clinics?

Kovner (1986) reports in interviews with 29 HCO managers and educators the following views regarding effective health care management and the education of health care managers. Health care managers have difficulty responding appropriately to a new environment of competition and purchaser price pressure; they have difficulty managing changing power relationships between physicians and governing boards; they have a lack of knowledge regarding efficient production of services of adequate qualtiy; and they have employers who make a low investment in continuing professional education and career development for managers.

Similar problems have confronted managers in other service industries facing rapid change, such as airlines and banks. Power relations problems require board leadership for effective responses. MBAs have a useful contribution to make to HCO management, particularly in the functional areas—marketing, finance, information systems, accounting—where expertise can be applied across sectors of the economy and the commitment of the functional specialist is to the function rather than to the sector. On the other hand, to develop successful agendas and networks in HCOs, managers require a knowledge of the health care sector that cannot be learned in business schools without specific health care programs. MBAs can learn on the job about the production of health care, quality assurance, health economics and reimbursement, and government regulations and medical politics, but they are not generally a good investment for HCOs short of scarce front-line management talent. Certainly, HCO managers require continuing training to cope with changing circumstances, and HCOs would probably benefit from devoting more resources to training managers relative to organizational objectives—rather than viewing such training as to be enjoyed by managers in vacation resorts as a fringe benefit of employment.

Two differences in managing public HCOs are legislative "ownership" of the programs and civil service regulations that constrain rather than facilitate organizational flexibility. To the extent that public HCOs provide services for which insurance does not pay to people who can not afford to pay either, they face less competitive pressure. Such services, particularly for low-income populations in large cities, include long-term psychiatric and nursing home care and acute care for substance abusers and AIDS patients. However, expectations need to be set in a similar way for public HCO managers as for managers of other types of HCOs. Managerial performance in public HCOs, as in other HCOs, needs to be improved; and this includes billing and collecting of revenues and even marketing of services as appropriate and certainly listening to customers and responding to their preferences.

References

Allison, R. F., & Dalston, J. W., "Governance of University-Owned Teaching Hospitals." *Inquiry, 19* (Spring), 11, 1982.

American Hospital Association. *Guide for Preparation of Constitution and By Laws for General Hospitals.* Chicago: AHA, 1981.

Brown, R. *Judgment in Administration.* New York: McGraw-Hill, 1966.

Burling, T., Lentz, E., & Wilson, R. *The Give and Take in Hospitals.* New York: G. P. Putnam's Sons, 1956.

Dayton, K. N. "Corporate Governance: The Other Side of the Coin." *Harvard Business Review, 84* (Jan-Feb), 34, 1984.

Drucker, P. F. "Managing the Public Service Institution." *The Public Interest, 33,* 46, 1973.

Gray, B. (ed.). *For Profit Enterprise in Health Care.* Washington, D.C.: Institute of Medicine, National Academy Press, 1986.

Griffith, J. R. "Measuring Hospital Performance." *Inquiry,* 3, 1978.

Hales, Colin P. What do Managers Do? A Critical Review of the Evidence, *Journal of Management Studies,* 23(1):88–115, 1986.

Himmelstein, D. U., & Woolhandler, S. "Cost without Benefit: Administrative Waste in U.S. Health Care." *New England Journal of Medicine,* 314(7), 441, 1986.

Hospital Corporation of America. *Annual Report.* Nashville, TN: HCA, 1984.

The Hospital Research & Educational Trust. *Current Issues in Governance.* Chicago: HRET, 1986.

Joint Commission on Accreditation of Hospitals. *Accreditation Manual for Hospitals.* Chicago: JCAH, 1989.

Kovner, A. R. "Improving the Effectiveness of Hospital Governing Boards." *Frontiers of Health Services Management,* 2 (August), 4, 1985.

Kovner, A. R. *Really trying: A career guide for the health service manager.* Ann Arbor, MI: Health Administration Press, 1984

Kovner, A. R. "Reflections in Health Management Education." *Journal of Health Administration Education,* 4(3) 359, 1986.

Kovner, A. R. *Really Managing:* The work of effective CEOs in large health organizations, Ann Arbor, MI: Health Administration Press, 1986.

Longest, B. B. *Management Practices for the Health Professional.* Reston, VA: Reston Publishing, 1980.

Mintzberg, H. *Power in and around Organizations.* Englewood Cliffs, N.J.: Prentice-Hall, 1983.

Pelligrino, E. T. "The Changing Matrix of Clinical Decision-Making." In B. Georgopoulos (ed.), *Organization Research in Health Institutions.* Ann Arbor, MI: Institute for Social Research, University of Michigan, 1972.

Perloff, E. "For the Trustee, Deepening Responsibilities." *Hospitals, 44,* 84, 1970.

Perrow, C. "Disintegrating Social Sciences." *Phi Delta Kappa, 63,* 684, 1982.

Peters, J. P., & Tseng, S. *Managing Strategic Change in Hospitals.* Chicago: American Hospital Publishing, 1983.

Pfeffer, J. "Size and Composition of Boards of Directors: The Organization and Its Environment." *Administrative Science Quarterly,* 17, 219, 1972.

Ritvo, R. A. "Adaptation to Environmental Change: The Board's Role." *Hospital & Health Services Administration,* 25 (Winter), 23, 1980.

Seay, J. D., & Vladeck, B. C. *Mission Matters.* New York: United Hospital Fund of New York, 1987.

Umbdenstock, R. *So You're on the Hospital Board* (2nd ed.). Chicago: American Hospital Publishing, 1983.

Umbdenstock, R. J. "Refinement of Board's Role Required." *Health Progress,* 68(1), 47, 1987.

Underwood, J. "How to Serve on a Hospital Board." *Harvard Business Review, 47,* 73, 1969.

Utah County v. Intermountain Health Care Inc., S. Ct. Utah, No. 17699, Slip Op., June 26, 1985.

Witt, J. *Building a Better Hospital Board.* Ann Arbor, MI: American College of Healthcare Executives, 1987.

17

Comparative Health Systems: A Policy Perspective

Victor G. Rodwin

Comparative analysis of health systems has produced a large literature that provides profiles of health care systems abroad.[1] There is even a two-volume bibliographic manual with appropriate taxonomies and summaries of relevant research (Elling). This chapter begins with an overview of general issues in the comparative study of health care systems. Next it assesses some common problems of health policy in three countries: France, Canada, and Britain. Finally, it analyzes the U.S. health system from a comparative perspective and examines the uses of comparative analysis, for Americans, in learning from abroad.

Three stages may be distinguished in the evolution of comparative health systems research (Dumbaugh & Neuhauser). During the first stage, which dominated until the mid-1960s, travelogues were written by physicians returning from overseas tours (Corson). During the second stage—still flourishing today—medical care systems were described from a variety of different perspectives.[2] During the third stage there has been an attempt to make the study of comparative health systems into a kind of social science. The research has focused largely on describing the organization of medical care and explaining variation on the basis

---

[1]The references at the end of this chapter provide a good bibliography of this literature. The recent books by Anderson (1989), Field, ed. (1989), de Kervasdoué, Kimberly and Rodwin (1984), Raffel (1985) and Saltman (1988) provide a good starting point for students.

[2]For examples of some classic works, see Milton Roemer (1977 and 1981) on aspects of health system organization around the world; John Fry's (1970) book on the medical care system in the Soviet Union, the United States, and the United Kingdom; Douglas-Wilson and McLachlan's (1974) collection of papers on international health prospects; Victor and Ruth Sidel's (1977) vignettes of the health care system in Sweden, Great Britain, the Soviet Union, and China. In addition, there are some case studies: Harry Eckstein (1959), Gordon Forsyth (1966), Rudolf Klein (1983), and Almont Lindsey (1962) on England; Victor and Ruth Sidel (1973) on China; Mark Field (1973); Gordon Hyde (1974) and Henry Sigerist (1947) on the Soviet Union, and Richard Weinerman (1969) on Eastern Europe.

of received theories within such disciplines as anthropology, sociology, political science, and economics.[3]

The social science approach to comparative health systems has the inherent defects of its virtues. To achieve a rigorous study design, it has classified descriptive data, elaborated hypotheses, and tested them against available evidence. The focus has been largely on cross-sectional comparisons of health services utilization and expenditures, thus narrowing the scope of research questions and eroding the ideals shared by stage 2 scholars, who were more motivated by the pragmatic concerns of improving the delivery of medical care. Social scientists tend to display more interest in the theoretical concerns of their disciplines than in social change. Nevertheless, a number of excellent case studies have been produced, and this has raised a number of important conceptual and methodological issues.

Conceptual Issues

The concept of health system is clearly central. And yet there is no fully satisfactory definition of this concept, for it is difficult to agree both on the boundaries of the system and on a definition of health. Blum (1981) provides a visual model of health, suggesting that health care services are merely one input into health among three others—heredity, behavior, and environment (Fig. 17.1). Weinerman (1971) defines the health system as "all of the activities of a society which are designed to protect or restore health, whether directed to the individual, the community, or the environment (p. 272)". Anderson (1972) has more concretely outlined the "boundaries of a relatively easily defined system with entry and exit points, hierarchies of personnel, types of patients"—in short, what he calls "the officially and professionally recognized 'helping' services regarding disease, disability, and death (p. 22)".

Viewing the concept of health system at a macrosociological level, Field (1973) proposes the following formal definition: "that societal mechanism that transforms generalized resources . . . into specialized outputs in the form of health services." He adds that "the 'health system' of any society is that social mechanism that has arisen or been devised to deal with the incapacitating aspects of illness, trauma, and (to some degree) premature mortality . . . the five D's: death, disease, disability, discomfort, and dissatisfaction (pp. 768, 772)".

Another approach to the concept of health system is to define it implicitly by postulating a causal model of it. Thus, drawing on Elling and Kerr's (1975) proposed framework for studying health systems, De Miguel (1975) outlines four

---

[3]For a good example of how anthropologists approach the comparative study of health systems, see Leslie (1978). For a sociological perspective, see Elling and Kerr (1975) or Light and Schuller (1986). For a political science approach, see Altenstetter (1978). For an economic approach, see Hu (1976) and Schweitzer (1978).

Figure 17.1 Inputs to Health

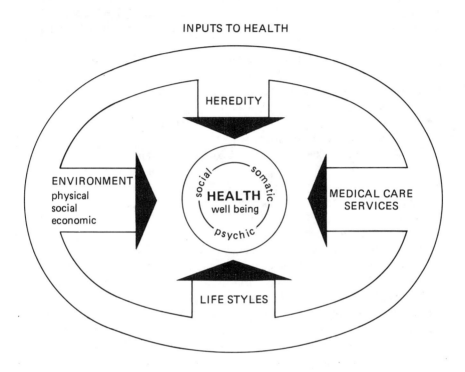

INPUTS TO HEALTH

HEREDITY

ENVIRONMENT
physical
social
economic

HEALTH
well being
social somatic psychic

MEDICAL CARE
SERVICES

LIFE STYLES

Source: Adapted from H. Blum, *Planning for Health* (2nd ed), New York: Human Sciences Press, 1981, p. 3.

subsystem levels that influence health status: individual, institutional, societal, and environmental. Such an approach allows one to analyze a health system by investigating the effects of a hierarchy of independent variables on the dependent variables, health status. It also raises questions about the most effective levels at which to effect system change.

Methodological Issues

The fundamental methodological issue in comparative health systems research involves devising a study design and selecting alternative systems that allow the analyst to hold some variables constant while manipulating experimental ones. In the area of health policy, for example, how does one evaluate the success of cost-containment efforts in health systems characterized by diverse patterns of financing and provider reimbursement? Quasi-experimental research designs would suggest matching two health systems on all but a few policy-related factors. But "matching," let alone a real experiment, is rarely feasible in policy research.

One response to this difficulty has been to match health systems on at least some criteria (e.g., levels of health resources) and then to call for "in-depth studies of contrasting cases" (Elling & Kerr). Another response has been to use the language of natural experiment and view "most similar systems" as laboratories in which to assess the effects of alternative policy options at home (Marmor, Bridges, & Hoffman).

Another methodological concern in the social science approach to comparative health systems research is whether the descriptive studies and data collected during stage 2 are actually comparable. If they are not, this casts great doubt on the utility of making international comparisons. If they are, qualifications must usually be made.

The most difficult methodological issues arise in evaluating health systems, for this involves specifying the relationship between the elements of a health system (inputs) and their impact on health (output). But how does one distinguish the impact of health services on health from the impacts of improvements in social services, income security, education, and transportation—not to mention the social and physical environment? This question raises the problem of devising indicators of health status. It also explains why, in his comparative study of the United States, Sweden, and England, Odin Anderson (1972) found it impossible to attribute differences in the usual health indices of morbidity and mortality to patterns of medical care organization in these countries. To evaluate health systems, it is necessary to agree on consistent definitions of health system inputs and to devise health status indicators to measure outputs. Such considerations raise a number of conceptual issues.

Learning from Abroad

Although there is a large literature on the comparative analysis of health systems, there are rarely attempts to draw lessons from comparative experience. Comparative studies of health policy are sparse. Most often, they describe national experience in a range of policy areas; only rarely do they interpret, let alone evaluate, this experience. Exceptions to this general rule are of interest because they have contributed at least three ideas that have implications for learning from abroad.

First is the idea of evolutionary progress in health systems. Medical sociologists such as Field (1973) and Mechanic (1976) have argued that health systems in Western industrialized nations are evolving in similar directions. Drawing on Field's typology, consisting of five systems—the private health system, the pluralistic one, the national health insurance (NHI) system, the national health service (NHS), and the socialized health service—such views would suggest that the direction of change in modern societies is from the system of Type 1 to that of Type 5 (Table 17.1). Unlike Field and Mechanic, who are not convinced that such change necessarily implies "progress," Milton Roemer (1977) describes similar trends as a march toward a health ideal.

The second idea, the notion of public policy learning, is methodological in nature. It is highlighted in Glaser's studies of health policy in Western Europe and Canada. *Paying the Doctor* (1970) analyzes systems of physician remuneration. *Health Insurance Bargaining* (1978) explains how alternative administrative arrangements affect the process of bargaining between the medical profession and the state. *Paying the Hospital* (1987) describes systems of hospital reimbursement and assesses the implications for the United States. Each of these studies starts with the presumption that the United States has many problems and that the policies and experience of Western Europe and Canada shed light on and provide a useful range of solutions.

The third idea focuses on understanding either the determinants of health policies or at least their effects. Leichter (1979), for example, analyzes the determinants of health policies in Britain, Germany, Japan, and the Soviet Union. Similarly, Altenstetter (1974) and Stone (1980) show how different structures and processes explain differences in policy between the United States and West Germany; and Hollingsworth (1986) attempts to relate differences in structure and performance by comparing the United States and Britain. This approach views "most similar systems" as laboratories in which to assess the effects of alternative policy options at home (Marmor et al., Teune). It is exemplified by Evans (1984) and Marmor and his colleagues (1978), who used this approach in their studies of Canada.

The idea of evolutionary progress in the development of health systems suggests that the United States can learn about future policy issues by studying nations whose systems are more advanced. Similarly, the idea that policy learning brings foreign solutions to bear on American problems is a variation on this theme. Finally, the idea of using comparative analysis to understand the determinants and effects of policies abroad can assist us in evaluating alternative policy options at home.

The ideas summarized above, indeed most of the literature in comparative health policy, often minimize or overlook the substantial problems of health systems abroad. An alternative, problem-oriented approach might be to reverse this emphasis. For example, another way to think about learning from abroad is

Table 17.1 The Evolution of Health Systems

Health System	Type 1: Private	Type 2: Pluralistic	Type 3: National health insurance	Type 4: National health service	Type 5: Socialized health service
General definition	Health care as item of personal consumption	Health care as predominantly a consumer good or service	Health care as an insured, guaranteed consumer good or service	Health care as a state-supported consumer good or service	Health care as a state-provided public service
Position of the physician	Solo entrepreneur	Solo entrepreneur and member of variety of groups, organizations	Solo entrepreneur and member of medical organizations	Solo entrepreneur and member of medical organizations	State employee and member of medical organizations
Role of professional associations	Powerful	Very strong	Strong	Fairly strong	Weak or nonexistent
Ownership of facilities	Private	Private and public	Private and public	Mostly public	Entirely public
Economic transfers	Direct	Direct and indirect	Mostly indirect	Indirect	Entirely indirect
Prototypes	U.S., Western Europe, Russia in 19th century	U.S. in 20th century	Sweden, France, Canada, Japan in 20th century	Great Britain in 20th century	Soviet Union in 20th century

Sources: V. G. Rodwin, *The Health Planning Predicament: France, Quebec, England, and the United States,* Berkeley: University of California Press, 1984, p. 245. Adapted from: M. G. Field, *Comparative Health Systems: Differentiation and Convergence.* Final Report under Grant No. HS-00272, Rockville, Md.: National Center for Health Services Research, 1978.

to begin with the recognition that most countries, irrespective of their particular health system, face serious common problems with regard to the efficient and equitable allocation of scarce health care resources.

Economists, for example, emphasize the problem of inefficiency in the allocation of health care resources. They point out that cost containment should not be confused with allocative efficiency in the use of health care resources, and they study the possibilities of obtaining more value for the money spent on health care. This applies not only with regard to improving health status but also with respect to altering input mixes in the provision of health services: taking advantage of cost-effective treatment settings (e.g. ambulatory surgery) and personnel (e.g. nurse practitioners).

Public health and medical care analysts criticize the lack of continuity of care between primary, secondary, and tertiary levels. Although health planners have called for redistributing resources away from hospitals to community-based ambulatory care services and public health programs, the allocation of resources within health regions has been notoriously biased in favor of the more costly technology-based medical care at the apex of the regional hierarchy (Fox, 1986; Rodwin, 1984). The consequence of this allocational pattern has been to weaken institutional capability for delivering primary care services. This has exacerbated the separation between primary, secondary, and tertiary levels of care, thus making it difficult for providers to assure that the right patient receives the right kind of care, in the right place, and for the right reason.

Consumers have noted the inflexibility of bureaucratic decision-making procedures and the absence of opportunities for exercising for what Hirschman (1970) calls "voice" in most health care organizations. Indeed, the problem of control and how it should be shared among consumers, providers, managers, and payers is at the center of most criticisms leveled against the current structure of health care in Western industrialized nations. In all of these systems, decisions about what medical services to provide, how and where they should be provided, by whom, and how often are separated from the responsibility for financing medical care.

Resource Allocation Problems: France, Canada, and Britain

Drawing on the problem-oriented approach presented above, this section assesses common problems with regard to the efficient and equitable allocation of scarce health care resources in France, Canada, and Britain. Outside the United States there are two principal methods of health care financing: compulsory insurance and general taxation. France represents a model national health insurance (NHI) system administered through a centralized social security system. Canada and Britain both rely on general taxation. But whereas Canada uses federal and provincial general tax revenues to finance a highly decentralized NHI system, Britain relies overwhelmingly on central government funds to finance a national health service (NHS).

France

France is noted for combining NHI with fee-for-service private practice in the ambulatory care sector and a mixed hospital sector of which two-thirds of all acute beds are in the public sector and one-third are in the private sector (Rodwin, 1981). Physicians in the ambulatory sector and in private hospitals (known as *cliniques*) are reimbursed on the basis of a negotiated fee schedule. Roughly 20% of all physicians have chosen to engage in extra billing beyond the negotiated fees; the remainder have agreed to accept the negotiated fees as payment in full. And physicians based in public hospitals—the principal teaching and research institutions—are reimbursed on a part-time or full-time salaried basis. *Cliniques* are reimbursed on the basis of a negotiated per diem fee. Public hospitals used to be reimbursed on a retrospective, cost-based, per diem fee, but they have received prospectively set "global" budgets since 1984.

There are several problems in this system. From a public health point of view, there is inadequate communication between full-time salaried physicians in public hospitals and solo-practice physicians working in the community. Although general practitioners in the fee-for-service sector have informal referral networks to specialists and public hospitals, there are no formal institutional relationships that assure continuity of medical care, disease prevention and health promotion services, posthospital follow-up care, and more generally systematic linkages and referral patterns between primary-, secondary-, and tertiary-level services.

From the point of view of economic efficiency criteria, there are additional problems in the French health care system. On the demand side, two factors encourage consumers to increase their use of medical care services: the uncertainty about the results of treatment and the presence of insurance coverage. To reduce the risk of misdiagnosis or improper therapy, physicians are always tempted to order more diagnostic tests. Since NHI covers most of the cost, there is no incentive—neither for the physician nor for the patient—to balance marginal changes in risk with marginal increases in costs. This results in excessive medical care utilization.

On the supply side, fee-for-service reimbursement of physicians provides incentives for them to increase their volume of services so as to raise their income. Likewise, per diem reimbursement of *cliniques* and hospitals creates incentives to increase patient lengths of stay. The recent imposition of global budgets in France has eliminated this problem but the budgets represent a blunt policy tool—one that tends to support the existing allocation of resources within the hospital sector and, possibly, to jeopardize the quality of hospital care. It is relatively easy for a hospital to receive an annual budget to maintain its ongoing activities but extremely difficult to receive additional compensation for higher service levels, institutional innovation, or improvements in the quality of care. Even with prospective budgets, hospitals naturally seek to maximize the level of their annual allocations and to resist budget cutbacks.

In summary, under French NHI, providers have no financial incentives to achieve savings while holding quality constant or even improving it. Nor are there incentives—in public hospitals, for example—to increase service activity in exchange for more income. Consumers have few incentives, other than minimal co-payments, to be economical in their use of medical care. And there are no incentives to move the French system away from hospital-centered services toward new organizational modalities.

Canada

Under Canadian NHI, although coverage for drugs is far less than in France, there are no co-payments; there is first-dollar coverage for hospital and medical services. Physicians in ambulatory care are paid predominantly on a fee-for-service basis, according to fee schedules negotiated between physicians' associations and provincial governments. In contrast to France, physicians in hospitals are most often paid on a fee-for-service basis, as in the United States.

There are few private, for-profit hospitals in Canada such as French *cliniques* and American proprietary or investor-owned institutions. Most acute-care hospitals in Canada are private, nonprofit institutions. But their operating expenditures are financed through the NHI system, and most of their capital expenditures are financed by the provincial governments. In the United States, Canada's health system is typically depicted as a model for NHI (Andreopoulos). Its financing, through a complex shared federal and provincial tax revenue formula, is more progressive than the European NHI systems financed on the basis of payroll taxes. Canada's levels of health status are high by international standards. And it has achieved notable success in controlling the growth of health care costs. What, then, are the problems in this system?

From the point of view of health care providers, there is, above all, a crisis of underfinancing. Physicians complain about low fee levels. Hospital administrators complain about draconian control of their budgets. And other health care professionals note that the combination of a physician "surplus" and excessive reliance on physicians prevents an expansion of their roles. Although Evans (1987) contends that Canadian cost-control policies cannot be shown to have jeopardized the quality of care, providers and administrators, alike, claim that there has been deterioration since the imposition of restrictive prospective budgets.

Leaving aside the issue of quality, the same issues discussed in the context of France are present in Canada with respect to economic efficiency. Neither the hospital physician nor the patient has an incentive to be economical in the use of health care resources. On the demand side, because patients benefit from what is perceived as "free" tax-financed first-dollar coverage, they have no incentive to choose cost-effective forms of care. For example, in the case of a demand for urgent care, there is no incentive for a patient to use community health centers rather than rush directly to the emergency room.

On the supply side, physicians lack incentives to make efficient use of hospitals, which are essentially a free good at their disposal. There are no incentives for altering input mixes to affect practice style. Nor are there incentives for providers to evaluate service levels and the kinds of therapy performed in relation to improving health status. It could be argued that these problems are common to all health systems, but they are especially acute in a system characterized by a bilateral monopoly that tends to support the status quo. On the one hand, providers organized in strong associations have strong monopoly power, which they use to defend their legitimate interests; on the other, the monopsony power of sole-source financing (NHI) keeps provider interests in check at the cost of not intervening in the organizational practice of medicine.

Stoddard (1984) has characterized the problems of the Canadian health system as "financing without organization." In his view, Canadian provinces "adopted a 'pay the bills' philosophy, in which decisions about service provision—which services, in what amounts, produced how, by whom, and where—were viewed as the legitimate domain of physicians and hospital administrators" (Stoddard, p. 3). The reason for this policy is that provincial governments were concerned about maintaining a good relationship with providers. This concern has not avoided tough negotiations and periodic confrontations. But there has been no effort to devise new forms of medical-care practice, for example, health maintenance organizations (HMOs) or new institutions to handle the growing burden of long-term care for the elderly. The side effect of Canadian NHI has been to support the separation of hospital and ambulatory care and to reinforce traditional organizational structures.

As in France or the United States, there are, in essence, two strategies for managing the Canadian health system and making adjustments. The first involves greater regulation on the supply side: even stronger controls on hospital spending, more rationing of medical technology, more hospital closures and mergers, and eventual prohibition of extra billing. The second involves increased reliance on market forces on the demand side: various forms of user charges such as co-payments and deductibles now advocated as forms of privatization. Neither strategy is likely to succeed on its own. The former will control health care expenditures in the short run, but it fails to affect practice styles. Its effectiveness runs the risk of exacerbating confrontation between providers and the state and jeopardizing health care needs. The latter deals with only part of the problem—the demand side—and neglects the issue of supply-side efficiency. It provides no mechanism by which consumer decisions can generate signals to providers to adopt efficient practice styles. Moreover, it is likely to raise the level of total (public and private) expenditures.

Britain

There are many models of an NHS in Europe, ranging from decentralized systems in Sweden, Norway, Finland, and Denmark to more centralized systems in Spain, Greece, Portugal, and Italy. Because the British NHS is one of the oldest and most thoroughly studied models, it stands as an exemplar. It is financed almost entirely through general revenue taxation and is accountable directly to the Department of Health and Social Security (DHSS) and Parliament. Access to health services is free of charge to all British subjects and to all legal residents. But despite the universal entitlement, Britons spend only 5.9% of their gross domestic product (GDP) on health care—one half of what Americans spend as a percentage of their GDP.

Although the NHS is cherished by most Britons, there are, nevertheless, some serious problems concerning both the equity and efficiency of resource allocation in the health sector. With regard to equity, in 1976 the Resource Allocation Working Party (RAWP) developed a formula for the allocation of NHS funds between regions (DHSS, 1976). The formula represents one of the most far-reaching attempts to allocate health care funds because it incorporates regional differences in measures of health status. Slow progress is now being made in redistributing the aggregate NHS budget along the lines of RAWP, but substantial inequities still remain, from the point of view of both spatial distribution and social class (Townsend & Davidson).

With regard to efficiency, the problems are even more severe because NHS resources are extremely scarce by international standards. Because there is less slack, the marginal costs of inefficiency are higher than in Western Europe or the United States. And because the NHS faces the same demands as other systems to make available new technology and to care for an increasingly aged population, British policymakers recognize that they must pursue innovations that improve efficiency. But there are numerous institutional obstacles in the way.

The tripartite structure of the NHS is itself a major source of inefficiency:

1. Regional Health Authorities (RHAs) are responsible for allocating budgets to hospitals in their regions. Hospital-based "consultants" are paid on a salaried basis, with distinguished clinicians receiving "merit awards," and all consultants have the right to see a limited number of private, fee-paying patients in "pay beds."
2. Outside the RHA budget are Family Practitioner Committees (FPCs) responsible for remunerating general practitioners (GPs), ophthalmologists, dentists, and pharmacists. The GPs are reimbursed on a capitation basis, with additional remuneration coming from special "practice

allowances" and fee-for-service payment for specific services (e.g., night visits and immunizations).

3. Separate from both the RHAs and the FPCs are the local authorities (LAs), which are responsible for the provision of social services, public health services, and certain community nursing services.

Such an institutional framework creates perverse incentives to shift borderline patients from GPs to hospital consultants, to the community, and back to the hospital. GPs, for example, have no incentive to minimize costs and can impose costs on RHAs by referring patients to hospital consultants or for diagnostic services. NHS managers can shift costs from the NHS to social security by sending elderly hospitalized patients to private nursing homes. And consultants can shift costs back onto the patient by keeping long waiting lists, thereby increasing demand for their private services. As in France and Canada, neither the patient nor the physician in Britain bears the costs of the decisions they make; it is the taxpayer who pays the bill.

Four recent strategies, all of them inadequate, have attempted to deal with this problem. The first came promptly with the arrival of the Thatcher government. After cautious attempts to denationalize the NHS by promoting a shift toward NHI and privatization, the Conservative government backed off when they realized that such an approach would not merely provoke strong political opposition but also would increase public expenditure and therefore conflict with their budgetary objectives (McLachlan & Maynard, 1982). Instead, the strategy was narrowed in favor of encouraging competition and market incentives in limited areas. To begin with, the government allowed a slight increase of private beds in NHS hospitals. In addition, it introduced tax incentives to encourage the purchase of private health insurance and the growth of charitable contributions. Also, the government encouraged local authorities to raise money through the sale of surplus property and to contract out to the private sector such services as laundry, cleaning, and catering.

The second response was the Griffiths Report, which resulted in yet another reorganization in the long history of administrative reform within the NHS. Roy Griffiths, the former director of a large English department store chain, introduced the concept of a general manager at the department (DHSS), regional, district, and unit levels. This manager is now presumably responsible for the efficient use of the budget of each level of the NHS. The problem, however, is that the tripartite structure of the system remains unchanged; and the general managers have very little information about least-cost strategies (across the tripartite structure) for generating improvements in health status.

The third response to the problem of improving efficiency has been to reduce the drug bill (Maynard). Since April 1985 the government has limited the list of reimbursable drugs and reduced the pharmaceutical industry's rate of return.

These measures will help contain the costs of the only open-ended budget within the NHS, but there is no evidence that they will have any impact on the efficiency of health care expenditures.

Finally, the fourth and most recent proposals for improving efficiency were published in a government White Paper, *Working for Patients* (1989). This report proposes a range of significant changes, all of which attempt to create internal markets, within the public sector, by giving providers incentives to treat more patients and having "money follow patients." On the demand side, the government proposes that instead of operating as monopoly suppliers of services, district health authorities be required to purchase services for the patients they serve. On the supply side, the government proposes that some of the larger NHS hospitals be transformed into independent self-governing NHS trusts. It is too early to evaluate these ideas, let alone the effects of the policies they generate. But it seems probable that they could result in far-reaching changes.

The U.S. Health System: A Comparative Perspective

How does the United States health care system measure up in comparison to health sector problems in France, Canada, and Britain? To answer this question, we will review the ways in which the U.S. health system differs from and resembles that of other Western industrialized nations. Let us examine this issue from the vantage point of three characteristics that typically distinguish the United States from Western Europe and Canada: (1) American values and popular opinion, (2) the structure of health care financing and organization, and (3) policy responses to health sector problems.

American Values and Popular Opinion

The prevailing image of American values and popular opinion is that of 19th-century liberalism, which has colored American perceptions of equity, of the proper role for government, and of citizenship. These perceptions represent a range of American values and popular opinions that distinguish the United States from Western Europe and Canada.

American attitudes about equity with regard to health care were formed in the 19th century as the country became populated by immigrant populations in urban centers. During this period the concept of the "truly needy" emerged (Rosner). Many Americans developed a sense of responsibility to come to their aid, but there were also harsher attitudes inspired by social Darwinist notions that distinguished between the "truly needy" and the "undeserving" or "unworthy" poor. Whereas in Western Europe broadly based socialist parties viewed poverty as an outcome of the economic system, in the United States there was an inclination to regard poverty as an individual problem. Hence, the greater attention to *equality of opportunity* in the United States as compared with *equality of result* in the more left-leaning European social democracies.

As far as the proper role of government is concerned, in contrast to Western Europe and Canada, the United States has a long history of antigovernment attitudes. The suspicion about excessive governmental authority and the attachment to individual liberties is a pervasive American value.

American perceptions of citizenship also present a striking contrast to Western European perceptions. In the United States individualist values, on the one hand, and social and ethnic heterogeneity, on the other hand, have resulted in more "fractionalized understandings of citizenship" (Klass). In Western Europe and Canada, the understandings of citizenship are grounded in notions of solidarity and universal entitlements. The difference is that Western Europe and Canada have largely succeeded in covering all of their citizens under some form of health insurance; the United States has not.

There is a general aversion among Americans to universal entitlements. As Reinhardt (1985) has observed, when Americans face a trade-off between establishing tax-financed entitlements and leaving the uninsured on their own, they prefer to do the latter. It would be misleading, however, to draw any conclusions about how generous Americans are or how much social welfare they provide based only on the image of liberalism outlined above. In contrast to Western Europe and Canada, Americans prefer to promote redistribution policies though local assistance and indirect subsidies to the voluntary sector via tax exemptions.

Clearly, in comparison to Western Europe and Canada, there are important differences in the United States with regard to values and popular opinion. But how much of a difference do these differences make?

The Structure of Health Care Financing and Organization

The prevailing image of the American health system is one of a privately financed, privately organized system with multiple payers. These characteristics derive, in large part, from the absence of a publicly mandated NHI program. In comparison with Western European nations, Japan and Canada, the United States is last with respect to the public share of total health expenditures (Table 17.2). Although the United States has the highest per capita health care expenditures—public and private combined (see Table 17.3)—and spends the highest percentage of its GDP on health care (Table 17.4), it retains the lowest share of public expenditure as a percentage of total health expenditures. (Table 17.4). Likewise, in comparing public health expenditures for the elderly as a percentage of gross national product (GNP) the United States spends the least. (Table 17.5).

The organization of health care in the United States is noted for being on the

**Table 17.2 Sources of Finance for Health Care
Expenditures: The Mix between
Public and Private in 1987 as a
Percentage of Total**

	Public	Private
Sweden	90.8	9.2
United Kingdom	86.4	13.6
Italy	79.2	20.8
West Germany	78.4	21.6
France	74.8	25.2
Canada	73.9	26.1
Netherlands	73.9	26.1
Australia	70.5	29.5
Switzerland	64.5	35.5
United States	40.0	60.0

Source: Organization for Economic Cooperation and Development: Health Data File. From *Health Care Financing Review,* 1989 Annual Supplement, Washington, D.C.: U.S. DHHS, 1990.

private end of the public/private spectrum. In comparison with Western Europe, the United States has one of the smallest public hospital sectors. In the organization of ambulatory care, American private fee-for-service practice corresponds to the norm, at least in comparison to NHI systems. However, the absence of an NHI program in the United States has resulted in a system of multiple payers and has encouraged a more pluralistic pattern of medical care organization and more innovative forms of medical practice—for example, multispecialty group practices, HMOs, ambulatory surgery centers, and preferred provider organizations (PPOs).

The United States is also different, in comparison to Canada and Western Europe, with regard to the ways in which health resources are used. For example, the United States has fewer hospital beds per thousand population than any Western European country or Canada (Table 17.6). The United States also has the lowest use of inpatient care per capita with the exception of Italy (Table 17.6). These data should not necessarily lead one to the conclusion that the United States is less prone to institutionalize patients than Western Europe or Canada. They probably reflect the size of the American nursing home industry, which has no equivalent in Western Europe and Canada, where a large portion of long-term care for the elderly is provided in hospitals.

These are ways in which the American health care system is different from that of Western Europe and Canada. But there are also some noteworthy points of similarity. For example, most health systems in industrially advanced nations are centered around the hospital. They allocate roughly one-half of total health care

Table 17.3 Total Health Care
Expenditures Per Capita in
1987 (at GDP Purchasing
Power Parities)

Country	US$
United States	2,051
Canada	1,483
Sweden	1,233
Switzerland	1,225
France	1,105
Germany	1,093
The Netherlands	1,041
Australia	939
Japan	915
Belgium	879
Italy	841
Denmark	792
United Kingdom	758
Spain	521
Greece	337

Source: (OECD). Schieber, G. and Poullier, J. "International Health Care Expenditure Trends: 1987", *Health Affairs* (8)3 Fall, 1989.

expenditures to the hospital sector. The United States corresponds to the norm in this regard (Table 17.7).

There is also a high degree of similarity among the United States, Canada, and Western Europe in the broad structure of health care financing and provider reimbursement (Figure 17.2). From the point of view of both consumers and providers, the essential feature of modern health care systems is the central role of third-party payment, by either government or health insurers. On the financing end, all health systems are supported either by general revenue taxes or by payroll taxes. On the payment end, the magnitude of third-party payment dwarfs that of out-of-pocket payment by consumers.

For the consumer, what matters with regard to health care financing is not the relative public and private mix but rather the relative portion of *direct* versus *indirect* third-party payment. To emphasize the large private portion of health care financing in the United States is misleading; for the more critical factor is that public and private health insurance are both forms of third-party payment. This amounted to 71.6% of national health expenditures in 1985 leaving consumers with direct out-of-pocket contributions equal to 28.4% of total health expenditures (Anderson, 1986). The most recent comparative analysis of consumers' out-of-pocket contributions to total health expenditures is based on 1975 data

Table 17.4 Health Care Expenditures, 1987

Country	Public health expenditures as % of total health expenditure	% Total expenditures on health in GDP
Australia	71.8	7.1
Austria	67.6	8.4
Belgium	76.9	7.2
Canada	74.8	8.6
Denmark	85.5	6.0
Finland	78.5	7.4
France	76.3	8.6
Germany	77.0	8.2
Ireland	87.0	7.4
Iceland	88.6	7.8
Italy	78.0	6.9
Japan	73.2	6.8
Luxembourg	91.6	7.5
Netherlands	77.8	8.5
New Zeland	82.5	6.9
Norway	97.6	7.5
Sweden	90.6	9.0
Switzerland	68.2	7.7
United Kingdom	86.6	6.1
United States	41.4	11.2
OECD average	76.0	7.5

GDP, gross domestic product.
Source: G. Schieber and J. P. Poullier, "International Health Care Expenditure Trends: 1987," *Health Affairs* (8)3, Fall, 1989.

Table 17.5 Public Expenditures for Health Care of the Elderly, 1980

Country	Public Expenditures as Percentage of GNP
United States	3.9
Canada	5.8
Denmark	6.4
France	6.1
Germany	6.2
Netherlands	6.5
Norway	5.8
Sweden	8.9
Switzerland	4.5
United Kingdom	5.2

GNP, gross national product.
Source: Adapted from U.S. Senate, Special Committee on Aging, *Long-Term Care in Western Europe and Canada: Implications for the United States,* Washington, D.C.: U.S. Government Printing Office, 1984.

Table 17.6 Hospital Beds and Use of Inpatient Care, 1987

OECD Countries	No. of Beds Per 1,000	Hospital Bed-Days Per Person Per Year
Australia	10.2	3.2 (1986)
Austria	10.8	3.3
Belgium	8.4	2.8 (1986)
Canada	16.1	2.0 (1985)
Denmark	6.3	1.9
Finland	13.6	4.2
France	10.7	3.3 (1986)
Germany	11.0	3.5
Iceland	14.5	4.0 (1986)
Italy	7.7	1.6
Japan	15.2	3.9 (1986)
Luxemburg	12.5	3.7 (1985)
Netherlands	11.8	3.8
New Zealand	9.2	2.1
Norway	15.7	4.9
Sweden	12.7	4.2
Switzerland	10.9	3.0
United Kingdom	6.8	2.1 (1986)
United States	5.3*	1.7 (1981)

*This figure includes beds for all hospitals registered with the American Hospital Association.
Source: Organization for Economic Cooperation and Development: Health Data File. *From Health Care Financing Review,* 1989 Annual Supplement, Washington, D.C.: U.S. DHHS, 1990.

(Maxwell, 1981). Once again, the United States is different (Figure 17.3). It has the highest share of direct out-of-pocket contributions by consumers. But even under French NHI, consumers contribute roughly 20% toward total health expenditures. The difference is not as large as the image of a private financing system would suggest.

The image of a private organizational structure in American health care is well founded. But that view, too, is incomplete. In spite of its *relatively* small size, there is an important role for the public sector in the United States—both in ambulatory services for the noninstitutionalized patient and in the provision of hospital services.

With regard to ambulatory care, there is a maze of special federal programs and a network of local government services largely for the poor. The services are provided either in county or municipal hospital emergency rooms, in local health

Table 17.7 Components of Health Spending, 1981 (Percentage of Total Health Spending)

	Spending as percentage of total			
Country	Institutional	Ambulatory	Pharmaceutical	Other
Australia	54.0	16.7	8.0	21.3
Belgium[a]	35.8	41.6	17.0	5.6
Canada[b]	55.1	21.8	9.4	13.7
Finland[a]	48.8	29.7	10.4	11.1
France[a]	46.2	26.0	15.7	12.1
Germany[b]	38.6	26.7	20.2	14.5
Ireland[pb]	71.8	11.5	7.0	9.7
Italy[a]	50.9	31.9	15.9	1.3
Luxembourg[pb]	32.5	21.5	12.0	34.0
Netherlands[a]	58.8	26.4	9.8	5.0
New Zealand[pe]	69.2	7.1	11.5	12.3
Norway[p]	69.9	15.3	7.2	7.6
Sweden[pa]	72.6	10.2	4.9	12.3
United Kingdom[pd]	58.5	10.0	9.9	21.6
United States[a]	47.5	27.8	6.7	16.0
Mean[e]	54.0	21.6	11.0	13.2

Sources: G. J. Schieber, "The Financing and Delivery of Health Care in OECD Countries: Past, Present and Future" (Tokyo: Joint Japanese/OECD Conference on Health and Pension Policies in the Context of Demographic Evolution and Economic Constraint, November 25–28, 1985). The data in the table are from *Measuring Health Care, 1960–1983*, Paris: OECD. 1985.
[a]1983.
[b]1982.
[c]1980.
[d]1979.
[e]Excludes Austria.
[p]Public spending by type of service as a percentage of total public spending on health.

departments, or in neighborhood health centers. As for hospitals, more than 30% of all acute-care institutions are owned and operated by governments. This includes the federal Veterans Administration hospitals and marine and military hospitals, as well as state and county hospitals. Although Medicare and Medicaid were intended to bring the poor into "mainstream medicine," (i.e., into the private sector), local county and municipal hospitals continue largely to serve the poor. These hospitals are a major source of care not only for Medicaid beneficiaries but also for more than half of the poverty population who do not meet

Figure 17.2 Health Care Financing and Provider Reimbursement

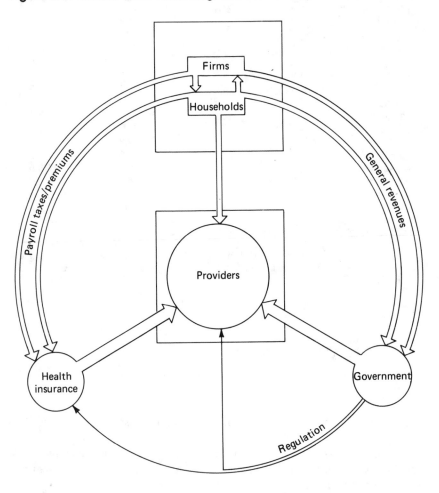

Figure 17.3 Direct Payment by Consumers in 1975, Excluding Voluntary Insurance, as a Percentage of Total Health Care Expenditures

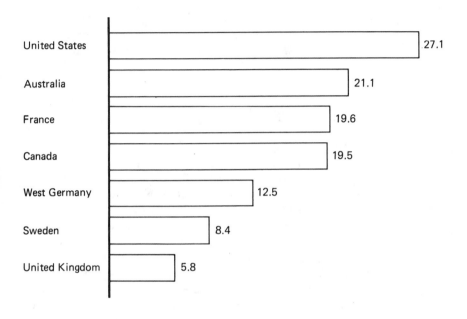

Source: Robert J. Maxwell, *Health and Wealth*, Lexington, Mass.: Lexington Books, D. C. Heath and Co., 1981. Reprinted by permission of the publisher.
Note: Information was not available for Italy, the Netherlands, and Switzerland.

Medicaid eligibility levels and consequently often do not have access to private physicians or voluntary hospitals.

To sum up, there are distinctive characteristics of health care financing and organization in the United States, but there are also striking points of similarity when compared with Western Europe and Canada. The distinctive characteristics include the absence of an NHI program, preferences for institutional flexibility, and innovative forms of medical care organization. The points of similarity—the coexistence of both public and private provision and third-party payment—are structural features of the American health system as well as those of most other health systems.

Policy Responses to Health Sector Problems

Abel-Smith (1985) argues that there is a growing divergence between Western European and American policy responses to the problem of containing health care costs. He suggests that Western Europe continues to rely on regulation whereas the United States seeks to promote competition and greater reliance on market forces. Abel-Smith points to three examples of these unique American policy responses to health sector problems: (1) the growth of deductibles, co-payments, and other cost-sharing mechanisms; (2) the trend toward making those who benefit from insurance actually pay the whole cost—this implies, for example, reducing tax deductions and thus providing incentives for employers and employees to shop more prudently for insurance coverage; and (3) the growth of competitive bidding as a mechanism of forcing competition between alternative providers.

There are some insights behind this caricature of the American policy response to health sector problems. But there is probably more regulation in the eastern states with "all-payer systems" (e.g., New York, New Jersey, and Maryland) than in Western Europe. Even in well-known "pockets of competition" (e.g., California, Arizona, and Minnesota) regulation is essential, if only to enforce the rules of the competitive game. The new Prospective Payment System (PPS) for Medicare provides a good illustration. Although one of its effects has been to intensify competition between hospitals, the use of diagnosis related groups (DRGs) for hospital reimbursement is actually a highly regulatory strategy of centralized price controls—one that falls well within Western European policy traditions.

In regulating physician activities, American policy has not backed off. Rather, since the creation of Physician Review Organizations (PROs) under PPS, the regulation of physician behavior in the United States is surely stronger than any emerging European equivalent, including the French and Canadian systems of medical profiles, which are among the most well developed outside of the United States.

Three characteristics distinguish American policy responses from those of Western Europe and Canada:

1. The United States has long been concerned about the dangers of monopoly power and has pursued (until the recent wave of mergers both inside and outside of the health sector) a strong antitrust policy. A notable case in point is recent Federal Trade Commission measures to curb the monopoly power of physicians and hospitals and to eliminate restraints on trade in health care by allowing advertising.[4] In the United States structural interests are not formally sanctioned and accepted as institutionalized counterparts for purposes of negotiating with the government. Instead, the more typical response of American health policy is to advocate proposals to fragment powerful groups that are presumed, as a consequence, to compete with one another.

2. Following directly from the first characteristic of the American policy response is the absence, in the United States, of institutional structures for negotiating between major groups of health care providers and the government or an NHI board of directors, or both. In contrast to the more adversarial American approach, which attempts to fragment both the medical profession and the hospital associations—a strategy of "divide and conquer"—the Western European and Canadian policy response consolidates the organization of provider groups and confronts them with countervailing organizations.

This important difference acts as a severe constraint, in the United States, on the possibilities of negotiating a national fee schedule for physicians or a uniform hospital payment system for *all* payers and hospitals. The constraint, however, has made it possible for individual payers (e.g., Medicare, Medicaid, and certain private insurance companies) to strike harder bargains with smaller groups and to foster competition and new organizational arrangements for medical care.

3. In contrast to Western European and Canadian strategies of comprehensive health care reform and strong centralized regulation, American strategies (with the exception of PPS for Medicare) are characterized by far greater decentralization and by more persistent social experimentation. Although major policy initiatives have usually come from the federal level, there is much discretion at the state level and a range of government programs at the county and municipal

---

[4]This change of policy was prompted by the 1977 U.S. Supreme Court decision in *Bates v. State Bar of Arizona*, 433 U.S. 350 (1977) allowing health care professionals to engage in advertising.

levels. When compared to unitary European states (e.g., France), American federalism provides a striking contrast. But even in comparison to other federal states, such as Canada and Germany, the United States is still characterized by more decentralization and experimentation in the policymaking process.

These three characteristics of American policy responses to health sector problems highlight the ways in which the United States is different from Western Europe and Canada. But if one compares the evolution of American health policy over the past four decades with that of Western Europe and Canada, there are also points of similarity.

For example, Brown (1985) identifies four American policy responses to health sector problems: (1) the subsidy strategy—government grants on the supply side; (2) the financing strategy—third-party financing on the demand side; (3) the reorganization strategy—government inducements to promote new organizations for delivering medical care; and (4) the regulatory strategy— government attempts to influence the "use, price and quality of services, and the size, location and equipment of facilities." Three of the four strategies—subsidy, financing, and regulatory—are equally good descriptors of the Western European and Canadian policy response to their health sector problems.

In the 1950s and 1960s, during the expansion phase of health care systems, there was extraordinary convergence among Western industrialized nations around both the subsidy and the financing strategies (de Kervasdoué, Kimberly, & Rodwin). In the mid-1970s and 1980s, during the containment phase, there was also convergence around the regulatory and reorganization strategies. Although one can point to examples of the reorganization strategy in all countries, Canada (particularly Quebec) and Western Europe have focused more on administrative reorganizations in the public sector, whereas the United States has encouraged reorganization in the private sector at the level of the delivery system. This is perhaps the most notable aspect of the American policy response to health sector problems.

The Uses of Comparative Analysis in Learning from Abroad

Given the ways in which the health sector in the United States resembles that of Western Europe and Canada and the ways in which it is exceptional, what inferences can one draw about the usefulness of comparative analysis for purposes of learning from abroad? If the United States is truly exceptional in the health sector, then one can argue that there is little to learn from Western Europe and Canada. Countries often rely on this "assumption of uniqueness" to reject ideas from abroad (Stone). To the extent that the United States is unexceptional, however, a case can be made for drawing lessons from comparative experience.

For example, there is a widely shared belief among American policymakers that a national program providing for universal entitlement to health care in the United States would result in runaway costs. In response to this presumption, nations that entitle all of their residents to a high level of medical care, while spending less on administration and on medical care than does the United States, are often held up as models. The Canadian health system is the most celebrated example. French NHI, a prototype of Western European continental health systems, is another case in point. Britain's NHS, although typically considered a "painful prescription" for the United States (Aaron & Schwartz), nevertheless assures first-dollar coverage for basic health services to its entire population and, as we have seen, spends less than half as much money, per capita, as the United States (Table 17.3).

All of these countries have produced some of the leading physicians and hospitals in the world. Judging by various measures of health status, they are in the same league as, or better than, the United States (Table 17.8). In Britain, *life expectancy at 60*—when medical care may have an important impact—is lower than in the United States. But in the United States over 15% of the population remains uninsured for health care services while spending, as a percentage of GDP, surpasses that of all industrially advanced nations (Table 17.4).

Should we adopt the Western European or Canadian models of health care financing and organization? Or should we maintain our present system and recognize that it is a manifestation of American exceptionalism, that is, of the ways in which the United States is fundamentally different from Western Europe and Canada? Both of these responses are probably inappropriate. The second response—that comparative analysis is not useful—insulates us from the experience of other nations. It smacks of ethnocentrism, makes us conservative, and thereby supports the status quo in the United States. The first response—that we should adopt the Western European or Canadian model—relies too heavily on the experience of those nations. It is misleading because, as we have seen, there are serious limitations in the Western European and Canadian health systems. Moreover, many of the present institutional arrangements of health care delivery in the United States are superior to those abroad.

The proliferation of medical technology combined with an aging demographic structure are trends common to all modern health care systems and have contributed to rising health care costs. Policymakers have responded largely by implementing systems with increasing control over expenditures on doctors' services as well as hospital budgets. Virtually no one in Canada or Western Europe views the American health system as a model to emulate. Even under the

Table 17.8 Health Care Expenditures and Health Status

Country	Health expenditures (1984) as % of GDP	Life expectancy (1980)				Infant mortality[a] (1983)
		At birth		At age 60		
		Males	Females	Males	Females	
France	9.1	70.1	78.3	17.2	22.3	.89
Canada	8.4	71.0	79.0	18.0	23.0	.85
Britain[b]	5.9	70.2	75.9	15.9	20.5	1.02
United States	10.7	69.6	76.7	17.2	22.4	1.09

[a]Infant mortality is expressed in death rates of infants below 1 year per 100 live births.
[b]All data are for the United Kingdom.
Sources: Data on health expenditures are from G. Schieber and J. P. Poullier, "International Health Care Spending," *Health Affairs,* Fall 1986. Data on life expectancy and infant mortality are from the Organization for Economic Cooperation and Development (OECD). *Measuring Health Care,* Paris: OECD 1985, Tables F.1 and F.2, p. 131.

government of Prime Minister Thatcher there is no significant challenge to the principle of a NHS in Britain (Klein; *Working for Patients*). Nor is there any question about eliminating NHI in such countries as France, Canada, Germany, Belgium, or the Netherlands.

Despite these attitudes, one striking aspect about how some common problems are currently being dealt with abroad is the extent to which a number of fashionable American themes have drifted north to Canada and across the Atlantic to Western Europe. In the context of the problems we identified earlier—inefficiency in the allocation of health care resources, lack of continuity between levels of care, and the absence of consumer "voice" in most health care organizations—the concept of an HMO, in combination with elements of market competition, has a certain appeal.

Since an HMO is, by definition, both an insurer and a provider of health services, it establishes a link between the financing and provision of health services. Because it is financed on the basis of prepaid capitation payments, its managers have an explicit budget as well as a clearly defined clientele. Moreover, since an HMO is responsible—on a contractual basis—for providing a broad range of primary-, secondary-, and tertiary-level services to its enrolled population, it has powerful incentives to provide these services in a cost-effective manner while simultaneously maintaining quality to minimize the risk of disenrollment.

The idea of introducing HMOs or similar kinds of health care organizations into national systems that provide universal entitlement to health care resembles in many ways the American experience of encouraging Medicare beneficiaries to enroll in federally qualified HMOs or competing medical plans (CMPs). The idea usually involves two reforms. It spurs policymakers to combine regulatory controls with competition on the supply side, and it encourages them to design market incentives for both providers and consumers of health care.

To the extent that the insertion of HMOs into NHI or NHS systems represents an American "solution" to *foreign* problems, it may provide a way in which Canada and Western Europe could learn from the United States (Rodwin, 1989). It may also, paradoxically, have more practical implications for the United States than simply transposing a European NHI or NHS system into the American context. For example, the insertion of HMOs into NHI or NHS systems might provide insights on how to implement Enthoven's NHI plan for the United States (Enthoven & Kronick).

Just how policy learning occurs as a result of studying health care systems abroad is not thoroughly understood. But there is no doubt that more policy research in the field of comparative health systems could potentially be helpful in learning from abroad.

References

Aaron, H. J., & Schwartz, W. B. *The Painful Prescription: Rationing Hospital Care.* Washington, D.C.: Brookings Institution, 1984.

Abel-Smith, B. "Who Is the Odd Man Out? The Experiences of Western Europe in Containing the Costs of Health Care." *Milbank Memorial Fund Quarterly: Health and Society. 63* (Winter), 1, 1985.

Altenstetter, C. *Health Policy-Making and Administration in West Germany and the United States.* Beverly Hills, CA.: Sage Publications, 1974.

Altenstetter, C. *Changing National-Subnational Relations in Health: Opportunities and Constraints* (DHEW Publication No. 6 NIH 78–182). Washington, D.C.: Government Printing Office, 1978.

Anderson, G. F. "National Medical Care Spending." *Health Affairs, 5* (Fall), 123, 1986.

Anderson, O. *Health Care: Can There Be Equity? The United States, Sweden, and England.* New York: John Wiley & Sons, 1972.

Anderson, O. *The Health Services Continuum in Democratic States.* Ann Arbor: Health Administration Press, 1989.

Andreopoulos, S. (ed.). *National Health Insurance: Can We Learn from Canada?* New York: John Wiley & Sons, 1975.

Blum, H. *Planning for Health.* New York: Human Sciences Press, 1981.

Brown, L. D. *Health Policy in the American Welfare State.* Paper prepared for the Ford Foundation Project on the Future of the Welfare State.

Corson, J. *Loiterings in Europe.* New York: Harper, 1948.

de Kervasdoué, J., Kimberly, J., & Rodwin, V. G. (eds.). *The End of an Illusion: The Future of Health Policy in Western Industrialized Nations.* Berkeley, CA.: University of California Press, 1984.

De Miguel, J. "A Framework for the Study of National Health Systems." *Inquiry, 12* (Suppl. 2), 10, 1975.

DHHS, *Sharing Resources for Health in England Report of the Resource Allocation Working Party.* London: Her Majesty's Stationary Office, 1976

Douglas-Wilson, I. and McLachlan, G., eds., *Health Service Prospects: An International Survey* (London: Nuffield Provincial Hospitals Trust, 1974).

Dumbaugh, K., & Neuhauser, D. "International Comparisons of Health Services: Where Are We?" *Social Science and Medicine, 13B,* 221, 1979.

Eckstein, H., *The English National Health Services: It's Origins, Structure & Achievements* (Cambridge, Harvard University Press, 1959).

Elling, R. H. *Cross-National Study of Health Systems: Political Economics and Health Care.* New Brunswick, N.J.: Transactions Books, 1980.

Elling, R. and Kerr, H., "Selection of Contrasting National Health Systems for In-depth Study," *Inquiry* Supplement to volume XII, 1975.

Elling, R., & Kerr, H. "Selection of Contrasting National Health Systems for In-Depth Study." *Inquiry, 12* (Suppl. 2), 25, 1975.

Enthoven, A. and Kronick, R., "A Consumer-Choice Health Plan for the 1990s," *New England J. of Medicine* (320) 2, January 12, 1989.

Evans, R. G. *Strained Mercy: The Economics of Canadian Health Care.* Toronto: Butterworths, 1984.

Evans, R. G. "Holding the Line: The Canadian Experience with Global Budgeting." In M. Berthod-Wurmser, V. Rodwin, et al. (eds.), *Systeme de sante, pouvoirs publics et financeurs: qui controle quoi?* Paris: Documentation Francaise, 1987.

Field, M., *Soviet Socialized Medicine* (New York, Free Press, 1967).

Field, M. G. "The Concept of 'Health Systems' at the Macrosociological Level." *Social Science and Medicine, 7* (October), 1973.

Field, M., *Success and Crisis in National Health Systems: A Comparative Approach.* New York: Routledge, 1989.

Forsyth, G., *Doctors and State Medicine: A Study of the British Health Service* (London: Pitman Medical, 1966).

Fox, D., *Health Policies, Health Politics.* Princeton: Princeton University Press, 1986.

Fry, J., *Medicine in Three Societies—Comparison of Medical Care in the USSR, USA, and UK* (New York: Elsevier, 1970).

Glaser, W. A. *Paying the Doctor: Systems of Remuneration and Their Effects.* Baltimore: Johns Hopkins University Press, 1970.

Glaser, W. A. *Health Insurance Bargaining: Foreign Lessons for Americans.* New York: Gardner Press, 1978.

Glaser, W. A. *Paying the Hospital.* San Francisco, CA.: Jossey Bass, 1987.

Hirschman, A. *Exit, Voice and Loyalty.* Cambridge, MA.: Harvard University Press, 1970.

Hollingsworth, J. R. *A Political Economy of Medicine: Great Britain and the United States.* Baltimore: The Johns Hopkins University Press, 1986.

Hu, T. *International Health Costs and Expenditures* (DHEW Pub. No. 78-184). Washington D.C.: U.S. Government Printing Office, 1976.

Hyde, G., *The Soviet Health Service: A Historical and Comparative Study* (London: Lawrence and Wilshardt, 1974).

Klass, G. "Explaining America and the Welfare State: An Alternative Theory." *British Journal of Political Science, 15,* 427, 1985.

Klein, R., *The Politics of the NHS* (London: Pitman Medical, 1983).

Klein, R. "Why Britain's Conservatives Support a Socialist Health Care System." *Health Affairs, 4* (Spring), 41, 1985.

Leichter, H. M. *A Comparative Approach to Policy Analysis: Health Care Policy in Four Nations.* Cambridge: Cambridge University Press, 1979.

Leslie, C. (ed.). "Theoretical Foundations for the Comparative Study of Medical Systems." *Social Science and Medicine, 12,* Special Issue 1978.

Light, D. and Schuller, A., eds. *Political Values and Health Care: The German Experience.* Cambridge: MIT Press, 1986.

Lindsey, A., *Socialized Medicine in England and Wales* (Chapel Hill: University of North Carolina Press, 1962).

Maxwell, R. J. *Health and Wealth,* Lexington, Mass.: Lexington Books, D.C. Heath and Co., 1981.

Marmor, T., Bridges, A., & Hoffman, W. "Comparative Politics and Health Policies: Notes on Benefits, Costs, Limits." In D. Ashford (ed.), *Comparing Public Policies.* Beverly Hills CA.: Sage Publications, 1978.

Maynard, A. *Annual Report on the National Health Service*. New York: Center for Health Economics, 1986.

McLachlan, G., & Maynard, A. (eds.). *The Public/Private Mix For Health: The Relevance and Effects of Change*. London: Nuffield Provincial Hospitals Trust, 1982.

Mechanic, D. "The Comparative Study of Health Care Delivery Systems." In *The Growth of Bureaucratic Medicine: An Inquiry into the Dynamics of Patient Behavior and the Organization of Medical Care* (Ch. 2). New York: John Wiley, 1976.

"Organization for Economic Cooperation and Development (OECD)." *Measuring Health Care, 1960–1983*. Paris, OECD, 1985.

Raffel, M. W., ed. *Comparative Health Systems*. Pennsylvania: The Pennsylvania State University Press, 1985.

Reinhardt, U. "Hard Choices in Health Care: A Matter of Ethics." In L. Etheredge et al. (eds.), *Health Care: How to Improve It and Pay for It*. Washington, D.C.: Center for National Policy, 1985.

Rodwin, V. G. "The Marriage of National Health Insurance and *La Médecine Libérale* in France: A Costly Union." *Milbank Memorial Fund Quarterly: Health and Society*, *59* (Winter), 16, 1981.

Rodwin, V. G. *The Health Planning Predicament: France, Quebec, England, and the United States*. Berkeley, CA.: University of California Press, 1984.

Rodwin, V. G. "New Ideas for Health Policy in France, Canada, and Britain." In Field, M., ed. *Success and Crisis in National Health Systems: A Comparative Approach*. New York: Routledge, 1989.

Roemer, M. I. *Comparative National Policies on Health Care*. New York: Marcel Dekker, 1977.

Roemer, M. and R., *Health Care Systems and Comparative Manpower Policies* (New York: Marcel Dekker, 1981).

Rosner, D. "Health Care for the 'Truly Needy': Nineteenth-Century Origins of the Concept." *Milbank Memorial Fund Quarterly: Health and Society*, 60 (Summer), 355, 1982.

Saltman, R., ed., *The International Handbook of Health Care Systems*. New York: Greenwood Press, 1988.

Schweitzer, S. *Policies for the Containment of Health Care Costs and Expenditures* (DHEW Publication No. 78-184). Washington, D.C.: U.S. Government Printing Office, 1978.

Sidel, V. and R., *Serve the People: Observations on Medicine in the People's Republic of China* (New York: Josiah Macy, 1973).

Sidel, V. and R., *A Healthy State: An International Perspective on the Crisis in United States Medical Care* (New York: Pantheon, 1977).

Sigerist, H., *Medicine & Health in the Soviet Union* (New York: Citadel Press, 1947).

Stodard, D. A. *Rationalizing the Health Care System*. Paper presented at the Ontario Economic Council Conference, Toronto, May 14–15, 1984.

Stone, D. A. "Drawing Lessons from Comparative Health Research." In R. A. Straetz, M. Liberman, & A. Sardell (eds.), *Critical Issues in Health Policy* (pp. 135–148). Lexington, MA: D.C. Heath, 1981.

Teune, H. "The Logic of Comparative Policy Analysis." In D. Ashford (ed.), *Comparing Public Policies*. Beverly Hills, CA.: Sage Publications, 1978.

Townsend, P., & Davidson, N. (eds.). *Inequalities in Health: The Black Report*. London: Penguin, 1982.

Weinerman, R. "Research on Comparative Health Systems." *Medical Care, 9:*3, 1971.

Weinerman, R. and J., *Social Medicine in Eastern Europe: Organization of Health Services and the Education of Medical Personnel in Czechoslovakia, Hungary, and Poland* (Cambridge: Harvard University Press, 1969).

Working for Patients. London: Her Majesty's Stationary Office, 1989.

18

Health Care Ethics

Dena J. Seiden

This chapter will cover the historical development of the field of bioethics, the various methodologies used in bioethics, the more important ethical principles and issues, and major topics of current interest in health care ethics. It will provide considerable detail about all of these topics but will not attempt an exhaustive discussion of each issue. It will occasionally discuss actual cases that are of importance in the development of biomedical ethics, but it will not use a case-study approach. Rather, the point is to give the reader an idea of the impetus for the rise of the field and of the current concerns in the field.

The discipline of health care ethics, sometimes known as bioethics or medical ethics, is a relatively recent development, with beginnings in the late 1960s and early 1970s. Though there was interest in the topic among both health care professionals and ethicists before that time, there was not a recognized group of scholars or practitioners or a literature that supported that interest. The change at the present time is startling for both intensity and depth. Medical ethical questions appear on the front pages of newspapers and on the evening news with regularity. Bioethical journals have become fixtures *(Hastings Center Report, Journal of Medical Ethics,* etc.), and the standard medical journals routinely carry articles on moral questions in virtually every issue (see particularly *The New England Journal of Medicine*). Degree-granting programs in the field have been established, and a national society for bioethical consultants has been formed, meeting for the first time in 1986. Despite this explosion of public, professional, and academic interest, health care institutions have been slow to hire ethicists as staff, often preferring a few ethics seminars through the year or the establishment of an ethics committee made up of professionals with fine intentions and little ethical training. As formal ethics teaching increasingly becomes part of the credentialing process for institutions, graduate school education, and residency training programs, it will be interesting to observe how the discipline and its practitioners are absorbed into the mainstream of institutional life.

Development of Health Care Ethics

Reason for Development

The quickening of interest in medical ethics *as a concept* began after World War II and the acknowledgment of the complicity of the German medical profession in the death camp exterminations and in medical and scientific "experiments" on prisoners, which were thought to be beyond any reasonable bounds of moral constraint (see Alexander, 1949; Declaration of Geneva, 1948; Declaration of Helsinki, 1964). There was general agreement among the world's medical associations that the profession had been corrupted and that strong national and international rules needed to be applied to the canons of scientific and medical experimentation on human beings and also to the way the profession should conduct itself despite political pressure.

Once these agreements and canons were in place, however, little more followed in the establishment of a discipline of health care ethics. But the seeds for such a development were sown in the 1950s and 1960s as a result of several factors. The first, seemingly nonmoral, was the rise and speed of innovation in medical technology, initially greeted as an unmitigated blessing and then looked upon somewhat as a sorcerer's apprentice type of problem. That is, the ability to prolong life through use of respirators, dialysis, artificial nutrition and hydration, though often dramatically effective, frequently resulted in prolonging a vegetative existence, which many people questioned as lacking meaning.

The second, derived from the earlier concerns with World War II medical atrocities but more truly generated by the preoccupation in the 1960s with individual rights and individual autonomy, was the ideal of patient autonomy, as opposed to the traditional beneficence model of the medical profession. The beneficence ideal has been dominant since at least the Hippocratic oath, with its statement "The regimen I adopt shall be for the benefit of my patients according to my ability and judgment" (Temkin & Temkin, 1967), in which the physician makes decisions without benefit of discussion or direction by the patient. The move toward patient autonomy directly challenged that posture, insisting that the patient be at least a partner in all decision making. Some ethicists believe that the patient should be the sole decision maker.

Notwithstanding the degree of autonomy desired, the ideal of individual autonomy became the basis for concrete health care policies, such as the Patient Bill of Rights (American Hospital Association), and a building block of health care ethics for such ideas as informed consent and the right to refuse treatment, of which more below. The ideal was given greater emphasis when startling incidents of patient mistreatment in the United States began to be revealed. Key among these were the following:

1. The U.S. Army's use of lysergic diethylamide acid (LSD) on unsuspecting volunteers during the 1950s and 1960s. Many of these servicemen suffered psychotic episodes and permanent psychiatric damage.

2. The Tuskegee syphilis experiments on black men in Alabama, which began in the 1930s and continued through the 1960s. The control group of black men were not treated for their disease, even when penicillin became available during the 1940s, and as a result many went blind, were institutionalized, and died. These men were never given the option of treatment for fear it would make the experiment less scientifically useful.

3. The Willowbrook hepatitis experiments on retarded children and adults in Staten Island, New York. Physicians and researchers at the institution injected the patients with a mild form of hepatitis, so as to have a controlled-population experiment, in an effort to discover a vaccine for the disease. The patients were not informed nor given the right to refuse the inoculation. Parents who wanted their children placed at Willowbrook were told admission was conditional upon their agreement to the inoculation. In consequence, this already sick population was given an additional sickness without consent and without therapeutic benefit to the patient.

These examples of medical arrogance and abrogation of individual rights gained widespread attention and underscored the need for patient autonomy and for the introduction of medical ethics into the profession in a formal way.

Finally, specific topics such as abortion, euthanasia, and the special problems of keeping alive multiply handicapped newborn infants fueled public and professional debate about when life begins and ends. These questions also led to great debate about the "sanctity" of life, as opposed to the "quality" of life. These ultimate questions have formed the central topics in current health care ethics.

Historical Development of the Field

Medical ethics began as a subset of the disciplines of ethics and philosophy and, to a lesser extent, that of the law. Given the issues and pressures described above, it has become a discipline of its own. Important ethicists such as Paul Ramsey and Joseph Fletcher began devoting time to medical ethics (Fletcher, 1960, 1966, 1979; Ramsey, 1971), among their other ethical concerns in the 1950s and 1960s. By the 1970s, thinkers such as James Childress, Tom Beauchamp, Daniel Callahan, Albert Jonsen (Beauchamp & Childress, 1983; Callahan, 1987a&b; Childress, 1970; Jonsen & Garland, 1976), and many others began to devote their full-time efforts to ethical problems in health care. At present there are hundreds of ethicists working in health care. In addition, it is estimated by the American Hospital Association that two-thirds of acute-care hospitals with more than 100 beds have some form of ethics committee.

That last fact highlights the movement of medical ethics out of academic centers and into the health care industry. As noted before, to date a great deal of this is more well-meant words than specific policies or case decisions. Yet there is a discernible movement into institutions, particularly multihospital institutions, such as the Sisters of Mercy, Kaiser Permanente Plan, Holy Cross Hospitals, and others.

Methodology

There are a number of methods used in analyzing medical problems from a moral perspective. One is to bring established ethical traditions and schools of thought to bear on current medical dilemmas and situations. These traditions and philosophical currents are generally both secular and religious, with the religious coming from the Judeo-Christian tradition, at least in the West. A second method is to examine cases or health care problems and policies against ethical standards, learning general ethical principles from the crossfire of discussion. A third method is to focus on health care ethical issues only, forgoing any attempt to learn the general ethical principles that have been collected over the last several millennia. A fourth method is to focus only on patient care cases or health care policies, assuming that the values generated in discussion will provide a sufficient ethical framework in which to judge the correct values of the dilemma. One ethicist has called this "practice become values" (Shinn, 1983).

Clearly, there are strengths and weaknesses in all of these methods. In the first, there is the difficulty of and resistance to learning basic philosophical tenets of the Western world. This is true for working health care professionals, whose training has tended to be in the sciences, as opposed to the humanities. It is true also for those in professional graduate schools and residency training programs, who tend toward either fiscal programs or experiential medical learning. It requires work on the part of both teacher and student to adapt such essentially different disciplines to forge a rigorous, thoughtful, hybrid discipline that combines such different needs as pure thought and immediate action. Ethics in a medical setting could easily sink into abstract contemplation of humanity's existential dilemmas, which would almost immediately alienate health care providers. Or it could become a second-rate litany of catch phrases (e.g., informed consent, patient autonomy) whose implications have not been fully explored and so lose the interest and respect of academics and of most intelligent people who have pondered these questions. The challenge is to keep both immediacy and ultimate meanings in the hybrid new discipline.

Ethical Principles and Issues

Principles

The Deontological Principle. This principle represents an ethical pole, an absolutist ethic that exists both as a principle in itself and also, in present times, as an extreme of ethical thought, against which other ethics can be measured.

The word *deontological* comes from the Greek *deon,* or duty. It is an ethic that relies on duty, on law, on rules that are based on a priori agreement on essential facts.

Deontological thought focuses on the "right"—which is different from "rights"—or what is "good." The right is what one *ought* to do and never deviate from. *Ought* is the key word here. If one follows the *ought,* without exception, the most moral decision will be reached. Importantly, within this ethic, one doesn't plan for consequences. Consequences are seen as truly unforeseeable. Life has too many permutations to allow for even a pretense of accurate prediction. Thus, one goes by the rules, the *ought,* the law. (Note the small *l* in law. We are talking about universal law, not categorical [e.g., civil, criminal] law.)

Overall, this is a highly individualistic ethic. The individual is the end of all action. In the words of Immanuel Kant, an 18th-century German philosopher and perhaps the foremost exponent of this ethic (Kant, 1949), each individual is in himself or herself the end of action and never the means. Here we see how well this ethic can be applied to clinical medicine. In clinical medicine, all efforts go to the individual, as there is no higher goal and no other goal for that moment in time. To do else would be to denigrate the almost sacred meaning of the individual. Moreover, as in clinical ethics, one goes by the *ought* and the rules. Medicine's *oughts* are its protocols for diseases and procedures. Deontological *oughts* are, as stated, the a priori laws, which are reached partially through reason.

The final point to keep in mind with this ethic is how firmly it is grounded in reason. It is reason, not emotion, that governs. There are many reasons for this; for instance, reason is thought of as more reliable than emotion. But the underlying point in favor of reason is that only men and women are capable of reason, and it is reason, that allows the free use of will, allowing us to choose between good and evil. Reason and free will are inextricable in this ethic.

The Utilitarian (Teleological) Principle. This principle represents the other ethical pole, the furthest opposite from the individualistic, deontological ethic. Originally called teleological (from the Greek *telos,* or end), in current parlance it has become, to all intents and purposes, synonymous with utilitarianism. By definition, it is an end-oriented ethic, with the end of human thought and action being human happiness. But it focuses on the mass happiness, as in utilitarian's most famous maxim, "the greatest good for the greatest number," as stated by J. S. Mill (1962). In this ethic, concern is for the group, the mass, the society as a whole or sometimes even the world.

Clearly, if concern is with the end point of thought and action for any group, this is an ethic that expects to be able to predict for consequences. Different utilitarians approach this in various ways, but all assume that reason (again a dominant theme in an ethical school of thought) can allow calculation on the part of some that will be beneficial for the many or, at best, calculation for the many that will be beneficial for the many.

Happiness itself was not conceptualized as a vulgar fleeting pleasure, which has undeservedly earned utilitarian ethicists the charge of being hedonists. Happiness can consist of many components, such as quiet contentment, intellectual pursuits, even health itself, important in bringing this ethic back to health care. Health for utilitarians is thought of as a basic good, necessary for happiness.

At least one prominent utilitarian active today, Joseph Fletcher (1966), has noted that this ethic depends on either a majority view of what is "the (ultimate) good" or at least an individual's view of what is the supreme good. (Remember here that "good" is different from "right," in that it finds its end in maximizing happiness. The deontologist will follow reason, the rule, and the right and not trust to happiness as too chimerical.) Fletcher notes that this leads at some point to a clash of overriding principles and that finally one principle must be defined as the supreme good in this ethic. Fletcher himself votes for love, the disinterested, non-self-regarding variety, but his underlying point holds, no matter what principle is used. The good must be defined. In a markedly pluralistic society such as our own, this is extremely difficult, if not impossible. Consider, for instance, the debate of the last 20 years over abortion, as to what is best for the society as a whole. The difficulty of defining the good becomes readily apparent. This is a major flaw in the utilitarian stance. Although a majority, perhaps even a temporary majority, may define the good, that leaves room for a minority to feel that some very bad things are happening to them and to their society. Their happiness is not being maximized, by their standards.

An example of how this could apply in health care would be a decision that a high-technology procedure, such as liver transplants, do not maximize the health and happiness of the majority of the population and that therefore such procedures should not be covered by insurance in this country. Rather, the same amount of money that would go for transplants should be used to provide a baseline "floor" of medical care for all Americans so that access for some definition of basic care could be achieved. This might well maximize the health and happiness of a majority. It would, however, leave those in need of transplants with an alternative of either dying or raising the funds for transplant by their own means, now estimated at from $120,000 to $140,000. Their happiness would be at risk. This example could be used in any number of other high-technology applications, for example, in vitro fertilization, which can benefit a small number of infertile women at considerable cost (and some risk). Can the money be better used to foster adoptions of "problem children" considered unadoptable or, going further, adoption of orphaned children from other countries, who live in dire straits? How would one ethically balance the greater happiness here? Obviously, these are complex, multifaceted issues, and the utilitarian solution, as well as the deontological solution, may simply not work in such complexity.

Other Ethical Schools of Thought

The Ethics of the Fitting. H. Richard Niebuhr, a 20th-century ethicist, is one of many ethicists who have tried to find a median point between the right and the good. In his 1963 book, *The Responsible Self,* he posited a four-point system for ethical decision making, aimed at the "fitting" ethical move. The ethical decision maker (1) must first be able to respond, then (2) must make an interpretation of the issues at stake, in terms of "what is being done to me, to us, to them," *not* what is my "law/right" or my "ultimate end," leading to (3) accountability, or taking into account the reactions of others, making the community's reactions part of the individual's decision. All of this leads to (4) social solidarity, when the decision is implemented, not as a completely final act but rather becomes part of a continuing discourse or interaction within the relevant community.

There are some major problems with this valiant attempt to get past the problem of totally opposed ethical opposites. One problem is that with all of the discussion, interaction, and taking into account of the community's values, the decision reached may merely be one of the common denominator. The decision may then be one with which no one is fully morally comfortable but with which all are somewhat quieted. Another even more potentially dangerous problem is that the values involved are derived from the community's values. If those values are distorted, there is no absolute corrective. This points to the reverse of the problem of having the absolutist values of either the deontological or teleological school. If there are no absolutes, no higher authority, law, or value system to which to appeal, then morals can become an infinite regression, without any ending or beginning moral point.

Max Weber: Supplements, Not Contrasts. Max Weber, a sociologist and political scientist of the early 20th century, was interested in ethical systems as well. In his treatise "Politics as a Vocation" (Weber, 1958), he wrote at length on the ethics of decision making and the need to take responsibility for the consequences of one's action. Weber called this "the ethics of responsibility" and was strong in support of this modality. He was highly condemnatory of what he called "the ethics of ultimate ends," condemning them as "political idiocy" and as being responsible for most of the bloody events then taking place in his native Germany.

In his criteria for ethical decision making, Weber relied on three characteristics: passion, an ability to abstract and to distance oneself from the problem, and a sense of responsibility. One cursory glance at his praise of the ethics of responsibility would seem to exclude "passion" as a desirable quality. But Weber stated that decisions are made "not with the head alone, but also with the heart." And because, for Weber, passion and the emotions are linked to the despised "ethics of ultimate ends," Weber had to come to an understanding and a synthesis of the place of both passion and absolutes.

Weber did this by postulating that the ethical, mature decision maker must continue with the ethics of responsibility, or being responsible for the consequences of one's actions, for as long as humanly possible. To do otherwise is to "intoxicate" oneself with "romantic sensations." Yet, even following along this path of reason and responsibility, one reaches a point where one says:

> Here I stand; I can do no other . . . and every one of us who is not spiritually dead must realize the possibility of finding himself [sic] at some time in the position. In so far as this is true, an ethic of ultimate ends and an ethic of responsibility are not absolute contrasts but rather supplements, which only in unison constitute a genuine human being. (p. 127)

Weber then admitted the necessity for some moral absolutes but only as a last resort and only when the absolute comes from the totality of the person. This ethic also has serious problems. By Weber's very definition of wringing the absolute out of oneself, he acknowledges that (a) it will be somewhat different for each person, and (b) an absolute will call forth the strongest and potentially most dangerous, irrational behavior from human beings. That is, of course, why he insists that the ethics of responsibility and the ethics of ultimate ends be supplements, not contrasts. Yet by admitting that it is for an absolute principle that people will stand fast, and not for a relative principle, he concedes the problem.

Absolutes in ethics and morality are exceedingly dangerous as they lead to nonnegotiable positions and to bitter and sometimes violent argument. Yet the alternative is a relativism that allows for no moral standing point, no appeal to an intrinsic or extrinsic higher authority, without which the moral dilemma is truly crucial and outside conventional morality. Weber's notion of supplements is useful as a possible way to escape these dangers, at least for a good deal of the time and for a good many situations.

The Doctrine of Double Effect. This doctrine was developed over centuries by Catholic theologians in an effort to make canon law more amenable to actual human predicaments. For instance, under this doctrine the removal of a uterus of a pregnant women may be justified, notwithstanding the Catholic opposition to abortion.

The doctrine of double effect attempts to justify certain actions that indirectly produce certain evil consequences, but it does this only after four basic principles have been justified.

1. The action, by itself and independently of its effect, must not be morally evil.
2. The evil effect must not be a means to producing the good effect.
3. The evil effect is sincerely not intended, but merely tolerated.
4. There is a proportionate reason for performing the action, despite its evil consequences.

This ethical system may be understood best in one of its classical illustrations. The case, which dates back many centuries is this: A woman, 9 months pregnant, has had an extremely difficult pregnancy. She wants very much to bring her child to term. She has been warned by the local physician not to exert herself. If she exerts herself, there is a real chance that she will lose the child she is carrying. She lives in a house on the river, and at the moment of moral decision is sunning herself by the river.

Suddenly, she hears the cries of a child, drowning in the river and screaming for help. There is no one else around. The *moral* question is can she run to help the drowning child? The point is not whether she wants to but whether, given the Catholic emphasis on protection of fetal life, she can run as a moral act.

Here is where the sophistication and precision of the doctrine of double effect can be shown. Going back to the first principle, the action, which is defined as *running,* is not "morally evil." For the second principle, the evil effect, the possible loss of the child in utero, is not the *means* of producing the good effect, the saving of the drowning child. Running is the means. In the third principle, the evil effect is clearly not intended, as the woman wants her child. For the fourth principle, there is, of course, a proportionate reason for performing the act, and that is the attempt to save the drowning child. The key principle and action in the above scenario, however, is the isolation of the evil effect from being the *means* of saving the drowning child. In using this kind of logic, formally called casuistry, secular and religious ethicists are able to respond to particular human situations while still holding to firm general principles.

The above certainly does not represent an endorsement of this method as a sure means of solving ethical dilemmas. Rather, it can be used to identify what is the moral dilemma, which is the first step in attempting to solve the problem. If there is a method being advocated among all of the above methods, perhaps it is the use of supplements, not contrasts, between absolutes and relativities.

Health Care Ethical Issues

Autonomy

Currently, the most important issue within health care ethics is that of individual autonomy. What this has come to mean is that the patient is the chief decision maker in all situations, regarding her/his medical care. The provider—physician, nurse, or other professional—may and should provide information as to the risks, benefits, and alternatives to a course of treatment, a procedure, or a medication. But according to the theory of autonomy, the patient makes the decision, up to and including the rejection of all forms of treatment, including lifesaving treatment. The professional must abide by the patient's wishes.

As explained in the section above, "Development of Health Care Ethics," this was an almost inevitable course of ethicists to follow. Both the fears and realities of medical excesses lead to a strong doctrine of individual autonomy. Certainly, the political climate of the 1960s and 1970s, with its emphasis on maximized individual rights, would also lead in such a direction. Further, a reaction against professional beneficence (see below) for a variety of reasons—the malpractice problem; excessive physician and hospital fees during the financially expansive Medicaid and Medicare years; fears of technology being used both for its own sake, without thought of what it might and might not do for the patient, simply to make money for those supplying it—led to individual patient autonomy as *the* central medical ethical principle. For good discussions of these ideas, Gerald Dworkin (1978, 1983), George Annas (1984) and Ruth Macklin (1986, 1987) have done superb work.

Most theories of individual patient autonomy are grounded in the work of Kant, discussed above, and his notion of each individual's being endowed with reason and free will and therefore unique in the universe. Each human being is a creature making his or her choices. Further, this theory holds that it diminishes the individual to have others make choices for him or her as this is, in effect, an insult to one's own reason and unique individuality.

However, there are limits to the position of full professional autonomy, both in reality and in theory. In reality, the patient is dependent on the health care professional for information, and no matter how scrupulous the professional is, it is difficult to keep professional biases out of the discussion. In addition, the professional knows a great deal more of the medical and scientific facts regarding the patient's situation, simply by virtue of years of study of the subject, which the patient has not had. Also, in reality, the patient may sometimes reject being given the option of choice, through fear, denial, or indecision. The cliche "Do whatever you think is best, Doc" is far from being history.

In terms of both reality and theory, there is a clearer limit on patient autonomy in asking for treatment than in rejecting treatment. Autonomy has been held to be grounded in *the right of privacy* in a number of legal decisions, notably in Roe versus Wade (1973), the landmark abortion decision. It has been held to be the basis for rejection of treatment in a number of the so-called right-to-die cases, beginning with the Karen Anne Quinlan case (*In re Quinlan,* 1976) and continuing with the major cases in the field (e.g., *In re Eichner* (1981), *In re Storar* (1981), *In re Spring* (1980), *Brophy vs. New England Sinai Hospital* (1986). In these and many like cases, the individual's right *not* to be treated has been based on privacy, or the freedom to do what one wants with his or her own body. Given the highly individualistic nature of American political, economic, social, and legal thought, it is natural to have reached this point. But does individual patient autonomy include the right to demand treatment, particularly treatment that may be useless to the individual?

A relatively benign example is the patient who demands antibiotics for a viral infection. In fact, antibiotics will not attack a viral infection, only a bacterial infection. Yet many patients have become so accustomed to getting a "shot" for the "flu" that anything less seems like shoddy care. Clearly, the right to demand this kind of useless treatment cannot be grounded in privacy. Can it and should it be grounded in some other notion of autonomy? (For a discussion of these and similar questions, see Brett and McCullough [1986].)

A less benign example, and one anchored in theory as well, is that complete patient autonomy may lead to a major consumption of resources by one individual or group of individuals, to the enormous detriment of the community as a whole. A few examples will make the point. A terminally ill patient may demand a large quantity of blood transfusions, which will minimally prolong his life. Yet the hospital or the region may be so short of blood as is now often the case, that to transfuse that individual at that rate may make it impossible to care for motor vehicle accident cases or other types of trauma cases for which transfusion is key. A patient or his or her family may demand that the patient remain in a critical care unit long after some definable clinical benefit can be achieved by the stay because they "want everything to be done" or because of fear or guilt or for other reasons. Yet the bed may be desperately needed for a patient who can clinically benefit from the stay in a critical care unit. Finally, the transfer of medical resources to the elderly population through the Medicare program in an era of deliberate cost containment has begun to raise serious questions about whether the remaining resources can adequately meet the needs of all other Americans. Some recent journal issues and books have begun to deal with this question (The Journal of Medicine and Philosophy, 13, [1], (see Daniels, 1988a, 1988b).

The basic question in relation to autonomy that arises from this is, how much can any person, elderly or not, demand in having their requests for aggressive, maximal treatment honored? This question particularly holds when the patient is terminal, but it may apply in other situations as well, when allocation of scarce resources is a serious problem. One author has gone so far as to suggest that, as an incentive, if people don't use their benefits themselves, they can transfer them to others (Hartwig, 1988). This is a new idea, which remains to be explored for moral and administrative problems. (For a general discussion about the limits of autonomy, and age as a criteria, see Callahan [1984, 1987]).

Professional Beneficence

The doctrine of professional beneficence is deeply embedded in medical history. It is part of the Hippocratic Oath, which states in part, "The regimen I adopt shall be for the benefit of my patients accortding to *my* [italics added] ability and judgment, and not for their hurt or for any wrong." Note that the patient has no say in the regimen adopted. The physician decides alone.

The roots of professional beneficence, sometimes less flatteringly called paternalism, lie very deep in medical history. The healing function and the priestly function have been combined in many societies, including our own. In biblical times, holy men were thought to be able to heal the sick by virtue of their ties to God. Jesus Christ healed by the laying on of hands or, in a more startling example, by having a hemorrhaging woman, unbeknownst to Him, touch the hem of His garments. In the Middle Ages, monks and priests practiced the art of healing as part of their role in keeping learning and knowledge alive but also, in part, in imitation of the example of Christ. Nuns nursed the sick in hospitals and elsewhere.

In many other cultures, in the past and continuing to the present, the healer was the local religious person, whose power derived from the deity of the culture. Often the healing ritual and the priestly ritual would be combined. It is worth noting that in the Hippocratic Oath, quoted above, the opening appeal by the Greek writers of the fourth century B.C. is to "Apollo *Physician* [italics added] and Aesculapias and Hygieia and Panaceia and the gods and goddesses, making them my witnesses, that I will fulfill according to my ability and judgment this oath and convenant." Again, there is the tie of the art of medicine to the reigning deities, to the extent of noting that one of the most powerful gods is himself a physician.

Given this background, the power of professional beneficence or paternalism is quite logical in the practice of medicine. Does not healing come from the highest authority, the most powerful Father of them all, at least for many people in the world? The switch into medical paternalism is an easy one to make, emotionally and psychologically.

Moreover, as noted in the "Informed Consents" section below, there is an internal logic to it. The physician and nurse do indeed know a great deal more medically and scientifically than the patient does, and their *medical* judgment is certainly more informed. As medicine has learned more and has become so specialized that physicians cannot claim much knowledge of each other's specialty, the reason for beneficence/paternalism appears even clearer. Physicians seem to be extraordinary people who know and can do extraordinary things, perhaps even cheat death itself. For ordinary patients to enter into a dialogue with people of such knowledge and skill seems foolish.

Of course, as the "Autonomy" section tried to make clear, this is not the case. The physician knows the medical facts and may empathize greatly with the patient's plight and feelings. But it is the patient's body and mind that is at stake, and thus the patient has the right to decide what to do after listening (one hopes) to sound advice. Moreover, as the most cursory reading of history shows, investing unchecked power in any group leads to abuse of power. Despite their long-standing ethical codes and traditions, this is as true of the medical profession as of any other profession.

Professional Autonomy

Given the struggle between individual patient autonomy and professional beneficence, what balance can be achieved? Many ethicists, including this one, think that the answer lies in professional autonomy. In a sense, this is giving to the health care professional the same dignity and respect accorded to the patient. It takes into account that the health care professional has striven to master a body of knowledge that allows for informed, discrete judgments. It also allows that health care professionals are human beings with feelings, beliefs, and values, not technicians who perform at the behest of patient, science, or employer.

One notable example of this is in the abortion situation. There are health care professionals who have strong beliefs against abortion. Most hospitals recognize this and do not assign such staff to areas where they will be dealing with abortions.

Equally compelling are cases in which the patient will be allowed to die by being taken off life-sustaining technological equipment. Some physicians and nurses feel very strongly that this is either tantamount to murder or against all medical ethics or both. Some feel, perhaps more strongly than the patient's own family, that this is the only possible course to end pointless and intractable suffering. In the first case, can medical staff be forced to terminate treatment? Clearly not, as to do so would be to violate their rights as individuals. In the second case, can medical staff override family wishes, perhaps even patient wishes, in their commendable desire to end suffering? Probably not, for to do so would violate individual rights and liberties. In both cases, the answer is probably for such professionals to be transferred off these cases and for professionals who are in agreement with the prevailing beliefs of the patients and family to take over in each case. This option should never be used as a subterfuge to allow health care professionals to abandon patients whom they do not wish to treat. The clearest current example of this is the way a few clinicians have declared that they will not treat AIDS patients because of fear of infection for themselves and their families and sometimes because of their dislike of the life-styles of the AIDS patients as well. The two examples of professional autonomy used above—disagreement over termination or continuance of treatment—cannot morally be used as reasons to refuse care because of health provider risk or discrimination.

Although some ethicists feel professional autonomy may be a way to bring back the discredited notion of professional beneficence, others feel that this may be a means of humanizing medicine. Health care professional training now focuses overwhelmingly on technology. By acknowledging that professionals have determining beliefs and values and making sure that the arena is open for them to act on those beliefs and values, the practice of medicine may become more cooperative, less adversarial, and more humane. The patient or surrogate still decides, within the bounds of reason, what is to be done with his or her mind and body, but the professional does not have to follow this dictate slavishly.

Societal Risk and Benefit

Medical ethics has tended to emulate medicine itself, in that the ethics have had an individualistic flavor, as has medicine. A great deal of this arises from the focus on individual autonomy, as discussed above. A less-noticed reason for the emphasis on individualism is that working ethicists, outside of think-tanks or academe, work on cases much the way medical staff do. That is to say, both groups focus intensely on one patient at a time. Even those ethicists outside the institutional malestrom tend to comment on specific cases involving specific individuals. To date, there are no public health ethicists, that is, ethicists whose concern is the health of large groups of people or whole societies.

There has been a small change in this tendency within the last few years as cost-containment has become a major theme in health care. Acknowledgment that resources are scarce forces consideration as to how these newly scarce resources may best be used to benefit society as a whole. The converse question is also raised: What is the risk to society of failing to use these resources appropriately or of using resources disproportionately for particular groups at the expense of other groups?

Other changes in the health care field have also forced reappraisal as to the good of society. The AIDS epidemic is key in this respect. Both the health professions and society as a whole are struggling to find the balance between protection of the AIDS-infected individual and the ability of society to have enough information to protect against the further spread of the disease. This has involved a reappraisal of the limits and benefits of confidentiality, as well as consideration of the protection of individuals against bigotry and discrimination.

The aging of the American population has also forced reconsideration of the use of resources. Medicare expenditures have continued to rise despite sustained efforts to control the increases. Nursing home care for the elderly consumes a large proportion of the Medicaid budget, originally intended for care for the poor. Numerous demographic studies show that the need for long-term care for the elderly will increase sharply as the baby boom generation of the 1940s and 1950s ages, and various proposals have been advanced to deal with the problem. They range from making long-term care a Medicare benefit to a tax increase for the population as a whole to support this service. The need for long-term care for the elderly is a reality, but the increasing allocation of resources to the health needs of the elderly can easily cut very deeply into the funds left for care of the rest of the population unless the society is willing to accept a substantial increase in the amount of national resources going into health care as a whole. It is unclear whether society is willing to do so, or what society wants to do about long-term care as a unique problem. Polls and studies are conflicting.

Finally, a classic example of difficulty in allocation of scarce resources has arisen in organ transplantation. There are far fewer donors for organs (livers, kidneys, hearts, etc.) than there are potential recipients. This is a problem in itself, but it is further complicated by many foreign nationals coming to the United States for transplants, as this country is using this technology so much more than any other country. There is thus a debate on whether or how many foreign nationals should be put on the waiting list for organs, instead of American citizens. Beyond this problem, and certainly more important, is how to justly allocate these scarce organs among those whose lives depend on the transplant. All too often, intense media publicity by distraught patients or their families has resulted in a patient being jumped from a low place on the waiting list to a top place, leaving those who have been waiting to wait still longer. This "jumping the list" has been fairly criticized as unjust. The current proposal is to have a national consortium, privately run, to deal with the allocation.

Beyond even this question is the ethically and politically difficult question of whether this country should be doing transplants at a rather rapid rate compared to other countries. Organ transplantation is extremely costly and benefits a relatively small number of patients, albeit very sick patients. Many ethicists and health care professionals argue that this money can be far better spent on basic public health services, preventive care, and health education. They further argue that such activities would diminish the need for organ transplantation as people learn better nutrition, adopt more useful exercise, or give up such damaging habits as smoking, drinking alcoholic beverages to excess, or the abuse of drugs. Those in favor of organ transplantation point to the enormous need of these very sick patients, who will surely die without the transplantation.

All of the above are examples of the vexing nature of the consideration of balancing risks and benefits to the society as a whole while still considering the individual as an important end point in himself or herself.

Meaning of Institutional Integrity and Survival

This chapter has been concerned with the great pressures on health care institutions and health care professionals to provide optimal care while limiting the cost of that care. It is an open question as to whether this can be done (Feldstein, 1988; McCarthy, 1988; Schramm & Gabel, 1988; Shortell & Hughes, 1988). It is difficult, in life, to have it all. However, such are the signals being given by patients, the government, insurers, and business to American health care.

Under these pressures, there is a strong incentive for hospitals, other health care institutions such as HMOs, and health care professionals to cut corners in a variety of ways. Hospitals may cut back on less visible but needed staff in an effort to hold down costs. HMOs may provide patients with fewer referrals to specialists or hold off on patient hospitalization past the point of patient safety. Physicians in a fee-for-service practice may turn a treatment or a procedure that can be accomplished in one visit into several, at risk and difficulty to the patient. Currently, with the emphasis on "managed care" ("Employers Test," 1988), the threat may be more in the other direction. Physicians who have promised an insurer or employer that they will deliver care at a set price per month per patient may simply not deliver care. This can be accomplished in a variety of ways. A physician can make the wait for an appointment so long that the patient will become discouraged or frightened and go elsewhere, paying the money out of pocket. Or the physician (or other professional) can minimize the difficulty a patient is having. Or the patient can be given a visit that is so short that nothing of much benefit can be discovered about or done for the patient.

Clearly, if an institution or a single health care professional does not survive professionally, no care at all can be given. This is almost always the reason given when care becomes shoddy or dangerous. The reasoning is that some care is better than no care at all. This is true to a point. At some point, however, the integrity of the institution or individual is so compromised that the care given is worse than no care because it prevents the patient from using an alternative source or even understanding that an alternative is available. This may be at the heart of the ethical dilemma for health care as both an industry and a profession in the immediate future. There is no fixed point at which any ethicist or, any person can say that the balance has tipped irretrievably. But it can and has, as in some notable scandals, and the danger must be taken seriously.

The Two-Tier System of Health Care

The two-tier system of health care refers to the lower classes receiving a lesser level of care than do the middle and upper classes. It also refers to the poor being treated in physically different settings than those for the well-to-do. The poor are treated in public hospitals and to a large extent in wardlike settings of private hospitals, whereas the well-to-do are treated in private hospitals, in more pleasant, small-room settings. The more serious problem is seen as the first one because the lower classes are treated by less-experienced staff in overcrowded and generally understaffed settings. Though a substantial number of poor people have had health insurance (i.e., Medicaid) since 1965, this has not substantially changed the situation. In part, this is because Medicaid is, of all insurance plans, the one that reimburses the most poorly, so hospitals and physicians claim that they cannot afford to treat these patients or to treat them as well as patients with better forms of insurance. But in part the phenomenon seems to be the result of the social stigma of poverty, racism, and the lesser amount of political power of the poor.

In a real sense, the two-tier system is almost a passé issue. What is evolving now is a multitier system, as different types of HMOs, preferred provider organizations, and employer self-insured managed-care plans, press workers into a variety of benefit programs with limited coverage. A middle-class patient may present with insurance that either does not cover his or her illness or covers it insufficiently. Because even many middle-class people cannot pay the cost of a serious illness, the institution or physician judges this type of patient to be a poor financial risk, and some tend to act in ways that are not to the medical benefit of the patient. They may refuse care, attempt to transfer the patient, or skimp on care, following the financial incentives. This sort of problem was traditional for the poor in the old two-tier system. What is new is the beginning of its extension to the working middle classes.

The ethical dimensions of this phenomenon are clear. The ethical issue is justice, or less dramatically put, the just and fair allocation of health resources in terms of manpower, technology, and access. The allocation has been traditionally made on the random factor of class and race. The injustice will be further deepened by the multilevel system now going into place, driven by the pressures of cost containment. Some philosophers from the egalitarian school have advocated a theoretical "veil of ignorance," behind which no one would know his or her advantages or disadvantages, as a means of combating the injustices of this system (Rawls, 1971). Others, from the libertarian school, have accepted the system as "unfortunate but not unfair" and part of the price for preserving our pluralistic society (Engelhardt, 1984).

Within the health care professions, there has been a longstanding tendency to decry the problem, but there has also been a lack of sustained effort to change the system. Within ethical circles, with the major exception of the libertarian stance noted above, the same tendency to deplore the system has consistently appeared. There have been a number of proposals to change the system, ranging from a national health service to a free-market competitive system where all would be given "vouchers" to purchase the best health care they can find. But as noted, the system has remained and is expanding to the middle class.

Major Topics in Health Care Ethics

To this point, we have discussed general ethical principles as they apply specifically to health care. But the field of bioethics has spawned a number of topics that are intrinsic to health and that have become key in understanding and appropriating the body of knowledge in the field. What follows will be a summary of such issues, including how they relate to the larger ethical principles discussed above.

Informed Consent

This is currently seen as the most central issue in bioethics. It rests on the general principle of individual autonomy and means that, with a patient who has some capacity to understand the information being given, no treatment, procedure, or medication can be given or done without the consent of the patient. Moreover, such consent must be in writing, or if the patient is not capable of that, such consent must be fully documented in the patient's medical record.

These statements may appear self-evident to a reader in the 1990s. Twenty years ago they were hardly thought of and almost never put into practice. Patients were sometimes told what would happen to them and that the procedure was based on sound medical judgment, and there the matter generally ended (see "Professional Beneficence" above). That this state of affairs should have existed is particularly unsettling, as no less a personage than Judge Benjamin Cardozo of the New York Court of Appeals, later to be a justice of the U.S. Supreme Court, had upheld the principle of informed consent in 1914. The decision was *Schloendorff v. Society of New York Hospital* (1914). It read, in part, that

> every human being of adult years and sound mind has a right to determine what shall be done with his own body; and a surgeon who performs an operation without his patient's consent commits an assault, for which he is liable in damages. . . . This is true except in cases of emergency where the patient is unconscious and where it is necessary to operate before consent can be obtained.

The Schloendorff ruling could have been narrowly held to apply to only surgery and surgical procedures. Yet even this was not done. It would be 50 years before the next two major court rulings would clarify the meaning, necessity, and force behind informed consent.

The first, *Cobbs v. Grant* (1972) was a response to the then current practice of defining what constituted informed consent by what everyone else practicing in a particular medical community did, rather than as a universal obligation. *Cobbs v. Grant* said, in part, that the necessity of obtaining informed consent prior to diagnosis and treatment of disease is not governed by "the standard of practice in the community; rather it is the duty imposed by law."

The second, *Canterbury v. Spence* (1972), dealt with standards of disclosure. Again, this had been something of a "standard practice" problem in that physicians and the courts had been using standard practice in a particular community as a sound rule for what could be disclosed. In addition, individual physicians had used as an indicator what *they* thought patients wanted to hear and were emotionally capable of hearing. *Canterbury v. Spence* changed to the ideal of the "reasonable person," who is defined as a composite or ideal of reasonable persons in society. The individual patient is not in question. Rather, the information the patient must be given is what the reasonable person would want to know.

The temper of the times, plus the universal claims of the decisions combined to make them much more acceptable than Justice Cardozo's decision in 1914. The idea of informed consent as a necessity in the clinician/patient or institution/patient relationship began to take hold. The difference between *simple* consent and *informed* consent became both clearer and more inflexible. Simple consent is a state in which patients are told what someone else thinks they can or want to comprehend and what the particular community, which may well be the medical community, believes the patient should know. The patient can then consent or refuse to consent, but refusal carries little weight if there is a good "medical" reason on the other side. Informed consent turns that situation on its head. The patient is *informed* by a clinician telling all a "reasonable" person would want to know, tells it in comprehensible, not obscure, medical language, and tells it out of a universally recognized obligation. Moreover, if a competent patient refuses in a nonemergency situation, that refusal carries over the clinician's wishes.

All this derives from the autonomy principle, though most ethicists would also argue that it derives somewhat from the principle of justice. The mechanics of informed consent require that this content arises from the clinician/patient or institution/patient relationship and presupposes reciprocity. Philosophically, ethically, and legally the person performing the procedure, prescribing the medication, or undertaking the treatment should obtain the consent; it should not be delegated to some lower level of staff. All this should be done in an absence of coercion, such as threats of abandonment, or of undue influence. It should be done in the patient's own language and should be understandable to the patient. This last point is more difficult than it sounds theoretically and practically. On the practical level, clinicians all too easily slip into "medicalese," and patients are often embarrassed to say that they do not understand what was said. On the theoretical level, there are a number of quite depressing studies (Cassileth et al., 1980) that show that the most understandable professionals attempting to give information to their patients in the simplest way, in an effort to obtain consent, are wildly misunderstood by their patients. Many patients, even after being told the contrary several times, stated that they believed that they had to sign the form, and a substantial number said they didn't know or even care what it was that they were signing. This is disconcerting. Nonetheless, the ideal and hope is to communicate the risks, benefits, and alternatives of what is being undertaken.

There are, of course, exceptions to the principle. One has already been discussed. The exceptions are as follows:

1. *Incapacity.* The patient is not capable, mentally, of understanding the conversation. This can be temporary or permanent. Obvious examples are patients who are severely mentally retarded, who arrive or slide into a comatose state, or who are minors (Curran & Beecher, 1969; Ramsey, 1971).

Even here it is essential to note that efforts should be made to communicate with the patient. Adolescent or even preadolescent minor children, for instance, may well be able to comprehend the situation and may have very strong feelings and beliefs about their care. Physicians, lawyers, and ethicists all disagree about what age is appropriate for beginning to involve children in their care, but there are few who would deny minors some say in their treatment.

Further, the mentally retarded or mentally ill may have degrees of capacities to understand their condition and be able to make decisions about much of their care. This section deliberately did not use the word *competence* as a condition that would constitute an exception to informed consent. Competence/incompetence are legal terms, and we are attempting to deal in matters of ethics, not the law. But within incompetency, a patient may still have the *capacity* to make decisions on matters as grave as surgery or chemotherapy for life-threatening conditions. The courts are currently attempting to decide if mentally ill patients can refuse medication that might alleviate their disease or the symptoms of their disease. The ethical community is divided on this question but tends toward allowing participation in decision making on this subject (Dworkin, 1983).

Finally, the patient who arrives in a stupor or becomes comatose may well improve and become lucid. At this point, it is incumbent on the clinician or institution to advise the patient of risks, benefits, and alternatives and to ask for consent, regardless of what may have gone before.

2. *Emergency treatment.* In emergency cases, ethics, the law, physicians, and common sense agree. When a patient presents in an emergency, life-threatening situation, and is not capable at that moment, because of pain or unconsciousness, of giving consent, the clinician may treat in the absence of consent. In fact, major operations may be performed with lack of consent if that is what is needed to save the patients's life. There are some in the communities mentioned above who will go further and say that even if a patient refuses consent after presenting in an emergency, life-threatening situation, the clinician may still treat. They base this on the terror, confusion, and misapprehension that often attend suddenly being about to die.

Where one stands on consent within the context of a life-threatening emergency depends in part on how strongly one believes in the autonomy principle and how strongly one believes in the beneficence principle. Beyond this, it is still somewhat subjective. If a patient is clearly so terrified of illness and death that communication is impossible, it may be ethically permissible to treat. However, if there is time, strong attempts should be made to communicate. The point in all of this is that if the clinician hesitates until the situation clarifies and the patient is able to give consent, it may well be too late to save the life of the patient. There are times when a minute's hesitation has the potential to be fatal. This exception is meant to deal with that situation.

3. *Waiver*. This exception is meant to apply to those patients who refuse to make a choice about the type of care they want or whether they want care at all. Colloquially put, this is the patient who says, "Whatever you say is fine, Doc." There are a number of reasons patients do this; among them are fear, denial, lifelong training to regard physicians as omniscient, indecision, and so on. If a patient indicates inaction along these lines, the patient's delegation of authority or waiver should be carefully documented in the patient's medical record. After recovery, some patients may deny that this was ever their stance.

4. *Therapeutic privilege*. This exception means that in the judgment of the clinician the patient is too sick to be able to hear the diagnosis, prognosis, risks, and so on. It generally also means that in the judgment of the clinician the patient's condition will worsen if such is discussed with the patient. This position is increasingly frowned upon by ethicists as a means of bringing the discredited professional beneficence doctrine back in the door.

A variation of it has, however, been brought back via the 1988 New York State Do Not Resuscitate law (State of New York Public Health Law, 1988). This law allows a physician to write a Do Not Resuscitate (DNR) order if "the attending physician determines that, to a reasonable degree of medical certainty, the adult with capacity would suffer immediate and severe injury from a discussion of CPR [cardiopulmonary resuscitation]." The attending physician may then write a DNR order after getting a concurring opinion from a second physician and also ascertaining the patient's wishes to the extent possible without having the discussion. Presumably, this is to be done by discussion with family and review of the patient's life-style for clues for beliefs on the issue of resuscitation. Again presumably, the physician objectively weighs the benefits and burdens to the patient, this last, of course, not being the patient's wishes but the physician's best thinking on the subject. The problems that arise by ascertaining the patient's wishes without discussion become enormous when there is no family to consult or a divided family, or when the patient is new to the physician and previous life-style is unclear or unknown. Then the physician can only rely on objective benefits and burdens, which have nothing to do with patient beliefs or wishes. It is this kind of situation that makes the use of therapeutic privilege such a dubious tool, at least for ethicists.

There are some rare cases in which the patient cannot bear to have any discussion or even hear the name of the disease he or she has. It was for these circumstances that the concept of therapeutic privilege was brought forth. However, most patients are generally glad to have someone finally tell them what is going on. They may be sad, grieving, or even distraught, but they are somewhat back in control and can plan for how they want to lead the lives that are left to them.

DNR Orders

The discussion above leads us to the topic of cardiopulmonary resuscitation (CPR) and ethical concerns about its use. Simply put, CPR is the welter of mechanical interventions that physicians, nurses, and technical medical personnel initiate when a patient's heart stops beating. This is probably the best-known and most-debated technology in public discussion.

There has been a medical tendency to automatically resuscitate a patient when his or her heart stops, regardless of the condition of that patient. The patient may have been in intractable pain and suffering or may have expressed a wish to die, given the miserable quality of life available; or the physician may know that resuscitation may "bring back" (from the dead) the patient in an even worse condition than the patient was in formerly. Yet all medical training has been aimed at the preservation of life, and despite all the above, the patient would be resuscitated or, to use the slang, "coded" (for code blue or code zero, as notifying the relevant staff that a patient's heart has stopped is called in many hospitals).

The public reaction against this practice has been very strong, and a shift has gradually come within the medical profession itself. In recent years, a substantial number of physicians have felt a repugnance at attempting CPR on a patient for whom they have no reasonable expectations. However, even these physicians have been reluctant to write a DNR order, or even communicate such an order to other personnel such as house staff and nurses, for fear of medical malpractice litigation against them. Until quite recently, most states have had neither legislation nor statute that would prevent such physicians from being sued for murder, assisted suicide, or the like. Some physicians in some hospitals have resorted to such methods as erasable blackboards to indicate which patients should not be resuscitated or have used multicolored dots on the patient's medical record for the same purpose. This is not only ludicrous but can lead to mistakes (e.g., the dots fall off). The same mistakes can happen with whispered verbal orders. A house officer going off duty, could inform the next shift that the *wrong* person was not to be resuscitated.

Some other ways around physicians' and nurses' fear of failing to resuscitate have been the "slow code" and the "show code." Since CPR depends on speed, if the code team takes its time getting to the area of a person in cardiac arrest whom nobody wants to resuscitate, the patient may well be past the point of no return by the time the team arrives. A "show code" is quite literally a show put on for the patient's relatives so that they will think that all possible is being done for their loved one, whereas, in reality, nothing of any significance is happening.

As mentioned, public repugnance against this charade, as well as against the actual practice of resuscitating hopelessly ill patients, began to build up in the late 1970s with the Karen Anne Quinlan case, though, in reality, that was a different type of case. However, it brutally served to make the point that technology could "keep alive" those who would prefer not to live in such conditions. It also became known, though more in the medical community than in the community at large, that statistics showed that chances for patients being able to leave the hospital, ever, after receiving CPR were very slim (Bedell & Delbanco, 1984).

It could be said that by the late 1980s, public consensus had switched away from CPR to DNR. This can be measured by the passage of a number of state laws designed to declare someone who is brain-dead legally dead: the California Natural Death Act (1976), the California Durable Power of Attorney Act (1985), the New York State DNR law (despite its peculiarity), and the report of the President's Commission for the Study of Ethical Problems in Medicine and Biomedical and Behavioral Research. These kinds of documents embody what has come to be the conventional wisdom, at least in this area of health care. That is, that the technology to "stop" death far outstrips our capacity to use it rationally and that there are many people who would prefer to die rather than live in states of dependency, pain, and disease. Furthermore, that at least as far as resuscitation is concerned, such people have the right not to be resuscitated and to be allowed to die. Furthermore, that this principle rests firmly on autonomy, privacy, and free will, which are governing principles not simply in medical ethics, or even ethics per se, but in the political system of the country. With the exception of a few groups (e.g., some right-to-life believers, Orthodox Jews, and some Native Americans), this would seem to be the prevailing view of the public, who in this case may be said to have pulled along the medical profession.

Forgoing Life-Sustaining Systems

Just as a discussion of informed consent led us to a discussion of DNR orders, so does a discussion of DNRs lead us to contemplate the use of other life-sustaining technology as an ethical problem. Some of this technology, such as the use of antibiotics to treat infections, goes back more than 40 years. Some is relatively new, such as the use of hyperalimentation or total parenteral nutrition (TPN) to feed patients who can no longer absorb sufficient nutrients to survive. The list of life-sustaining technologies includes, but is not limited to, antibiotics, artificial nutrition and hydration, dialysis, drugs, surgery, cancer chemotherapy, ventilation, the insertion and changing of catheters and other "lines," and transplants. The same questions apply here as in a discussion of DNR orders. Is life itself sacred and to be maintained at all costs as the ultimate good? Or is quality of life to be taken seriously despite its subjective nature? When a certain quality of life can no longer be maintained, which may differ enormously from person to person and from group to group, does the considerable array of current technology *have* to be used to forestall death or perhaps merely prolong the dying process? What indices, if any, can be used for quality of life to universalize these questions, rather than leave them so subjective that practice may vary in hospitals a mile from each other?

One source many students may think of as unlikely has addressed some of these questions. In 1957, the Roman Catholic pope, Pius XII (1958), speaking to a group of anesthesiologists, said that "extraordinary" means do not have to be used to keep alive those who are surely dying. Reiterating and clarifying this in 1980, Pope John Paul II spoke of the "benefits and burdens" of treatment and stated that, when the burdens have outweighed the benefits to the individual patient, treatment is no longer obligatory and may cease. This weighing of benefits and burdens is not only a Catholic mode of ethical thinking but a general ethical method. The change that many modern ethicists might bring to it, though, is that when the patient's condition is extraordinary, all treatment is extraordinary. In such an extreme condition, there is no ordinary treatment.

Consider the case of a patient who has survived a severe heart attack and a stroke and is now in a persistent vegetative state. The patient develops a pneumonia, which could be treated by antibiotics. In the modern world, antibiotics fall under the rubric of ordinary treatment. But the patient has lost all higher brain functions and cannot relate to himself or to others. The point of life, beyond biological life, has arguably been lost. The patient's condition is thus extraordinary, and so the treatment is also extraordinary. The concept of what is "ordinary" changes as the patient's condition changes.

There is not as yet a clear consensus from society in general or from the health care professions as to the issue of the sanctity of life versus the quality of life in cases of forgoing life-sustaining treatment. Most health care ethicists feel strongly that the quality issue is the dominant issue, but even among this group, there are various beliefs as to the definitions of quality. Some feel that it is consciousness or the ability to reason (Fletcher, 1979; Saint Augustine, 1963, 1984). Some believe, as noted above, that quality of life lies in the ability to relate to oneself and to others. Those who believe in God add a third relationship, the ability to relate to God (McCormick, 1974). Some believe that quality is found in the ability to derive some pleasure and happiness from life, by the sick individual's own definition.

There are some in the medical profession and in the public at large who point to the dreadful historical consequences of making decisions on the qualities of lives lived, as happened with the Nazis. These people hold that the sanctity of life is the central point and that to do anything other than maximally preserve life is to make a pact with the devil. The phrase "playing God with people's lives" is often heard in this context. People who hold these beliefs also generally oppose the issuance of DNR orders.

The fallacy in the "playing God with people's lives" argument is that the practice of medicine has always involved rigorous, sometimes brutal interventions in people's lives. From the beginning of the practice of medicine, strong drugs were used to halt disease. Certainly, harsh practices such as "bleeding" the patient and surgery that included amputations were carried out without benefit of anesthesia. These drugs, practices, and procedures often killed the patient. Their purpose, though, was to cure disease and prolong life, and so they were generally accepted. But the usual understanding of "playing God" is direct intervention in people's lives (and in the case of health care, intervention in their disease process), and withholding or withdrawing treatment continues in this same line. It doesn't alter the overall thrust of medicine. It rather acknowledges the limits of technology, which have always been present. Withholding or withdrawing treatment intervenes to end suffering or, allows the illness to claim what it has already claimed, that is, the patient's meaningful life.

There are a fair number of signals that this view is becoming a consensus view in the health care professions and in the larger community as well. Many recent court decisions, in differing states (*Brophy v. New England Sinai Hospital,* 1986; *Delio, v. Westchester County Medical Center,* 1987; *In the Matter of Conroy,* 1985; *In the Matter of Jobes,* 1987), have held that withdrawing life-sustaining treatment is in the best interests of the patient. In all of these cases, the patient has been unable to express his or her own wishes at the time. Still, the courts have found for withdrawing treatment. In the case of a conscious patient who can state wishes and desires, the courts have shown unanimity that such a patient can have a request for cessation of treatment honored, even including a stated wish to die because of deeply distressing circumstances (*Bouvia v. Superior Court,* 1986). In another setting, the American Medical Association's Council on Judicial and Ethical Affairs (AMA, 1986) allowed the cessation of feeding a patient by artificial means, when to do so would simply prolong the dying process. There has been little direct polling on these issues, but those health care organizations that have done so have found a considerable willingness to forgo treatment by their patients when the case is hopeless.

The distinction between withholding and withdrawing treatment is often made by many professionals. Ethically, there is no difference between not starting a treatment and stopping one that has already begun. The principle is whether the treatment will be or has been of benefit or burden to the patient. However, there is a clear emotional difference between not starting a treatment and stopping a treatment. In stopping a treatment, the professional also breaks the emotional bond with the patient, and this is difficult to do. Family members often feel the same way. However, unless one is permitted to stop a treatment, in reality, one could never start a treatment, for fear that it would continue pointlessly after all hope for recovery had been lost.

The other emotional sticking point seems to be around difficulty in not feeding a patient by artificial means. What appears to be at stake here is the symbolic value of eating and drinking in everyday life. A common theme here is "I can't stop feeding the patient because that's a natural part of life." There is also a fear that the patient will suffer hunger and thirst. As to the former complaint, the idea of the natural act, it is again important to remember that it is the patient's condition that matters, not the type of treatment. If the patient is being maintained in a hopeless situation by artificial feeding, that is neither natural nor ordinary. As for the second problem, the fear of hunger and thirst, if the patient shows any sign of either, the patient should be fed and hydrated (with consent, of course). However, patients in a persistent vegetative state or permanent loss of consciousness do not experience these sensations. For the sake of patient dignity, and also for the feelings of family and staff, the patient's mouth can be kept moistened after artificial hydration has been withdrawn.

This is a lengthy topic, and this section has only touched on some major issues. Many institutions have worked out elaborate protocols for different levels of care for different types of patients (e.g., general nursing care for those in a persistent vegetative state). Readers are referred to Wanzer et al. (1984) and Meisel et al. (1986) for further exploration of this subject.

Multiply Handicapped Newborns

Once again, the previous discussion leads to an extension of an ethical question. The question is when, if ever, should a child born with multiple anomalies be allowed to die, rather than being treated. Although the issue contains many of the same ethical points as in the discussion of forgoing life-sustaining treatment for adults, it differs in the following ways. One, the infant can never express wishes, and the decision makers cannot be guided by previous wishes. Two, the infant is at the beginning of life and has had no experience of life. It is emotionally more difficult to terminate life in such circumstances. Three, diagnosis and prognosis are often less clear than with adult patients, and this creates a hesitation to make any irrevocable moves. Four, the tests of quality for an adult, whether they be rationality or ability to relate, simply do not apply. Perhaps the only tests of quality that can apply are estimates of the potential for consciousness and relationship and, more surely, whether the infant appears to be enjoying or finding pleasure in babyhood.

The questions came to the fore with some highly publicized cases in the early 1980s. In the first, a child with Down's syndrome and an esophageal fistula was not treated for the fistula, which is easily corrected by surgery. His parents made the decision not to treat on the basis of his Down's syndrome, and the obstetrician concurred. The local district attorney sued, but the child died before the case could be heard. This case, the Baby Doe case, created a sensation, and the federal government responded with regulations that demanded the aggressive treatment of *every* infant born, regardless of handicap. The government created severe penalties for noncompliance, and a new federal office, nicknamed the

"Baby Doe squad," was staffed around the clock to monitor such cases and receive complaints. The American Academy of Pediatrics and later the American Medical Association successfully sued in federal court to rescind these regulations. Less stringent regulations are presently in effect that attempt to leave the bulk of the decision making with the parents and attending physician (Public Law 98-457, 1984).

While the double suit was continuing, the second of the well-publicized cases arose. This was a spina bifida infant with hydroencephaly, whose parents, in consultation with physicians and clergy, decided against proposed treatment for the condition. A local right-to-life lawyer sued on behalf of the child (University Hospital, 1984). The federal government then intervened, though unsuccessfully. The Supreme Court ruled against the government on the narrow ground of medical record confidentiality, leaving open the larger question of what parties may make what kinds of decisions for minor children and infants (Otis Bowen v. AHA, 1986). The case, named the Baby Jane Doe case, ended somewhat inconclusively. The parents eventually allowed some treatment, and the child surprisingly, spontaneously made some improvement. Baby Jane Doe eventually left the hospital to live with her parents.

The only area of consensus within the issues involving treatment of newborns with multiple anomalies is possibly that of anencephalic infants. That there are no documented survivors for this condition and that the infants normally die within a few days to a month has led to an understanding that anencephalic infants will not be placed on respirators. Yet even this virtual unanimity has been displaced by a new issue. Brain tissue of anencephalic infants can be transplanted into adult patients ill with Parkinson's disease. One consequence is a policy of placing the infants on respirators until their tissue can be used. Another consequence is that mothers who are diagnosed as carrying such infants in utero are choosing to carry such children to term to "redeem" their pregnancy. Another issue involving anencephalic infants is similar: the use of their organs for transplantation into otherwise viable infants. The ethical question is to what degree, if any, may anencephalic infants be used as organ donors if there is no benefit to them in being kept alive until transplant is possible. There is little agreement here. The traditional touchstone, suggested by Paul Ramsey (1971), has been that all research and treatment of a child must benefit that child. In the face of this traditional claim, the problem of anencephalic infants as donors to adults or children remains an ethical conundrum.

The issues involved in the cases of infants born with multiple anomalies have proved so difficult ethically and emotionally that at the present time most are being decided on a case-by-case basis. There is no agreement on who, among the various parties (parents, physicians, the state, the infant, the adult *in potentia*), should make the decisions and no agreement on what method the parties should use for their decision making. There is little agreement on how long to wait before questions on diagnosis and prognosis become clear, except for a tentative accord to immediately resuscitate infants born without the ability to breathe on their own, until consultation with parents can take place. There is some belief that Down's syndrome and other indications of mental retardation are in themselves insufficient reason not to treat. However, that perception is somewhat mitigated by the abortion issue (see below). The reader who wishes to pursue these issues further should refer to articles by Shaw (1973), Duff and Campbell (1973), and Lantos (1987).

Perhaps the most difficult and exciting issue is that the threshold of what defines a salvageable infant is constantly being thrust backward. A child with a birth weight of 750 grams or even lower is now considered a salvageable child, as is with great effort, an infant born at 20 weeks. Given that the technology is changing and improving at almost miraculous speed, the challenge is to arrive at an ethic that can rationalize care. The principle of benefit and burden is applicable in this area, but understanding what is technologically possible for various diseases, birth weights, and gestational ages and understanding long-term prognoses will be key before further progress can be made ("Imperiled Newborns," 1987).

One useful addition may be the infant care review committees that the revised federal regulation suggested and that 80% of American hospitals have now established. These are, in effect, ethics committees for decisions on infants, and it is hoped that they will contain a broad spectrum of views and varying types of members. The committees mainly review issues on a case-by-case basis, but the combined experience of these committees may provide a framework for deciding the pressing moral issues on a policy basis.

Abortion

The question of legalization of abortion was to a degree settled legally by the Supreme Court decision in *Roe v. Wade* in 1973. The decision, in brief, held that abortion was solely in the province of the mother-to-be for the first trimester and was a matter for consultation between the mother-to-be and her physician until the end of the second trimester. Abortion was not permitted through the third trimester, on the usual grounds of the interest of the state in the preservation of life and with the usual exceptions, such as abortion to save the life of the mother. The clinical ground on which the Court made its decision was viability, that is, whether the child could survive outside the body of the mother at a given point. In 1973, 6 months was not an unreasonable time to set for viability. The moral and legal reasoning was based on the doctrine of privacy in this case, that the decision of the woman on what to do with her body was a question of her privacy. A number of ethicists believe that autonomy would have been a stronger moral reason than privacy, which has traditionally fallen in many areas when challenged by the rights of others.

The question of viability has been sharply altered, as seen in the previous discussion on salvageable infants. As mentioned, it is now possible, with enormous effort and great expenditure, to salvage infants at 20 weeks, which is four weeks before "viability" in *Roe v. Wade*. The development of fetal surgery, which allows the correction of some congenital defects in utero, also challenges the point of viability, as these procedures may allow for the possibility of a healthy infant at an age when abortion is still legally permissible. Finally, the developing doctrine of *fetal rights*, a prolonged discussion of which is beyond the scope of this chapter, has raised difficult questions of what rights the fetus may have in utero (Murray, 1987; Robertson & Schulman, 1987). Some examples of this doctrine are the right to a mother who refrains from or alters unhealthy behavior or even the right to be born if the mother has declared her intention of bringing the child to term. All of these developments since 1973 have called into question, for some, the very basis of the thinking in *Roe v. Wade*. Strong proponents of the theory that a women has the sole right to control what is in her body largely remain highly supportive of *Roe v. Wade*.

It is important to remember, however, that although the Supreme Court decision settled the legal questions on abortion, the political and ethical questions were not settled. Those who opposed the decision, for religious and other reasons, opposed it from the date it was issued. They have continued to oppose the decision legally, with legislative campaigns to overturn it by Constitutional amendment, by marches, petitions, and publicity, and they have opposed it by illegal means, such as the bombing of abortion clinics. This is certainly not meant to link all of the opponents of legalized abortion together in one camp, including those who use violent means. Rather, it is to reinforce how strongly this decision was opposed by large segments of the population, even at the moment when the Court's definition of viability made medical sense. Many of those who oppose legalized abortion see the procedure as legalized murder. They believe this because they believe that an embryo becomes human at the moment of conception or perhaps at the moment of individuation. Some will extend this to the moment of "quickening" or the fetus's first movements in the uterus. But to its opponents, abortion is the taking of human life.

To its proponents, the issue is intrinsic to women's rights. They point to the long and bloody history of illegal abortion, in which many women who felt unable to bring a child to term died in unsanitary and brutal procedures. They point out that many more suffered irreparable harm to their health from such procedures. They believe that this situation was allowed to continue because the value of women was historically low and because it allowed men to control the reproductive process. For these advocates, abortion is central to women's gaining control of the reproductive process and, with it, taking control of their own lives from male rule. They go further, to point out that our society continues to value neither women nor children, in their view, as shown by the lack of support for universal child health care and lack of focus on the particular needs of children in the society. For this view (Harrison, 1983), the antiabortion position is a sham, as it is not children's lives that are at stake but rather power in the society.

Obviously, such diametrically opposed views have had difficulty finding any meeting ground or, in the ethical parlance we have used, any balance. Each side has won some political victories. The antiabortion people won a Supreme Court ruling that Medicaid funds could not be used to pay for abortions, but many states have funded abortions for poor women from their tax funds. The proabortion forces have fought back several strong challenges to the overall ruling in the legislature.

As there is no moral consensus within the nation on when life begins or on what the meaning of that life is in utero, so there can yet be no consensus on abortion as an ethical and political problem. There is no clearer case in health care of how personal morality affects health care decisions. One's perceptions and beliefs on the very meaning of life and on the place of women and children in the society have determined and will continue to determine how this issue is handled by American society. There will undoubtedly be further Supreme Court decisions changing and/or clarifying *Roe v. Wade,* beyond the 1989 *Webster v. Missouri Reproductive Health Services* which allowed states to ban abortions by public employees in public institutions. Several are on the docket as of this writing. (See also Noonan, 1970; Thomson, 1971; Warren, 1973.)

Confidentiality

The ideal of confidentiality is one that is deeply held in the practice of medicine. Once again, this is a precept that is found in the Hippocratic oath: "Whatever things I see or hear concerning the life of men, in my attendance on the sick or even apart therefrom, which ought not to be noised abroad, I will keep silence thereon, counting such things to be as sacred secrets." An influential volume published at the beginning of the 19th century, Thomas Percival's *Medical Ethics* (1927), orders that "professional visits should be used with discretion and with the most scrupulous regard to fidelity and honour." The American Medical Association (1980) stated that "a physician shall safeguard patient confidences within the constraints of the law." The American College of Physicians (1984) goes further, saying that a physician may break the law to protect a patient if the physician is prepared to accept the consequences of such behavior.

The ethics on which all of this rests are again autonomy, privacy, and the protection of the individual. Interestingly, there is another ethic at work in protecting confidentiality, and that is utilitarian. The thinking here is that if patients cease to trust their physicians, they will not go for treatment, and that society as a whole would be harmed by such behavior (e.g., outbreaks of epidemics, untreated mental illness).

Clearly, all health care professionals, by the nature of their work, hear and see things that patients do not wish known (eg., sexually transmitted diseases, genetic chronic diseases). Until fairly recently, the standard of confidentiality has remained strong in the health care community, though tested by such problems as teenage drug use. (For example, does the treating pediatrician tell the parents of a teenager's drug use, over the patient's objections?) But the question began to become more pointed over the use of confidentiality in the case of mentally ill, violence-prone patients and has now become a national debate with the rise of the AIDS epidemic.

The issue of confidentiality regarding violent, mentally ill patients came to a turning point with the Tarasoff case, (*Tarasoff v. Regents of the University of California,* 1976). Prosenjit Poddar killed Tatiana Tarasoff on October 27, 1969. They were both students at the University of California at Berkeley, and Mr. Poddar had been seeing a campus psychologist over the issue of his unrequited love for Miss Tarasoff. After 9 or 10 sessions, Mr. Poddar confided that he had purchased a gun and intended to use it against a woman who could be readily identified as Miss Tarasoff. The psychologist, Dr. Moore, asked the campus police to detain Mr. Poddar, which they did. They found him rational and warned him to stay away from Miss Tarasoff. Dr. Moore consulted with his superior, Dr. Powelson, Director of the department of psychiatry, who ordered that all records of the case be destroyed and that Poddar *not* be placed in a treatment and evaluation facility. Mr. Poddar then killed Miss Tarasoff, after ingratiating himself with her brother in order to find out when she was returning from a summer vacation.

Miss Tarasoff's parents sued Dr. Moore, Dr. Powelson, and the Regents of the University of California, who were ultimately responsible for all services at the university. Their belief was that they and Miss Tarasoff's brother, as the people most directly concerned with Miss Tarasoff's welfare, should have been warned. In a hotly disputed and narrowly split decision, they won their case. In a sentence that became famous among ethicists and psychiatrists, the majority opinion held that "the protective privilege ends where the public peril begins." The opinion stated that the therapist "owes a legal duty not only to his patient, but also to his patient's would-be victim" and that "professional inaccuracy in predicting violence cannot negate the therapist's duty to protect the threatened victim." The majority did not state, however, whom they felt should have been warned by Dr. Moore or Dr. Powelson. The dissenting opinion held that the majority opinion would destroy the practice of psychiatry because without strict confidentiality those needing assistance would be deterred from seeking it; further, that patients who are in treatment would no longer confide in their therapists should it become known that their thoughts might be told to others. The minority held that the majority had not only invaded individual rights but also had increased the possibility of increased violence due to patient reluctance to fantasize and of unnecessary civil commitment as the likely alternative when a third party is warned of impending danger.

The Tarasoff decision has been used by both sides in the dispute over whether to warn the sexual or drug-using contacts of patients who test positive for the human immunodeficiency virus HIV, the AIDS virus that they are in danger of contracting the virus from their contacts. Most HIV-positive patients are cooperative in warning contacts whom they know. Some, however, refuse to do so, putting these contacts at great risk. The sentence from *Tarasoff*, "The protective privilege ends where the public peril begins," is often used by advocates of breaking confidentiality to warn contacts over the objections of the patient. These advocates argue that the public peril is clear and that the contacts are at risk of their lives. Moreover, unknowing individuals may spread disease to others. Whereas if they knew of their danger, they might take protective measures or abstain from sex or drugs. Thus, keeping silent, they argue, means an intolerable risk to the whole of society by means of a fatal illness for which there is no cure. These people are making an essentially utilitarian argument from "the greatest good for the greatest number." Those who favor keeping confidentiality in all circumstances take issue as to whether the utilitarians are correct in their premises, much less their ethics. Echoing the minority opinion in *Tarasoff*, they claim that if those who are HIV-positive know that their physicians will inform their contacts, the patients will go underground and never receive either counseling or treatment. Thus, the epidemic will spread more rapidly. This premise remains unproved. It is interesting to note that with regard to *Tarasoff*, a study published 10 years after the final decision found that there had been no diminution of the practice of psychiatry as a result of the decision (Mills, Sullivan, & Eth, 1987). However, the very real cases of discrimination against HIV-positive people, wherein they have lost jobs, homes, and insurance because of their health status, gives credence to the possibility of such people hiding their status from the health care system.

The other argument that advocates of absolute confidentiality make also mirrors that of the minority *Tarasoff* opinion; that is, that privacy is a right, based on individual autonomy (Bok, 1983). Therefore, no one, including health care professionals, has the right to violate it. This is harking back to deontology as an ethical touchstone.

Given that the medical profession is actively debating these issues and that several state legislatures have also become involved, it is likely that there will soon be both a societal and professional consensus on this issue. The most basic part of it appears to be taking shape as the right (not the obligation) to warn *known* others if their contacts refuse to do so. New York State is among several states that has passed legislation that would free physicians from liability should they warn known contacts. However, there is no officially sanctioned move afoot as yet to attempt to track down fleeting or anonymous contacts and warn them of danger. This has been the standard means of treating sexually transmitted diseases in the United States in the 20th century, so it would not be surprising if the position taken eventually includes this traditional public health function as well. As the epidemic progresses, it will put confidentiality, among many other principles, under severe strain.

Allocation of Scarce Resources

The problem of the allocation of scarce resources is a new topic in American health care. The problem itself is not new, as resources are by definition finite. But the topic itself has not been under discussion in American health care for two reasons. The first reason is that Americans have historically rationed health care by level of socioeconomic status (see "The Two-Tier System of Health Care" above). The second reason is that, other than using income as a measure, the United States has not rationed or even allocated care by planning. Attempts such as the Health Services Agencies (HSAs) of the 1970s have failed for a variety of reasons beyond the scope of this chapter. (The HSAs were health planning agencies established by Congress to coordinate health care within states, cities, and localities.) When faced with a rationing or allocation problem beyond income, the American health care system has expanded. This has been possible because the overall economy has been expanding, because the public wanted increased access and technology, and because various interested groups mobilized successfully to continue the expansion (e.g., those in need of renal dialysis).

As noted previously, in the 1980s the situation changed. The economy found itself under pressure from other countries, such as West Germany and Japan, whose prices were more competitive than American prices. American business claims that, at least in part, this is because of the huge costs of health care benefits to workers, dependents, and retirees. Therefore, American business began strong efforts to contract their portion of the health care budget. In addition, the federal government claimed, at the beginning of the 1980s, that the Medicare trust fund would soon be depleted (Office of the Actuary, 1984), and in response, the government also began efforts to contract the costs of their share of the health care budget. The insurance industry claimed that it was experiencing heavy losses from the health care section of its business and also began contraction. Resource allocation thus began to appear as a debatable topic, under the pressure of all these cost-containment efforts, along with the specific fear that quality of care would suffer as funds diminished.

Moreover, health care inflation continued to be at least double that of the general inflation rate throughout the 1980s. And the proportion of the gross national product that is consumed by health care services went to over 11% by the end of 1988, compared with around 6.5% 11 years previously. Though a variety of polls indicate that the American people are willing to pay that and more for optimal health care for themselves and their neighbors, the triad of business, insurance industry, and federal government views these numbers with alarm and dismay.

The debate on allocation of resources has also been heightened by the advent of managed care, itself partly an outgrowth of cost-containment efforts. In HMOs, and to a lesser extent in preferred provider organizations, the budget is fixed, generally on a yearly basis. Therefore, expensive treatments for a few patients or for a group of patients with a particular disease can mean that the organization may have to cut back on routine care for the remainder of its members/patients. Setting aside the problem of financial incentives for undertreatment, with which some charge the managed care organizations, expensive, repeated treatments raise serious questions of resource allocation. This is a new problem for the American health care system, accustomed as it is to third-party billing in a fee-for-service setting and the consequent lack of a fixed budget (Levinson, 1987; Reagan, 1987).

Finally, the finitude of resources has been dramatically demonstrated by the questions inherent in organ transplantation, as noted in the "Societal Risk and Benefit" section. The principle of justice has been the dominant ethical theme in considerations of organ transplantation, both in questions of who gets the transplanted organs and what proportion of the national health care dollar will go to support these services. But the consideration of justice is, in fact, the principal theme in the allocation of resources, tempered by compassion. Now that the allocation problem is moving into the open, it will be a sure test of a democratic society to determine how ethics can affect the political and economic processes of resource allocation.

Equity of Access

Any discussion of allocation of resources is based on the idea of equity of access. Without access to the health care system, it is not possible to receive care at all. Equity of access can be defined as all people having the right and ability to receive similar treatment for similar conditions. Some moral limitations on access are arguable—that is, the distinction between "basic" medical needs and "felt" medical needs. An example of a basic medical need could be asthma control programs for children. An example of a felt medical need could be cosmetic surgery (e.g., face-lifting). The distinction between basic needs and felt needs, however, is often more difficult to make. There are those, for instance, who believe that treatment for infertility is a basic medical need. There are those who believe it is only a felt medical need. There are those who believe that it is not a problem for health care, but rather a societal problem of the imbalance between infertile couples and children already available for adoption, or a problem of narcissism. When definition of need itself is controversial, it is more difficult to define equity of access. However, there are broad categories of need, such as primary, emergency, and critical care, that most ethicists agree demand equity of access.

There are any number of impediments to equity at present. Income problems have been discussed, as have the cost-containment efforts that have deepened the problems of socioeconomic status. The two-tier and now the multi-tier health care system have been explored, and this is one of the bases of inequity. But there are other barriers as well. Approximately 38 million Americans are estimated to have no health care insurance of any type. Estimates on the number of other Americans with drastically inadequate health care range from 18 million to 40 million. Though public facilities funded by tax monies are available to these people, the facilities are overcrowded and understaffed. A small number of underinsured people find their way into private hospitals, but decreasingly, as cost pressures cause "dumping" of such patients into the public facilities.

Another barrier is geographic. People in rural areas may be truly isolated from any facilities or physicians, when these areas are financially unattractive places in which to practice. People in urban slums may have difficulty in achieving access for the same reasons; that is, many hospitals and physicians find that they cannot stay in business in such areas and depart for more financially rewarding locations.

In addition, in what is overall a complex organized system but for the individual is often a fragmented, confusing system, it is difficult for patients to find out what kind of care they need and then locate that care. In an era of medical specialization, the lack of primary care may itself be a barrier to access. The information necessary to understand how to use the system is most easily possessed by those within the system. The individual patient, without the guide of a primary care practitioner, may be unable to reach care, even if insured.

Equity of access is a key ethical problem, as it is almost impossible to discuss fair distribution, or indeed any distribution, without it (President's Commission, 1983).

AIDS

The AIDS epidemic contains almost all current dilemmas in ethics within it. These, as will be detailed below, include such matters as confidentiality, resource allocation, and physician responsibility to patients. The epidemic can be seen ethically in the words of Albert Camus, writing in *The Plague,* as coming for the "bane and enlightenment of men," the possible enlightenment being the focus the epidemic beings to vital moral questions.

AIDS is an infectious disease caused by a retrovirus that is capable of replicating in the body and causing the destruction of the body's immune system. Thus, the individual becomes prey to opportunistic infections that the body could otherwise protect itself against. The AIDS virus (HIV) is effectively transmitted by sexual contact between men, from men to women, and, somewhat less effectively, from women to men. Transmission is also blood-borne, thus putting those who share syringes for intravenous drug use at risk. It also leaves at risk those who have been transfused with large amounts of blood, such as hemophiliacs, though since 1985 the blood banks have effectively cleaned their supplies from the HIV virus. Perinatal transmission is also possible, from infected mothers to their infants in utero, during parturition, or during postpartum breast-feeding. Infection is also possible from accidental injuries, such as needle-sticks to health care workers during the course of caring for an HIV-positive patient. Such cases have been few, however. There is reason to believe that a single inoculation of HIV is unlikely to transmit the virus, though recent evidence from the Fourth and Fifth International Conferences on AIDS leaves that less clear than previously. It is still believed that the most effective means of AIDS transmission is receptive anal intercourse with multiple partners.

AIDS is a fatal disease for which there is neither cure nor vaccine. The pandemic contains most of the issues of health care ethics within it. The discussion of confidentiality touched on one such issue. The issue of mandatory versus voluntary screening for the HIV virus is a spin-off from that issue, though there is more involved than simply confidentiality. The issue, so far unresolved, is whether to institute a mandatory testing program for groups at high risk, such as homosexuals, bisexuals, and intravenous drug abusers, for groups society may especially want to protect, such as expectant mothers, or for the entire society.

Those in favor of mandatory testing on any of the above levels give many reasons for their advocacy. They state the value of tracking the disease epidemiologically. They claim it will alert health care workers to take extra precautions to guard against risk of infection. They claim it will give either the government or various other institutions the opportunity to offer help to these individuals. They say it will alert those who unsuspectingly have the virus to change behavior patterns in ways that can protect others.

Those who oppose mandatory testing, particularly at the broad level of the whole of society, raise strong civil liberties objections to the concept. They point out that there are few guarantees in most states against discrimination against HIV-positive people and that individuals who test positively can easily be subject to punitive action. Some take that thought a step further, fearing the HIV-positive people would be quarantined or subject to criminal sanctions for transmission of the disease. They emphasize that so far the disease has affected those people already at the margins of society, such as homosexuals, bisexuals, and illegal drug users, and that the concerns and protection of marginal peoples are historically quickly discarded. They also state that such a program will cost enormous amounts of money, yielding little in the way of hard results and a great deal in the way of false positives. The lack of hard results would come about because the homosexual and bisexual communities largely already assume infection and have moved to take precautions, as evidenced by the falling rates of other sexually transmitted diseases in these groups. The false positives are a problem because such incorrect knowledge could harm or destroy a person's life, before the misinformation was corrected.

Those opposed to mandatory testing often oppose it for particular groups as well, such as expectant mothers and patients about to undergo surgery. As to the former, once again, they believe testing to be a violation of individual autonomy and privacy and a dangerous invitation for future invasions. As to hospitalized patients awaiting surgery, they cite the Centers for Disease Control (CDC) standards, which are, in essence, that every patient be treated as an AIDS patient so that full precautions are taken on every patient (Bayer et al., 1986).

Other ethical issues that have been discussed in other contexts above are the use of life-prolonging technologies and the allocation of resources. The question of the use of life-prolonging technologies for an invariably fatal and degenerative disease adds even more tension to the problem than it normally generates. There are a considerable number of AIDS patients who refuse technologies, such as respirators, from virtually the onset of the disease. This may produce tension with medical staff who believe that the patient could have months or even years of meaningful life if the patient accepted technological help. On the other hand, there are patients who will request major interventions when all hope is gone and there can be no clinical benefit from the intervention. Many health care professionals find it difficult to deny such interventions, however, to young patients, the very sort of patient for whom they historically have used the most aggressive treatments. Another issue along these lines is the use of experimental and/or very expensive drugs for AIDS patients or for patients who are HIV-positive. Patients will often request these drugs before there is approval from the Food and Drug Administration and/or reason to believe that patients will benefit from the drugs. There is thus resistance to ordering such drugs, yet patients will demand them as a last chance at life, however unrealistic this seems.

The ethical and emotional issues can become confused in this situation. At least one ethical issue involved here is the allocation of resources, and there are a welter of emotions regarding HIV-positive patients that complicate the allocation issue. For instance, there are many in society who believe that the life-style choices of homosexuals and illegal drug abusers have brought the punishment of AIDS upon its victims. Whether this is divinely inspired wrath or a secular settling of scores, such people would not choose to allocate much in the way of treatment for AIDS patients. Yet on the other side, there are also many in society who feel that AIDS is a horrendous additional burden for those already carrying the onus of bigotry and that considerable resources should be apportioned to the afflicted. This problem will deepen in the years to come, as the epidemic increases and the dollar amounts to pay for care increase as well.

Another ethical problem is the response of the health care community to the risk inherent in caring for AIDS patients. Presently, there are over 1,000 health care workers who have accidentally exposed themselves to HIV from needlestick injuries, blood splashes, contact through open skin lesions, and the like. They are being followed by the CDC, and to date only about 18 have become HIV-positive. Yet there is considerable fear and resentment in the medical community and, from a very small number of professionals, a refusal to treat AIDS patients.

There has been an extensive discussion of this question, and there is a clear professional consensus that the duty to treat must overcome all hesitation caused by fear of infection. This stand has been embraced by the American Medical Association, the American College of Physicians, and the American Hospital Association, among others. All have pointed to the long-standing tradition in medicine of caring for the sick at great personal risk. Many have also pointed out that freedom from risk of infection is a very new development in the history of medicine and that professionals were routinely at risk until the development of antibiotics, which is as recent as the 1940s (Pellegrino, 1987; Zuger & Miles, 1987).

This certainly does not exhaust the list of ethical problems that the AIDS epidemic has brought about. There is, for instance, the question of what role the health care professions should take to protect their patients when society has not provided such protections (e.g., antidiscrimination laws). There is the problem of finding some means of dealing with those, such as prostitutes, who have a better than average chance of being HIV-positive and who continue to practice their trade, as well as what to do with those who patronize them. For those interested in this area, there are a number of works on the AIDS epidemic dealing with the study of the ethical problems involved ("AIDS," 1988; Gostin & Curran, 1986; Macklin, 1986; Osborn, 1988; Steinbock, 1986; Steinbrook et al., 1986). "AIDS. The Responsibilities of Health Professionals: A Special Supplement," Hastings Center Report, 1988).

Ethics of Managers in Health Care

The health care administrator has been gaining power steadily through the last few decades, for reasons made clear in other chapters. This has been particularly true during the 1980s as a result of funding changes, the physician surplus, and the determination of government, business, and the insurance industry to cut health costs, (making the administrator the point man in the effort). The balance of power has shifted dramatically from the physician to the manager and will continue to do so in the foreseeable future. This shift also entails a change in outlook. Clinicians tend toward an individualistic ethic, centered on the patient they are caring for at that moment. Managers tend to look at the institution's needs as a whole, by both training and inclination (Seiden, 1982, 1985).

Managers were perhaps not well prepared for the power they would have thrust upon them or would assume, and they have certainly not been prepared for the ethical responsibilities that power entails. As has been pointed out in this chapter, physicians have a tradition of ethics that extends back at least 2,500 years. Managers have been trained to think of budgets, staffing, reimbursements and development with a conspicuous lack of moral tradition to center these activities. This is a considerable problem, as power without morality inevitably degenerates into abuse.

Managerial training programs infrequently include training in ethics. A reversal of this in the undergraduate and graduate schools seems an obvious place to begin educating managers-to-be to the moral implications of their work. But that strategy leaves unchanged the current generation of working managers, and that is an unacceptable solution. The American College of Health Care Executives revised its Code of Ethics in 1987 to try to delineate the moral responsibilities of managers. This is a beginning, but formulated codes from voluntary organizations cannot change thought processes geared to "the bottom line." In-service training on a continuing basis, substantial regional and local conferences on topics of interest, such as resource allocation, and a serious literature on managerial ethics are all needs that should be fulfilled for the good of the health care professions and the patients that are its charge (Darr, 1984).

Further, since managers now have great power, they cannot follow ethical trends but should rather take the lead in establishing policies and protocols on ethical issues in their institutions. To do this, they must involve all of the constituencies related to their institutions: physicians, nurses, ancillary personnel, patients, community members affected by their institutions, and so on. Once policies are in place, institutions can begin to act on individual cases within a given framework, and, except in emergency cases, patients can find out beforehand an institution's stance on questions that concern them and act accordingly. For instance, if an individual with a terminal disease knows before entering a hospital that the staff is committed to the most aggressive measures for treatment, that patient can choose to enter that hospital or find another, in accordance with individual preferences.

In a time of fierce competitive pressures, when the impetus to cut corners is very great, managers must come to a new understanding of the moral implications of their role. A major role can be as an advocate for the community's health. It is not a difficult step to take that bias to a consideration of what best serves the community. This would give administrators a new, moral role that could protect against the inroads that cost-containment pressure may make on delivery of good care (Wesbury, 1983).

This differs from the roles of both clinicians and patients. Patients are generally concerned with their health and perhaps how that health or lack of it will affect family and friends. The clinician is similarly concerned, and also concerned with collegial relationships, referrals, consultants, and the various pressures of operating a practice or participating in a group practice or HMO (Veatch, 1981). The manager of necessity is concerned with the entire institution or program, and, as mentioned, it is an easy jump from that concern to acting as advocate for the health of the community. However, to do all of this, managers will have to seriously reassess their education, training, and career pressures and begin to think in new ways.

These are matters that affect all health care professionals and all society (American Journal of Nursing, 1977). In a very real sense, how we decide these issues will shape the type of civilization we become. If the moral implications of medicine are ignored, glossed over, or trampled upon, the civilization will be deeply harmed. Though medical ethics is a new discipline, it arose because the problems and the challenges were there. It will be instructive to see how all branches of the professions, in concert with the community, act to adapt ancient and modern theories to very new concerns.

References

"AIDS: The Responsibilities of Health Professionals" [Special supplement]. *Hastings Center Report, 18*(2), April/May 1988.

Alexander, L. "Medical Science under Dictatorship." *New England Journal of Medicine, 241*(2), 1949.

American College of Physicians. *Ethics Manual,* 1984.

American Hospital Association. *Patient Bill of Rights.*

American Medical Association. *Proceedings of the Judicial Council.* Chicago: Author, 1980.

American Medical Association. *Proceedings of the Council on Judicial and Ethical Affairs.* Chicago: Author, 1986.

Annas, G., "Prisoner in the ICU: The Tragedy of William Bartling." *Hastings Center Report, 16*(4), December, 1984.

Annas, G. & Densberger, J. "Competence to Refuse Medical Treatment: Autonomy vs. Paternalism." *Toledo Law Review, 15*(561), 1984.

Bayer, R. et al. "HIV Antibody Screening: An Ethical Framework for Evaluating Proposed Programs." *Journal of the American Medical Association, 256*(13), 1986.

Beauchamp, T., & Childress, J. *Principles of Biomedical Ethics.* New York: Oxford University Press, 1983.

Bedell, S. & Delbanco, T. "Choices about Cardiopulmonary Resuscitation in the Hospital." *New England Journal of Medicine, 310*(17), 1984.

Bok, S. "The Limits of Confidentiality." In *Secrets: On the Ethics of Concealment and Revelation,* 1983.

Bouvia v. Superior Court, 1986, 179 Cal. App. 3d 1127.

Brett, A. S., & McCullough, L. B. "When Patients Request Specific Interventions: Defining the Limits of the Physician's Obligations." *New England Journal of Medicine, 315*; 1347–1351), 1986.

Brophy, v. New England Sinai Hospital, 479 N.E. 2d 626 (Mass. 1986).

California Natural Death Act. California Hospital Association, December 1976.

Callahan, D. "Autonomy: A Moral Good, Not a Moral Obsession." *Hastings Center Report, 15*(1), April 1984.

Callahan, D. *Setting Limits: Medical Goals in an Aging Society,* New York: Simon and Schuster, 1987. (a)

Callahan, D. "Terminating Treatment: Age as a Standard." *Hastings Center Report 17*(5), Oct./Nov. 1987. (b)

Camus, A., The Plague, Vintage Books, N.Y., 1972, p. 287.

Canterbury v. Spence, 464 Federal Reporter, 1972.

Cassileth, B., et al. "Informed Consent—Why Are Its Goals Imperfectly Realized?" *New England Journal of Medicine, 302*(16), 1980.

Childress, J. "Who Shall Live When Not All Can Live." *Soundings, 43*(1), Winter 1970.

Cobbs v. Grant, S. F. 22887, Sup. Court, Calif., 1972.

Curran, W. & Beecher, H. "Experimentation in Children: A Reexamination of Legal Ethical Principles." *Journal of the American Medical Association, 10*(1), 1969.

Daniels, N. *Am I My Parent's Keeper?* New York: Oxford University Press, 1988. (a)

Daniels, N. (Ed.). "Justice between Generations and Health Care for the Elderly" [Special issue]. *Journal of Medicine and Philosophy, 13*(1), February 1988. (b)

Darr, K. "Administrative Ethics and the Health Services Manager." *Hospital and Health Services Administration, 29*(2), 1984.

Declaration of Geneva. Adopted by the General Assembly of The World Medical Association, Geneva, Switzerland, September 1948. Amended by the 22nd World Medical Assembly, Sydney, Australia, August 1968.

Declaration of Helsinki. Adopted by the 18th World Medical Assembly, Helsinki, Finland, 1964. Revised by the 29th World Medical Assembly, Tokyo, Japan, 1975.

Delio v. Westchester County Medical Center, N.Y. Sup. Ct. App. Div. 1987, 516 N.Y.S. 2d 677.

Duff, R., & Campbell, A. G. M. "Moral and Ethical Dilemmas in the Special Care Nursery." *New England Journal of Medicine, 289*(17), 1973.

Durable Power of Attorney for Health Care. California Civil Code Sections 2410-2443, January 1, 1985.

Dworkin, G. "Moral Autonomy." In H. Engelhardt, Jr., & D. Callahan, (Eds.), *Science and Sociality,* Hastings, N.Y.: The Hastings Center, 1978.

Dworkin, G. "Autonomy and Informed Consent." *President's Commission for the Study of Ethical Problems in Medicine and Biomedical and Behavioral Research,* Appendix F, Washington, D.C.: Government Printing Office, 1983.

"Employers Test New Ways to Shift Risk on Health Costs." *New York Times,* June 27, 1988.

Engelhardt, H. T. "Shattuck Lecture: Allocating Scarce Medical Resources and the Availability of Organ Transplantation." *New England Journal of Medicine, 316* July 5, 1984.

"Ethics." *American Journal of Nursing,* Chicago: American College of Physicians, May 1977.

Feldstein, P., et al. "Private Cost Containment: The Effects of Utilization Review Programs on Health Care Use and Expenditures." *New England Journal of Medicine, 318*(20), 1988.

Fletcher, J. *Morals and Medicine.* Boston: Little, Brown, 1960.

Fletcher, J. *Situation Ethics: The New Morality.* Philadelphia: Westminster Press, 1966.

Fletcher, J. *Humanhood: Essays in Biomedical Ethics.* Buffalo, N.Y.: Prometheus Books, 1979.

Francis, D., & Chin, J. "The Prevention of Acquired Immunodeficiency Syndrome in the United States." *Journal of the American Medical Association, 257*(10), 1987.

Gostin, L., & Curran, W. "The Limits of Compulsion in Controlling AIDS." *Hastings Center Report, 16*(6), December 1986.

Harrison, B. *Our Right to Choose,* New York: Beacon Press, 1983.

Hartwig, J. "Donating Your Health Care Benefits." *Hastings Center Report, 18*(2), April/May 1988.

Hirsch, D., & Enlow, R. "The Effects of the Acquired Immune Deficiency Syndrome on Gay Lifestyle and the Gay Individual." *Annals of the New York Academy of Science,* 1985.

"Imperiled Newborns" [Special issue]. *Hastings Center Report, 17*(6), December 1987.

In re Eichner (Brother Fox), Court of Appeals, 52 N.Y.S. 2d 266 (1981).

In re Quinlan, 70 N.J. 10, 355 A. 2d 647, cert. denied, 429 U.S. 922 (1976).

In re Spring, (Mass. 1980) 405 N.E.2d 115.

In re Storar, 420 N.E.2d 64 (NY 1981).

In the matter of Conroy, N.J. 1985, 486 A 2d 1209.

In the matter of Jobes, N.J. Supr. Court, No. A-108/109, 1987.

Jonsen, A., & Garland, M. *Ethics of Newborn Intensive Care,* San Francisco and Berkeley: University of California, 1976.

Kant, I. "Metaphysical Foundations of Morals." In C. J. Freidrich (ed.), *The Philosophy of Kant.* New York: Modern Library, 1949.

Kass, L. "Regarding the End of Medicine and the Pursuit of Health." *The Public Interest, 40,* Summer 1975.

Lantos, J. "Baby Doe Five Years Later: Implications for Child Health." *New England Journal of Medicine, 317*(7), 1987.

Levinson, D. "Toward Full Disclosure of Referral Restrictions and Financial Incentives by Prepaid Health Plans." *New England Journal of Medicine, 817*(27), 1987.

Macklin, R. "Predicting Dangerousness and the Public Health Response to AIDS." *Hastings Center Report, 16*(6), December 1986.

Macklin, R. *Mortal Choices: Bioethics in Today's World.* New York: Pantheon Books, 1987.

Matthews, G., & Neslund, V. "The Initial Impact of AIDS on Public Health Law in the United States—1986." *Journal of the American Medical Association, 257*(3), 1987.

McCarthy, C. "DRGs—Five Years Later." *New England Journal of Medicine, 318*(25), 1988.

McCormick, R. "To Save or Let Die." *Journal of the American Medical Association, 229*(2), 1974.

McKinlay, J. & McKinlay, S. "The Questionable Contribution of Medical Measures to the Decline of Mortality in the United States in the Twentieth Century." *Milbank Memorial Quarterly, 55*(4), 1977.

Meisel, A., et al. "Hospital Guidelines for Deciding about Life-Sustaining Treatment: Dealing with Health Limbo." *Critical Care Medicine, 14*(3), 1986.

Mill, S. "Utilitarianism." In A. Smullyan et al., (Eds.), *Introduction to Philosophy.* Belmont, CA: Wadsworth, 1962.

Mills, M., et al. "The Acquired Immunodeficiency Syndrome: Infection Control and Public Health Law." *New England Journal of Medicine, 314*(14), 1986.

Mills, M., Sullivan, G., & Eth, L. "Prohibiting Third Parties: A Decade after Tarasoff." *American Journal of Psychiatry, 144*(1), 1987.

Murray, T. "Moral Obligations to the Not-Yet-Born: The Fetus as Patient." *Clinics in Perinatology,* June 1987.

Niebuhr, H. *The Responsible Self: An Essay in Christian Moral Philosophy.* New York: Harper and Row, 1963.

Noonan, J. *The Morality of Abortion: Legal and Historical Perspectives.* Cambridge, MA: Harvard University Press, 1970.

Office of the Actuary. *1984 Annual Report of the Board of Trustees of the Federal Hospital Insurance Trust Fund.* Washington, DC: Health Care Financing Administration, 1984.

Osborn, J. "AIDS: Politics and Science." *New England Journal of Medicine, 318*(7), 1988.

Otis, Bowen v. American Hospital Association et al., U.S. Supreme Court 106 S. Ct. 2101, No. 84-15-9, June 9, 1986.

Pellegrino, E. "Altruism, Self-Interest and Medical Ethics." *Journal of the American Medical Association, 258*(14), 1987.

Percival, T. *Medical Ethics* (C. D. Leake, Ed.). Baltimore: Williams and Wilkins, 1927.

Pope Pius XII. "The Prolongation of Life." In *The Pope Speaks* (Vol. 4, pp. 393–398), 1958.

President's Commission for the Study of Ethical Problems in Medicine and Biomedical and Behavioral Research. *Summing Up,* Washington, D.C.: Government Printing Office, 1983.

Ramsey, P. *The Patient as Person.* New Haven, CT: Yale University Press, 1971.

Rawls, J. *A Theory of Justice.* Cambridge, MA: Harvard University Press, 1971.

Reagan, M. "Physicians as Gatekeepers." *New England Journal of Medicine, 817*(27), 1987.

Roe v Wade, 410 U.S. 113, 93 Supreme Court 705, 35 L.E.D. 2d 147, 1973.

Robertson, J. & Schulman, J. "Pregnancy and Prenatal Harm to Offspring: The Case of Mothers with PKU." *Hastings Center Report, 117*(4), Aug./Sept. 1987.

Saint Augustine. "On the Trinity." In J. Burnaby (Ed.), *Augustine: Later Works.* Philadelphia: Westminster Press, 1963.

Saint Augustine. *Confessions, Book 10.* New York: Penguin Books, 1984.

Schloendorff v. Society of New York Hospital, 211 N.Y. 125, 127, 129; 1914.

Schramm, C., & Gabel, J. "Prospective Payment: Some Retrospective Observations." *New England Journal of Medicine, 318*(25), 1988.

Seiden, D. "Ethics for Hospital Administrators." *Hospital and Health Services Administration, 28*(2), 1982.

Seiden, D. "Diminishing Resources, Critical Choices." *Commonweal, 112*(5), 1985.

Shaw, A. "Dilemmas of Informed Consent in Children." *New England Journal of Medicine, 289*(17), 1973.

Shinn, R. *Forced Options: Social Decisions for the 21st Century.* San Francisco: Harper and Row, 1983.

Shortell, S., & Hughes, E. F. X. "The Effects of Regulation, Competition and Ownership on Mortality Rates among Hospital Inpatients." *New England Journal of Medicine, 318*(17), 1988.

State of New York Public Health Law, Article 29-B, Statute 413-A, April 1, 1988.

Steinbock, B. "Patient vs. Public: Whose Right Is It Anyway." *Medical Ethics, 1*(5), December 196.

Steinbrook, R., et al. "Preferences of Homosexual Men with AIDS for Life-Sustaining Treatment." *New England Journal of Medicine, 314,* 457–460, 1986.

Tarasoff v. Regents of the University of California, 17 Cal. 3d 425, 1976.

Temkin, O., & Temkin, C. L. (Eds.). *Ancient Medicine: Selected Papers of Ludwig Edelstein.* Baltimore: Johns Hopkins University Press, 1967.

Thomson, J. J. "A Defense of Abortion." *Philosophy and Public Affairs, 1*(1), 1971.

University Hospital, State of New York at Stony Brook, U.S. Court of Appeals of the Second Circuit, No. 679, February 23, 1984.

U.S. Child Abuse Protection and Treatment Amendments of 1984, Public Law 98-457.

Veatch, R. "Nursing Ethics, Physician Ethics and Medical Ethics." *Law, Medicine and Health Care,* October 1981.

Wanzer, S., et al. "The Physician's Responsibility toward Hopelessly Ill Patients." *New England Journal of Medicine, 310*(15), 1984.

Warren, M. A. "On the Moral and Legal Status of Abortion." *The Monist, 57*(1), 1973.

Weber, M. "Politics as a Vocation." In H. H. Gerth & C. W. Mills (Eds.), *Max Weber: Essays in Sociology.* New York: Galaxy, 1958.

Wesbury, S. "Ethics and Hospital Decision Making." *Michigan Hospitals, 19*(4), 1983.

Zuger, A., & Miles, S. "Physicians, AIDS and Occupational Risk." *Journal of the American Medical Association, 258*(14), 1987.

19

Futures

Anthony R. Kovner

Forecasting is an old art and a recent science. It has involved everything from Joseph's interpretation of the Pharaoh's dreams to econometric models and political scenarios. There are many methods for predicting the future. One is the extrapolation of a past trend. Cyclical trends such as consumer control of health care, are particularly amenable to this method. In the mid-1800s the health care consumer was dominant, but by the middle of the 20th century the physician had gained control. Since the 1970s, however, the consumer has begun to gain dominance again.

Another type of forecasting deals with predicting technological inventions that create breakthroughs and are followed by major developments. Such a breakthrough was the discovery of the microbial cause of disease; another, more recent breakthrough has been the discovery of the impact of environmental factors on disease causation. With this second type of forecast, a trend is likely to come slowly at first while the concept or idea develops and spreads; then the trend will gather momentum, moving into a phase where the development is exponential. Later the trend will flatten at a new level.

The Rand Corporation developed a forecasting technique called Delphi, in which large numbers of observers' opinions are polled and responded to, and projections are made with less bias than results from the predictions of individuals or small groups. Several Delphi studies have been done in health care, and it is perhaps instructive to review two such studies conducted in 1967 (Bender et al.) and 1974 (McLaughlin & Sheldon). Table 19.1 presents certain projections taken from these studies. Some of the projections, such as widespread use of physician assistants, have been borne out in the 1980s. Others, such as "never" for a "second class" system for medical care in the "wake of a wave of health centers, clinics, and prepayment systems," have come to pass. Still others, such as "solo practice virtually disappeared except by doctors over 50 years of age" has not taken place, as of 1990.

Table 19.1 Effects of Internal and External Forces on the Elements of the System

	Time Implemented
Technology	
Transmission of genetic information[a]	1980 ± 5 years
Electronic control of human behavior[a]	never
Chemical control of human behavior[a]	never
Use of computer for information storage and retrieval[a]	1978 + 10 years
Development of Mechanical Heart[a]	1988 + 5 to 10
Genetic control[b]	1990–1994
Computer record bank covering 80% of U.S. population[b]	1987
Government	
De facto federal control of psychiatric and medical facilities	1980–1994
Medical industry	1975–1984
12% GNP[b]	1994
20% GNP[b]	
Uniform geographic districts for political and public health education and all human service industries	Never
Physicians	
Few if any physicians in solo practice[a]	1993 ± 6 years
Solo practice virtually disappeared except in doctors over 50[b]	1981
Physicians undergo compulsory reexam[b]	1984
Other health practitioners	
Other health care systems workers in independent practice[a]	1993–1995
Widespread use of physicians assistants[b]	1975–1979
Organization	
Direct public participation in decision making with "real time" polling[b]	1985
A "second class" system for medical care in wake of a wave of health centers clinics and prepayment systems[b]	Never
Broad community participation in all medical institutions[b]	1980–1989

[a]Bender et al. (1967)—90% probability
[b]McLaughlin and Sheldon (1974).
Samuel P. Martin and Anthony R. Kovner, Futures, in Kovner, Anthony R. & Samuel P. Martin (eds.) Community Health & Medical Care, New York: Arvine Stratton 1978, pp. 413–442, pp 415

Vladeck (1987) notes that in 1982 experts were predicting that the trend toward increasing control of hospitals by national investor-owned corporations would reach a peak of 50 to 60% by the year 2000. Almost no one believes this in 1990, as the major national chains have closed or sold off almost one-third of their facilities, and several small hospital companies have lost great amounts of money or have gone into bankruptcy.

In a January 1985 study conducted for the Health Insurance Association of America, based on interviews with 40 "nationally recognized leaders in health care," Arthur D. Little and Company (1985) made the following predictions for the health care system in the mid-1990s:

- Health care will increasingly be perceived as an economic good subject to the influence of supply, demand, and price.
- Government and business purchasers of health care will intensify efforts to contain costs, which will dominate the health care agenda.
- The health system in 1995 will be highly competitive and, to some degree, regulated.
- Regulation is most likely at the state level, varying from state to state.
- Evaluation of cost-containment strategies will be aided by a major improvement in the availability of information on health care utilization, cost, and quality.
- Consumers will increasingly accept responsibility for their own health care.
- There will be more health services for the aged, increasing public pressure for protection against the costs of long-term care; a variety of emerging specialized services; a shift from inpatient to ambulatory care; and more care delivered in managed-care systems.
- A limited "safety net" will provide some guarantee of access to care.
- A "tiered" system of care will be recognized and accepted.
- Cost containment and overcapacity will combine to change the way hospitals function.
- The growing surplus of physicians amid pressure for cost containment will change the nature of physician practice (e.g., more physicians will be salaried, and the use of midlevel practitioners will be inhibited).
- Health maintenance organizations (HMOs) and other capitation arrangements will experience explosive growth.
- Negotiated provider contracts will be based on services and management efficiency rather than on price discounts.
- Cost increases will taper off.

Similar predictions for 1995 were made by 1,600 "national health care leaders and astute observers" in a study conducted by Arthur Andersen and Co. and the American College of Health Care Executives (1987):

- Growth in the elderly population will affect the health care system in 1995 more than any other issue.
- Adequate quality for all should drive health policy, but budgetary concerns will be the primary driving force behind federal health policy through 1995.

- A majority of all panelists believe there will not be a comprehensive national health policy by 1995.
- Health care's share of the gross national product (GNP) will exceed 12%.
- Rationing of health services will be the top medical ethics issue.
- Elderly consumers will exercise increased influence on U.S. health care policy.
- Ethical and legal issues surrounding AIDS will be addressed (61% of all respondents predict a cure for AIDS by 1995).
- Length of stay and admissions to hospitals will continue to decline.
- 700 of the nation's hospitals will close by 1995 (75–84 per year).
- Preferred provider organizations (PPOs), and HMOs will continue to grow.

In 1988, Amara and his co-workers, of the Institute for the Future, singled out trends most likely to change health care by the year 2000 by describing two different scenarios of "tough choices" and "health and wealth" depending on the amount of resources available to the health sector. Key driving forces included aging of the population, more sophisticated consumers, cost pressures from payers, pluralism and diversity of the system, new technologies, excess capacity, growth in health care expenditures, and government as a steering agent. Structural shifts from 1985 forward to the year 2000 were predicted to include growth of managed care, more salaried physicians with less autonomy, fewer hospital admissions and more ambulatory care, increased intensity of inpatient care, decline in medical school applicants, increasing concentration of medical research dollars, and a growth in the cost of health benefits administration and the net cost of insurance (Amara et al.)

My own predictions, with rationales, for the next 5 years are as follows:

Prediction 1: There will be no national health insurance.

Rationale: Americans' preferences for pluralism and diversity, plus distrust of government, will combine with the perceived high cost/benefit ratio of such insurance relative to other national expenditure needs to prevent adoption of any national insurance program.

Prediction 2: Fewer larger groups of health care providers will compete for capped purchaser dollars in increasingly organized local markets.

Rationale: There are economies of scale in the marketing, production, and financing of health care. Certain organizations can provide certain services better and cheaper than others and will be so perceived by increasingly sophisticated purchasers.

Prediction 3: Consumers will use less medical care per capita on an age-adjusted basis.

Rationale: Budgets will increasingly be limited, based on purchaser preferences, as validated by consumers and providers. More of each health-benefit dollar will be spent on cost-effective treatment and prevention. Less of each dollar will be spent on services that do not predictably improve health outcomes.

Prediction 4: State regulation will increase regarding cost, quality, and access to health care.

Rationale: Access to care will become a political issue for populations in rural areas and inner cities, as will the uneven quality of care in these areas. States will also face increased costs for Medicaid beneficiaries and state government employees. The federal government will not supersede state government on these matters.

Prediction 5: The power of physicians to shape and benefit from decision making in health care will diminish.

Rationale: Managers, including clinician-managers, will have more power relative to practicing physicians and nurses. This will result from less per capita utilization of health services, more physicians per capita, and more pervasive standards regarding clinical process and outcome.

An oversimplified model of some of these predictions and relationships is shown in Figure 19.1.

Important factors that will influence the shape of health care in the future include population demographics, disease patterns, information systemization, and medical technology.

Figure 19.1 Forecasted Health Sector Pressures and Responses, 1988–1993.

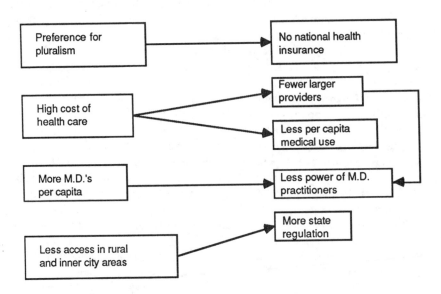

Demographics: Age and Income

By the year 2000 the number of Americans aged 75 and over is expected to increase by 48%; and the number aged 85 and over by 83%. Already persons 65 and over account for more than 40% of inpatient days in general hospitals and more than 30% of all physician visits. At the same time there is a shrinking number and percentage of adolescents and young adults. It has been estimated that from 1985 to 2000 the number of persons between the ages of 18 and 24 in the United States will decrease by 14% while the number of persons 25 to 34 falls by 13%. The impact of these trends is expected to be increasing political pressure to provide national health insurance for long-term care and a shortage of younger health workers to provide care, especially on nights and weekends.

Another demographic trend is the increasing growth of a minority, low-income underclass population in large cities. This population has special health problems but has equally important other problems relating to jobs, education, and housing, all of which have received little national attention during the Reagan years. Per Arthur D. Little's prediction of a tiered system in 1985, different levels of services to consumers based on income seems to have been recognized and accepted in the United States, circa 1988.

Patient Preferences and Values

As Americans have become more educated, they have acquired higher expectations for health care and for the physician. When expectations are not met, there is great disenchantment. Physicians are sued frequently for their failure to cure. Patients want to know more about health care and to participate more fully in decisions regarding it, including the right to die.

The past 60 years has been characterized by a shift from the extended family to the nuclear family. Now, even the nuclear family is showing great strain. There is one divorce for every two marriages. Working mothers have become the norm rather than the exception, and many single parents, both male and female, are heading households. Mobility of the population (20% of the population moves each year) also has contributed to the instability of the family and family neighborhood structure.

One impact of these trends has been to move more responsibility for health care away from the family and toward the educational system or employer. Schools are more responsible for student competency with regard to knowledge about health and health care, and they provide on-site services from nutrition to family planning. Employers provide health benefits ranging from health insurance, day care, and exercise classes to managment of long-term care for workers' parents.

The Information Revolution

According to Griffith (1987), by the middle of the 21st century, patient care in hospitals will be highly computerized:

> [T]he doctor will guide an electronic system which suggests a plan of care for each patient based on analysis of both the patient's history and detailed data about specific treatment options. Forecasts of all patients' needs will be available to each patient service unit. Systems will optimize schedules, order supplies, and prompt completion of the original assignment and follow-up of any unexpected occurrence. Complete records will be available to establish expectations and monitor performance for the doctor and the nurse. [p. 330]

As of 1985 the processing ability of the computer has far exceeded its use in practice. The computer has had much wider acceptance in finance and billing for services than in patient care. But computers are being used increasingly in analyzing treatment in relation to outcome and in developing standards for diagnosis and treatment.

Near-term (3–5 yrs) directions for expanded computer capability are in areas of revenue control, budgeting and accounting control, clinical review, final product cost accounting and risk management (Griffith). Information systems can increasingly break down revenues by services rendered and by payer, employer, and insurance group. Expenses can be allocated increasingly to a larger number of cost centers, and flexible budgeting can be implemented for varying volumes of service.

Medical records are increasingly being automated, with larger and more detailed patient abstracts integrated with cost and revenue data. Many health care organizations (HCOs) have implemented quality of care review while the patient is currently undergoing treatment. Such review adds to the cost of care. For example, in 1988 the Lutheran Medical Center, a 550-bed hospital in New York City, had 20 staff members dedicated to quality assurance, at a cost of $650,000 per year.

Other near-term trends include movement toward final-product cost accounting, by which services for groups of patients requiring regular treatment can be budgeted at alternating levels of demand; and risk management, by which all untoward incidents can be aggregated and analyzed from incident reports.

New Technology

New technology in health care will be developed and increasingly assessed. Among examples of such technology and assessments are periodic findings of studies conducted by the National Center for Health Services Research (NCHSR) and Health Care Technology Assessment. For example, findings released in 1987 on the efficiency and uses of fully automated blood pressure monitoring, cochlear (inner ear) implant devices for the deaf, and continuous positive airway pressure for treating obstructive sleep apnea in adults were as follows:

- Although safe and accurate, automated blood pressure monitoring's role in blood pressure measurement other than during sleep "has yet to be clearly differentiated" from that of the traditional manual method and of semiautomatic monitoring.
- Cochlear implant devices (surgically inserted special hearing devices) are "considered to be safe and to help patients by restoring auditory sensation and speech detection and by improving voice modulation."
- Continuous positive airway pressure (PAP) provides even levels of air pressure from a flow generator through the nose to counteract obstructed sleep apnea (OSA) in which a sleeping person's respiratory airflow stops for 10 seconds or more. PAP "appears to reduce signs and symptoms of OSA and in appropriately selected patients, may completely prevent upper airway obstruction during sleep."

These assessments are conducted by NCHSR relative to coverage under Medicare. The Health Care Financing Administration decides on whether new technologies are reimbursable based in large part on NCHSR's assessment of safety and effectiveness. One of the weaknesses of diagnosis related group (DRG) reimbursement under Medicare is the lack of responsiveness in rate changes to new technology, thereby discouraging its introduction.

The last 30 years have seen great advances in technology and the development of the belief that all problems can be solved by the engineering biological science approach. This approach was eminently successful with antibiotics for the acute infectious diseases and neuropharmacological agents for nervous disorders; but despite new diagnostic advances such as lasers and magnetic resonance imaging, technology has not yet been able to combat chronic diseases. Although confidence is being strained, it is still strong.

With regard to predictions of clinical advances, 23 experts were invited by *Medical World News* ("Tomorrow's Medicine") in 1976 to predict what two or three useful clinical advances in their specialty would become conventional medical practice within the next 25 years. Examples of the predictions are as follows:

Oncology

1. Enzyme or radioimmunoassay detection of people at high risk   1985
   of cancer

2. More careful screening of environment for carcinogens by   1990
   bacterial and mammalian cell systems
3. Interruption of carcinogenic process in high risk individuals   2000

Bioengineering

1. Clinical use of implantable artificial bladder, heart, kidneys,   1990
   pancreas, and liver
2. Instrumentation for home use with information relayed by   1990
   telephone or telemetry to physician base for analysis with
   treatment prescribed by phone
3. Completely computerized general health care centers for treat-   1990
   ment of mass populations

Neurology

1. Nonnarcotic treatment of pain   1980
2. Prevention or treatment of multiple sclerosis, perhaps by vac- 1990
   cine
3. Chemical treatment of malignant brain tumor   2000

Coile (1988) has made a more updated assessment for the 1990s, with the following forecasts, among others: biosensors will be implanted in the chronically ill to provide a continuous stream of physiological data and alert caregivers if health status falters; drug-dispensing pumps will provide more precise and self-regulating drug therapy to diabetics and chronic-disease patients and will relieve problems of overmedication and missed dosages; self-care robots will provide support in daily living to the disabled; and many forms of cancer will yield to genetically engineered drugs, blocking the damaging spread of defective cells by chemically altering the cellular structure.

Politics of Health Care Costs

Blendon and Altman (1987) summarized the major themes drawn from 15 national opinion polls regarding health care costs. Conducted between 1981 and 1984, the polls showed the following:

- Rising health care costs do not rank very high on a list of most important problems now facing the nation.

- Most Americans are concerned about their own, not business's or the government's, health cost problem.
- People are happier with the status quo than one might think.
- Most Americans do not see themselves as having any responsibility for creating the problem of health care costs.
- The view of practicing physicians are often more influential with the public than the opinions of groups proposing change, such as government officials and business and labor leaders.
- Although the majority of Americans see the deficit as a major threat to the nation, they do not see cutting federal health outlays as the most desirable way to reduce it.

The above conclusions appear to be challenged by the 1988 Harris poll referred to in Chapter 1. According to this survey, Americans are now significantly less happy with their health care system than either the British or the Canadians are with theirs (Blendon). According to Blendon, Americans say "they want a fundamental break with their current health care policies and a much more central role played by the central government in remedying America's health problems." I believe that in the early 1990s no such break will occur because of the limited political power of the uninsured. Rather, it is much more likely that long-term care for the elderly will be federally financed because of their political power.

American Culture

Consumerism, a force in the late 1960s, continues to grow. Government and business purchasers intervene on behalf of consumers and influence client–provider behavior. Increasingly purchasers of care are steering their beneficiaries by paying in full only for care given by providers who are preferred in terms of quality and price.

Income distribution in the United States has become more inequitable. Instead of increasing purchasing power of the poor, who have a greater need for health services, the next few years may see increased governmental activity in restricting choice of providers for beneficiaries of public programs. Higher income is associated with increased demand for care and hospitalization, often leading to overutilization of services. Affluence itself can influence disease patterns as a result of life-style.

After a period of 35 years of unbridled health care cost expansion, there has developed among purchasers a serious concern for cost and benefit. There is increasingly serious scrutiny of the cost of medical services. This is being accomplished through evaluation of the quality of health services and some control of ineffective utilization. There is strong demand to prove the effectiveness of hospitalization, laboratory tests, and medications.

Large corporations meet most of our needs, and this ethos has an impact on health care in three ways. First, hospitals and clinics are increasingly being organized and managed like large corporations. Second, health care has become a promising market for large and small corporations. Third, large corporations see health care costs for their employees as one of their largest and most rapidly increasing expenditures.

An example of what corporations are doing to control health care costs is General Motors's Informed Choice Plan, which went into effect in April 1985. Workers were given a choice of three types of coverage: a traditional fee-for-service plan (with strict utilization controls), HMOs, and PPOs. In 1984, GM spent $2.35 billion on employee health benefits, and the objective of the new plan was to save the company money. In the first 9 months, enrollment in the managed-care plans increased significantly. HMO enrollment among GM employees and retirees rose from 70,000 to an estimated 123,000, and PPO enrollment—nonexistent before the contract—climbed to almost 75,000. Add in an estimated 330,000 dependents, and the total equals nearly 24% of those eligible for health insurance benefits.

Government has increasingly seen health care costs as something to be controlled for its beneficiaries and employees rather than for its own sake. And health care has increasingly been viewed as an economic good, access to which is available to poor people only on limited terms, that is, through Medicaid or through local charity; and some 35 million to 40 million Americans lack adequate health insurance.

Effect of External Forces on the Elements of the Health Care System

The major forces described previously are producing significant changes in the health care industry. Rather than health care being the fiefdom of the physician, it is becoming the domain of the consumer and the corporation. A mature, sophisticated, technological society cannot accept on faith the physician's assurance of the effectiveness and quality of the care provided. When quality control of health care is so important to so many individuals, some wonder why government has not taken more responsibility in this area. A number of movements are afoot to assure quality control. Some are implemented in the name of quality and outcome measurements. Legislation for quality control has had the same history as legislation for payment systems. The legislative mandate is opposed with extreme vigor, but when it is passed, its force is diverted by the medical providers to their control and ultimately to their benefit. Efforts to control and assure quality of care will increase during the next 5 years.

Within the health care industry, as in all industries, there is a demand for freedom of information. Increased data availability in the doctor's office and in the hospital involving quality of care has created greater demand for disclosure, more openness and availability of the data. Most importantly, such availability can alter doctor and hospital behavior.

Government

Health care remains politicized. Politicians seek election or reelection based in part on their position on health issues, whether national health insurance on the Massachusetts model, treatment of AIDS patients, health care for the homeless, the amount of Medicare rate increases, or the quality of care in public hospitals.

Government participation in health care has changed. It used to consist of limited provision of services to the poor, services for government employees, administration of communicable disease programs, statistics compilation, licensing, and financing of research and construction. It now also consists of financing the bulk of health care for the elderly and the poor and extensive regulation of quality and cost in these programs. At the same time, governmental provision of direct care, at all levels, is diminishing.

Government initiatives in the early 1970s included stimulation of HMOs, Professional Standards Review Organizations (PSROs), certificate-of-need legislation, and research in health care delivery. This was accompanied by cutbacks in the ambitious direct service programs of the 1960s, such as neighborhood health and community mental health centers. More recently there have been attempts to control the increase in the governmental cost of the Medicare and Medicaid programs, to stabilize the basic research expenditures of the National Institutes of Health, and to slow hospital construction and the supply of physicians.

In 1978, Kovner and Martin predicted inaccurately that the next 3 to 5 years would see national health insurance for medical care, the establishment of a national council for health services policy similar to the Council of Economic Advisors, and the establishment of a national center to evaluate medical procedures and tests equivalent to the Food and Drug Administration. We also stated that government attempts to directly proscribe the behavior of providers, such as PSROs; rate setting; and certificate-of-need legislation were bound to fail, as these created counterpressures to "beat the system" rather than altering basic incentives. This reaction on the part of health care providers would be similar to that of producers in other heavily regulated industries. The first response is frequently to enact regulation, and it is often counterproductive. Through political influence and campaign contributions, the regulated often become the regulators. Of course, we based our predictions on a rationality in public affairs that, we should have been aware, often belies reality.

No one in 1980 could predict the AIDS epidemic, which has had a major impact on the American population since 1982. In 1988 on any given day in New York City, for example, approximately 1,500 inpatient beds are occupied by patients with AIDS or AIDS-related illnesses. The already significant demands that AIDS places on the health care system will only increase in the next 5 to 10 years, perhaps substantially. The government has spent millions of dollars on AIDS research and services that do not yet meet the need or cure the disease.

Through DRG reimbursement, the federal government did pursue an incentives policy that alters provider behavior not only by provision of rewards but also by changing cognitive patterns as to what is acceptable. I see increased governmental regulation in the area of quality of care such as that undertaken recently in New York State, where all hospitals must meet strict criteria in quality assurance programs, state investigations of quality are frequent, limitations on house staff working hours have been enacted, and proposals have been made for recredentialing physicians.

Unfortunately, improved planning and regulation in government is constrained, especially at the state and local level, by the lack of accountability for the performance of its own bureaucracy. The uneven quality of state government may result in increased federalizing of the regulatory system, either directly or indirectly, by means of incentives to reward or punish performance by state bureaucracies.

The federal government will continue to support medical and nursing research and some part of medical and nursing education. The health care industry will continue to meets its capital expenditures by long-term debt financing in the capital market. The debt is amortized over a long period by devoting a part of the service cost to capital debt. Local mechanisms to secure the loans and develop taxfree status for the bonding mechanism have become widespread.

Clinicians

Physicians are being challenged from inside and outside the health care system. The physician's place within the system has narrowed and moved toward the purely curing role of the technician, as other professionals encompass the care, cure, and support functions. Physicians are increasingly employed by large HCOs and supervised by physician-managers with special management training.

The 1970s witnessed an increasing attack on the authority of the physician: by the patient for a lack of responsiveness to personal and primary care needs, by the taxpayer for a lack of concern in controlling medical care costs, and by increasing numbers of other professionals regarding their remuneration and power relative to the physician.

The 1980s witnessed increasing competition between physicians and hospitals. Services that had been provided primarily in hospitals, such as ambulatory surgery and rehabilitation, were now provided by physicians on an outpatient, freestanding basis.

There is increasing skepticism concerning the efficiency of physicians and their capacity to allocate resources. They are being criticized for performing unnecessary surgical procedures, overprescribing, and faulty labeling of the mentally ill and inability to treat them effectively. There is evidence that additional expenditure on medical technology is becoming less productive, and it might be more productive to influence consumers to better utilize the medical care system and to lead healthier lives. There is criticism of the maldistribution of physicians by specialty (i.e., too many surgeons and not enough primary care doctors) and by location (i.e., too many doctors in big cities and not enough in small towns). Increasingly, the public prefers that decisions over resource allocation in the medical care industry be taken out of the hands of physicians. As the organizations in which physicians work increase in size, complexity, and bureaucratization, the power of practicing physicians to allocate resources dwindles compared to that of governing boards, chiefs of services, and key managers.

Despite the influence of physician organizations such as the AMA, the individual doctor is yielding some of his prerogatives to organizational imperatives. Under physician guidance, but with a healthy input from other professions, some medical care tasks have been specified and clustered and are being performed by less trained, less educated, and less expensive, workers. Increasingly, physicians are using physician extenders, even to work in hospitals as extensions of the physician office and under physician supervision. How these extenders relate to nursing is an area of conflict. The division of labor will increasingly be negotiated among physicians, nurses, social workers, pharmacists, and other professionals and evaluated continually and jointly by them. In such negotiations physicians will play a major but not an exclusive part. The responsibility base will shift from the single individual physician to a wider and more shared base.

Part of the idealism of the health care professional is a strong commitment to individual patients as opposed to whole populations or the interests of society. The essence of clinical training is concern for the individual. Customer responsiveness is often ignored within the health care system; patients want professionals to listen more attentively to what they are saying. As a result of competitive pressures, the level of personalized services is expected to improve.

Two major movements challenge physician dominance within HCOs: the professionalization of other health care disciplines and the unionization of non-professional workers. As other health care professionals receive more extensive education, they develop organizations that challenge the dominance of physicians. Some groups have claimed to have a mandate and have set up independent licensing and accreditation programs, openly challenging physician control. Nurses, psychologists, and social workers have established independent practices, seeing patients without physician referral and supervision and charging a fee for their services. These kinds of practices have grown. However, both physician and nonphysician professionals will meet with an anti-elitism movement in society.

Nonprofessional workers are growing strong and moving toward organization, lobbying, collective bargaining, and strikes. They have been concerned with working conditions, authority, and role, as well as with compensation.

The two-tiered economic system in medicine, well-compensated physicians and the other poorly compensated workers, is rapidly crumbling. Extension of minimum wages and collective bargaining has had an impact on narrowing the gap. This trend will increase with the rapid growth of a middle management in HCOs made up of professional managers and managerial professionals.

Ten years ago we inaccurately predicted an increasing rationalization of health manpower (Kovner & Martin). We said that tasks will be specified, clustered—into job categories and career lattices, with corresponding development of educational lattices—implemented, and standardized. This would be reflected in shortened educational programs for many occupations. For example, the psychiatrist may not need the same amount of anatomy and physiology as the specialist in internal medicine. As of 1990, I do not see these hoped for improvements in the next 5 years either. Nor is there likely to be dramatic changes in education for health care workers, such as increased common core courses cutting across professional and other program boundaries, increased on-the-job and in-service education, and credentialing. There has been increased emphasis on continuing education programs after graduation and to a much lesser extent on relicensing. And the next 5 years will see greater recognition and legitimization given at the work place to the necessity for continuing education programs.

HCOs

The forces described previously are propelling the health care system toward a corporate ethos. Institutionalization is resulting in radical changes in client and provider relations as well as in interpersonal and interprofessional functions. With this has come the development of sophisticated personnel systems, labor relations staff, financing staff, and management information systems. Marketing staffs have been developed not only to aid in recruiting clients but also to plan strategies for new services. These trends will increase.

The forces are changing the locus of care. There is increasing effort to centralize care in geographical proximity, such as having clinics and professional buildings near hospitals. Some hospitals have provided practitioners with space and services within or adjacent to the hospital. In this way, the solo practitioner can gain some of the advantages of the group. Cooperative efforts in administrative and professional staffing have shifted from the ad hoc to planned and shared bases. One can expect to see these arrangements increase and the patterns become more formal.

Greater efforts will be made to integrate care so as to avoid unnecessary and wasteful duplication. Agencies will not be developed to avoid the duplication of facilities, nor will they require a physician or group to obtain a franchise before opening a practice. Some of this regionalization and franchising will be operated by large HCOs, but I do not see much unnecessary and wasteful duplication being avoided during the next 5 years unless an even more rapid spread of prepaid insurance and preferred provider plans forces other providers out of business.

HCOs will continue to grow larger and more complex. As the pressures for accountability increase, these will focus on top management. To adapt effectively to outside pressures, internal activities will increasingly be organized into responsibility centers, as in business, with subordinate managers held responsible for results. Whether internal activities are grouped by departments, or occupations, or by divisions across occupations or in some combination, i.e., matrix management, managers will be held accountable increasingly for results. Private enterprise will continue to expand into the health care industry. Chains will once again increase their hospital operations. Insurance companies will expand their HMO development and growth efforts. The ability of the nonprofit and public organization to survive under increasing competition will be determined by their capability to obtain results. The future will see a massive struggle of solo practitioners and small groups to survive in competition with other organizational forms. There has been no stampede toward multidisciplinary group practice, but there is a solid trend. The concept of group practice will be much more acceptable to the medical student and resident of the 1990s than for those of the 1980s (especially to those in two-career marriages), and many project this as their practice goal. Vigorous competition has developed in some locations between solo practitioners and medical care foundations and between independent and group practice associations and HMOs maintenance organizations. The early 1990s will see such competition continue.

Hospitals. The hospital has been the focus of organization in the health care field, and hospitals will try to keep this leadership role. The main response of the American Hospital Association (AHA) in the 1970s to public pressures for cost equality control was the development of hospital franchising as a keystone of national health insurance. Under the AHA Ameriplan, hospitals would have been franchised to oversee the delivery of all medical care in a geographic area and would have been held accountable by government for their effectiveness in controlling quality and cost. Of course, the hospital, not the medical society nor the group practice would have been the hub of the system; and competition among hospitals would have decreased, or at least would not have been fostered in a given geographical area. Ameriplan did not come to pass, but may be revived by hospital groups, partly in response to challenges to their tax exempt status, by demonstrating their benefit to designated communities which they serve.

The next 5 years will see an enormous struggle on the part of hospital leaders to maintain their margin of leadership and to place the health care mandate in the hospital industry. Additional hospitals will move into prevention and chronic care to supplement their present acute-disease focus.

The traditional primary concerns of hospital governing boards have been not to operate at a deficit and to keep the physicians contented. Under DRG reimbursement and competitive pressures, hospital top management is becoming increasingly concerned with performance in relation to costs. This concern has manifested itself in more formal relationships—both vertically with other providers, such as medical groups and nursing homes, and horizontally with other hospitals to share supporting services (purchasing, public relations, fund raising, data processing) or medical care programs, such as consolidation of obstetrics departments at one hospital and pediatrics departments at another.

The main response to financial problems by several state hospital associations has been to urge transfer payments or special taxes to provide for uncompensated care. State governments, of course, may consider limiting hospital revenues as part of the negotiations. This is what has happened in several northeastern states during the 1970s and 1980s.

Linkages are being developed between major organizations in health care. Hospitals are developing and fostering home care programs and extended-care facilities; they are merging to form larger conglomerates. In the absence of mergers, HCOs are collaborating to provide each other with viable services. This has been most evident in the area of obstetrics, where a declining census has motivated closure of services. Shared facilities also are also being developed. Thus, there is a major trend for hospitals to develop cooperative arrangements and mergers.

Chronic-Care Organizations. The aging of the population will lead to an increase of chronic disease. Studies have shown that people over 65 have, on the average, four chronic conditions. The needs in chronic care represent the primary future tasks of the health service enterprise. Many think these needs will be too vast for doctors and nurses, and our present "system" will have to be replaced with a better system; and some expect it to be organized primarily on a social rather than a medical model.

In the past 20 years, one approach to responding to these needs has been the integration of chronic-care with acute-care services, thereby enabling some resources to be diverted to chronic care. The establishment in general hospitals of units for the mentally ill and those suffering from additive disease and alcoholism can be viewed in this light, as can the medical supervision by hospitals or group practices of patients in nursing homes and homes for the mentally retarded. Another controversial approach has been the deinstitutionalization of the chronically ill through the development of drug, home, and ambulatory care centers.

The next 5 years are not expected to yield significant and continuing technological advances in chronic care. There will be increasing focus on output measures of disability or discomfort and in evaluation of methods for alleviating these conditions. Tasks will increasingly be analyzed and more sensibly allocated so that valuable medical resources will not be squandered and so that providers with less formal education can do valuable work of acceptable quality and be proportionately remunerated. There may be some scaling down of goals where technology is not cost-effective. For example, humane care rather than curative treatment may serve as the official goal of certain chronic care institutions.

There will be additional efforts to employ the chronically ill. During the past 20 years employment opportunities for the mentally retarded have expanded. Traditionally, ex-alcoholics have worked with alcoholics and ex-narcotics addicts with addicts. There may be more emphasis on other approaches in line with innovations on behaviorist therapies. As behavior is modified, many of the chronically ill can become increasingly employable.

There is currently a stigma attached to the chronically ill and dying, which also extends to those who work in such organizations. Whether additional funding and greater integration with the rest of the medical care system has been erasing this stigma is difficult to discern. Clearly, the results achieved by chronic-care organizations will be determined to a greater extent by the cultural values and resource allocations of those who are unlikely to be current clients of the system. Chronic-care organizations cannot respond effectively without additional resources or without scaling down their tasks to do what can realistically be done. More than any other area in health care, chronic care needs additional research support concerning new ways of health care delivery and managerial innovation. It needs to develop and implement successful findings and demonstrations on a large scale. I believe that during the next 5 years such suppprt will increasingly be forthcoming.

HMOs and PPOs. The growth of HMOs and PPOs has been rapid during the 1980s. The number of HMOs and their total enrollment increased from 265 HMOs and 10,827,000 enrollees in 1982 to 595 plans and 23,663,000 enrollees in 1986. Faster growth is occurring in individual practice association HMOs, which contract with private physicians for services; growth is somewhat slower in staff models in which HMOs contract with or employ physician groups. Enrollment in PPOs grew from 1.3 million Americans in health plans eligible to the PPO services in 1984 to 16.5 million in 1986. Unlike HMOs, PPOs allow patients the freedom to use providers that have not contracted with the PPO. The fundamental strategy is to use financial incentives such as volume discounts to steer patients to cost-effective providers.

What has taken place is regulation of providers by purchasers, with measures such as prior approval screening, use of PPOs and HMOs, and restructuring of benefit plans to shift health costs from employers to employees. Purchasers are beginning to grapple with quality issues as well. In the next 5 years they will be increasingly designing incentives to weigh against the choice of what are perceived to be low-quality providers and assessing the quality of services provided to their beneficiaries. They will attempt to identify outliers—hospitals and physicians that are clearly better or worse than most others in regard to medical outcomes achieved for certain procedures—and they will increasingly steer beneficiaries toward certain providers and away from others.

I believe that more care for more Americans will be purchased by health care purchasing organizations as employers and their agents buy services from fewer providers increasingly organized in local markets. The nation will not see the formation of national health care firms with large chunks of the market, as in the auto industry, but in many cities there will be fewer larger groups of providers contracting with purchasers. And the national corporations such as Humana and Kaiser-Permanente and Prudential also will increase in size and have increased market share.

Educational and Credentialing Organizations

Education in the health care professions, particularly in the medical profession, has been directed toward their own interests, with little or no societal responsibility. As Ebert (1985) writes, other than substantial change in distribution of residencies toward primary care, "the medical education establishment has changed little in other ways, except to become increasingly dependent on income from fee-for-service high technology medicine."

Ebert and Ginzberg (1988) assert that "the existing medical educational system is not providing the types of physicians who will be able to meet the health care needs of the public and to function in the newly emerging modes of health care delivery." They recommend shortening medical education by combining the last 2 years of medical school and the first 2 years of graduate medical education as implemented by consortia of medical schools in a geographic area. For specialties other than general medicine, pediatrics, and family medicine, in which education would be completed at the end of medical school, those intending to specialize would spend 3 rather than 4 years in medical school. A stipend would be paid for medical students during the last 2 years of clinical training as it currently exists in graduate medical education. Ebert and Ginzberg note that at present there is no consensus for such reform. Given the average indebtedness of 82% of medical school graduates of $33,500 in 1986, and perceptions of oversupply by state and federal legislators, I would expect to see demonstrations funded toward implementing these recommendations in pilot programs over the next 5 years.

Although there has been an increasing oversupply of physicians, there is a growing shortage of nurses and other skilled health occupations, such as physical therapists and lab and x-ray technicians. Aiken and Mullinix (1987) explain the hospital nursing shortage in terms of three reasons: sicker hospitalized patients, who require more care than in years past; more budgeted nursing positions; unfavorable changes in nurses' wages relative to other workers with comparable educational requirements and job responsibilities. Between 1983 and 1987 enrollment in nursing schools has dropped by 20%, and the number of new nurses graduating annually is predicted to fall from a high of 82,700 in 1985 to 68,700 or less by 1995 (see Chapter 5, this volume; Aiken & Mullinix).

Characteristically, health care professionals are educated in separate schools, and there are no career ladders between professions, so it would take less time for a nurse or physical therapist to become a doctor than it would a college graduate. After education in separate schools of medicine, nursing, social work, dentistry, physical therapy, public health, and others, graduates are required to work together taking care of patients. Understandably, there is considerable conflict regarding who is supposed to do what for whom. Productivity is therefore lower than might be the case if expectations took adequate account of which professionals can and should do which tasks and take what responsibilities for the patient at what costs and quality. It is predicted that no significant changes will take place regarding joint training of health professionals. More government monies will be allocated to increasing the supply of nurses who will be paid more, especially if they assume more responsibility and continue to work nights and weekends.

The direction that medical schools will take in the service area is not clear. Their past record has not always been exemplary as providers of high-quality care, particularly in the ambulatory care area. There has been some outside pressure and a good deal of inside entrepreneurship to make the medical school hospitals the hub of the medical care system as well as the tertiary-care center. The assumption of responsibility for comprehensive medical care for a segment of population has had mixed success when it has been placed in the hands of educational institutions. Leading educators can be found on both sides of the question, but it has become less likely that medical schools will exert leadership in this area as purchasers become more desirous of cheaper prices and more customized services for their beneficiaries.

Credentialing in the health professions has been the province of the professions. It has had little or no governmental or consumer input and has been one more mechanism by which the professional controls access to the professions and the market. This control is being eroded by governmental and consumer forces. Accreditation of educational programs by the educator and the profession without concern for the greater public good will not last much longer. Already, accrediting bodies have nonprofessional representatives, and governmental bodies will begin to demand more consumer concern. During the next 5 years accrediting agencies will still be dominated by providers rather than by consumers.

Licensure should undergo similar shifts. The present restrictions across state lines are archaic. Nursing professions have found methods of breaking down state barriers. I do not see licensing of institutions rather than individuals in the next 5 years. Since institutions are corporate units and can assume responsibility for their practice, it is possible that hospitals, clinics, and groups could be licensed to practice and assume responsibility for their actions. But professional groups have mustered strong forces against accrediting institutions regarding the practice of clinicians within them, rather than the individual clinicians themselves. I predict that the professions will continue to be successful in resisting this change.

Certification has been another area of professional control. There have been no restrictions by government on criteria for certification or on numbers of specialists certified. Certification standards may have been more responsive to physician and hospital needs for inexpensive helping hands than to societal needs for qualified practitioners. Again, governmental and consumer forces outside the profession, as well as forces within the system, have been largely unsuccessful on this issue.

Pressures outside and inside the industry are being directed toward recertification and relicensure to ensure that the health professional continues to maintain a level of competence. This will be implemented in more states during the next 5 years. Unfortunately, there is no assurance that such procedures will result in proper patient care. Undoubtedly, as quality of care becomes of wider concern and measurement capability increases, the work of individual physicians is being scrutinized and the examination of knowledge is giving way to measurement of process and outcome in practice. If quality of process and outcome in practice is measured, relicensure and certification will no longer be necessary. This may be increasingly implemented by state legislators dissatisfied with the pace of private sector improvements.

In the 1900s the AMA had a leadership role in organizing and advocating change in medical care systems. Their position since World War I and particularly in the last 30 years, however, has been to oppose all change that might tend to weaken the physician's autonomy and control over the medical care industry. Such a stance has proved eminently successful, not only in halting or slowing legislation for change but also in channeling whatever change occurred to the massive benefit of the nation's physicians. For example, Medicare, which was bitterly and expensively opposed by the AMA, has resulted in some shift in the delivery of medical services from the under-65 population to those over 65, at a tremendous inflation in medical care prices and at a tremendous increase in physician incomes. Formal AMA opposition to the magnitide and quality of change described here is expected to continue, and lobbying by other professional organizations, such as the American Nurses Association, is expected to increase in order to achieve like rewards for their constituents. Neither organization will achieve the power that the AMA had circa 1950–1975 because of the now increased power of purchaser organizations.

Legislation concerning peer review of physician care has been channeled into control by Professional Review Organizations (PROs) rather than hospitals and other organizations that deliver the care. These organizations seem to have achieved a level of acceptance within medicine and by HCOs and will probably continue to carry out these functions as long as they retain the confidence of government and other purchasers who largely pay their bills. Similar organizations will not be created for other clinicians, such as nurses and social workers, as it is expected that physicians will continue to dominate the decision-making process with respect to diagnosis and treatment, particularly in acute care.

Summary and Conclusions

The author has attempted to predict future directions in the American health care delivery system, not so much because of confidence that they will happen but rather to focus discussion on key issues, the constraints that surround them, and the opportunities for resolving them.

American preferences for pluralism and diversity and distrust of government are likely to continue into the 1990s. Health care will be provided increasingly by large organizations. Because of cost pressures, Americans will use less medical care per capita on an age-adjusted basis. Government increasingly will regulate the cost of, quality and access to health care. And the power of physicians to shape and benefit from the delivery system will diminish relative to other providers and to consumers.

Health is the ideal all persons strive for. And health care is the reality which not all persons can afford. The challenge is to gain more of the elusive ideal without forgoing meaningful work and relationships and sufficient food, clothing, and shelter, all of which affect health and are affected by it.

References

Aiken, L. H., & Mullinix, C. F. "The Nurse Shortage: Myth or Reality." *New England Journal of Medicine, 317*(10), 641, 1987.

Amara, R., Ian, M. J., & Schmid, G. *Looking Ahead at American Health Care.* Washington, D.C.: McGraw-Hill, 1988.

Arthur Andersen & Co. & American College of Health Care Executives. *The Future of Health Care: Changes & Choices.* Chicago: Author; 1987.

Bender, A. D., Strack, A. E., Ebrigh, G. W., & VanHaunulter, X. X. *A Delphic Study of the Future of Medicine.* Philadelphia: Smith, Kline, and French Laboratories, 1967.

Blendon, R. J. "Three Systems: A Comparative Survey." *Health Management Quarterly, 11*(1), 2, 1989.

Blendon, R. J., & Altman, D. E. "Public Opinion and Health Care Costs." In C. Schramm (ed.), *Health Care and Its Costs.* New York: W. W. Norton, 1987.

Coile, R. C., Jr. "The Promise of Technocracy: A Technoforecast for the 1990s." *Healthcare Executive,* November–December, 1988, p. 22.

Ebert, R. H. "The Medical School Revisited." *Health Affairs, 4*(2), 47, 1985.

Ebert, R. H., & Ginzberg, E. "The Reform of Medical Education." *Health Affairs, 7,* (Suppl. 2), 5, 1988.

Griffith, J. *The Well Managed Community Hospital.* Ann Arbor, MI: Health Administration Press, 1987.

Jonas, S. (ed.). *Health Care Delivery in the United States* (3d ed.). New York: Springer Publishing Co., 1986.

Kovner, A. R., & Martin S. P. (eds.). *Community Health and Medical Care.* New York: Grune and Stratton, 1978.

Little, A. D. *The Health Care System in the Mid-1990's* Boston: 1985.

McLaughlin, C. P., & Sheldon, A., *The Future and Medical Care: A Health Manager's Guide to Forecasting.* Cambridge, MA: Ballinger, 1974.

National Center for Health Services Research and Health Care Technology Assessment. *Research Activities.* Rockville, MD: Department of Health and Human Services (No. 92). 1987.

"Tomorrow's Medicine." *Medical World News,* January 24, 1988, p. 55

Vladeck, B. *President's Letter.* New York: United Hospital Fund, 1987.

Appendix

Abbreviations

AAMC	Association of American Medical Colleges
AAN	American Academy of Nursing
AARP	American Assocation of Retired Persons
ACHE	American College of Healthcare Executives
ACP	American College of Physicians
ADAMHA	Alcohol, Drug Abuse, and Mental Health Administration
ADL	Activities of Daily Living
AFDC	Aid to Families with Dependent Children
AHA	American Hospital Association
AIDS	Acquired Immune Deficiency Syndrome
ALOS	Average Length of Stay
AMA	American Medical Association
ANA	American Nurses Assocation
APA	American Psychiatric Association
APHA	American Public Health Association
AUPHA	Association of University Programs in Health Administration
BCHS	Bureau of Community Health Services
BHP	Bureau of Health Professions
CAT	Computerized Axial Tomography (scanner)
CBO	Congressional Budget Office
CCMC	Committee on the Costs of Medical Care
CCU	Coronary Care Unit
CDC	Centers for Disease Control
CEO	Chief Executive Officer
CEU	Continuing Education Unit
CFO	Chief Financial Officer

CFR	Code of Federal Regulations
CHAMPUS	Civilian Health and Medical Program of the Uniformed Services
CHC	Community Health Center
CHP	Comprehensive Health Planning
CME	Continuing Medical Education
CMHC	Community Mental Health Center
CON	Certificate of Need
CORF	Comprehensive Outpatient Rehabilitation Facility
COTH	Council of Teaching Hospitals
CPI	Consumer Price Index
CPR	Cardiopulmonary Resuscitation
DAF	Discretionary Adjustment Factor
DHHS	Department of Health and Human Services
DME	Durable Medical Equipment
D.O.	Doctor of Osteopathy
DRG	Diagnosis Related Group
EMS	Emergency Medical Services
EPA	Environmental Protection Agency
ER	Emergency Room
ESP	Economic Stabilization Program
FDA	Food and Drug Administration
FEHBP	Federal Employees Health Benefits Program
FHA	Federal Housing Authority
FMC	Foundation for Medical Care
FMG	Foreign Medical Graduate
FTE	Full-time Equivalent
FY	Fiscal Year
GAO	General Accounting Office
GHI	Group Health Insurance
GMENAC	Graduate Medical Education National Advisory Committee
GNP	Gross National Product
HANES	Health and Nutrition Examination Survey
HCA	Hospital Corporation of America
HCFA	Health Care Financing Administration
HDS	Hospital Discharge Survey
HHS	Health and Human Services (Department of)
HIAA	Health Insurance Association of America
HIS	Health Interview Survey
HIV	Human Immunodeficiency Virus
HMO	Health Maintenance Organization
HRA	Health Resources Administration

HRSA	Health Resources and Services Administration
HSA	Health Systems Agency
ICDA	International Classification of Diseases, Adapted
ICF	Intermediate Care Facility
ICU	Intensive Care Unit
IHS	Indian Health Service
IOM	Institute of Medicine
IPA	Individual Practice Association
JCAHO	Joint Commission on Accreditation of Healthcare Organizations
LOS	Length of Stay
LPN	Licensed Practical Nurse
MCH	Maternal and Child Health
M.D.	Medical Doctor
MI	Myocardial Infarction
MICU	Medical Intensive Care Unit
MRI	Magnetic Resonance Imaging
NAHC	National Association for Home Care
NAMCS	National Ambulatory Care Survey
NCHS	National Center for Health Statistics
NCHSR	National Center for Health Services Research
NHC	Neighborhood Health Center
NHI	National Health Insurance
NHP	National Health Plan
NHS	National Health Service
NHSC	National Health Service Corps
NIH	National Institutes of Health
NIMH	National Institute of Mental Health
NIOSH	National Institute of Occupational Safety and Health
NLN	National League for Nursing
NMR	Nuclear Magnetic Resonance
OEO	Office of Economic Opportunity
OHMO	Office of Health Maintenance Organizations
OMB	Office of Management and Budget
OPD	Outpatient Department
OSHA	Occupational Safety and Health Administration
OT	Occupational Therapy
OTA	Office of Technology Assessment
PA	Physician's Assistant
PAC	Political Action Committee
PAS	Professional Activity Study
PHS	Public Health Service

PGP	Prepaid Group Practice
PPO	Preferred Provider Organization
PPS	Prospective Payment System
PRO	Peer Review Organization
PROPAC	Prospective Payment Assessment Commission
PSRO	Professional Standards Review Organization
PT	Physical Therapy
QA	Quality Assurance
RCT	Randomized Clinical Trial
RMP	Regional Medical Program
RN	Registered Nurse
RRA	Registered Records Administrator
RUG	Resource Utilization Group
SCH	Sole Community Hospital
SDS	Same Day Surgery
SHMO	Social Health Maintenance Organization
SICU	Surgical Intensive Care Unit
SNF	Skilled Nursing Facility
SSA	Social Security Administration
STD	Sexually Transmitted Disease
TEFRA	Tax Equity and Fiscal Responsibility Act
Title XVIII	(Medicare)
Title XIX	(Medicaid)
USDA	United States Department of Agriculture
USDHEW	United States Department of Health, Education and Welfare
USDHHS	United States Department of Health and Human Services
USFMG	United States Foreign Medical Graduate
USPHS	United States Public Health Service
VA	Veterans Administration
VNA	Visiting Nurse Association
WHO	World Health Organization

Index

Springer publishing company

AN INTRODUCTION TO THE U.S. HEALTH CARE SYSTEM - *Second Edition*
Milton I. Roemer

In this expanded and updated revised edition of his widely used text, Dr. Roemer clarifies the basic structure and operation of the U.S. health care system. His concise description serves as a unique introduction for professionals in the health care and social science fields. Among the key topics explored in greater depth are health insurance, ambulatory care, public health, nursing, market dynamics, and ethical issues. Major recent accomplishments of the system are summarized along with persistent difficulties. 1986 / 176pp / $15.95

MANAGEMENT IN NURSING:
An Experiential Approach that Makes Theory Work for You
Elaine L. La Monica

This is a comprehensive textbook for management and leadership courses in nursing. Drawing on state-of-the-art research in business, educational administration, and organizational psychology, the author demonstrates that creative application of theory increases management effectiveness in the nursing service and aids in the professional development of all nurses.

Sections of the book include simulation exercises (e.g., case presentations and multimedia activities) that illustrate the content of each topic and provide learners with an opportunity to observe experience.

This text evolves from the author's experience in teaching management and leadership courses. It is also intended as a resource for graduate administration nursing students, practicing nurses, learners in service and continuing education programs, and nursing faculty. 1990 / 464pp / $37.95